DEDICATION

To our families, friends, and loved ones, who supported and assisted in the task of assembling this guide.

and

To the contributors to this and future editions, who took time to share their knowledge, insight, and humor for the benefit of students.

FIRST AID FOR THE®

USMLE STEP 2 CK

Seventh Edition

TAO LE, MD, MHS
Assistant Clinical Professor of Medicine and Pediatrics
Chief, Section of Allergy and Immunology
Department of Medicine
University of Louisville

VIKAS BHUSHAN, MD
Diagnostic Radiologist

HERMAN SINGH BAGGA, MD
Resident, Department of Urology
University of California, San Francisco

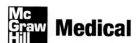 **Medical**

New York / Chicago / San Francisco / Lisbon / London / Madrid / Mexico City
Milan / New Delhi / San Juan / Seoul / Singapore / Sydney / Toronto

First Aid for the® USMLE Step 2 CK, Seventh Edition

1 2 3 4 5 6 7 8 9 0   QWD/QWD   12 11 10 9

ISBN-13: 978-0-07-162354-4
MHID: 0-07-162354-X
ISSN: 1532-320X

NOTICE

Medicine is an ever-changing science. As new research and clinical experience broaden our knowledge, changes in treatment and drug therapy are required. The authors and the publisher of this work have checked with sources believed to be reliable in their efforts to provide information that is complete and generally in accord with the standards accepted at the time of publication. However, in view of the possibility of human error or changes in medical sciences, neither the authors nor the publisher nor any other party who has been involved in the preparation or publication of this work warrants that the information contained herein is in every respect accurate or complete, and they disclaim all responsibility for any errors or omissions or for the results obtained from use of the information contained in this work. Readers are encouraged to confirm the information contained herein with other sources. For example and in particular, readers are advised to check the product information sheet included in the package of each drug they plan to administer to be certain that the information contained in this work is accurate and that changes have not been made in the recommended dose or in the contraindications for administration. This recommendation is of particular importance in connection with new or infrequently used drugs.

This book was set in Electra LH by Rainbow Graphics.
The editor was Catherine A. Johnson.
The production supervisor was Phil Galea.
Production management was provided by Rainbow Graphics.
Quebecor Dubuque was printer and binder.

This book is printed on acid-free paper.

McGraw-Hill books are available at special quantity discounts to use as premiums and sales promotions, or for use in corporate training programs. To contact a representative please e-mail us at bulksales@mcgraw-hill.com.

CONTENTS

SECTION 3   TOP-RATED REVIEW RESOURCES   545

CONTRIBUTING AUTHORS

Steven Chen

Johns Hopkins University School of Medicine
Class of 2010
Hematology/Oncology; Emergency Medicine

Allen Omid Eghrari

Johns Hopkins University School of Medicine
Class of 2009
Neurology; Epidemiology; Ethics

Seth Goldstein, MPhil

Johns Hopkins University School of Medicine
Class of 2009
Gastrointestinal; Musculoskeletal

Kristin H. Kan

Johns Hopkins University School of Medicine
Class of 2010
Endocrinology; Infectious Disease

Kenta Nakamura

University of California, San Francisco
Class of 2010
Cardiovascular; Pulmonary

Pushpa Raja

Johns Hopkins University School of Medicine
Class of 2009
Dermatology; Psychiatry

Marcela Smid, MA, MS

University of California, San Francisco
Class of 2009
Obstetrics; Gynecology

Darcy Weidemann

Johns Hopkins University School of Medicine
Class of 2009
Pediatrics; Renal/Genitourinary

WEB CONTRIBUTOR

Lauren Rothkopf, MD

Resident
Department of Internal Medicine
Beth Israel Deaconess Medical Center

FACULTY REVIEWERS

Tammy Brady, MD, MHS

Assistant Professor, Nephrology
Johns Hopkins University School of Medicine

Barish Edil, MD

Assistant Professor, Surgery and Oncology
Johns Hopkins University School of Medicine

Meg Gerstenblith, MD

Resident, Department of Dermatology
Johns Hopkins University School of Medicine

Emily Gower, PhD

Assistant Professor, Epidemiology and Ophthalmology
Director, Clinical Research Unit, Wilmer Eye Institute
Johns Hopkins University School of Medicine

Karen E. Hauer, MD

Director of Internal Medicine Clerkships
Professor of Medicine, Gold Headed Cane Endowed
    Education Chair
University of California, San Francisco, Department of Medicine

Christina Hines, MD, PhD

Resident, Department of Psychiatry and Behavioral Science
Johns Hopkins University School of Medicine

Julianna Jung, MD

Assistant Professor, Emergency Medicine
Johns Hopkins University School of Medicine

Matthew Kim, MD

Assistant Professor, Endocrinology
Johns Hopkins University School of Medicine

Kristi Mizelle, MD

Clinical Fellow, Rheumatology
Johns Hopkins University School of Medicine

Margaret R. Moon, MD, MPH

Assistant Professor, General Pediatrics and Adolescent Medicine
Johns Hopkins University School of Medicine
Core Faculty, Johns Hopkins Berman Institute of Bioethics

David Newman-Toker, MD, PhD

Assistant Professor, Neurology and Otolaryngology
Johns Hopkins University School of Medicine

Ben Ho Park, MD, PhD

Associate Professor, Oncology
The Sidney Kimmel Comprehensive Cancer Center at Johns Hopkins

Stanley G. Rockson, MD

Chief of Consultative Cardiology
Allan and Tina Neill Professor of Lymphatic Research and Medicine
Director, Stanford Center for Lymphatic and Venous Disorders
Professor of Medicine, Stanford University School of Medicine

Maunank R. Shah, MD

Fellow, Infectious Diseases
Johns Hopkins University School of Medicine

Jade Tan, MD

Fellow, Pediatrics
Johns Hopkins University School of Medicine

Dilys Walker, MD

Assitant Clinical Professor, Obstetrics, Gynecology and Reproductive
    Sciences
University of California, San Francisco

With the seventh edition of *First Aid for the USMLE Step 2 CK*, we continue our commitment to providing students with the most useful and up-to-date preparation guide for the USMLE Step 2 CK. The seventh edition represents a thorough revision in many ways and includes:

- A revised and updated exam preparation guide for the USMLE Step 2 CK. Includes updated study and test-taking strategies for the FRED v2 computer-based testing (CBT) format.
- Revisions and new material based on student experience with the 2008 and 2009 administrations of the USMLE Step 2 CK.
- Concise summaries of more than 300 heavily tested clinical topics written for fast, high-yield studying.
- Topics that integrate clinically relevant high-yield basic science facts from *First Aid for the USMLE Step 1*.
- A "rapid review" that tests your knowledge of each topic.
- A high-yield collection of more than 120 glossy photos similar to those appearing on the USMLE Step 2 CK exam.
- A completely revised, in-depth guide to clinical science review and sample examination books.

The seventh edition would not have been possible without the help of the many students and faculty members who contributed their feedback and suggestions. We invite students and faculty to continue sharing their thoughts and ideas to help us improve *First Aid for the USMLE Step 2 CK*. (See How to Contribute, p. xv.)

Louisville	Tao Le
Los Angeles	Vikas Bhushan
San Francisco	Herman Singh Bagga

ACKNOWLEDGMENTS

This has been a collaborative project from the start. We gratefully acknowledge the thoughtful comments, corrections, and advice of the many medical students, international medical graduates, and faculty who have supported the authors in the continuing development of *First Aid for the USMLE Step 2 CK*.

For support and encouragement throughout the process, we are grateful to Thao Pham, Selina Franklin, and Louise Petersen. Thanks also to those who supported the authors through the revision process.

Thanks to our publisher, McGraw-Hill, for the valuable assistance of their staff. For enthusiasm, support, and commitment to this challenging project, thanks to our editor, Catherine Johnson. For outstanding editorial work, we thank Andrea Fellows. A special thanks to Rainbow Graphics, especially David Hommel and Susan Cooper, for remarkable editorial and production work, and to Silas Wang for creating the web survey. Thanks to Elizabeth Sanders and Ashley Pound for the interior design.

For contributions and corrections, we thank Hany Al-Khedr, Ariel Brandwein, Jonathan Dayan, Tim Elder, Hana Gheith, Anna Guidry, Scott Hudson, Manorama Joisha, Shep Nickel, Andres O'Daly, Niraj Patel, Raj Patel, Rajesh Reddy, Rocio Rius, Shane Smith, Lindsay Stephenson, and Qi Zhuo. Thanks to Kashif Ahmad, Rachel Biller, Clarissa Chaisson-McRae, Benjamin Chen, Yu Chen, Ryan Childers, Alice Ching, Benjamin Cohen, Kinjal Desai, Sam Desai, Shilpa Desai, Nabil Ejaz, Aisha Ejaz, Christian Escobar, Joshua Evans, Caroline Foust-Wright, Rebecca Franklund, Stacey Gandhi, Christoph Gelsdorf, Ted Gerstenblith, Rozalina Grubina, Chen He, Boris Heifets, Danya Heller, Kurt Hofmann, Homaira Hossain, Lisa Huynh, Jason Hymas, Kristen Johnson, David Jolley, Kyle Bradford Jones, Rina Khatri, Albert Kim, Jared Klein, Peter Knoll, Heather Kuntz, Daniel Lee, Kachiu Lee, Adina Leon, Jeni Linn, Florence Loo, David Mark, Laura Medford-Davis, Patcharica Meteesatien, Judith Oh, Laureen Ojalvo, Cara Pensabene, Marisa Quattrone, Carrie Ann Ranum, Pawan Rawal, Rabia Razi, Abhiram Reddy, Analiz Rodriguez, Jon Russell, Natasha Shapiro, Jeremy Sparrow, Jesse Stringer, Lakshmi Sukumaran, Jeffrey Tomasini, Nathan Trayner, Jonathan Tresley, Jenny Tristano, Sasha Turok, Ravi Venkatesh, Jing Wang, Mark Wang, and Ying Zhang for submitting book reviews.

Louisville	Tao Le
Los Angeles	Vikas Bhushan
San Francisco	Herman Singh Bagga

HOW TO CONTRIBUTE

To continue to produce a high-yield review source for the Step 2 CK exam, you are invited to submit any suggestions or corrections. We also offer paid internships in medical education and publishing ranging from three months to one year (see below for details). Please send us your suggestions for

- Study and test-taking strategies for the Step 2 CK exam.
- New facts, mnemonics, diagrams, and illustrations.
- Low-yield topics to remove.

For each entry incorporated into the next edition, you will receive a $10 gift certificate, as well as personal acknowledgment in the next edition. Diagrams, tables, partial entries, updates, corrections, and study hints are also appreciated, and significant contributions will be compensated at the discretion of the authors. Also let us know about material in this edition that you feel is low yield and should be deleted.

The preferred way to submit entries, suggestions, or corrections is via our blog:

www.firstaidteam.com

Otherwise, please send entries, neatly written or typed or on disk (Microsoft Word), to:

First Aid for the USMLE Step 2 CK
914 North Dixie Avenue, Suite 100
Elizabethtown, KY 42701
Attention: Contributions

NOTE TO CONTRIBUTORS

All entries become property of the authors and are subject to editing and reviewing. Please verify all data and spellings carefully. In the event that similar or duplicate entries are received, only the first entry received will be used. Include a reference to a standard textbook to facilitate verification of the fact. Please follow the style, punctuation, and format of this edition if possible.

INTERNSHIP OPPORTUNITIES

The author team is pleased to offer part-time and full-time paid internships in medical education and publishing to motivated physicians. Internships may range from three months (e.g., a summer) up to a full year. Participants will have an opportunity to author, edit, and earn academic credit on a wide variety of projects, including the popular *First Aid* series. Writing/editing experience, familiarity with Microsoft Word, and Internet access are desired. For more information, e-mail a résumé or a short description of your experience along with a cover letter to the authors at their e-mail address.

Guide to Efficient Exam Preparation

▶ INTRODUCTION

The United States Medical Licensing Examination (USMLE) Step 2 allows you to pull together your clinical experience on the wards with the numerous "factoids" and classical disease presentations that you have memorized over the years. Whereas Step 1 stresses basic disease mechanisms and principles, Step 2 places more emphasis on clinical diagnosis and management, disease pathogenesis, and preventive medicine. The Step 2 exam is now composed of two parts:

- The Step 2 Clinical Knowledge examination (Step 2 CK)
- The Step 2 Clinical Skills examination (Step 2 CS)

The USMLE Step 2 CK is the second of three examinations that you must pass in order to become a licensed physician in the United States. The computerized Step 2 CK is a one-day (nine-hour) multiple-choice exam.

Students are also required to take the Step 2 CS, which is a one-day live exam in which students examine 12 standardized patients. For more information on this examination, please refer to *First Aid for the USMLE Step 2 CS*. Information about the Step 2 CS format and about eligibility, registration, and scoring can be found at www.nbme.org.

The information found in this section as well as in the remainder of the book will address only the Step 2 CK.

▶ USMLE STEP 2 CK–COMPUTER-BASED TESTING BASICS

How Will the CBT Be Structured?

The Step 2 CK is a computer-based test (CBT) administered by Prometric, Inc. It is a one-day exam with approximately 368 questions divided into eight 60-minute blocks of 46 questions each, administered in one nine-hour testing session. A new form of testing software called **FRED v2** is now being used by the USMLE. FRED v2 may be different from the Step 1 exam you took in that it offers improved **highlight** and **strike-out** features as well as the ability to make **brief notes** to yourself. The format of display for normal lab values has also changed, and now particular lab values can be searched for, which is quicker than scrolling through lengthy lists of normal values. Additionally, a calculator application has been made available to allow you to do basic calculations. Finally, "sequential item sets" have been introduced to the exam. These are sets of multiple-choice questions that are related and must all be answered in order without skipping a question in the set along the way. As you answer questions in a given set, the previous answers become locked and cannot be changed. These are the only questions on the USMLE exam that are locked in such a way. There will be no more than five "sequential item sets" within each USMLE Step 2 CK exam.

During the time allotted for each block on the USMLE Step 2 CK, the examinee can answer test questions in any order as well as review responses and change answers (with the exception of responses within the "sequential item sets" described above). However, under no circumstances can examinees go back and change answers from previous blocks. Once an examinee finishes a block, he or she must click on a screen icon in order to continue to the next block. Time not used during a testing block will be added to your overall break time, but it cannot be used to complete other testing blocks. Expect to spend up to nine hours at the test center.

Testing Conditions: What Will the CBT Be Like?

Even if you're familiar with computer-based testing and the Prometric test centers, FRED v2 is a new testing format that you should access from the USMLE CD-ROM or Web site (www.usmle.org) and try out prior to the exam.

If you familiarize yourself with the FRED v2 testing interface ahead of time, you can skip the 15-minute tutorial offered on exam day and add those minutes to your allotted break time of 45 minutes.

For security reasons, examinees are not allowed to bring personal electronic equipment into the testing area—which means that watches (even analog), cellular telephones, and electronic paging devices are all prohibited. Food and beverages are prohibited as well. Examinees are given laminated writing surfaces for note taking, but these must be returned after the examination. The testing centers are monitored by audio and video surveillance equipment.

You should become familiar with a typical question screen. A window to the left displays all the questions in the block and shows you the unanswered questions (marked with an "i"). Some questions will contain figures or color illustrations adjacent to the question. Although the contrast and brightness of the screen can be adjusted, there are no other ways to manipulate the picture (e.g., zooming or panning). Larger images are accessed with an **"exhibit"** button. The examinee can also call up a window displaying normal **lab values.** You may **mark** questions to review at a later time by clicking the check mark at the top of the screen. The **annotation** feature functions like the provided erasable dry boards and allows you to jot down notes during the exam. Play with the **highlighting/strike-out** and annotation features with the vignettes and multiple answers.

You should also do a few practice blocks to get a feel for which tools actually help you process questions more efficiently and accurately. If you find that you are not using the marking, annotation, or highlighting tools, then **keyboard shortcuts** can save you time over using a mouse.

What Does the CBT Format Mean for Me?

With the exception of the new features described earlier, the CBT format is the same format as that of the USMLE Step 1. If you are uncomfortable with this testing format, spend some time playing with a Windows-based system and pointing and clicking icons or buttons with a mouse.

The USMLE also offers students an opportunity to take a simulated test, or practice session, at a Prometric center. The session is divided into three one-hour blocks of 50 test items each. The 143 Step 2 CK sample test items that are available on the CD-ROM or on the USMLE Web site (www.usmle.org) are the same as those used at CBT practice sessions. **No new items are presented.** The cost is about $42 for U.S. and Canadian students but is higher for international students. The student receives a printed percent-correct score after completing the session. No explanations of questions are provided. You may register for a practice session online at www.usmle.org.

The goal of the Step 2 CK is to apply your knowledge of medical facts to clinical scenarios you may encounter as a resident.

Keyboard shortcuts:
A–E–Letter choices.
Enter or Spacebar–Move to next question.
Esc–Exit pop-up Lab and Exhibit windows.
Alt-T–Countdown timers for current session and overall test.

How Do I Register to Take the Exam?

Information on Step 2 CK format, content, and registration requirements can be found on the USMLE Web site. To register for the exam in the United States and Canada, apply online at the National Board of Medical Examiners (NBME) Web site (www.nbme.org). A printable version of the application is also available on this site. The preliminary registration process for the USMLE Step 2 CK is as follows:

- Complete a registration form and send your examination fees to the NBME (online).
- Select a three-month block in which you wish to be tested (e.g., June/July/August).
- Attach a passport-type photo to your completed application form.
- Complete a Certification of Identification and Authorization Form. This must be signed by an official at your medical school (e.g., the registrar's office) to verify your identity. This form is valid for five years, allowing you to use only your USMLE identification number for future transactions.
- Send your certified application form to the NMBE for processing. (Applications may be submitted more than six months before the test date, but examinees will not receive their scheduling permits until six months prior to the eligibility period.)
- The NBME will process your application within 4–6 weeks and will send you a slip of paper that will serve as your scheduling permit.
- Once you have received your scheduling permit, decide when and where you would like to take the exam. For a list of Prometric locations nearest you, visit www.prometric.com.
- Call Prometric's toll-free number or visit www.prometric.com to arrange a time to take the exam.
- The Step 2 CK is offered on a year-round basis except for the first two weeks in January. For the most up-to-date information on available testing days at your preferred testing location, refer to www.usmle.org.

The scheduling permit you receive from the NBME will contain the following important information:

- Your USMLE identification number.
- The eligibility period in which you may take the exam.
- Your "scheduling number," which you will need to make your exam appointment with Prometric.
- Your candidate identification number, or CIN, which you must enter at your Prometric workstation in order to access the exam.

Because the exam is scheduled on a "first-come, first-served" basis, you should be sure to call Prometric as soon as you receive your scheduling permit.

Prometric has no access to the codes and will not be able to supply these numbers, so **do not lose your permit!** You will not be allowed to take the Step 2 CK unless you present your permit along with an unexpired, government-issued photo identification that contains your signature (e.g., driver's license, passport). Make sure the name on your photo ID exactly matches the name that appears on your scheduling permit.

What If I Need to Reschedule the Exam?

You can change your date and/or center within your three-month period without charge by contacting Prometric. If space is available, you may reschedule up to five days before your test date. If you need to reschedule outside your initial three-month period, you can apply for a single three-month extension (e.g., April/May/June can be extended through July/August/September) after your eligibility period has begun (visit www.nbme.org for more information). This extension currently costs $50. For other rescheduling needs, you must submit a new application along with another application fee.

What About Time?

Time is of special interest on the CBT exam. Here is a breakdown of the exam schedule:

Tutorial	15 minutes
60-minute question blocks (46 questions per block)	8 hours
Break time (includes time for lunch)	45 minutes
Total test time	9 hours

The computer will keep track of how much time has elapsed during the exam. However, the computer will show you only how much time you have remaining in a given block. Therefore, it is up to you to determine if you are pacing yourself properly.

The computer will not warn you if you are spending more than the 45 minutes allotted for break time. **If you do exceed the 45-minute break time, the time to complete the last block of the test will be reduced.** However, you can elect not to use all of your break time, or you can gain extra break time either by skipping the tutorial or by finishing a block ahead of the allotted time.

New Security Measures

In early 2009, the NBME initiated a new check-in/check-out process that includes electronic capture of your fingerprints and photograph. These measures are intended to increase security by preventing fraud, thereby safeguarding the integrity of the exam. The new procedures also decrease the amount of time needed to check in and out of the examination throughout the day, thus maximizing your break time.

If I Leave During the Exam, What Happens to My Score?

You are considered to have started the exam once you have entered your CIN onto the computer screen. In order to receive an official score, however, you must finish the entire exam. This means that you must start and either finish or run out of time for each block of the exam. If you do not complete all the question blocks, your exam will be documented on your USMLE score transcript as an incomplete attempt, but no actual score will be reported.

The exam ends when all blocks have been completed or time has expired. As you leave the testing center, you will receive a written test-completion notice to document your completion of the exam.

What Types of Questions Are Asked?

The Step 2 CK is an integrated exam that tests understanding of normal conditions, disease categories, and physician tasks. Almost all questions on the exam are case based. A substantial amount of extraneous information may be given, or a clinical scenario may be followed by a question that could be answered without actually requiring that you read the case. It is your job to determine which information is superfluous and which is pertinent to the case at hand. Content areas include internal medicine, OB/GYN, pediatrics, preventive services, psychiatry, surgery, and other areas relevant to the provision of care under supervision. Physician tasks are distributed as follows:

- Promoting preventive medicine and health maintenance (15–20%)
- Understanding the mechanisms of disease (20–35%)
- Establishing a diagnosis (25–40%)
- Applying principles of management (15–25%)

Most questions on the exam have a **single best answer,** but some **matching sets** call for multiple responses (the number to select will be specified). The part of the vignette that actually asks the question—the stem—is usually found at the end of the scenario and generally relates to the physician task. From student experience, there are a few stems that are consistently addressed throughout the exam:

- What is the most likely diagnosis? (40%)
- Which of the following is the most appropriate initial step in management? (20%)
- Which of the following is the most appropriate next step in management? (20%)
- Which of the following is the most likely cause of . . . ? (5%)
- Which of the following is the most likely pathogen . . . ? (3%)
- Which of the following would most likely prevent . . . ? (2%)
- Other (10%)

Other exam tips are as follows:

- Note the age and race of the patient in each clinical scenario. When ethnicity is given, it is often relevant. Know these well (see high-yield facts), especially for more common diagnoses.
- Be able to recognize key facts that distinguish major diagnoses.
- Questions often describe clinical findings rather than naming eponyms (e.g., they cite "audible hip click" instead of "positive Ortolani's sign").
- Questions about acute patient management (e.g., trauma) in an emergency setting are common.

The cruel reality of the Step 2 CK is that no matter how much you study, there will still be questions you will not be able to answer with confidence. If you recognize that a question cannot be solved in a reasonable period of time, make an educated guess and move on; you will not be penalized for guessing. Also bear in mind that 10–20% of the USMLE exam questions are "experimental" and will not count toward your score.

How Long Will I Have to Wait Before I Get My Scores?

The USMLE reports scores 3–4 weeks after the examinee's test date. During peak periods, however, reports may take up to six weeks to be scored. Official information concerning the time required for score reporting is posted on the USMLE Web site, www.usmle.org.

How Are the Scores Reported?

Like the Step 1 score report, your Step 2 CK report includes your pass/fail status, two numeric scores, and a performance profile organized by discipline and disease process (see Figures 1-1A and 1-1B). The first score is a three-digit scaled score based on a predefined proficiency standard. In 2009, the required passing score was 184, which required answering 60–70% of questions correctly. The second score scale, the two-digit score, defines 75 as the minimum

UNITED STATES MEDICAL LICENSING EXAMINATION™

USMLE Step 2 is administered to students and graduates of U.S. and Canadian medical schools by the
NATIONAL BOARD OF MEDICAL EXAMINERS® (NBME®)
3750 Market Street, Philadelphia, Pennsylvania 19104-3190.
Telephone: (215) 590-9700

STEP 2 SCORE REPORT

Schmoe, Joe T	USMLE ID: 1-234-567-8
Anytown, CA 12345	Test Date: August 2008

The USMLE is a single examination program for all applicants for medical licensure in the United States; it has replaced the Federation Licensing Examination (FLEX) and the certifying examinations of the National Board of Medical Examiners (NBME Parts I, II and III). The program consists of three Steps designed to assess an examinee's understanding of and ability to apply concepts and principles that are important in health and disease and that constitute the basis of safe and effective patient care. **Step 2** is designed to assess whether an examinee possesses the medical knowledge and understanding of clinical science considered essential for the provision of patient care under supervision, including emphasis on health promotion and disease prevention. The inclusion of Step 2 in the USMLE sequence ensures that attention is devoted to principles of clinical science that undergird the safe and competent practice of medicine. Results of the examination are reported to medical licensing authorities in the United States and its territories for use in granting an initial license to practice medicine. The two numeric scores shown below are equivalent; each state or territory may use either score in making licensing decisions. These scores represent your results for the administration of Step 2 on the test date shown above.

PASS	This result is based on the minimum passing score set by USMLE for Step 2. Individual licensing authorities may accept the USMLE-recommended pass/fail result or may establish a different passing score for their own jurisdictions.

200	This score is determined by your overall performance on Step 2. For recent administrations, the mean and standard deviation for first-time examinees from U.S. and Canadian medical schools are approximately 208 and 23, respectively, with most scores falling between 140 and 260. A score of 170 is set by USMLE to pass Step 2. The standard error of measurement (SEM)‡ for this scale is approximately six points.

82	This score is also determined by your overall performance on the examination. A score of 82 on this scale is equivalent to a score of 200 on the scale described above. A score of 75 on this scale, which is equivalent to a score of 170 on the scale described above, is set by USMLE to pass Step 2. The SEM‡ for this scale is one point.

‡Your score is influenced both by your general understanding of clinical science and the specific set of items selected for this Step 2 examination. The standard error of measurement (SEM) provides an estimate of the range within which your scores might be expected to vary by chance if you were tested repeatedly using similar tests.

267PU007

NOTE: Original score report has copy-resistant watermark.

FIGURE 1-1A.   Sample Score Report—Front Page

INFORMATION PROVIDED FOR EXAMINEE USE ONLY

The Performance Profile below is provided solely for the benefit of the examinee.

These profiles are developed as assessment tools for examinees only and will not be reported or verified to any third party.

USMLE STEP 2 PERFORMANCE PROFILES

PHYSICIAN TASK PROFILE	Lower Performance	Borderline Performance	Higher Performance
Preventive Medicine & Health Maintenance			xxxxxxxxxxxx*
Understanding Mechanisms of Disease			xxxx*
Diagnosis			xxxxx*
Principles of Management			xxxxxxxxxx*

NORMAL CONDITIONS & DISEASE CATEGORY PROFILE

	Lower Performance	Borderline Performance	Higher Performance
Normal Growth & Development; Principles of Care			xxxxxxxxxxxxxxxxx*
Immunologic Disorders			xxxxxxxxxxxxx*
Diseases of Blood & Blood Forming Organs			xxxxxxxxxx*
Mental Disorders			xxxxxxxxxxx*
Diseases of the Nervous System & Special Senses			xxxxxxxxxx*
Cardiovascular Disorders		xxxxxxxxxxxxxxxx	
Diseases of the Respiratory System			xxxxxxxxxxxx*
Nutritional & Digestive Disorders			xxxxxxxxxx*
Gynecologic Disorders			xxxxxxxxxxx*
Renal, Urinary & Male Reproductive Systems			xxxxxxxxxx*
Disorders of Pregnancy, Childbirth & Puerperium			xxxxxxxxxxxxxxxxxx*
Musculoskeletal, Skin & Connective Tissue Diseases			xxxxxxxxx*
Endocrine & Metabolic Disorders			xxxxxxxxxxxxx*

DISCIPLINE PROFILE

	Lower Performance	Borderline Performance	Higher Performance
Medicine			xxx*
Obstetrics & Gynecology			xxxxxxxxxxx*
Pediatrics			xxxxxxxx*
Psychiatry			xxxxxxxxxxxx*
Surgery			xx*

The above Performance Profile is provided to aid in self-assessment. The shaded area defines a borderline level of performance for each content area; borderline performance is comparable to a HIGH FAIL / LOW PASS on the total test.

Performance bands indicate areas of relative strength and weakness. Some performance bands are wider than others. The width of a performance band reflects the precision of measurement: narrower bands indicate greater precision. An asterisk indicates that your performance band extends beyond the displayed portion of the scale. Small differences in the location of bands should not be over interpreted. If two bands overlap, the performance in the associated areas should not be interpreted as significantly different.

This profile should not be compared to those from other Step 2 administrations.

Additional information concerning the topics covered in each content area can be found in the *USMLE Step 2 General Instructions, Content Description, and Sample Items.*

007PU267

FIGURE 1-1B.   Sample Score Report—Back Page

passing score (equivalent to a score of 184 on the first scale). This score is not a percentile. Any adjustments in the required passing score will be available on the USMLE Web site.

▶ **DEFINING YOUR GOAL**

The first and most important thing to do in your Step 2 CK preparation is define how well you want to do on the exam, as this will ultimately determine the extent of preparation that will be necessary. The amount of time spent in preparation for this exam varies widely among medical students. Possible goals include the following:

- **Simply passing.** This goal meets the requirements for becoming a licensed physician in the United States. However, if you are taking the Step 2 CK in a time frame in which residency programs will see your score, you should strive to do as well as or better than you did on Step 1.
- **Beating the mean.** This signifies an ability to integrate your clinical and factual knowledge to an extent that is superior to that of your peers (between 200 and 220 for recent exam administrations). Others redefine this goal as achieving a score one SD above the mean (usually in the range of 220–240). Highly competitive residency programs may use your Step 1 and Step 2 (if available) scores as a screening tool or as selection criteria (see Figure 1-2). International medical graduates (IMGs) should aim to beat the mean, as USMLE scores are likely to be a selection factor even for less competitive U.S. residency programs.
- **Acing the exam.** Perhaps you are one of those individuals for whom nothing less than the best will do—and for whom excelling on standardized exams is a source of pride and satisfaction. A high score on the Step 2 CK might also represent a way to strengthen your application and "make up" for a less-than-satisfactory score on Step 1, especially if you are taking the exam in the fall before applying for residency.
- **Evaluating your clinical knowledge.** In many ways, this goal should serve as the ultimate rationale for taking the exam, since it is technically the reason the exam was initially designed. The case-based nature of the Step 2 CK differs significantly from the more fact-based Step 1 exam in that it more thoroughly examines your ability to recognize classic clinical presentations, deal with acute emergent situations, and follow the step-by-step thought processes involved in the treatment of particular diseases.

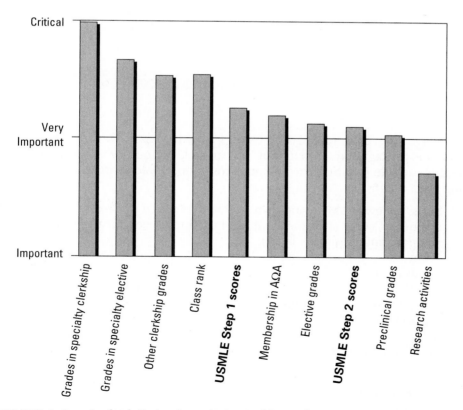

FIGURE 1-2. Academic Factors Important to Residency Directors

The Step 2 CK is an opportunity to consolidate your clinical knowledge and prepare for internship.

■ **Preparing for internship.** Studying for the USMLE Step 2 CK is an excellent way to review and consolidate all of the information you have learned in preparation for internship, especially if the exam is taken in the spring.

When to Take the Exam

With the CBT, you now have a wide variety of options regarding when to take the Step 2 CK. Here are a few factors to consider:

■ **The nature of your objectives,** as defined above.
■ **The specialty to which you are applying.** Some competitive residency programs may request your Step 2 CK scores, so you should consider taking the exam in the fall. If you already have a strong application and do not need Step 2 CK scores for residency applications, taking the exam in the fall could potentially hurt your application if you do poorly.
■ **Prerequisite to graduation.** If passing the USMLE Step 2 CK is a prerequisite to graduation at your medical school, you will need to take the exam in the fall or winter.
■ **Proximity to clerkships.** Many students feel that the core clerkship material is fresher in their minds early in the fourth year, making a good argument for taking the Step 2 CK earlier in the fall.
■ **The nature of your schedule.**
■ **Considerations for MD/PhD students.** Some state licensure bodies require that medical licensure occur within seven years of matriculating into medical school. However, the typical pathway for MD/PhD students consists of two years of preclinical work in medical school, 3–4 years of graduate work with research, and finally returning to medical school for clinical work. MD/PhD students typically exceed the seven-year limit. Depending on the state in which licensure is sought, such students may need to petition their licensure body for an exception to this rule.

▶ STUDY RESOURCES

Quality Considerations

Although an ever-increasing number of USMLE Step 2 CK review books and software packages are available on the market, the quality of this material is highly variable (see Section 3). Some common problems include the following:

■ Some review books are too detailed to be reviewed in a reasonable amount of time or cover subtopics that are not emphasized on the exam (e.g., a 400-page anesthesiology book).
■ Many sample question books have not been updated to reflect current trends on the Step 2 CK.
■ Many sample question books use poorly written questions, contain factual errors in their explanations, give overly detailed explanations, or offer no explanations at all.
■ Software for boards review is of highly variable quality, may be difficult to install, and may be fraught with bugs.

Clinical Review Books

Many review books are available, so you must decide which ones to buy by evaluating their relative merits. Toward this goal, you should weigh different opinions from other medical students against each other; read the reviews and ratings in Section 3 of this guide; and examine the various books closely in the bookstore. Do not worry about finding the "perfect" book, as many subjects simply do not have one.

There are two types of review books: those that are stand-alone titles and those that are part of a series. Books in a series generally have the same style, and you must decide if that style is helpful for you and optimal for a given subject.

The best review book for you reflects the way you like to learn. If a given review book is not working for you, stop using it no matter how highly rated it may be.

Texts and Notes

Most textbooks are too detailed for high-yield boards review and should be avoided. When using texts or notes, engage in active learning by making tables, diagrams, new mnemonics, and conceptual associations whenever possible. If you already have your own mnemonics, do not bother trying to memorize someone else's. Textbooks are useful, however, to supplement incomplete or unclear material.

Commercial Courses

Commercial preparation courses can be helpful for some students, as they offer an effective way to organize study material. However, multiweek courses are costly and require significant time commitment, leaving limited time for independent study. Also note that some commercial courses are designed for first-time test takers, students who are repeating the examination, or IMGs.

Practice Tests

Taking practice tests can serve multiple functions for examinees, including the following:

- Provide information about strengths and weaknesses in your fund of knowledge.
- Add variety to your study schedule.
- Serve as the main form of study.
- Improve test-taking skills.
- Familiarize examinees with the style of the USMLE Step 2 CK exam.

Students report that many practice tests have questions that are, on average, shorter and less clinically oriented than those on the current Step 2 CK. Step 2 CK questions demand fast reading skills and the application of clinical facts in a problem-solving format. Approach sample examinations critically, and do not waste time with low-quality questions until you have exhausted better sources.

Use practice tests to identify concepts and areas of weakness, not just facts that you missed.

After you have taken a practice test, try to identify concepts and areas of weakness, not just the facts that you missed. Use this experience to motivate your study and to prioritize the areas in which you need the most work. Analyze the pattern of your responses to questions to determine if you have made systematic errors in answering questions. Common mistakes include reading too much into the question, second-guessing your initial impression, and misinterpreting the question.

NBME/USMLE Publications

We strongly encourage students to use the free materials provided by the testing agencies and to study the following NBME publications:

- **USMLE *Bulletin of Information*.** This publication provides you with nuts-and-bolts details about the exam (included on the Web site www.usmle.org; free to all examinees).
- **USMLE *Step 2 Computer-Based Content and Sample Test Questions*.** This is a hardcopy version of the test questions and test content also found on the CD-ROM or at www.usmle.org.
- **NBME Test Delivery Software (FRED) and Tutorial.** This includes 143 valuable practice questions. The questions are available on the USMLE CD-ROM and on the USMLE Web site. Make sure you are using the new version of FRED and not the older Prometric version.
- **USMLE Web site (www.usmle.org).** In addition to allowing you to become familiar with the CBT format, the sample items on the USMLE Web site provide the only questions that are available directly from the test makers. Student feedback varies as to the similarity of these questions to those on the actual exam, but they are nonetheless worthwhile to know.

▶ TEST-DAY CHECKLIST

Things to Bring with You to the Exam

- Be sure to bring your scheduling permit and a photo ID with signature. (You will not be admitted to the exam if you fail to bring your permit, and Prometric will charge a rescheduling fee.)
- Remember to bring lunch, snacks (for a little "sugar rush" on breaks), and fluids.
- Bring clothes to layer to accommodate temperature variations at the testing center.
- Earplugs will be provided at the Prometric center.

▶ TESTING AGENCIES

National Board of Medical Examiners (NBME)
Department of Licensing Examination Services
3750 Market Street
Philadelphia, PA 19104-3102
(215) 590-9500
www.nbme.org

USMLE Secretariat
3750 Market Street
Philadelphia, PA 19104-3190
(215) 590-9700
www.usmle.org

Educational Commission for Foreign Medical Graduates (ECFMG)
3624 Market Street
Philadelphia, PA 19104-2685
(215) 386-5900
Fax: (215) 386-9196
www.ecfmg.org
e-mail: info@ecfmg.org

Federation of State Medical Boards (FSMB)
P.O. Box 619850
Dallas, TX 75261-9850
(817) 868-4041
Fax: (817) 868-4000
www.fsmb.org
e-mail: usmle@fsmb.org

Special Situations

▶ First Aid for the International Medical Graduate

▶ First Aid for the Student with a Disability

"International medical graduate" (IMG) is the term now used to describe any student or graduate of a non-U.S., non-Canadian, non–Puerto Rican medical school, regardless of whether he or she is a U.S. citizen. The old term "foreign medical graduate" (FMG) was replaced because it was misleading when applied to U.S. citizens attending medical schools outside the United States.

The IMG's Steps to Licensure in the United States

If you are an IMG, you must go through the following steps (not necessarily in this order) to become licensed to practice in the United States. You must complete these steps even if you are already a practicing physician and have completed a residency program in your own country.

- Complete the basic sciences program of your medical school (equivalent to the first two years of U.S. medical school).
- Take the USMLE Step 1. You can do this while still in school or after graduating, but in either case your medical school must certify that you completed the basic sciences portion of your school's curriculum before taking the USMLE Step 1.
- Complete the clinical clerkship program of your medical school (equivalent to the third and fourth years of U.S. medical school).
- Take the USMLE Step 2 Clinical Knowledge (CK) exam. If you are still in medical school, you must have completed two years of school.
- Take the Step 2 Clinical Skills (CS) exam.
- Graduate with your medical degree.
- Then, send the ECFMG a copy of your degree and transcript, which they will verify with your medical school.
- Obtain an ECFMG certificate. To do this, candidates must accomplish the following:
  - Graduate from a medical school that is listed in the International Medical Education Directory (IMED). The list can be accessed at www.ecfmg.org.
  - Pass Step 1, the Step 2 CK, and the Step 2 CS within a seven-year period.
  - Have your medical credentials verified by the ECFMG.
- The standard certificate is usually sent two weeks after all the above requirements have been fulfilled. You must have a valid certificate before entering an accredited residency program, although you may begin the application process before you receive your certification.
- Apply for residency positions in your field of interest, either directly or through the Electronic Residency Application Service (ERAS) and the National Residency Matching Program, or NRMP ("the Match"). To be entered into the Match, you need to have passed all the examinations necessary for ECFMG certification (i.e., Step 1, the Step 2 CK, and the Step 2 CS) by the rank order list deadline (February 24, 2010, for the 2010 Match). If you do not pass these exams by the deadline, you will be withdrawn from the Match.
- Obtain a visa that will allow you to enter and work in the United States if you are not already a U.S. citizen or a green-card holder (permanent resident).
- If required for IMGs by the state in which your residency is located, obtain an educational/training/limited medical license. Your residency program may assist you with this application. Note that medical licensing is the pre-

More detailed information can be found in the latest edition of the ECFMG Information Booklet, *available at www. ecfmg.org/pubshome.html.*

Applicants may apply online for the USMLE Step 2 CK or Step 2 CS or request an extension of the USMLE eligibility period at www. ecfmg.org/usmle/index.html or www.ecfmg.org/usmle/ step2cs/index.html.

rogative of each individual state, not of the federal government, and that states vary with respect to their laws about licensing (although all 50 states recognize the USMLE).

- In order to begin your residency program, make sure your scores are valid.
- Once you have the ECFMG certification, take the USMLE Step 3 during your residency, and then obtain a full medical license. Once you have a license in any state, you are permitted to practice in federal institutions such as VA hospitals and Indian Health Service facilities in any state. This can open the door to "moonlighting" opportunities and possibilities for an H1B visa application. For details on individual state rules, write to the licensing board in the state in question or contact the FSMB.
- Complete your residency and then take the appropriate specialty board exams in order to become board certified (e.g., in internal medicine or surgery). If you already have a specialty certification in your home country (e.g., in surgery or cardiology), some specialty boards may grant you six months' or one year's credit toward your total residency time.
- Currently, many residency programs are accepting applications through ERAS. For more information, see *First Aid for the Match* or contact:

ECFMG/ERAS Program
P.O. Box 11746
Philadelphia, PA 19101-0746
(215) 386-5900
e-mail: eras-support@ecfmg.org
www.ecfmg.org/eras

The USMLE and the IMG

The USMLE is a series of standardized exams that give IMGs a level playing field. It is the same exam series taken by U.S. graduates even though it is administered by the ECFMG rather than by the NBME. This means that passing marks for IMGs for Step 1, the Step 2 CK, and the Step 2 CS are determined by a statistical process that is based on the scores of U.S. medical students. For example, to pass Step 1, you will probably have to score higher than the bottom 8–10% of U.S. and Canadian graduates.

Timing of the USMLE

For an IMG, the timing of a complete application is critical. It is extremely important that you send in your application early if you are to garner the maximum number of interview calls. A rough guide would be to complete all exam requirements by August of the year in which you wish to apply. This would translate into sending both your score sheets and your ECFMG certificate with your application.

In terms of USMLE exam order, arguments can be made for taking the Step 1 or the Step 2 CK exam first. For example, you may consider taking the Step 2 CK exam first if you have just graduated from medical school and the clinical topics are still fresh in your mind. However, keep in mind that there is substantial overlap between Step 1 and Step 2 CK topics in areas such as pharmacology, pathophysiology, and biostatistics. You might therefore consider taking the Step 1 and Step 2 CK exams close together to take advantage of this overlap in your test preparation.

USMLE Step 1 and the IMG

What Is the USMLE Step 1? It is a computerized test of the basic medical sciences that consists of 336 multiple-choice questions divided into seven blocks.

Content. Step 1 includes test items in the following content areas:

- Anatomy
- Behavioral sciences
- Biochemistry
- Microbiology and immunology
- Pathology
- Pharmacology
- Physiology
- Interdisciplinary topics such as nutrition, genetics, and aging

Significance of the Test. Step 1 is required for the ECFMG certificate as well as for registration for the Step 2 CS. Since most U.S. graduates apply to residency with their Step 1 scores only, it may be the only objective tool available with which to compare IMGs with U.S. graduates.

Official Web Sites. www.usmle.org and www.ecfmg.org/usmle.

Eligibility. Both students and graduates from medical schools that are listed in IMED are eligible to take the test. Students must have completed at least two years of medical school by the beginning of the eligibility period selected.

Eligibility Period. A three-month period of your choice.

Fee. The fee for Step 1 is $710 plus an international test delivery surcharge (if you choose a testing region other than the United States or Canada).

Retaking the Exam. In the event that you failed the test, you can reapply and select an eligibility period that begins at least 60 days after the last attempt. You cannot take the same Step more than three times in any 12-month period. You cannot retake the exam if you passed. The minimum score to pass the exam is 75 on a two-digit scale. To pass, you must answer roughly 60–70% of the questions correctly.

Statistics. In 2007, only 70% of ECFMG candidates passed Step 1 on their first attempt, compared with 95% of U.S. and Canadian medical students and graduates. Of note, 1994–1995 data showed that USFMGs (U.S. citizens attending non-U.S. medical schools) performed 0.4 SD lower than IMGs (non-U.S. citizens attending non-U.S. medical schools). Although their overall scores were lower, USFMGs performed better than IMGs on behavioral sciences. In general, students from non-U.S. medical schools perform worst in behavioral science and biochemistry (1.9 and 1.5 SDs below U.S. students) and comparatively better in gross anatomy and pathology (0.7 and 0.9 SD below U.S. students). Although derived from data collected in 1994–1995, these data may help you focus your studying efforts.

Tips. Although few if any students feel totally prepared to take Step 1, IMGs in particular require serious study and preparation in order to reach their full potential on this exam. It is also imperative that IMGs do their best on Step 1, as a poor score on Step 1 is a distinct disadvantage in applying for most residencies. Remember that if you pass Step 1, you cannot retake it in an attempt to improve your score. Your goal should thus be to beat the mean, because you can then assert with confidence that you have done better than average for U.S. students. Good Step 1 scores will also lend credibility to your residency application and help you get into highly competitive specialties such as radiology, orthopedics, and dermatology.

Commercial Review Courses. Do commercial review courses help improve your scores? Reports vary, and such courses can be expensive. Many IMGs decide to try the USMLE on their own and then consider a review course only if they fail. Just keep in mind that many states require that you pass the USMLE within three attempts. (For more information on review courses, see Section IV.)

USMLE Step 2 CK and the IMG

What Is the Step 2 CK? It is a computerized test of the clinical sciences consisting of 368 multiple-choice questions divided into eight blocks. It can be taken at Prometric centers in the United States and several other countries.

Content. The Step 2 CK includes test items in the following content areas:

- Internal medicine
- Obstetrics and gynecology
- Pediatrics
- Preventive medicine
- Psychiatry
- Surgery
- Other areas relevant to the provision of care under supervision

Significance of the Test. The Step 2 CK is required for the ECFMG certificate. It reflects the level of clinical knowledge of the applicant. It tests clinical subjects, primarily internal medicine. Other areas that are tested are surgery, obstetrics and gynecology, pediatrics, orthopedics, psychiatry, ENT, ophthalmology, and medical ethics.

Official Web Sites. www.usmle.org and www.ecfmg.org/usmle.

Eligibility. Students and graduates from medical schools that are listed in IMED are eligible to take the Step 2 CK. Students must have completed at least two years of medical school. This means that students must have completed the basic medical science component of the medical school curriculum by the beginning of the eligibility period selected.

Eligibility Period. A three-month period of your choice.

Fee. The fee for the Step 2 CK is $710 plus an international test delivery surcharge (if you choose a testing region other than the United States or Canada).

Retaking the Exam. In the event that you fail the Step 2 CK, you can reapply and select an eligibility period that begins at least 60 days after the last attempt. You cannot take the same Step more than three times in any 12-month period. You cannot retake the exam if you passed.

Statistics. In 2006–2007, 79% of ECFMG candidates passed Step 2 on their first attempt, compared with 96% of U.S. and Canadian candidates.

Tips. It's better to take the Step 2 CK after your internal medicine rotation because most of the questions on the exam give clinical scenarios and ask you to make medical diagnoses and clinical decisions. In addition, because this is a clinical sciences exam, cultural and geographic considerations play a greater role than is the case with Step 1. For example, if your medical education gave you ample exposure to malaria, brucellosis, and malnutrition but little to alcohol withdrawal, child abuse, and cholesterol screening, you must work to familiarize yourself with topics that are more heavily emphasized in U.S. medicine. You must also have a basic understanding of the legal and social aspects of U.S. medicine, because you will be asked questions about communicating with and advising patients.

USMLE Step 2 CS and the IMG

What Is the Step 2 CS? The Step 2 CS is a test of clinical and communication skills administered as a one-day, eight-hour exam. It includes 10–12 encounters with standardized patients (15 minutes each, with 10 minutes to write a note after each encounter). Test results are valid indefinitely.

Content. The Step 2 CS tests the ability to communicate in English as well as interpersonal skills, data-gathering skills, the ability to perform a physical exam, and the ability to formulate a brief note, a differential diagnosis, and a list of diagnostic tests. The areas that are covered in the exam are as follows:

- Internal medicine
- Surgery
- Obstetrics and gynecology
- Pediatrics
- Psychiatry
- Family medicine

Unlike the USMLE Step 1, Step 2 CK, or Step 3, there are no numerical grades for the Step 2 CS—it's simply either a "pass" or a "fail." To pass, a candidate must attain a passing performance in **each** of the following three components:

- Integrated Clinical Encounter (ICE): includes Data Gathering, Physical Exam, and the Patient Note
- Spoken English Proficiency (SEP)
- Communication and Interpersonal Skills (CIS)

According to the NBME, the most common component failed by IMGs on the Step 2 CS is the CIS component.

Significance of the Test. The Step 2 CS is required for the ECFMG certificate. It has eliminated the Test of English as a Foreign Language (TOEFL) as a requirement for ECFMG certification.

Official Web Site. www.ecfmg.org/usmle/step2cs.

Eligibility. Students must have completed at least two years of medical school in order to take the test. That means students must have completed the basic medical science component of the medical school curriculum at the time they apply for the exam.

Fee. The fee for the Step 2 CS is $1200.

Scheduling. You must schedule the Step 2 CS within **four months** of the date indicated on your notification of registration. You must take the exam within 12 months of the date indicated on your notification of registration. It is generally advisable to take the Step 2 CS as soon as possible in the year before your Match, as often the results either come in late or arrive too late to allow you to retake the test and pass it before the Match.

Retaking the Exam. There is no limit to the number of attempts you can make to pass the Step 2 CS. However, you cannot retake the exam within 60 days of a failed attempt, and you cannot take it more than three times in a 12-month period.

Test Site Locations. The Step 2 CS is currently administered at the following five locations:

- Philadelphia, PA
- Atlanta, GA
- Los Angeles, CA
- Chicago, IL
- Houston, TX

For more information about the Step 2 CS exam, please refer to *First Aid for the Step 2 CS*.

USMLE Step 3 and the IMG

What Is the USMLE Step 3? It is a two-day computerized test in clinical medicine consisting of 480 multiple-choice questions and nine computer-based case simulations (CCS). The exam aims at testing your knowledge and its application to patient care and clinical decision making (i.e., this exam tests if you can safely practice medicine independently and without supervision).

Significance of the Test. Taking Step 3 before residency is critical for IMGs seeking an H1B visa and is also a bonus that can be added to the residency application. Step 3 is also required to obtain a full medical license in the United States and can be taken during residency for this purpose.

Official Web Site. www.usmle.org.

Fee. The fee for Step 3 is $690 (the total application fee can vary among states).

Eligibility. Most states require that applicants have completed one, two, or three years of postgraduate training (residency) before they apply for Step 3 and permanent state licensure. The exceptions are the 13 states mentioned below, which allow IMGs to take Step 3 at the beginning of or even before residency. So if you don't fulfill the prerequisites to taking Step 3 in your state of choice, simply use the name of one of the 13 states in your Step 3 application. You can take the exam in any state you choose regardless of the state that you mentioned on your application. Once you pass Step 3, it will be recognized by all states. Basic eligibility requirements for the USMLE Step 3 are as follows:

- Obtaining an MD or DO degree (or its equivalent) by the application deadline.
- Obtaining an ECFMG certificate if you are a graduate of a foreign medical school or are successfully completing a "fifth pathway" program (at a date no later than the application deadline).
- Meeting the requirements imposed by the individual state licensing authority to which you are applying to take Step 3. Please refer to www.fsmb.org for more information.

The following states do not have postgraduate training as an eligibility requirement to apply for Step 3:

- Arkansas
- California
- Connecticut
- Florida
- Louisiana
- Maryland
- Nebraska*
- New York
- South Dakota
- Texas
- Utah*
- Washington
- West Virginia

* Requires that IMGs obtain a "valid indefinite" ECFMG certificate.

The Step 3 exam is not available outside the United States. Applications can be found online at www.fsmb.org and must be submitted to the FSMB.

Residencies and the IMG

In the residency Match, the number of U.S.-citizen IMG applications has grown for the past few years, while the percentage accepted has been stable (see Table 1-1). More information about residency programs can be obtained at www.ama-assn.org.

TABLE 1-1. IMGs in the Match

APPLICANTS	2006	2007	2008
U.S.-citizen IMGs	2,435	2,694	2,969
% U.S.-citizen IMGs accepted	51	50	52
Non-U.S.-citizen IMGs	6,442	6,992	7,335
% non-U.S.-citizen IMGs accepted	49	46	42
U.S. graduates (non-IMGs)	15,008	15,206	15,242
% U.S. graduates accepted	94	93	94

The Match and the IMG

Given the growing number of IMG candidates with strong applications, you should bear in mind that good USMLE scores are not the only way to gain a competitive edge. However, USMLE Step 1 and Step 2 CK scores continue to be used as the initial screening mechanism when candidates are being considered for interviews.

Based on accumulated IMG Match experiences over recent years, here are a few pointers to help IMGs maximize their chances for a residency interview:

- **Apply early.** Programs offer a limited number of interviews and often select candidates on a first-come, first-served basis. Because of this, you should aim to complete the entire process of applying for the ERAS token, registering with the Association of American Medical Colleges (AAMC), mailing necessary documents to ERAS, and completing the ERAS application before September (see Figure 1-3). Community programs usually send out interview offers earlier than do university and university-affiliated programs.
- **U.S. clinical experience helps.** Externships and observerships in a U.S. hospital setting have emerged as an important credential on an IMG application. Externships are like short-term medical school internships and offer hands-on clinical experience. Observerships, also called "shadowing," involve following a physician and observing how he or she manages patients. Externships are considered superior to observerships, but having either of them is always better than having none. Some programs require students to have participated in an externship or observership before applying. It is best to gain such an experience before or at the time you apply

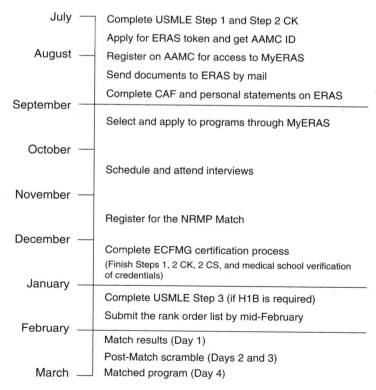

July	Complete USMLE Step 1 and Step 2 CK
	Apply for ERAS token and get AAMC ID
August	Register on AAMC for access to MyERAS
	Send documents to ERAS by mail
	Complete CAF and personal statements on ERAS
September	Select and apply to programs through MyERAS
October	
	Schedule and attend interviews
November	
	Register for the NRMP Match
December	Complete ECFMG certification process (Finish Steps 1, 2 CK, 2 CS, and medical school verification of credentials)
January	Complete USMLE Step 3 (if H1B is required)
	Submit the rank order list by mid-February
February	Match results (Day 1)
	Post-Match scramble (Days 2 and 3)
March	Matched program (Day 4)

FIGURE 1-3. **IMG timeline for application.**

to various programs so that you can mention it on your ERAS application. If such an experience or opportunity comes up after you apply, be sure to inform the programs accordingly.

■ **Clinical research helps.** University programs are attracted to candidates who show a strong interest in clinical research and academics. They may even relax their application criteria for individuals with unique backgrounds and strong research experience. Publications in well-known journals are an added bonus.

■ **Time the Step 2 CS well.** Most program directors would like to see a passing score on Step 1, Step 2 CK, and Step 2 CS before they rank an IMG on their rank order list in mid-February. There have been too many instances in which candidates have relinquished a position on the rank order list—and have thus lost a potential match—either because of delayed CS results or because they have been unable to retake the exam on time following a failure. Therefore, it is advisable to take the Step 2 CS as early as possible in the application year.

■ **U.S. letters of recommendation (LORs) help.** LORs from clinicians practicing in the United States carry more weight than recommendations from home countries.

■ **Step up the Step 3.** If H1B visa sponsorship is desired, aim to have Step 3 results by January of the Match year. In addition to the visa advantage you will gain, an early and good Step 3 score may benefit IMGs who have been away from clinical medicine for a while as well as those who have low scores on Step 1 and Step 2 CK.

■ **Verify medical credentials in a timely manner.** Do not overlook the medical school credential verification process. The ECFMG certificate arrives only after credentials have been verified and after you have passed Step 1, Step 2 CK, and Step 2 CS, so you should keep track of the process and keep checking with ECFMG from time to time about your status.

■ **Schedule interviews with pre-Matches in mind.** Schedule interviews with your favorite programs first. This will leave you better prepared to make a decision in the event that you are offered a pre-Match position.

Visa Options for the IMG

If you are living outside the United States, you will need to apply for a visa that will allow you lawful entry into the United States in order to take the Step 2 CS and/or do your interviews for residency. A B1 or B2 visitor visa may be issued by the U.S. consulate in your country. Citizens of some countries may have to undergo an additional security check that could take up to six months. Upon your entry into the United States, either the B1 or, more commonly, the B2 will be issued on your I-94. Both visas allow you a limited period within which to stay in the United States (2–6 months) in order to take the exam. If the given period is not sufficient, you may apply for an extension before the expiration of your I-94.

Documents that are recommended to facilitate this process include the following:

■ The Step 2 CS admission permit and a letter from the ECFMG (which explains why the applicant must enter the United States)
■ Your medical diploma
■ Transcripts from your medical school

- Your USMLE score sheets
- A sponsor letter or affidavit of support stating that you (if you are sponsoring yourself) or your sponsor will bear the expense of your trip and that you have sufficient funds to meet that expense
- An alien status affidavit

Individuals from certain countries may be allowed to enter the United States for up to 90 days without a visa under the Visa Waiver Program. See www.uscis.gov.

As an IMG, you will need a visa to work or train in the United States unless you are a U.S. citizen or a permanent resident (i.e., hold a green card). Two types of visas enable you to accept a residency appointment in the United States: J1 and H1B. Most sponsoring residency programs (SRPs) prefer a J1 visa. Above all, this is because SRPs are authorized by the Department of Homeland Security (DHS) to issue a Form DS-2019 directly to an IMG. By contrast, SRPs must complete considerable paperwork, including an application to the Immigration and Labor Department, to apply to the DHS for an H1B visa on behalf of an IMG.

The J1 Visa

Also known as the Exchange Visitor Program, the J1 visa was introduced to give IMGs in diverse specialties the chance to use their training experience in the United States to improve conditions in their home countries. As mentioned above, the DHS authorizes most SRPs to issue Form DS-2019 in the same manner that I-20s are issued to regular international students in the United States.

To enable an SRP to issue a DS-2019, you must obtain a certificate from the ECFMG indicating that you are eligible to participate in a residency program in the United States. First, however, you must ask the Ministry of Health in your country to issue a statement indicating that your country needs physicians with the skills you propose to acquire from a U.S. residency program. This statement, which must bear the seal of your country's government and must be signed by a duly designated government official, is intended to satisfy the U.S. Secretary of Health and Human Services (HHS) that there is such a need. The Health Ministry in your country should send this statement to the ECFMG (or they may allow you to mail it to the ECFMG).

How can you find out if the government of your country will issue such a statement? In many countries, the Ministry of Health maintains a list of medical specialties in which there is a need for further training abroad. You can also consult seniors in your medical school. A word of caution: If you are applying for a residency in internal medicine and internists are not in short supply in your country, it may help to indicate an intention to pursue a subspecialty after completing your residency training.

The text of your statement of need should read as follows:

> Name of applicant for visa: _____. There currently exists in _____ (your country) a need for qualified medical practitioners in the specialty of _____. (Name of applicant for visa) has filed

a written assurance with the government of this country that he/she will return to _____ (your country) upon completion of training in the United States and intends to enter the practice of medicine in the specialty for which training is being sought.

Stamp (or seal and signature) of issuing official of named country. Dated _____

To facilitate the issuing of such a statement by the Ministry of Health in your country, you should submit a certified copy of the agreement or a contract from your SRP in the United States. The agreement or contract must be signed by you and the residency program official responsible for the training.

Armed with Form DS-2019, you should then go to the U.S. consulate closest to the residential address indicated in your passport. As for other nonimmigrant visas, you must show that you have a genuine nonimmigrant intent to return to your home country. You must also show that all your expenses will be paid.

When you enter the United States, bring your Form DS-2019 along with your visa. You are usually admitted to the United States for the length of the JI program, designated as "D/S," or duration of status. The duration of your program is indicated on the DS-2019.

In the wake of the terrorist attacks of September 11, 2001, a number of new regulations have been introduced to improve the monitoring of exchange visitors during their time in the United States. All SRPs and students are currently required to register with the Student and Exchange Visitor Program (SEVP) via the Student and Exchange Visitor Information System (SEVIS). SEVIS allows the DHS to maintain up-to-date information (e.g., enrollment status, current address) on exchange visitors. SEVIS Form DS-2019 is used for visa applications, admission, and change of status. Contact your SRP or check www.uscis.gov for the most current information.

Duration of Participation. The duration of a resident's participation in a program of graduate medical education or training is limited to the time normally required to complete such a program. If you would like to get an idea of the typical training time for the various medical subspecialties, you may consult the *Directory of Medical Specialties*, published by Marquis Who's Who for the American Board of Medical Specialties. The authority charged with determining the duration of time required by an individual IMG is the State Department. The maximum amount of time for participation in a training program is ordinarily limited to seven years unless the IMG has demonstrated to the satisfaction of the ECFMG and the State Department that his or her home country has an exceptional need for the specialty in which he or she will receive further training. An extension of stay may be granted in the event that an IMG needs to repeat a year of clinical medical training or needs time for training or education to take an exam required for board certification.

Requirements after Entry into the United States. Each year, all IMGs participating in a residency program on a JI visa must furnish the Attorney General of the United States with an affidavit (Form I-644) attesting that they are in good standing in the program of graduate medical education or training in which they are participating and that they will return to their home countries upon completion of the education or training for which they came to the United States.

Restrictions under the J1 Visa. No later than two years after the date of entry into the United States, an IMG participating in a residency program on a J1 visa is allowed one opportunity to change his or her designated program of graduate medical education or training if his or her director approves that change.

The J1 visa includes a condition called the "two-year foreign residence requirement." The relevant section of the Immigration and Nationality Act states:

> Any exchange visitor physician coming to the United States on or after January 10, 1977, for the purpose of receiving graduate medical education or training is automatically subject to the two-year home-country physical presence requirement of section 212(e) of the Immigration and Nationality Act, as amended. Such physicians are not eligible to be considered for section 212(e) waivers on the basis of "No Objection" statements issued by their governments.

The law thus requires that a J1 visa holder, upon completion of the training program, leave the United States and reside in his or her home country for a period of at least two years. Currently, the American Medical Association (AMA) is advocating that this period be extended to five years.

An IMG on a J1 visa is ordinarily not allowed to change from a J1 to most other types of visas or (in most cases) to change from J1 to permanent residence while in the United States until he or she has fulfilled the foreign residence requirement. The purpose of the foreign residence requirement is to ensure that an IMG uses the training he or she obtained in the United States for the benefit of his or her home country. The U.S. government may, however, waive the two-year foreign residence requirement under the following circumstances:

- If you as an IMG can prove that returning to your country would result in "exceptional hardship" to you or to members of your immediate family who are U.S. citizens or permanent residents;
- If you as an IMG can demonstrate a "well-founded fear of persecution" due to race, religion, or political opinions if forced to return to your country;
- If you obtain a "no objection" statement from your government; or
- If you are sponsored by an "interested governmental agency" or a designated state Department of Health in the United States.

Applying for a J1 Visa Waiver. IMGs who have sought a waiver on the basis of the last alternative have found it beneficial to approach the following potentially "interested government agencies":

- **The Department of Health and Human Services.** Recently, HHS has expanded its role in reviewing J1 waiver applications. HHS's considerations for a waiver have classically been as follows: (1) the program or activity in which the IMG is engaged is "of high priority and of national or international significance in an area of interest" to HHS; (2) the IMG must be an "integral" part of the program or activity "so that the loss of his/her services would necessitate discontinuance of the program or a major phase of it";

and (3) the IMG "must possess outstanding qualifications, training, and experience well beyond the usually expected accomplishments at the graduate, postgraduate, and residency levels and must clearly demonstrate the capability to make original and significant contributions to the program." Under these criteria, HHS waivers are granted to physicians working in high-level biomedical research.

New rules will also allow HHS to review J1 waiver applications from community health centers, rural hospitals, and other health care providers. In the past, the U.S. Department of Agriculture (USDA) served as the interested federal government agency that reviewed waiver applications to allow foreign doctors to serve in rural underserved communities outside Appalachia, while the Appalachian Regional Commission (ARC) played that role for Appalachian communities. The USDA is no longer handling applications for J1 waivers. HHS will now review waiver applications for primary care practitioners and psychiatrists who have completed residency training within one year of application to practice in designated Health Professional Shortage Areas (HPSAs), Medically Underserved Areas and Populations (MUA/Ps), and Mental Health Professional Shortage Areas (MHPSAs). HHS waiver applications should be mailed to Joyce E. Jones, Executive Secretary, Exchange Visitor Waiver Review Board, Room 639-H, Hubert H. Humphrey Building, Department of Health and Human Services, 200 Independence Avenue, S.W., Washington, D.C. 20201; phone (202) 690-6174.

■ **The Department of Veterans Affairs.** With more than 170 health care facilities located in various parts of the United States, the VA is a major employer of physicians in this country. In addition, many VA hospitals are affiliated with university medical centers. The VA sponsors IMGs working in research, patient care (regardless of specialty), and teaching. The waiver applicant may engage in teaching and research in conjunction with clinical duties. The VA's latest guidelines (issued on June 22, 1994) provide that it will act as an interested government agency only when the loss of an IMG's services would necessitate the discontinuance of a program or a major phase of it and when recruitment efforts have failed to locate a U.S. physician to fill the position.

The procedure for obtaining a VA sponsorship for a J1 waiver is as follows: (1) the IMG should deal directly with the Human Resources Department at the local VA facility; and (2) the facility must request that the VA's chief medical director sponsor the IMG for a waiver. The waiver request should include the following documentation: (1) a letter from the director of the local facility describing the program, the IMG's immigration status, the health care needs of the facility, and the facility's recruitment efforts; (2) recruitment efforts, including copies of all job advertisements run within the preceding year; and (3) copies of the IMG's licenses, test results, board certifications, IAP-66 or SEVIS DS-2019 forms, and the like. The VA contact person in Washington, D.C., should be contacted by the local medical facility rather than by IMGs or their attorneys.

■ **The Appalachian Regional Commission.** ARC sponsors physicians in certain places in the eastern and southern United States—namely, in Alabama, Georgia, Kentucky, Maryland, Mississippi, New York, North Carolina, Ohio, Pennsylvania, South Carolina, Tennessee, Virginia, and West Virginia. Since 1992, ARC has sponsored approximately 200 primary care IMGs annually in counties within its jurisdiction that have been designated as HPSAs by HHS.

In accordance with its February 1994 revision of its J1 waiver policies, ARC requires that waiver requests initially be submitted to the ARC contact person in the state of intended employment. Contact information for each state can be found on the ARC Web site (www.arc.gov). If the state concurs, a letter from the state's governor recommending the waiver must be addressed to Anne B. Pope, the federal cochair of ARC. The waiver request should include the following: (1) a letter from the facility to Ms. Pope stating the proposed dates of employment, the IMG's medical specialty, the address of the practice location, an assertion that the IMG will practice primary care for at least 40 hours per week in the HPSA, and details as to why the facility needs the services of the IMG; (2) a J1 Visa Data Sheet; (3) the ARC federal cochair's J1 Visa Waiver Policy and the J1 Visa Waiver Policy Affidavit and Agreement with the notarized signature of the IMG; (4) a contract of at least three years' duration; (5) evidence of the IMG's qualifications, including a résumé, medical diplomas and licenses, and IAP-66 or SEVIS DS-2019 forms; and (6) evidence of unsuccessful attempts to recruit qualified U.S. physicians within the preceding six months. Copies of advertisements, copies of résumés received, and reasons for rejection must also be included. ARC will not sponsor IMGs who have been out of status for six months or longer.

Requests for ARC waivers are then processed in Washington, D.C. (ARC, 1666 Connecticut Avenue, N.W., Washington, D.C. 20009). ARC is usually able to forward a letter confirming that a waiver has been recommended to the requesting facility or attorney within 30 days of the request.

- **The Department of Agriculture.** At the time of publication, the USDA is no longer sponsoring J1 waivers. The scope of the HHS J1 waiver program has been expanded to fill the gap.

- **State Departments of Public Health.** There is no application form for a state-sponsored J1 waiver. However, regulations specify that an application must include the following documents: (1) a letter from the state Department of Public Health identifying the physician and specifying that it would be in the public interest to grant him or her a J1 waiver; (2) an employment contract that is valid for a minimum of three years and that states the name and address of the facility that will employ the physician and the geographic areas in which he or she will practice medicine; (3) evidence that these geographic areas are located within HPSAs; (4) a statement by the physician agreeing to the contractual requirements; (5) copies of all IAP-66 or SEVIS DS-2019 forms; and (6) a completed U.S. Information Agency (USIA) Data Sheet. Applications are numbered in the order in which they are received, since only 30 physicians per year may be granted waivers in a particular state under the Conrad State 30 program. Individual states may elect to participate or not to participate in this program.

The H1B Visa

Since 1991, the law has allowed medical residency programs to sponsor foreign-born medical residents for H1B visas. There are no restrictions on changing the H1B visa to any other kind of visa, including permanent resident status (green card), through employer sponsorship or through close relatives who are U.S. citizens or permanent residents. It is advisable for SRPs to apply for H1B visas as soon as possible in the official year (beginning October 1) when the new quota officially opens up.

According to the Web site www.immihelp.com, as of October 17, 2000, the following beneficiaries of approved H1B petitions are exempt from the H1B annual cap:

- Beneficiaries who are in J1 nonimmigrant status in order to receive graduate medical education or training, and who have obtained a waiver of the two-year home residency requirement;
- Beneficiaries who are employed at, or who have received an offer of employment at, an institution of higher education or a related or affiliated nonprofit entity;
- Beneficiaries who are employed by, or who have received an offer of employment from, a nonprofit research organization;
- Beneficiaries who are employed by, or who have received an offer of employment from, a governmental research organization;
- Beneficiaries who are currently maintaining, or who have held within the last six years, H1B status, and are ineligible for another full six-year stay as an H1B; and
- Beneficiaries who have been counted once toward the numerical limit and are the beneficiary of multiple petitions.

H1B visas are intended for "professionals" in a "specialty occupation." This means that an IMG intending to pursue a residency program in the United States with an H1B visa needs to clear all three USMLE Steps before becoming eligible for the H1B. The ECFMG administers Steps 1 and 2, whereas Step 3 is conducted by the individual states. You will need to contact the FSMB or the medical board of the state where you intend to take Step 3 for details (see p. 21, USMLE Step 3 and the IMG).

H1B Application. An application for an H1B visa is filed not by the IMG but rather by his or her employment sponsor—in your case, by the SRP in the United States. If an SRP is willing to do so, you will be told about it at the time of your interview for the residency program.

Before filing an H1B application with the DHS, an SRP must file an application with the U.S. Department of Labor affirming that the SRP will pay at least the normal salary for your job that a U.S. professional would earn. After receiving approval from the Labor Department, your SRP should be ready to file the H1B application with the DHS. The SRP's supporting letter is the most important part of the H1B application package; it must describe the job duties to make it clear that the physician is needed in a "specialty occupation" (resident) under the prevalent legal definition of that term.

Most SRPs prefer to issue a SEVIS Form DS-2019 for a J1 visa rather than file papers for an H1B visa because of the burden of paperwork and the attorney costs involved in securing approval of an H1B visa application. Even so, a sizable number of SRPs are willing to go through the trouble, particularly if an IMG is an excellent candidate or if the SRP concerned finds it difficult to fill all the available residency slots (although this is becoming rarer with continuing cuts in residency slots). If an SRP is unwilling to file for an H1B visa because of attorney costs, you could suggest that you would be willing to bear the burden of such costs. The entire process of getting an H1B visa can take anywhere from 10 to 20 weeks.

H1B Premium Processing Service. According to the Web site www.myvisa. com, the DHS offers the opportunity to obtain processing of an H1B visa application within 15 calendar days. Within 15 days of receiving Form I-907, the DHS will mail you a notice of approval, request for evidence, intent to deny, or notice of investigation for fraud or misrepresentation. If the notice requires the submission of additional evidence or indicates an intent to deny, a new 15-day period will begin upon delivery to the DHS of a complete response to the request for evidence or notice of intent to deny. The fee for this service is $1000. With this service, the total time needed to obtain an H1B visa has become significantly shorter than that required for the J1.

Although an H1B visa can be stamped by any U.S. consulate abroad, it is advisable that you have it stamped at the U.S. consulate where you first applied for a visitor visa to travel to the United States for interviews.

A Final Word

IMGs should also be aware of a new program called the National Security Entry-Exit Registration System, which aims to tighten up homeland security by keeping closer tabs on nonimmigrants residing in or entering the United States on temporary visas.

Male citizens or nationals of specific countries who are already residing in the United States may be required to report to a designated DHS office for registration, which includes being fingerprinted, photographed, and interviewed under oath. The official list of countries includes Bangladesh, Egypt, Indonesia, Jordan, Kuwait, Pakistan, Saudi Arabia, Afghanistan, Algeria, Bahrain, Eritrea, Lebanon, Morocco, North Korea, Oman, Qatar, Somalia, Tunisia, the United Arab Emirates, Yemen, Iran, Iraq, Libya, Sudan, and Syria. Different registration deadlines and criteria have been assigned to citizens of the above-mentioned countries, so please refer to www.uscis.gov for details.

If you are entering the United States, you may be registered at the port of entry if you are (1) a citizen or national of Iran, Iraq, Libya, Sudan, or Syria; (2) a nonimmigrant who has been designated by the State Department; or (3) any other nonimmigrant identified by immigration officers at airports, seaports, and land ports of entry in accordance with new regulation 8 CFR 264.1(f)(2). If you will be staying in the United States for more than 30 days, you will then be required to register in person at a DHS district office within 30 days for an interview and will be required to reregister annually.

Once you are registered, certain special procedures will apply. If you leave the United States for any reason, you must appear in person before a DHS inspecting officer at a preapproved airport, seaport, or land port and leave the United States from that port on the same day. If you change your address, employment, or school, you must report to the DHS in writing within 10 days using Form AR-11 SR. If any of these regulations are not followed, you may be considered out of status and subject to arrest, detention, fines, and/or removal from the United States, and any further application for immigration may be affected.

For the most up-to-date information regarding policies and procedures, please consult www.uscis.gov.

Summary

Despite some significant obstacles, a number of viable methods are available to IMGs who seek visas to pursue a residency program or eventually practice medicine in the United States. There is no doubt that the best alternative for an IMG is to obtain an H1B visa to pursue a medical residency. However, in cases where an IMG joins a residency program with a J1 visa, there are some possibilities for obtaining waivers of the two-year foreign residency requirement, particularly for those who are willing to make a commitment to perform primary care medicine in medically underserved areas.

Resources for the IMG

- **ECFMG**
  3624 Market Street
  Philadelphia, PA 19104-2685
  (215) 386-5900
  Fax: (215) 386-9196
  www.ecfmg.org

  The ECFMG telephone number is answered only between 9:00 A.M. and 12:30 P.M. and between 1:30 P.M. and 5:00 P.M. Monday through Friday EST. The ECFMG often takes a long time to answer the phone, which is frequently busy at peak times of the year, and then gives you a long voicemail message—so it is better to write or fax early than to rely on a last-minute phone call. Do not contact the NBME, as all IMG exam matters are conducted by the ECFMG. The ECFMG also publishes an information booklet on ECFMG certification and the USMLE program, which gives details on the dates and locations of forthcoming USMLE and English tests for IMGs together with application forms. It is free of charge and is also available from the public affairs offices of U.S. embassies and consulates worldwide as well as from Overseas Educational Advisory Centers. You may order single copies of the handbook by calling (215) 386-5900, preferably on weekends or between 6 P.M. and 6 A.M. Philadelphia time, or by faxing to (215) 387-9963. Requests for multiple copies must be made by fax or mail on organizational letterhead. The full text of the booklet is also available on the ECFMG's Web site at www.ecfmg.org.

- **FSMB**
  P.O. Box 619850
  Dallas, TX 75261-9850
  (817) 868-4000
  Fax: (817) 868-4099
  www.fsmb.org

  The FSMB has a number of publications available, including *The Exchange, Section I*, which gives detailed information on examination and licensing requirements in all U.S. jurisdictions. The cost is $30. (Texas residents must add 8.25% state sales tax.) To obtain these publications, submit the online order form. Payment options include Visa or MasterCard. Alternatively, write to Federation Publications at the above address. All orders must be prepaid with a personal check drawn on a U.S. bank, a cashier's check, or a money order payable to the FSMB. Foreign orders must be accompanied by an international money order or the equivalent, payable in U.S. dollars through a U.S. bank or a U.S. affiliate of a foreign bank. For Step 3 inquiries, the telephone number is (817) 868-4041. You may e-mail the FSMB at usmle@fsmb.org or write to Examination Services at the address above.

- Immigration information for IMGs is available from the sites of Siskind Susser, a firm of attorneys specializing in immigration law: www.visalaw.com/IMG/resources.html.
- Another source of immigration information can be found on the Web site of the law offices of Carl Shusterman, a Los Angeles attorney specializing in medical immigration law: www.shusterman.com.
- International Medical Placement Ltd., a U.S. company specializing in recruiting foreign physicians to work in the United States, has a site at www.intlmedicalplacement.com.
- Two more useful Web sites are www.myvisa.com and www.immihelp.com.
- *First Aid for the International Medical Graduate*, 2nd ed., by Keshav Chander (2002; 313 pages; ISBN 9780071385329), is an excellent resource written by a successful IMG. The book includes interviews with successful IMGs and students gearing up for the USMLE, complete "getting settled" information for new residents, and tips for dealing with possible social and cultural transition difficulties. The book provides useful advice on the U.S. curriculum, the health care delivery system, and ethical issues—and the differences IMGs should expect. Dr. Chander points out the weaknesses often found in IMG hopefuls and suggests ways to improve their performance on standardized tests as well as on academic and clinical evaluations. As a bonus, the guide contains information on how to get good fellowships after residency. The bottom line is that this is a reassuring guide that can help IMGs boost their confidence and proficiency. A great "first of its kind" that will empower IMGs with information that they need to succeed.

Other books that may be useful and of interest to IMGs are as follows:

- *International Medical Graduates in U.S. Hospitals: A Guide for Program Directors and Applicants*, by Faroque A. Khan and Lawrence G. Smith (1995; ISBN 9780943126418).
- *Insider's Guide for the International Medical Graduate to Obtain a Medical Residency in the U.S.A.*, by Ahmad Hakemi (1999; ISBN 9781929803002).

The USMLE provides accommodations for students with documented disabilities. The basis for such accommodations is the Americans with Disabilities Act (ADA) of 1990. The ADA defines a disability as "a significant limitation in one or more major life activities." This includes both "observable/physical" disabilities (e.g., blindness, hearing loss, narcolepsy) and "hidden/mental disabilities" (e.g., attention-deficit hyperactivity disorder, chronic fatigue syndrome, learning disabilities).

To provide appropriate support, the administrators of the USMLE must be informed of both the nature and the severity of an examinee's disability. Such documentation is required for an examinee to receive testing accommodations. Accommodations include extra time on tests, low-stimulation environments, extra or extended breaks, and zoom text.

Who Can Apply for Accommodations?

Students or graduates of a school in the United States or Canada that is accredited by the Liaison Committee on Medical Education (LCME) or the American Osteopathic Association may apply for test accommodations directly from the NBME. Requests are granted only if they meet the ADA definition of a disability. If you are a disabled student or a disabled graduate of a foreign medical school, you must contact the ECFMG (see below).

Who Is Not Eligible for Accommodations?

Individuals who do not meet the ADA definition of disabled are not eligible for test accommodations. Difficulties not eligible for test accommodations include test anxiety, slow reading without an identified underlying cognitive deficit, English as a second language, and learning difficulties that have not been diagnosed as a medically recognized disability.

Understanding the Need for Documentation

Although most learning-disabled medical students are all too familiar with the often exhausting process of providing documentation of their disability, you should realize that **applying for USMLE accommodation is different from these previous experiences.** This is because the NBME determines whether an individual is disabled solely on the basis of the guidelines set by the ADA. Previous accommodation does not in itself justify provision of an accommodation, so be sure to review the NBME guidelines carefully.

Getting the Information

The first step in applying for USMLE special accommodations is to contact the NBME and obtain a guidelines and questionnaire booklet. This can be obtained by calling or writing to:

Testing Coordinator
Office of Test Accommodations
National Board of Medical Examiners
3750 Market Street

Philadelphia, PA 19104-3102
(215) 590-9700

Internet access to this information is also available at www.nbme.org. This information is also relevant for IMGs, since the information is the same as that sent by the ECFMG.

Foreign graduates should contact the ECFMG to obtain information on special accommodations by calling or writing to:

ECFMG
3624 Market Street
Philadelphia, PA 19104-2685
(215) 386-5900

When you get this information, take some time to read it carefully. The guidelines are clear and explicit about what you need to do to obtain accommodations.

▶ NOTES

Database of High-Yield Facts

The seventh edition of *First Aid for the USMLE Step 2 CK* contains a revised and expanded database of clinical material that student authors and faculty have identified as high yield for boards review. The facts are organized according to subject matter, whether medical specialty (e.g., Cardiovascular, Renal) or high-yield topic (e.g., Ethics) in medicine. Each subject is then divided into smaller subsections of related facts. Individual facts are generally presented in a logical approach, from basic definitions and epidemiology to **History/Physical Exam, Diagnosis,** and **Treatment.** Lists, mnemonics, and tables are used when helpful in forming key associations.

The content is mostly useful for reviewing material already learned. This section is not ideal for learning complex or highly conceptual material for the first time. Black-and-white images appear throughout the text. In some cases, reference is made to the "clinical image" section at the end of Section 2, which contains full-color glossy plates of histology and patient pathology by topic. At the end of Section 2, we also feature a Rapid Review chapter of key facts and classic associations to cram a day or two before the exam.

The Database of High-Yield Facts is not comprehensive. Use it to complement your core study material and not as your primary study source. The facts and notes have been condensed and edited to emphasize the essential material. Work with the material, add your own notes and mnemonics, and recognize that not all memory techniques work for all students.

We update Section 2 biannually to keep current with new trends in boards content as well as to expand our database of high-yield information. However, we must note that inevitably many other high-yield entries and topics are not yet included in our database.

We actively encourage medical students and faculty to submit entries and mnemonics so that we may enhance the database for future students. We also solicit recommendations of additional tools for study that may be useful in preparing for the examination, such as diagrams, charts, and computer-based tutorials (see How to Contribute, p. xv).

Disclaimer

The entries in this section reflect student opinions of what is high yield. Owing to the diverse sources of material, no attempt has been made to trace or reference the origins of entries individually. We have regarded mnemonics as essentially in the public domain. All errors and omissions will be gladly corrected if brought to the attention of the authors, either through the publisher or directly by e-mail.

Cardiovascular

To evaluate patients for cardiac abnormalities, methodically assess the ECG for rate, rhythm, axis, intervals, waveforms, and chamber enlargement (see Figures 2.1-1 and 2.1-2).

Rate

The normal heart rate is 60–100 bpm. A rate < 60 bpm is bradycardia; > 100 bpm is tachycardia.

Rhythm

Look for sinus rhythm (P before every QRS and QRS after every P), irregular rhythms, junctional or ventricular rhythms (no P before a QRS), and ectopic beats.

Axis

- **Normal:** An upright (positive) QRS in leads I and II (–30 degrees to +105 degrees).
- **Left-axis deviation:** An upright QRS in lead I and a downward (negative) QRS in lead II (< –30 degrees).
- **Right-axis deviation:** A downward QRS in lead I and an upright QRS in lead II (> +105 degrees).

Quickly estimate heart rate by counting the number of large boxes subtended by two consecutive QRS complexes, as follows: 300-150-100-75-60-50-30 bpm.

An upright QRS in leads I and II—the "double thumbs-up" sign—signifies a normal axis.

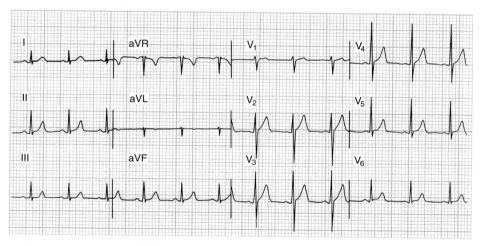

FIGURE 2.1-1. Normal electrocardiogram from a healthy subject.

Sinus rhythm is present with a heart rate of 75 bpm. The PR interval is 0.16 sec; the QRS interval (duration) is 0.08 sec; the QT interval is 0.36 sec; QT_c is 0.40 sec; and the mean QRS axis is about +70 degrees. The precordial leads show normal R-wave progression with the transition zone (R wave = S wave) in lead V_3. (Reproduced, with permission, from Fauci AS et al. *Harrison's Principles of Internal Medicine*, 17th ed. New York: McGraw-Hill, 2008: Fig. 221-7.)

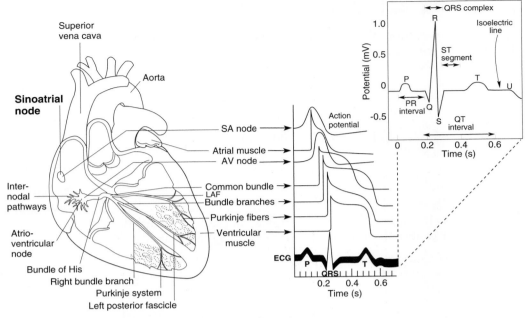

SA node "pacemaker" inherent dominance with slow phase of upstroke
AV node - 100-msec delay - atrioventricular delay

FIGURE 2.1-2. **Electrocardiogram measurements.**

<table>
<tr><td>

To distinguish between LBBB and RBBB—

WiLLiaM MaRRoW:

W pattern of QRS in V_1–V_2 and **M** pattern of QRS in V_3–V_6 for **L**BBB

M pattern of QRS in V_1–V_2 and **W** pattern of QRS in V_3–V_6 for **R**BBB

</td></tr>
</table>

Intervals

- **Normal:** PR interval between 120 and 200 msec and QRS < 100 msec.
- **Atrioventricular (AV) block:** PR interval > 200 msec, or P with no QRS afterward.
- **Left bundle branch block (LBBB):** QRS duration > 120 msec; no R wave in V_1; wide, tall R waves in I, V_5, and V_6.
- **Right bundle branch block (RBBB):** QRS duration > 120 msec; RSR′ complex ("rabbit ears"); qR or R morphology with a wide R wave in V_1; QRS pattern with a wide S wave in I, V_5, and V_6.
- **Long QT syndrome:** QTc > 440 msec. An underdiagnosed congenital disorder that predisposes to ventricular tachyarrhythmias.

Ischemia/Infarction

- **Ischemia:** Inverted T waves; poor R-wave progression in precordial leads; ST-segment changes (elevation or depression).
- **Transmural infarct:** Significant Q waves (> 40 msec or more than one-third of the QRS amplitude). ST elevation; T-wave inversion; the presence of possible impending infarction based on plaque instability.

Chamber Enlargement

- **Atrial hypertrophy:** Right atrial abnormality if P-wave amplitude in lead II is < 2.5 mm; left atrial abnormality if P-wave width in lead II is > 120 msec, or if terminal negative deflection in V_1 is > 1 mm in amplitude and > 40 msec in duration.

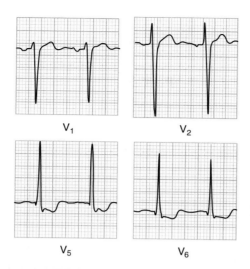

V₁   V₂

V₅   V₆

FIGURE 2.1-3.   Left ventricular hypertrophy.

Shown are leads V_1, V_2, V_5, and V_6. S wave in V_2 + R wave in V_5 = 55 mm. Note ST changes and T-wave inversion in V_5 and V_6, suggesting strain. (Reproduced, with permission, from Gomella LG et al. *Clinician's Pocket Reference*, 11th ed. New York: McGraw-Hill, 2006: Fig. 19-27.)

- **Left ventricular hypertrophy (LVH;** see Figure 2.1-3):
  - **Cornell criteria:** Amplitude of R in aVL + S in V_3 > 28 mm in men or > 20 mm in women.
  - **Sokolow-Lyon criteria:** S in V_1 + R in V_5 or V_6 > 35 mm.
- **Right ventricular hypertrophy (RVH):** Right-axis deviation and an R wave in V_1 > 7 mm.

▶ **CARDIAC PHYSICAL EXAM**

Key exam findings that can narrow the differential include the following:

- **Jugular venous distention** (JVD, > 7 cm above sternal angle): Suggests right heart failure, pulmonary hypertension, volume overload, tricuspid regurgitation, or pericardial disease.
  - **Hepatojugular reflux:** Fluid overload; impaired right ventricular compliance.
  - **Kussmaul's sign (↑ in JVP with inspiration):** Right ventricular infarction, postoperative cardiac tamponade, tricuspid regurgitation, constrictive pericarditis.
- **Systolic murmurs:**
  - **Aortic stenosis:** Harsh systolic ejection murmur; radiation to carotids.
  - **Mitral regurgitation:** Holosystolic murmur; radiation to axillae or to carotids.
  - **Mitral valve prolapse:** Midsystolic or late-systolic click.
  - **Flow murmur:** Very common, and does not imply cardiac disease.
- **Diastolic murmurs:** Always abnormal.
  - **Aortic regurgitation:** Early decrescendo murmur.
  - **Mitral stenosis:** Mid- to late, low-pitched murmur.

- **Gallops:**
  - **S₃ gallop:** Dilated cardiomyopathy (floppy ventricle), mitral valve disease; often normal in younger patients and in high-output states (e.g., pregnancy).
  - **S₄ gallop:** Hypertension, diastolic dysfunction (stiff ventricle), aortic stenosis; often normal in younger patients and athletes.
- **Edema:**
  - **Pulmonary:** Left heart failure.
  - **Peripheral:** Right heart failure and biventricular failure, peripheral venous disease, constrictive pericarditis, tricuspid regurgitation, hepatic disease, lymphedema; also nephrotic syndrome, hypoalbuminemia, and drugs.
- **Peripheral pulses:**
  - ↑: Compensated aortic regurgitation, coarctation (arms > legs), patent ductus arteriosus.
  - ↓: Peripheral arterial disease.
  - **Pulsus paradoxus** (↓ systolic BP with inspiration): Pericardial tamponade; also asthma and COPD, tension pneumothorax, foreign body in airway.
  - **Pulsus alternans** (alternating weak and strong pulses): Cardiac tamponade, impaired left ventricular systolic function; poor prognosis.
  - **Pulsus parvus et tardus** (weak and delayed pulse): Aortic stenosis.

> **ARRHYTHMIAS**

Bradyarrhythmias and Conduction Abnormalities

Table 2.1-1 outlines the etiologies, clinical presentation, and treatment of common bradyarrhythmias and conduction abnormalities.

Tachyarrhythmias

Tables 2.1-2 and 2.1-3 outline the etiologies, clinical presentation, and treatment of common supraventricular and ventricular tachyarrhythmias.

> **CONGESTIVE HEART FAILURE (CHF)**

Defined as a clinical syndrome caused by the inability of the heart to pump enough blood to maintain fluid and metabolic homeostasis. Risk factors include coronary artery disease (CAD), hypertension, cardiomyopathy, valvular heart disease, and diabetes. The American Heart Association/American College of Cardiology (AHA/ACC) guidelines classify heart failure according to clinical syndromes, but alternative classification systems include functional severity, left-sided vs. right-sided failure, and systolic vs. diastolic failure (see Tables 2.1-4 through 2.1-7).

TABLE 2.1-1.   Bradyarrhythmias and Conduction Abnormalities

TYPE	ETIOLOGY	SIGNS/SYMPTOMS	ECG FINDINGS	TREATMENT
Sinus bradycardia	Normal response to cardiovascular conditioning; can also result from sinus node dysfunction or from β-blocker or calcium channel blocker (CCB) excess.	May be asymptomatic, but may also present with lightheadedness, syncope, chest pain, or hypotension.	Ventricular rate < 60 bpm; normal P wave before every QRS complex.	None necessary if asymptomatic; atropine may be used to ↑ heart rate; pacemaker placement is the definitive treatment in severe cases.
First-degree AV block	Can occur in normal individuals; associated with ↑ vagal tone and with β-blocker or CCB use.	Asymptomatic.	PR interval > 200 msec.	None necessary.
Second-degree AV block (Mobitz I/ Wenckebach)	Drug effects (digoxin, β-blockers, CCBs) or ↑ vagal tone; sinoatrial conduction disease; right coronary ischemia or infarction.	Usually asymptomatic.	Progressive PR lengthening until a dropped beat occurs; PR interval then resets.	Stop the offending drug. Atropine or pacemaker placement as clinically indicated.
Second-degree AV block (Mobitz II)	Results from fibrotic disease of the conduction system or from acute, subacute, or prior myocardial infarction (MI).	Occasionally syncope; frequent progression to third-degree AV block.	Unexpected dropped beat(s) without a change in PR interval.	Pacemaker placement.
Third-degree AV block (complete)	No electrical communication between the atria and ventricles.	Syncope, dizziness, acute heart failure, hypotension, cannon A waves.	No relationship between P waves and QRS complexes.	Pacemaker placement.
Sick sinus syndrome (SSS)/ tachycardia-bradycardia syndrome	A heterogeneous disorder consisting of abnormalities in supraventricular impulse generation and conduction that lead to intermittent supraventricular tachy- and bradyarrhythmias.	2° to tachycardia or bradycardia; may include syncope, palpitations, dyspnea, chest pain, TIA, and stroke.		The most common indication for pacemaker placement.

TABLE 2.1-2. Supraventricular Tachyarrhythmias

Type	Etiology	Signs/Symptoms	ECG Findings	Treatment
Atrial				
Sinus tachycardia	Normal physiologic response to fear, pain, and exercise. Can also be 2° to hyperthyroidism, volume contraction, infection, or pulmonary embolism.	Palpitations, shortness of breath.	Ventricular rate > 100 bpm; normal P waves before every QRS complex.	Treat the underlying cause.
Atrial fibrillation (AF)	**Acute AF— PIRATES:** **P**ulmonary disease **I**schemia **R**heumatic heart disease **A**nemia/**A**trial myxoma **T**hyrotoxicosis **E**thanol **S**epsis **Chronic AF—** hypertension, CHF.	Often asymptomatic, but may present with shortness of breath, chest pain, or palpitations. Physical exam reveals irregularly irregular pulse.	No discernible P waves, with variable and irregular QRS response.	Estimate risk of stroke using CHAD2 score. Anticoagulation if > 48 hours (to prevent CVA); rate control (CCBs, β-blockers, digoxin, amiodarone). Initiate cardioversion only if new onset (< 48 hours) or if transesophageal echocardiogram (TEE) shows no left atrial clot, or after 3–6 weeks of warfarin treatment with satisfactory INR (2–3). See the Hematology chapter for more information on warfarin.

TABLE 2.1-2. Supraventricular Tachyarrhythmias (continued)

TYPE	ETIOLOGY	SIGNS/SYMPTOMS	ECG FINDINGS	TREATMENT
Atrial flutter	Circular movement of electrical activity around the atrium at a rate of 300 times per minute.	Usually asymptomatic, but can present with palpitations, syncope, and lightheadedness.	Regular rhythm; "sawtooth" appearance of P waves can be seen. Atrial rate is usually 240–320 bpm with varying degrees of blockade.	Anticoagulation and rate control. Cardiovert according to AF criteria.
Multifocal atrial tachycardia	Multiple atrial pacemakers or reentrant pathways; COPD, hypoxemia.	May be asymptomatic.	Three or more unique P-wave morphologies; rate > 100 bpm.	Treat the underlying disorder; verapamil or β-blockers for rate control and suppression of atrial pacemakers (not very effective).

AV junction

TYPE	ETIOLOGY	SIGNS/SYMPTOMS	ECG FINDINGS	TREATMENT
Atrioventricular nodal reentry tachycardia (AVNRT)	A reentry circuit in the AV node depolarizes the atrium and ventricle nearly simultaneously.	Palpitations, shortness of breath, angina, syncope, lightheadedness.	Rate 150–250 bpm; P wave is often **buried in** QRS or shortly after.	Carotid massage, Valsalva, or adenosine can stop the arrhythmia. Cardiovert if hemodynamically unstable.
Atrioventricular reciprocating tachycardia (AVRT)	Circular movement of an impulse between the AV node and the atrium through a bypass tract. Seen in Wolff-Parkinson-White syndrome.	Palpitations, shortness of breath, angina, syncope, lightheadedness.	A retrograde P wave is often seen **after** a normal QRS.	Same as that for AVNRT.
Paroxysmal atrial tachycardia	Rapid ectopic pacemaker in the atrium (not sinus node).	Palpitations, shortness of breath, angina, syncope, lightheadedness.	Rate > 100 bpm; P wave with an unusual axis **before** each normal QRS.	Adenosine can be used to unmask underlying atrial activity.

HIGH-YIELD FACTS

CARDIOVASCULAR

TABLE 2.1-3. **Ventricular Tachyarrhythmias**

TYPE	ETIOLOGY	SIGNS/SYMPTOMS	ECG FINDINGS	TREATMENT
Premature ventricular contraction (PVC)	Ectopic beats arise from ventricular foci. Associated with hypoxia, electrolyte abnormalities, and hyperthyroidism.	Usually asymptomatic, but may lead to palpitations.	Early, wide QRS not preceded by a P wave. PVCs are usually followed by a compensatory pause.	Treat the underlying cause. If symptomatic, give β-blockers or occasionally other antiarrhythmics.
Ventricular tachycardia (VT)	Can be associated with CAD, MI, and structural heart disease.	Nonsustained VT is often asymptomatic; sustained ventricular tachycardia can lead to palpitations, hypotension, angina, and syncope. Can progress to VF.	Three or more consecutive PVCs; wide QRS complexes in a regular rapid rhythm; AV dissociation.	Cardioversion and antiarrhythmics (e.g., amiodarone, lidocaine, procainamide).
Ventricular fibrillation (VF)	Associated with CAD and structural heart disease. Also associated with cardiac arrest (together with asystole).	Syncope, absence of blood pressure, pulselessness.	Totally erratic wide-complex tracing.	Immediate electrical cardioversion and ACLS protocol.
Torsades de pointes	Associated with long QT syndrome, proarrhythmic response to medications, hypokalemia, and congenital deafness.	Can present with sudden cardiac death; typically associated with palpitations, dizziness, and syncope.	Polymorphous QRS; VT with rates between 150 and 250 bpm.	Correct hypokalemia; withdraw offending drugs. Give magnesium initially and cardiovert if unstable.

TABLE 2.1-4. AHA/ACC Classification and Treatment of CHF

STAGE	DESCRIPTION	TREATMENT
A	Patients who are at high risk of developing CHF because of the presence of risk factors, but who have no identified structural or functional abnormalities and no signs or symptoms of CHF.	Manage treatable risk factors (hypertension, smoking, hyperlipidemia, obesity, exercise, alcohol abuse). ACEIs can be used in patients with atherosclerotic vascular disease, DM, or hypertension.
B	Patients with structural heart disease (e.g., a history of MI, left ventricular systolic dysfunction, or valvular disease) who have never had symptoms of CHF.	ACEIs, β-blockers.
C	Patients with structural heart disease who have prior or current symptoms of CHF (shortness of breath, fatigue, ↓ exercise tolerance).	Treatment includes diuretics, ACEIs, β-blockers, digitalis, and dietary salt restriction.
D	Patients with marked symptoms of CHF at rest despite maximal medical therapy.	Treatment options include mechanical assist devices, heart transplantation, continuous IV inotropic drugs, and hospice care for end-stage patients.

TABLE 2.1-5. NYHA Functional Classification of CHF

CLASS	DESCRIPTION
I	No limitation of activity; no symptoms with normal activity.
II	Slight limitation of activity; comfortable at rest or with mild exertion.
III	Marked limitation of activity; comfortable only at rest.
IV	Confined to complete rest in bed or chair, as any physical activity brings on discomfort; symptoms present at rest.

TABLE 2.1-6. Left-Sided vs. Right-Sided Heart Failure

LEFT-SIDED CHF SYMPTOMS	RIGHT-SIDED CHF SYMPTOMS
Dyspnea predominates	**Fluid retention predominates**
Left-sided S_3/S_4 gallop	Right-sided S_3/S_4 gallop
Bilateral basilar rales	JVD
Pleural effusions	Hepatojugular reflex
Pulmonary edema	Peripheral edema
Orthopnea, paroxysmal nocturnal dyspnea	Hepatomegaly, ascites

TABLE 2.1-7. Comparison of Systolic and Diastolic Dysfunction

	SYSTOLIC DYSFUNCTION	DIASTOLIC DYSFUNCTION
Patient age	Often < 65 years of age.	Often > 65 years of age.
Comorbidities	Dilated cardiomyopathy, valvular heart disease.	Restrictive or hypertrophic cardiomyopathy; renal disease or hypertension.
Physical exam	Displaced PMI, S_3 gallop.	Sustained PMI, S_4 gallop.
CXR	Pulmonary congestion, cardiomegaly.	Pulmonary congestion, normal heart size.
ECG/echocardiography	Q waves, ↓ EF (< 40%).	LVH, normal EF (> 55%).

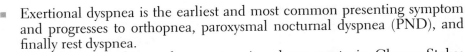

Systolic Dysfunction

Heart failure caused by systolic dysfunction is defined as a ↓ EF (< 50%) and ↑ left ventricular end-diastolic volumes. It is caused by inadequate left ventricular contractility or ↑ afterload. The heart compensates for low EF and ↑ preload through hypertrophy and ventricular dilation (Frank-Starling law), but the compensation ultimately fails, leading to ↑ myocardial work and worsening systolic function.

HISTORY/PE

The most common cause of right-sided heart failure is left-sided heart failure.

- Exertional dyspnea is the earliest and most common presenting symptom and progresses to orthopnea, paroxysmal nocturnal dyspnea (PND), and finally rest dyspnea.
- Chronic cough, fatigue, lower extremity edema, nocturia, Cheyne-Stokes respirations, and/or abdominal fullness may be seen.
- Look for signs to distinguish left- from right-sided heart failure (see Table 2.1-6).

DIAGNOSIS

- CHF is a **clinical syndrome** whose diagnosis is based on signs and symptoms.
- Exam reveals parasternal lift, an elevated and sustained left ventricular impulse, and an S_3/S_4 gallop.
- **CXR:** Cardiomegaly, cephalization of pulmonary vessels, pleural effusions, vascular plumpness, and prominent hila.
- **Echocardiogram:** ↓ EF and ventricular dilation.
- **Lab abnormalities:** BNP > 500, ↑ creatinine, ↓ sodium.
- **ECG:** Usually nondiagnostic, but MI or AF may precipitate acute exacerbations.

TREATMENT

Diuretics are for symptomatic relief only and confer no mortality benefit.

- **Acute:**
  - Correct underlying causes such as arrhythmias, myocardial ischemia, and drugs (e.g., CCBs, antiarrhythmics, NSAIDs, alcohol, thyroid and valvular disease, high-output states).
  - Diurese aggressively with loop and thiazide diuretics (see Table 2.1-8).

TABLE 2.1-8. Types of Diuretics

Class	Examples	Site of Action	Mechanism of Action	Side Effects
Loop diuretics	Furosemide, ethacrynic acid, bumetanide, torsemide	Loop of Henle	↓ $Na^+/K^+/2Cl^-$ cotransporter; ↓ urine concentration; ↑ Ca^{2+} excretion.	Ototoxicity, hypokalemia, hypocalcemia, dehydration, gout.
Thiazide diuretics	HCTZ, chlorothiazide, chlorthalidone	Early distal tubule	↓ NaCl reabsorption leading to ↓ diluting capacity of nephron; ↓ Ca^{2+} excretion.	Hypokalemic metabolic alkalosis, hyponatremia, hyperglycemia, hyperlipidemia, hyperuricemia, hypercalcemia.
K^+-sparing agents	Spironolactone, triamterene, amiloride	Cortical collecting tubule	Spironolactone is an aldosterone receptor antagonist; triamterene and amiloride block Na^+ channels.	Hyperkalemia, gynecomastia, hirsutism, sexual dysfunction.
Carbonic anhydrase inhibitors	Acetazolamide	Proximal convoluted tubule	$NaHCO_3$ diuresis ↓ total body $NaHCO_3$.	Hyperchloremic metabolic acidosis, neuropathy, NH_3 toxicity, sulfa allergy.
Osmotic agents	Mannitol	Proximal tubule	Creates ↑ tubular fluid osmolarity, leading to ↑ urine flow.	Pulmonary edema, dehydration. Contraindicated in anuria and CHF.

- Give ACEIs to all patients who can tolerate them. If a patient cannot tolerate ACEIs, consider an angiotensin receptor blocker (ARB). β-blockers should not be used during decompensated CHF but should be started once the patient is euvolemic.
- Treat acute pulmonary congestion with **LMNOP** (see mnemonic).
- **Chronic:**
  - Control comorbid conditions (e.g., diabetes, hypertension, obesity) and limit dietary sodium and fluid intake.
  - Long-term β-blockers and ACEIs/ARBs together help prevent neurohormonal remodeling of the heart. All of these agents ↓ mortality for New York Heart Association (NYHA) class II–IV patients.
  - Daily ASA and a statin are recommended for ischemic heart disease to prevent further ischemic events.
  - Chronic diuretic therapy (loop diuretics +/– thiazide) can prevent volume overload.
  - Low-dose spironolactone ↓ mortality risk when given with ACEIs and loop diuretics in patients with left ventricular systolic dysfunction and NYHA class III–IV heart failure. Monitor for hyperkalemia.
  - Anticoagulate patients with AF and those with a history of previous embolic events or a mobile left ventricular thrombus. Consider an implantable biventricular cardiac defibrillator (ICD) in patients with both an EF < 30% and CAD.

> *Acute CHF management—*
>
> **LMNOP**
>
> **L**asix
> **M**orphine
> **N**itrates
> **O**xygen
> **P**osition (upright)

Loops lose calcium, whereas thiazides save it.

■ CHF that is unresponsive to maximal medical therapy may require a mechanical left ventricular assist device or cardiac transplantation.

Diastolic Dysfunction

Defined by ↓ ventricular compliance with normal systolic function. The ventricle has either impaired active relaxation (2° to ischemia, aging, and/or hypertrophy) or impaired passive filling (scarring from prior MI; restrictive cardiomyopathy). Left ventricular end-diastolic pressure ↑, cardiac output remains essentially normal, and EF is normal or ↑.

HISTORY/PE

Associated with stable and unstable angina, shortness of breath, dyspnea on exertion, arrhythmias, MI, heart failure, and sudden death.

TREATMENT

■ Diuretics are first-line therapy (see Table 2.1-8).
■ Maintain rate and BP control via β-blockers, ACEIs, ARBs, or CCBs.
■ Digoxin is not useful in these patients.

► CARDIOMYOPATHY

Myocardial disease; categorized as dilated, hypertrophic, or restrictive (see Table 2.1-9).

Dilated Cardiomyopathy

The most common cardiomyopathy. Left ventricular dilation and systolic dysfunction (low EF) must be present for diagnosis. Most cases are idiopathic, but known 2° causes include alcohol, myocarditis, postpartum status, drugs (doxorubicin, AZT, cocaine), endocrinopathies (thyroid dysfunction, acromegaly, pheochromocytoma), infection (coxsackievirus, HIV, Chagas' disease, parasites), genetic factors, and nutritional disorders (wet beriberi). The two most common causes of 2° dilated cardiomyopathy are ischemia and long-standing hypertension.

TABLE 2.1-9. Differential Diagnosis of Cardiomyopathies

	DILATED	HYPERTROPHIC	RESTRICTIVE
Major abnormality	Impaired contractility	Impaired relaxation	Impaired elasticity
Left ventricular cavity size (end diastole)	↑↑	↓	↑
Left ventricular cavity size (end systole)	↑↑	↓↓	↑
Ejection fraction (EF)	↓↓	↑ or ↔	↓ or ↔
Wall thickness	↓, variable	↑↑	↑, variable

HISTORY/PE

- Often presents with gradual development of CHF symptoms.
- Exam often reveals displacement of the left venticular impulse, JVD, an S₃/S₄ gallop, or mitral/tricuspid regurgitation.

DIAGNOSIS

- Echocardiography is diagnostic.
- ECG may show nonspecific ST-T changes, low-voltage QRS, sinus tachycardia, and ectopy. LBBB is common.
- CXR shows an enlarged, balloon-like heart and pulmonary congestion.

TREATMENT

- Address the underlying etiology (e.g., stop all alcohol use, treat endocrine disorders).
- Treat symptoms of CHF with diuretics, and prevent disease progression with ACEIs, β-blockers, and aldosterone antagonists. Consider anticoagulation to ↓ thrombus risk only if AF or an intraventricular thrombus is present. Digoxin is a second-line agent; avoid CCBs in CHF.
- Consider an ICD if EF < 35%.

An S₃ gallop signifies the end of rapid ventricular filling in the setting of fluid overload and is associated with dilated cardiomyopathy.

Hypertrophic Cardiomyopathy

LVH results in impaired left ventricular relaxation and filling (diastolic dysfunction). Hypertrophy frequently involves the interventricular septum, leading to left ventricular outflow tract obstruction and impaired ejection of blood. The congenital form, hypertrophic obstructive cardiomyopathy (HOCM), is inherited as an autosomal-dominant trait in 50% of HOCM patients and is the most common cause of sudden death in young, healthy athletes in the United States. Other causes of marked hypertrophy include hypertension and aortic stenosis.

Hypertrophic cardiomyopathy is the most common cause of sudden death in young, healthy athletes in the United States.

HISTORY/PE

- Patients may be asymptomatic but may also present with syncope, dyspnea, palpitations, angina, or sudden cardiac death.
- Exam often reveals a sustained apical impulse, an S₄ gallop, and a systolic ejection crescendo-decrescendo murmur that ↑ with ↓ preload (e.g., Valsalva maneuver, squatting).
- Obstruction is worsened by ↑ myocardial contractility or by ↓ left ventricular filling (e.g., exercise, Valsalva maneuvers, vasodilators, dehydration).

DIAGNOSIS

- Echocardiography is diagnostic and shows an asymmetrically thickened left ventricular wall and dynamic obstruction of blood flow.
- ECG may show signs of LVH.
- CXR may reveal left atrial enlargement (LAE) 2° to mitral regurgitation.

TREATMENT

- β-blockers are initial therapy for symptomatic relief; CCBs are second-line agents.

An S₄ gallop signifies a stiff, noncompliant ventricle and ↑ "atrial kick" and may be associated with hypertrophic cardiomyopathy.

- Surgical options for HOCM include dual-chamber pacing, partial excision or catheter ablation of the myocardial septum, ICD placement, and mitral valve replacement.
- Patients should avoid intense athletic competition and training.

Restrictive Cardiomyopathy

Defined as ↓ elasticity of myocardium leading to impaired diastolic filling without significant systolic dysfunction (a normal or near-normal EF). It is caused by infiltrative disease (amyloidosis, sarcoidosis, hemochromatosis) or by scarring and fibrosis (2° to radiation or doxorubicin).

HISTORY/PE

Signs and symptoms of left-sided and right-sided heart failure occur, but symptoms of right-sided heart failure (JVD, peripheral edema) often predominate.

DIAGNOSIS

- CXR, MRI, and cardiac catheterization may be helpful, but echocardiography is key to diagnosis and reveals rapid early filling with a normal or near-normal EF.
- Cardiac biopsy may reveal fibrosis or evidence of infiltration.
- ECG frequently shows LBBB.

TREATMENT

Therapeutic options are limited and generally are palliative only. Medical treatment includes cautious use of diuretics for fluid overload, vasodilators to ↓ filling pressure, and anticoagulation if not contraindicated.

▶ CORONARY ARTERY DISEASE (CAD)

Clinical manifestations of CAD include stable and unstable angina, shortness of breath, dyspnea on exertion, arrhythmias, MI, heart failure, and sudden death. Risk factors include DM, a family history of premature CAD, smoking, dyslipidemia, abdominal obesity, hypertension, and male gender.

Angina Pectoris

Substernal chest pain 2° to myocardial ischemia (O_2 supply and demand mismatch). Prinzmetal's (variant) angina mimics angina pectoris but is caused by vasospasm of coronary vessels. It classically affects young women at rest in the early morning and is associated with ST-segment elevation in the absence of cardiac enzyme elevation.

HISTORY/PE

- The classic triad consists of substernal chest pain or pressure (often described as a heaviness or pressure without pain), usually precipitated by stress or exertion and relieved by rest or nitrates.
- Pain can radiate to the left arm, jaw, and neck and may be associated with shortness of breath, nausea/vomiting, diaphoresis, or lightheadedness.
- Examination of patients experiencing stable angina is generally unremarkable. Look for carotid and peripheral bruits suggesting atherosclerosis and hypertension.

Major risk factors for CAD include age, male gender, hyperlipidemia, DM, hypertension, obesity, a family history, and smoking.

The classic triad of angina consists of substernal chest pain that is provoked by exertion and relieved by rest or nitrates.

DIAGNOSIS

- Rule out pulmonary, GI, or other cardiac causes of chest pain.
- Angina may be diagnosed from the history alone, but significant ST-segment changes on exercise stress test with ECG monitoring is diagnostic of CAD.
- Women and diabetics classically experience "silent" ischemic events and present "atypically"; for this reason, it is necessary to maintain a high index of suspicion in this patient population.

TREATMENT

- Treat acute symptoms with ASA, O_2 and/or IV nitroglycerin, and IV morphine, and consider IV β-blockers. The efficacy of nondihydropyridine CCBs (diltiazem, verapamil) and ACEIs has also been validated.
- Patients with a suspected MI must be admitted and monitored until acute MI is ruled out by serial cardiac enzymes.
- Treat chronic symptoms with nitrates, ASA, and β-blockers; CCBs are second-line agents for symptomatic control only.
- Initiate risk factor reduction (e.g., smoking, cholesterol, hypertension). Hormone replacement therapy is not protective in postmenopausal women.

Women, diabetics, the elderly, and post–heart transplant patients may have atypical, clinically silent MIs.

Only ASA and β-blockers have been shown to have a mortality benefit in the treatment of angina.

▶ ACUTE CORONARY SYNDROMES

A spectrum of clinical syndromes caused by plaque disruption or vasospasm that leads to acute myocardial ischemia.

Unstable Angina/Non-ST-Elevation Myocardial Infarction (NSTEMI)

Unstable angina describes chest pain that is new onset, is accelerating (i.e., occurs with less exertion, lasts longer, or is less responsive to medications), or occurs at rest; it is distinguished from stable angina by patient history. It signals the presence of possible **impending infarction** based upon plaque instability. In contrast, **NSTEMI** indicates myocardial necrosis marked by elevations in **troponin I, troponin T, or CK-MB**.

Think unstable angina if chest pain is new onset, accelerating, or occurring at rest.

DIAGNOSIS

- Patients should be risk stratified according to the TIMI (Thrombolysis in Myocardial Infarction study) criteria to determine the likelihood of adverse cardiac events (see Table 2.1-10).
- Unstable angina is not associated with elevated cardiac markers, but ST changes may be seen on ECG and are indicative of high-risk occlusions.
- NSTEMI is diagnosed by serial cardiac enzymes and ECG.

TREATMENT

- Acute treatment of symptoms is the same as that for stable angina. Clopidogrel, unfractionated heparin or enoxaparin, and glycoprotein IIb/IIIa inhibitors (e.g., eptifibatide, tirofiban, abciximab) should also be considered.
- Patients with chest pain refractory to medical therapy, a TIMI score of ≥ 3, a troponin elevation, or ST changes > 1 mm should be given heparin and scheduled for angiography and possible revascularization (percutaneous coronary intervention [PCI] or CABG).

TABLE 2.1-10. **TIMI Risk Score for Unstable Angina/NSTEMI**

CHARACTERISTICS	POINT	RISK OF CARDIAC EVENTS (%) WITHIN 14 DAYS		
		RISK SCORE	DEATH OR MI	DEATH, MI, OR URGENT REVASCULARIZATION
History				
Age ≥ 65 years	1	0/1	3	5
≥ 3 CAD risk factors (family history, DM, tobacco, hypertension, ↑ cholesterol)	1	2	3	8
Known CAD (stenosis > 50%)	1	3	5	13
ASA use in past seven days	1	4	7	20
Presentation		5	12	26
Severe angina (≥ 2 episodes within 24 hours)	1	6/7	19	41
ST deviation ≥ 0.5 mm	1	Higher-risk patients (risk score ≥ 3) benefit more from enoxaparin (vs. unfractionated heparin), glycoprotein IIb/IIIa inhibitors, and early angiography.		
+ cardiac marker	1			
Risk score—total points	(0–7)			

ST-Elevation Myocardial Infarction (STEMI)

Defined as ST-segment elevations and cardiac enzyme release 2° to prolonged cardiac ischemia and necrosis.

HISTORY/PE

- Presents with acute-onset substernal chest pain, commonly described as a pressure or tightness that can radiate to the left arm, neck, or jaw.
- Associated symptoms may include diaphoresis, shortness of breath, light-headedness, anxiety, nausea/vomiting, and syncope.
- Physical exam may reveal arrhythmias, new mitral regurgitation (ruptured papillary muscle), hypotension (cardiogenic shock), and evidence of new CHF (rales, peripheral edema, S_3 gallop).
- The best predictor of survival is left ventricular EF.

DIAGNOSIS

- **ECG:** Look for ST-segment elevations or new LBBB. ST-segment depressions in leads V_1–V_2 can also be reciprocal change indicating infarction in the posterior wall.

- **Sequence of ECG changes:** Peaked T waves → ST-segment elevation → Q waves → T-wave inversion → ST-segment normalization → T-wave normalization over several hours to days.
- **Cardiac enzymes:** Troponin I is most sensitive; CK-MB is more specific. Both can take up to six hours to rise after the onset of chest pain (see Figure 2.1-4).
- **ST-segment abnormalities:**
  - ST-segment elevation in leads **II, III**, and **aVF** is consistent with an **inferior MI** involving the RCA/PDA and LCA (see Figure 2.1-5).
  - ST-segment elevation in leads V_1–V_4 usually indicates an **anterior MI** involving the LAD and diagonal branches (see Figure 2.1-6).
  - ST-segment elevation in leads **I, aVL**, and V_5–V_6 points to a **lateral MI** involving the LCA.
  - ST-segment depression in leads V_1–V_2 can be "reciprocal change" indicative of an acute infarct in the posterior wall.

TREATMENT

- Six key medications should be considered: ASA, β-blockers, clopidogrel, morphine, nitrates, and O_2.
- If the patient is in heart failure or in cardiogenic shock, do not give β-blockers; instead, give ACEIs, provided that the patient is not hypotensive.
- **Emergent angiography and PCI** should be performed; if possible, the patient should undergo PCI for the lesion thought to be responsible for STEMI.

Common causes of chest pain include GERD, angina, esophageal pain, musculoskeletal disorders (costochondritis, trauma), and pneumonia.

Other causes of ST-segment elevation (often diffuse across multiple leads) include acute pericarditis, LVH, LBBB, and a normal variant (e.g., "early repolarization").

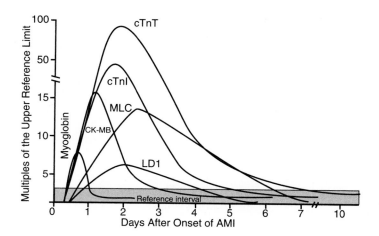

FIGURE 2.1-4. **Typical pattern of serum marker elevation after an acute MI.**

CK-MB = creatine kinase, MB isoenzyme; cTnI = cardiac troponin I; cTnT = cardiac troponin T; LD1 = lactate dehydrogenase isoenzyme 1; MLC = myosin light chain. (Reproduced, with permission, from Tintinalli JE et al. *Tintinalli's Emergency Medicine: A Comprehensive Study Guide*, 6th ed. New York: McGraw-Hill, 2004: Fig. 49-1.)

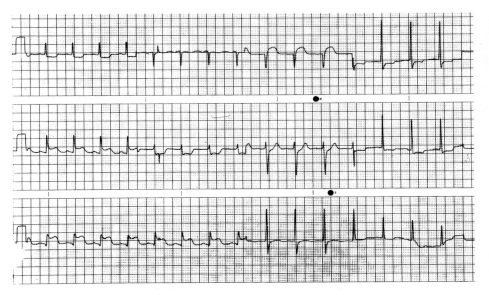

FIGURE 2.1-5. Inferior wall MI.

In this patient with acute chest pain, the ECG demonstrated acute ST-segment elevation in leads II, III, and aVF with reciprocal ST-segment depression and T-wave flattening in leads I, aVL, and V_4–V_6. (Reproduced, with permission, from Stobo J et al. *The Principles and Practice of Medicine*, 23rd ed. Stamford, CT: Appleton & Lange, 1996: 20.)

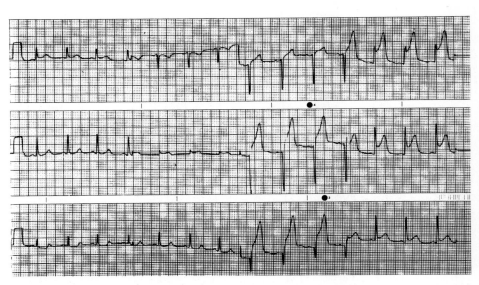

FIGURE 2.1-6. Anterior wall MI.

This patient presented with acute chest pain. The ECG showed acute ST-segment elevation in leads aVL and V_1–V_6, and hyperacute T waves. (Reproduced, with permission, from Stobo J et al. *The Principles and Practice of Medicine*, 23rd ed. Stamford, CT: Appleton & Lange, 1996: 19.)

- If the patient presents within three hours, PCI cannot be performed within 90 minutes, and there are no contraindications to thrombolysis (e.g., a history of hemorrhagic stroke or recent ischemic stroke, severe heart failure, or cardiogenic shock), thrombolysis with tPA, reteplase, or streptokinase should be performed instead of PCI.
- In the setting of three-vessel disease, left main coronary artery disease, discrete lesions not amenable to PCI, or diffuse disease with good target vessels, **PCI should be attempted immediately** for the lesion thought to be responsible for STEMI; the patient is a candidate for CABG afterward.
- Long-term treatment includes ASA, ACEIs, β-blockers, high-dose statins, and clopidogrel (if PCI was performed). Modify risk factors with dietary changes, exercise, and tobacco cessation.

> *Indications for CABG—*
>
> **DUST**
>
> **D**epressed ventricular function
> **U**nable to perform PCI (diffuse disease)
> **S**tenosis of left main coronary artery
> **T**riple-vessel disease

COMPLICATIONS

- Arrhythmia is the most common complication and cause of death following acute MI; lethal arrhythmia is the most common cause of death following acute MI.
- Less common complications include reinfarction, left ventricular wall rupture, VSD, pericarditis, papillary muscle rupture (with mitral regurgitation), left ventricular aneurysm or pseudoaneurysm, and mural thrombi.
- Dressler's syndrome, an autoimmune process occurring 2–10 weeks post-MI, presents with fever, pericarditis, pleural effusion, leukocytosis, and ↑ ESR.
- A timeline of common post-MI complications is as follows:
    - **First day:** Heart failure (treat with nitroglycerin and diuretics).
    - **2–4 days:** Arrhythmia, pericarditis (diffuse ST elevation with PR depression).
    - **5–10 days:** Left ventricular wall rupture (acute pericardial tamponade causing electrical alternans, pulseless electrical activity), papillary muscle rupture (severe mitral regurgitation).
    - **Weeks to months:** Ventricular aneurysm (CHF, arrhythmia, persistent ST elevation, mitral regurgitation, thrombus formation).

▶ HYPERCHOLESTEROLEMIA

Total cholesterol > 200 mg/dL, LDL > 130 mg/dL, triglycerides > 500 mg/dL, and HDL < 40 mg/dL are risk factors for CAD. Etiologies include obesity, DM, alcoholism, hypothyroidism, nephrotic syndrome, hepatic disease, Cushing's disease, OCP use, high-dose diuretic use, and familial hypercholesterolemia.

HISTORY/PE

- Most patients have **no specific signs or symptoms.**
- Patients with extremely high triglyceride or LDL levels may have xanthomas (eruptive nodules in the skin over the tendons), xanthelasmas (yellow fatty deposits in the skin around the eyes), and lipemia retinalis (creamy appearance of retinal vessels).

DIAGNOSIS

- Conduct a fasting lipid profile for patients > 20 years of age and repeat **every five years** or sooner if elevated.
- Total serum cholesterol > 200 mg/dL on two different occasions is diagnostic of hypercholesterolemia.

Dyslipidemia:

- LDL > 130 mg/dL or
- HDL < 40 mg/dL

TABLE 2.1-11. ATP III Guidelines for Risk Stratification of Hypercholesterolemia

RISK CATEGORY	LDL GOAL	LDL TO START LIFESTYLE MODIFICATION	LDL TO CONSIDER DRUG THERAPY
CAD or CAD risk equivalents[a]	< 100 mg/dL (or < 70)	> 100 mg/dL	> 130 mg/dL
2+ risk factors[b]	< 130 mg/dL	> 130 mg/dL	> 160 mg/dL
0–1 risk factor[b]	< 160 mg/dL	> 160 mg/dL	> 190 mg/dL

[a] CAD risk equivalents = symptomatic carotid artery disease, peripheral arterial disease, abdominal aortic aneurysm, diabetes.

[b] Risk factors = cigarette smoking, hypertension, low HDL (< 40 mg/dL), a family history of premature CAD, and age (men > 45 years; women > 55 years). An HDL > 60 mg/dL counts as a "negative" risk factor and removes one risk factor from the total score.

- LDL > 130 mg/dL or HDL < 40 mg/dL, even if total serum cholesterol is < 200 mg/dL, is diagnostic of dyslipidemia.

TREATMENT

- Based on risk stratification (see Table 2.1-11). Risk factors include diabetes (considered a CAD risk equivalent), smoking, hypertension, HDL < 40 mg/dL, age > 45 (males), age > 55 (females), and early CAD in first-degree relatives (males < 55 and females < 65).
- The **first intervention** should be a **12-week trial of diet and exercise** in a patient with no known atherosclerotic vascular disease. Commonly used lipid-lowering agents are listed in Table 2.1-12.

▶ HYPERTENSION

Defined as a systolic BP > 140 mmHg and/or a diastolic BP > 90 based on three measurements separated in time (see Table 2.1-13). Classified as 1° or 2°.

The BP goal in uncomplicated hypertension is < 140/< 90. For diabetics or patients with renal disease, the goal is < 130/< 80.

1° (Essential) Hypertension

Hypertension with no identifiable cause. Represents 95% of cases of hypertension. Risk factors include a family history of hypertension or heart disease, a high-sodium diet, smoking, obesity, race (blacks > whites), and advanced age.

HISTORY/PE

- Hypertension is asymptomatic until complications develop.
- Patients should be evaluated for end-organ damage to the brain (stroke, dementia), eye (cotton-wool exudates, hemorrhage), heart (LVH), and kidney (proteinuria, chronic kidney disease). Renal bruits may signify renal artery stenosis as the cause of hypertension.

DIAGNOSIS

- Conduct cardiovascular, neurologic, ophthalmologic, and abdominal exams.
- Obtain a UA, BUN/creatinine, CBC, and electrolytes to assess the extent of end-organ damage.

TABLE 2.1-12. Lipid-Lowering Agents

Class	Examples	Mechanism of Action	Effect on Lipid Profile	Side Effects
HMG-CoA reductase inhibitors (statins)	Atorvastatin, simvastatin, lovastatin, pravastatin, rosuvastatin	Inhibit the rate-limiting step in cholesterol synthesis.	↓ LDL, ↓ triglycerides	↑ LFTs, myositis, warfarin potentiation.
Lipoprotein lipase stimulators (fibrates)	Gemfibrozil	↑ lipoprotein lipase, leading to ↑ VLDL and triglyceride catabolism.	↓ triglycerides, ↑ HDL	GI upset, cholelithiasis, myositis, ↑ LFTs.
Cholesterol absorption inhibitors	Ezetimibe (Zetia)	↓ absorption of cholesterol at the small intestine brush border.	↓ LDL	Diarrhea, abdominal pain. Can cause angioedema.
Niacin	Niaspan	↓ fatty acid release from adipose tissue; ↓ hepatic synthesis of LDL.	↑ HDL, ↓ LDL	Skin flushing (can be prevented with ASA), paresthesias, pruritus, GI upset, ↑ LFTs.
Bile acid resins	Cholestyramine, colestipol, colesevelam	Bind intestinal bile acids lead to ↓ bile acid stores and ↑ catabolism of LDL from plasma.	↓ LDL	Constipation, GI upset, LFT abnormalities, myalgias. Can ↓ absorption of other drugs from the small intestine.

TABLE 2.1-13. JNC-7 Classification and Management of Hypertension

BP Classification	Systolic BP (mmHg)		Diastolic BP (mmHg)	Lifestyle Modification	Drug Therapy with No Comorbidities
Normal	< 120	and	< 80	Encourage	
Prehypertension	120–139	or	80–89	Yes	No antihypertensive drug indicated.
Stage 1 hypertension	140–159	or	90–99	Yes	Thiazide diuretics for most patients; ACEIs, ARBs, β-blockers, CCBs, or a combination may be considered.
Stage 2 hypertension	≥ 160	or	≥ 100	Yes	Two-drug combination for most patients (usually a thiazide diuretic plus an ACEI, an ARB, a β-blocker, or a CCB).

HIGH-YIELD FACTS

CARDIOVASCULAR

TREATMENT

- Rule out 2° causes of hypertension, particularly in younger patients.
- Begin with lifestyle modifications (e.g., weight loss, smoking cessation, salt reduction). Weight loss is the single most effective lifestyle modification. The BP goal in otherwise healthy patients is < 140/< 90. The goal in diabetics or patients with renal disease with proteinuria is < 130/< 80.
- Diuretics (which are inexpensive and particularly effective in African-Americans), ACEIs, and β-blockers (which are beneficial for patients with CAD) have been shown to ↓ mortality in uncomplicated hypertension. They are first-line agents unless a comorbid condition requires another medication (see Table 2.1-14).
- Periodically test for end-organ complications, including renal (BUN, creatinine, urine protein-to-creatinine ratio) and cardiac (ECG evidence of hypertrophy) complications.

> **Treatment of hypertension—**
>
> **ABCD**
>
> **A**CEIs/**A**RBs
> β-blockers
> **C**CBs
> **D**iuretics

2° Hypertension

Hypertension 2° to an identifiable organic cause. See Table 2.1-15 for the diagnosis and treatment of common causes.

> **Causes of 2° hypertension—**
>
> **CHAPS**
>
> **C**ushing's syndrome
> **H**yperaldosteronism (Conn's syndrome)
> **A**ortic coarctation
> **P**heochromocytoma
> **S**tenosis of renal arteries

Hypertensive Crises

A spectrum of clinical presentations in which elevated BPs lead to end-organ damage.

HISTORY/PE

Presents with end-organ damage revealed by chest pain (ischemia or MI), back pain (aortic dissection), or changes in mental status (hypertensive encephalopathy).

DIAGNOSIS

- **Hypertensive urgency:** Diagnosed on the basis of an elevated BP with only mild to moderate symptoms (headache, chest pain, syncope) and without end-organ damage.
- **Hypertensive emergency:** Diagnosed by a significantly elevated BP with signs or symptoms of impending end-organ damage such as ARF, intracra-

Hypertensive crises are diagnosed on the basis of the extent of end-organ damage, not BP measurement.

TABLE 2.1-14. Treatment of 1° Hypertension with Comorbid Conditions

CONDITION	TREATMENT
Heart failure	Thiazide diuretics, β-blockers, ACEIs, ARBs, aldosterone antagonists.
Post-MI	β-blockers, ACEIs, aldosterone antagonists.
High CVD risk	Thiazide diuretics, β-blockers, ACEIs, CCBs.
Diabetes	Thiazide diuretics, β-blockers, ACEIs, ARBs, CCBs.
Chronic kidney disease	ACEIs, ARBs.
Recurrent stroke prevention	Thiazide diuretics, ACEIs.

TABLE 2.1-15. Common Causes of 2° Hypertension

	DESCRIPTION	MANAGEMENT
1° renal disease	Often unilateral renal parenchymal disease.	Treat with ACEIs, which slow the progression of renal disease.
Renal artery stenosis	Especially common in patients < 25 and > 50 years of age with recent-onset hypertension. Etiologies include fibromuscular dysplasia (usually in younger patients) and atherosclerosis (usually in older patients).	Diagnose with MRA or renal artery Doppler ultrasound. May be treated with angioplasty or stenting. Consider ACEIs as adjunctive or temporary therapy in unilateral disease. (In bilateral disease, ACEIs can accelerate kidney failure by preferential vasodilation of the efferent arteriole.) Open surgery is a second option if angioplasty is not effective or feasible.
OCP use	Common in women > 35 years of age, obese women, and those with long-standing use.	Discontinue OCPs (effect may be delayed).
Pheochromocytoma	An adrenal gland tumor that secretes epinephrine and norepinephrine, leading to episodic headache, sweating, and tachycardia.	Diagnose with urinary metanephrines and catecholamine levels or plasma metanephrine. Surgical removal of tumor after treatment with both α-blockers and β-blockers.
Conn's syndrome (hyperaldosteronism)	Most often 2° to an aldosterone-producing adrenal adenoma. Causes the triad of hypertension, unexplained hypokalemia, and metabolic alkalosis.	Surgical removal of tumor.
Cushing's syndrome	Due to an ACTH-producing pituitary tumor, an ectopic ACTH-secreting tumor, or cortisol secretion by an adrenal adenoma or carcinoma. (See the Endocrinology chapter for more details.)	Surgical removal of tumor.
Coarctation of the aorta	See the Pediatrics chapter.	Surgical repair.

nial hemorrhage, papilledema, or ECG changes suggestive of ischemia or pulmonary edema.

■ **Malignant hypertension:** Diagnosed on the basis of progressive renal failure and/or encephalopathy with papilledema.

TREATMENT

■ **Hypertensive urgencies:** Can be treated with oral antihypertensives (e.g., β-blockers, clonidine, ACEIs) with the goal of gradually lowering BP over 24–48 hours (see Tables 2.1-16 and 2.1-17).

■ **Hypertensive emergencies:** Treat with IV medications (labetalol, nitroprusside, nicardipine) with the goal of lowering mean arterial pressure by no more than 25% over the first two hours to prevent cerebral hypoperfusion or coronary insufficiency.

TABLE 2.1-16. Major Classes of Antihypertensive Agents

CLASS	AGENTS	MECHANISM OF ACTION	SIDE EFFECTS
Diuretics	Thiazide, loop, K+ sparing	↓ extracellular fluid volume and thereby ↓ vascular resistance.	Hypokalemia (not with K+ sparing), hyperglycemia, hyperlipidemia, hyperuricemia, azotemia.
β-adrenergic blockers (β-blockers)	Propranolol, metoprolol, nadolol, atenolol, timolol, carvedilol, labetalol	↓ cardiac contractility and renin release.	Bronchospasm (in severe active asthma), bradycardia, CHF exacerbation, impotence, fatigue, depression.
Centrally acting adrenergic agonists	Methyldopa, clonidine	Inhibit the sympathetic nervous system via central α$_2$-adrenergic receptors.	Somnolence, orthostatic hypotension, impotence, rebound hypertension.
α$_1$-adrenergic blockers	Prazosin, terazosin, phenoxybenzamine	Cause vasodilation by blocking actions of norepinephrine on vascular smooth muscle.	Orthostatic hypotension.
CCBs	Dihydropyridines (nifedipine, felodipine, amlodipine), nondihydropyridines (diltiazem, verapamil)	↓ smooth muscle tone and cause vasodilation; may also ↓ cardiac output.	**Dihydropyridines:** Headache, flushing, peripheral edema. **Nondihydropyridines:** ↓ contractility.
Vasodilators	Hydralazine, minoxidil	↓ peripheral resistance by dilating arteries/arterioles.	**Hydralazine:** Headache, lupus-like syndrome. **Minoxidil:** Orthostasis, hirsutism.
ACEIs	Captopril, enalapril, fosinopril, benazepril, lisinopril	Block aldosterone formation, reducing peripheral resistance and salt/water retention.	Cough, rashes, leukopenia, hyperkalemia.
ARBs	Losartan, valsartan, irbesartan	Block aldosterone effects, reducing peripheral resistance and salt/water retention.	Rashes, leukopenia, and hyperkalemia but no cough.

▶ PERICARDIAL DISEASE

Results from acute or chronic pericardial insults; may lead to pericardial effusion.

Pericarditis

Inflammation of the pericardial sac. Can compromise cardiac output via tamponade or constrictive pericarditis. Most commonly idiopathic, although known etiologies include viral infection, TB, SLE, uremia, drugs, radiation, and neoplasms. May also occur after MI (either within days after MI or as a delayed phenomenon, i.e., Dressler's syndrome) or open heart surgery.

TABLE 2.1-17. Antihypertensive Agents for Specific Patient Populations

POPULATION	AGENT
Diabetes with proteinuria	ACEIs or ARBs.
CHF	β-blockers, ACEIs or ARBs, diuretics (including spironolactone).
Isolated systolic hypertension	Diuretics are preferred; long-acting dihydropyridines.
MI	β-blockers without intrinsic sympathomimetic activity; ACEIs.
Osteoporosis	Thiazide diuretics.
BPH	α_1-adrenergic blockers.

HISTORY/PE

- May present with pleuritic chest pain, dyspnea, cough, and fever.
- Chest pain tends to worsen in the supine position and with inspiration.
- Exam may reveal a pericardial friction rub, elevated JVP, and pulsus paradoxus (a ↓ in systolic BP > 10 mmHg on inspiration).

DIAGNOSIS

- CXR, ECG, and echocardiogram to rule out MI and pneumonia.
- ECG changes include diffuse ST-segment elevation and PR-segment depressions followed by T-wave inversions (see Figure 2.1-7).
- Pericardial thickening or effusion may be evident on echocardiography.

TREATMENT

- Address the underlying cause (e.g., corticosteroids/immunosuppressants for SLE, dialysis for uremia) or symptoms (e.g., ASA for post-MI pericarditis, ASA/NSAIDs for viral pericarditis). Avoid corticosteroids within a few days after MI, as they can predispose to ventricular wall rupture.
- Pericardial effusions without symptoms can be followed, but evidence of tamponade requires pericardiocentesis, with continuous drainage as needed.

Cardiac Tamponade

Excess fluid in the pericardial sac, leading to compromised ventricular filling and ↓ cardiac output. The condition is more closely related to the rate of fluid formation than to the size of the effusion. Risk factors include pericarditis, malignancy, SLE, TB, and trauma (commonly stab wounds medial to the left nipple).

HISTORY/PE

- Presents with fatigue, dyspnea, anxiety, tachycardia, and tachypnea that can rapidly progress to shock and death.

Causes of pericarditis—

CARDIAC RIND

Collagen vascular disease
Aortic dissection
Radiation
Drugs
Infections
Acute renal failure
Cardiac (MI)
Rheumatic fever
Injury
Neoplasms
Dressler's syndrome

Look for signs of PERICarditis—

Pulsus paradoxus
ECG changes
Rub
Increased JVP
Chest pain

Beck's triad can diagnose acute cardiac tamponade:

- *JVD*
- *Hypotension*
- *Distant heart sounds*

HIGH-YIELD FACTS

CARDIOVASCULAR

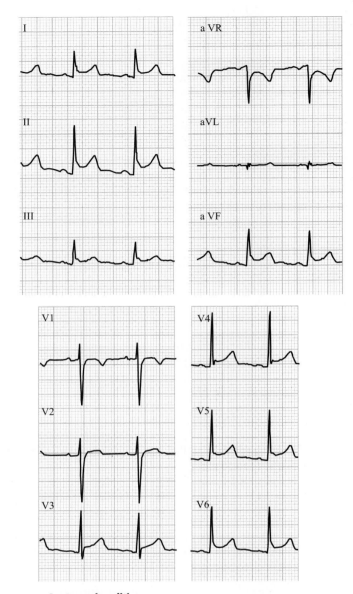

FIGURE 2.1-7. Acute pericarditis.

Diffuse ST-segment elevations in multiple leads not consistent with any discrete coronary vascular territory and PR-segment depressions. (Reproduced, with permission, from Gomella LG et al. *Clinician's Pocket Reference*, 11th ed. New York: McGraw-Hill, 2006: Fig. 19-34.)

- Examination of a patient with acute tamponade may reveal Beck's triad (hypotension, distant heart sounds, and JVD), a narrow pulse pressure, pulsus paradoxus, and Kussmaul's sign (JVD on inspiration).

DIAGNOSIS

- Echocardiogram shows right atrial and right ventricular diastolic collapse. CXR shows an enlarged, globular heart.
- If present on ECG, electrical alternans is diagnostic.

TREATMENT

- Aggressive volume expansion with IV fluids.
- Urgent pericardiocentesis (aspirate will be nonclotting blood).
- Decompensation may warrant balloon pericardiotomy and pericardial window.

▶ VALVULAR HEART DISEASE

Until recently, rheumatic fever (which affects the mitral valve more often than the aortic valve) was the most common cause of valvular heart disease in U.S. adults; the leading cause is now mechanical degeneration. Subtypes are listed in Table 2.1-18 along with their etiologies, presentation, diagnosis, and treatment.

▶ VASCULAR DISEASE

Aortic Aneurysm

Aortic aneurysms are most commonly **associated with atherosclerosis.** Most are abdominal, and > 90% originate below the renal arteries.

HISTORY/PE

- **Usually asymptomatic** and discovered incidentally on exam or radiologic study.
- Risk factors include hypertension, high cholesterol, other vascular disease, a family history, smoking, gender (males > females), and age.
- Exam demonstrates a **pulsatile abdominal mass or abdominal bruits.**
- Ruptured aneurysm leads to hypotension and severe, tearing abdominal pain that radiates to the back.

Aortic aneurysm is most often associated with atherosclerosis, while aortic dissection is commonly linked to hypertension.

DIAGNOSIS

Abdominal ultrasound for diagnosis or to follow an aneurysm over time. CT may be useful to determine the precise anatomy.

TREATMENT

- In asymptomatic patients, monitoring is appropriate for lesions < 5 cm.
- Surgical repair is indicated if the lesion is > 5.5 cm (abdominal), > 6 cm (thoracic), or smaller but rapidly enlarging.
- Emergent surgery for symptomatic or ruptured aneurysms.

Aortic Dissection

A transverse tear in the intima of a vessel that results in blood entering the media, creating a false lumen and leading to a hematoma that propagates longitudinally. **Most commonly 2° to hypertension.** The most common sites of origin are above the aortic valve and distal to the left subclavian artery. Most often occurs at 40–60 years of age, with a greater frequency in males than in females.

TABLE 2.1-18.   Types of Valvular Heart Disease

TYPE	ETIOLOGY	HISTORY	EXAM/DIAGNOSIS	TREATMENT
Aortic stenosis	Most often seen in the elderly. Unicuspid and bicuspid valves can lead to symptoms in childhood and adolescence.	May be asymptomatic for years despite significant stenosis. Once symptomatic, usually progresses from angina to syncope to CHF to death within five years. **Cx** (also indications for valve replacements): **ACS**—**A**ngina, **C**HF, **S**yncope.	**PE:** Pulsus parvus et tardus (weak, delated carotid upstroke) and a single or paradoxically split S$_2$ sound; systolic murmur radiating to the carotids. **Dx:** Echocardiography.	Valve replacement. Balloon valvuloplasty can bridge patients to aortic valve replacement but is not definitive treatment.
Aortic regurgitation	**Acute:** Infective endocarditis, aortic dissection, chest trauma. **Chronic:** Valve malformations, rheumatic fever, connective tissue disorders. **Causes:** **CREAM**— **C**ongenital **R**heumatic damage, **E**ndocarditis, **A**ortic dissection/ **A**ortic root dilatation, **M**arfan's syndrome.	**Acute:** Rapid onset of pulmonary congestion, cardiogenic shock, and severe dyspnea. **Chronic:** Slowly progressive onset of dyspnea on exertion, orthopnea, and PND.	**PE:** Blowing diastolic murmur at the left sternal border, mid-diastolic rumble (Austin Flint murmur), and midsystolic apical murmur. Widened pulse pressure causes de Musset's sign (head bob with heartbeat), Corrigan's sign (water-hammer pulse), and Duroziez's sign (femoral bruit). **Dx:** Echocardiography.	Vasodilator therapy (dihydropyridines or ACEIs) for isolated aortic regurgitation until symptoms become severe enough to warrant valve replacement.
Mitral valve stenosis	The most common etiology continues to be rheumatic fever.	Symptoms range from dyspnea, orthopnea, and PND to infective endocarditis and arrhythmias.	**PE:** Opening snap and mid-diastolic murmur at apex; pulmonary edema. **Dx:** Echocardiography.	Antiarrhythmics (digoxin, β-blockers) for symptomatic relief; mitral balloon valvotomy and valve replacement are effective for severe cases.
Mitral valve regurgitation	Primarily 2° to rheumatic fever or chordae tendineae rupture after MI.	Patients present with dyspnea, orthopnea, and fatigue.	**PE:** Holosystolic murmur radiating to axillae. **Dx:** Echocardiography will demonstrate regurgitant flow; angiography can assess the severity of disease.	Antiarrhythmics if necessary (AF is common with LAE; nitrates and diuretics to ↓ preload).

- Sudden tearing/ripping pain in the anterior chest in ascending dissection; interscapular back pain in descending dissection.
- The patient is typically hypertensive. If a patient is hypotensive, consider pericardial tamponade, hypovolemia from blood loss, or acute MI from involvement of the coronary arteries.
- **Asymmetric pulses and BP measurements** are indicative of aortic dissection.
- Signs of pericarditis or pericardial tamponade may be seen; a murmur of aortic regurgitation may be heard if the aortic valve is involved with a proximal dissection. **Neurologic deficits** may be seen if the **aortic arch or spinal arteries** are involved.

DIAGNOSIS

- ECG, CXR (shows widening of the mediastinum, cardiomegaly, or new left pleural effusion). CT angiography is the gold standard of imaging.
- TEE can provide details of the thoracic aorta, the proximal coronary arteries, the origins of arch vessels, the presence of a pericardial effusion, and aortic valve integrity.
- There are two systems of classification for aortic dissection:
    - **DeBakey system:** Classifies dissections as involving both the ascending and descending aorta (type I), confined to the ascending aorta (type II), or confined to the descending aorta (type III).
    - **Stanford system:** Classifies dissection of the ascending aorta as type A and all others as type B.

Ascending aortic dissections are surgical emergencies, but descending dissections can often be treated medically.

TREATMENT

- Monitor and medically manage BP and heart rate as necessary.
- Do not give thrombolytics.
- If the dissection involves the ascending aorta, it is a surgical emergency; descending dissections can often be managed with BP and heart rate control.

Deep Venous Thrombosis (DVT)

Clot formation in the large veins of the extremities or pelvis. The classic **Virchow's triad** of risk factors includes venous stasis (e.g., from plane flights, bed rest, or incompetent venous valves in the lower extremities), endothelial trauma (injury to the lower extremities), and hypercoagulable states (e.g., malignancy, pregnancy, OCP use).

Virchow's triad: hemostasis, trauma (endothelial damage), hypercoagulability.

HISTORY/PE

- Presents with unilateral lower extremity pain, erythema, and swelling.
- **Homans' sign** is calf tenderness with passive foot dorsiflexion (poor sensitivity and specificity for DVT).

DIAGNOSIS

Doppler ultrasound; spiral CT or V/Q scan may be used to evaluate for pulmonary embolism (see Figure 2.1-8).

A negative D-dimer test can be used to rule out the possibility of pulmonary embolism in low-risk patients.

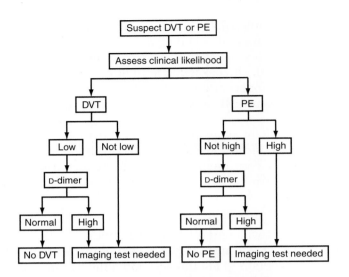

FIGURE 2.1-8. Algorithm for diagnostic imaging of DVT and PE.

(Reproduced, with permission, from Fauci AS et al. *Harrison's Principles of Internal Medicine*, 17th ed. New York: McGraw-Hill, 2008: Fig. 256-1.)

TREATMENT

- Initial anticoagulation with IV unfractionated heparin or SQ low-molecular-weight heparin followed by PO warfarin for a total of 3–6 months.
- Consider an IVC filter in patients with contraindications to anticoagulation.
- Hospitalized patients should receive DVT prophylaxis consisting of exercise as tolerated, anti-thromboembolic stockings, and SQ unfractionated heparin or low-molecular-weight heparin.

Peripheral Arterial Disease

Occlusion of the blood supply to the extremities by atherosclerotic plaque. The lower extremities are most commonly affected. Clinical manifestations depend on the vessels involved, the extent and rate of obstruction, and the presence of collateral blood flow.

HISTORY/PE

The 6 P's of acute ischemia:

Pain
Pallor
Pulselessness
Paralysis
Paresthesia
Poikilothermia

- Presents with intermittent claudication (reproducible leg pain that occurs with walking and is always relieved with rest). As the disease progresses, pain occurs at rest and affects the distal extremities. Dorsal foot ulcerations may develop 2° to poor perfusion. A painful, cold, numb foot is characteristic of critical limb ischemia.
- **Aortoiliac disease:** Associated with Leriche's syndrome (buttock claudication, ↓ femoral pulses, male impotence).
- **Femoropopliteal disease:** Calf claudication; pulses below the femoral artery are absent.
- **Acute ischemia:** Most often caused by embolization from the heart; acute occlusions commonly occur at bifurcations distal to the last palpable pulse. May also be 2° to cholesterol atheroembolism ("blue toe syndrome").

- **Severe chronic ischemia:** Lack of blood perfusion leads to muscle atrophy, pallor, cyanosis, hair loss, and gangrene/necrosis.

DIAGNOSIS

- Carefully palpate pulses and auscultate for bruits.
- Measurement of ankle and brachial systolic BP (ankle-brachial index, or ABI) can provide objective evidence of atherosclerosis (rest pain usually occurs with an ABI < 0.4). A high ABI can indicate calcification of the arteries.
- Doppler ultrasound helps identify stenosis and occlusion. Doppler ankle systolic pressure readings that are > 90% of brachial readings are normal.
- Arteriography and digital subtraction angiography are necessary for surgical evaluation.

TREATMENT

- Control underlying conditions (e.g., DM, other cardiac risk factors); eliminate tobacco and institute careful hygiene and foot care. Exercise helps develop collateral circulation.
- ASA, cilostazol, and thromboxane inhibitors may improve symptoms; anticoagulants may prevent clot formation.
- Angioplasty and stenting have a variable success rate that is dependent on the area of occlusion.
- Surgery (arterial bypass) or amputation can be employed when conservation treatment fails.
- Avoid β-blockers in peripheral arterial disease 2° to B2-mediated peripheral vasoconstriction.

Lymphedema

Disruption of the lymphatic circulation that results in peripheral edema and chronic infection of the extremities. Often a complication of surgery involving lymph node dissection. In underdeveloped countries, parasitic infection can lead to lymphatic obstruction, resulting in edema. Congenital malformations of the lymphatic system, such as Milroy's disease, can present with lymphedema in childhood.

HISTORY/PE

- Postmastectomy patients present with unexplained swelling of the upper extremity.
- Immigrants present with progressive swelling of the lower extremities bilaterally with no cardiac abnormalities (i.e., filariasis).
- Children present with progressive, bilateral swelling of the extremities.

DIAGNOSIS

Diagnosis is clinical. Rule out other causes of edema, such as cardiac and metabolic disorders.

TREATMENT

- Directed at symptom management, as no curative treatment exists. Agents such as diuretics are ineffective and relatively contraindicated.
- Exercise, massage therapy, and pressure garments to mobilize and limit fluid accumulation may be of help.

- Maintain vigilance for cellulitis with prompt gram-⊕ antibiotic coverage for infection.

A sudden, temporary loss of consciousness and postural tone 2° to cerebral hypoperfusion. Etiologies are either cardiac or noncardiac:

- **Cardiac:** Valvular lesions, arrhythmias, pulmonary embolism, cardiac tamponade, aortic dissection.
- **Noncardiac:** Orthostatic/hypovolemic hypotension, neurologic (TIA, stroke), metabolic abnormalities, neurocardiogenic syndromes (e.g., vasovagal/micturition syncope), psychiatric.

Cardiac syncope is associated with one-year sudden cardiac death rates of up to 40%.

HISTORY/PE

- Rule out many potential etiologies. Triggers, prodromal symptoms, and associated symptoms should be investigated.
- Cardiac causes of syncope are typically associated with very brief or absent prodromal symptoms, a history of exertion, lack of association with changes in position, and/or a history of cardiac disease.

DIAGNOSIS

Depending on the suspected etiology, Holter monitors or event recorders (arrhythmias), echocardiograms (structural abnormalities), and stress tests (ischemia) can be useful diagnostic tools.

TREATMENT

Tailored to the etiology.

Dermatology

The skin consists of three layers: the epidermis, the dermis, and subcutaneous tissue (see Figure 2.2-1). Table 2.2-1 describes pertinent components of the epidermis, the dermis, and the various skin appendages.

► **COMMON TERMINOLOGY**

Table 2.2-2 outlines terms frequently used to describe common manifestations of dermatologic disease.

► **ALLERGIC AND IMMUNE-MEDIATED DISORDERS**

Hypersensitivity Reactions

Table 2.2-3 outlines the types and mechanisms of hypersensitivity reactions. Descriptions of common allergic and immune-mediated disorders follow.

Atopic Dermatitis (Eczema)

A **relapsing** inflammatory skin disorder that is common in infancy and presents differently in different age groups. It is characterized by **pruritus** that leads to **lichenification** (see Figure 2.2-2).

HISTORY/PE

- Atopic dermatitis is commonly associated with asthma and allergic rhinitis.
- Patients are at ↑ risk of 2° bacterial and viral infection.
- Triggers include climate, food, contact with allergens or physical or chemical irritants, and emotional factors.

Eczema is the "itch that rashes."

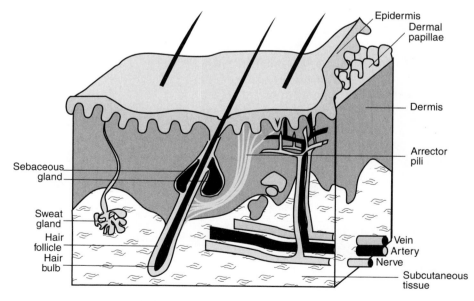

FIGURE 2.2-1.   Layers of the skin.

(Adapted, with permission, from Hardman JG et al. *Goodman and Gilman's The Pharmacological Basis of Therapeutics*, 10th ed. New York: McGraw-Hill, 2001: 1805.)

TABLE 2.2-1. **Components of Skin Layers**

EPIDERMIS	DERMIS	SKIN APPENDAGES
Keratinocytes	Fibroblasts (synthesize collagen, elastin, and ground substance)	Nails (nail matrix, nail fold, nail plate, nail bed)
Melanocytes		
Langerhans cells	Mast cells	Hair complex (hair follicles, sebaceous glands, apocrine glands)
Merkel cells	Monocytes/macrophages	
	Vessels/lymphatics	
	Nerves	Eccrine gland
	Smooth muscle	

TABLE 2.2-2. **Common Terms Used to Describe Skin Lesions**

TERM	DEFINITION
Macule	A flat lesion that differs in color from surrounding skin (< 1 cm in diameter).
Papule	An elevated solid lesion that is generally small (< 5 mm in diameter).
Patch	A small, circumscribed area differing in color from the surrounding surface (> 1 cm in diameter).
Plaque	An elevated solid lesion (> 5 mm in diameter).
Cyst	An epithelial-lined sac containing fluid or semisolid material.
Vesicle	A fluid-filled, very small (< 0.5-mm), elevated lesion.
Bulla	A large vesicle (> 5 mm).
Wheal (or hive)	An area of localized edema that follows vascular leakage and usually disappears within hours.
Erosion	A circumscribed, superficial depression resulting from the loss of some or all of the epidermis.
Ulcer	A deeper depression resulting from destruction of the epidermis and upper dermis.
Scale	Abnormal shedding or accumulation of stratum corneum in flakes.
Crust	A hardened deposit of dried serum, blood, or purulent exudates.
Lichenification	Thickening of the epidermis.
Scar	A healing defect of the dermis (the epidermis alone heals without a scar).

TABLE 2.2-3. Types and Mechanisms of Hypersensitivity Reactions

TYPE	MECHANISM	COMMENTS
Type I	**Anaphylactic and atopic:** Antigen cross-links IgE on presensitized mast cells and basophils, triggering the release of vasoactive amines (i.e., histamine). Reaction develops rapidly after antigen exposure as a result of preformed antibody. Examples include anaphylaxis, asthma, urticarial drug reactions, and local wheal and flare.	First and Fast (anaphylaxis). Types I, II, and III are all antibody, or B-cell, mediated.
Type II	**Cytotoxic:** IgM and IgG bind to antigen on an "enemy" cell, leading to lysis (by complement) or phagocytosis. Examples include autoimmune hemolytic anemia, Rh disease (erythroblastosis fetalis), Goodpasture's syndrome, and rheumatic fever.	Cy-**2**-toxic. Antibody and complement lead to membrane attack complex (MAC).
Type III	**Immune complex:** Antigen-antibody complexes activate complement, which attracts neutrophils; neutrophils release lysosomal enzymes. Examples include polyarteritis nodosa, immune complex glomerulonephritis, SLE, and rheumatoid arthritis.	Imagine an immune complex as three things stuck together: antigen-antibody complement. Includes many glomerulonephritides and vasculitides.
	Serum sickness: An immune complex disease (type III) in which antibodies to the foreign proteins are produced (takes five days). Immune complexes form and are deposited in membranes, where they fix complement (leading to tissue damage). More common than Arthus reaction.	Most serum sickness is now caused by drugs (not serum). Fever, urticaria, arthralgias, proteinuria, and lymphadenopathy occur 5–10 days after antigen exposure.
	Arthus reaction: A local subacute antibody-mediated hypersensitivity (type III) reaction. **Intradermal injection of antigen** induces antibodies, which form antigen-antibody complexes in the skin. Characterized by edema, necrosis, and activation of complement. Examples include hypersensitivity pneumonitis and thermophilic actinomycetes.	Antigen-antibody complexes cause the Arthus reaction.
Type IV	**Delayed (cell-mediated) type:** Sensitized T lymphocytes encounter antigen and then release lymphokines (leading to macrophage activation). Examples include TB skin tests, transplant rejection, and contact dermatitis (e.g., poison ivy, poison oak).	**4th** and last—**delayed.** Cell mediated, not antibody mediated; therefore, it is not transferable by serum.

HIGH-YIELD FACTS

DERMATOLOGY

- Clinical manifestations by age group are as follows:
  - **Infants:** Erythematous, weeping, pruritic patches on the face, scalp, and diaper area.
  - **Children:** Dry, scaly, pruritic, excoriated patches in the flexural areas and neck.
  - **Adults:** Lichenification and dry, fissured skin, often limited to the hands.

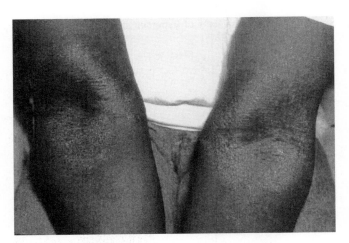

FIGURE 2.2-2. Atopic dermatitis.

Hyperpigmentation, lichenification, and scaling are seen in the antecubital fossae. (Courtesy of Robert Swerlick, MD, as published in Fauci AS, Braunwald E, Kasper DL, et al. *Harrison's Principles of Internal Medicine*, 17th ed. New York: McGraw-Hill, 2008.)

DIAGNOSIS

Diagnosis is made clinically. Patients may have mild eosinophilia and ↑ IgE. Rule out seborrheic dermatitis, contact dermatitis, pityriasis rosea, drug eruption, and cutaneous T-cell lymphoma.

TREATMENT

- Prophylactic measures include use of nondrying soaps, application of **moisturizers,** and avoidance of known triggers.
- Treat with topical corticosteroids (avoid systemic steroids in light of their side effect profile), PUVA, and topical immunomodulators (e.g., tacrolimus, pimecrolimus).
- Topical corticosteroids should not be used for longer than 2–3 weeks.

Contact Dermatitis

A type IV hypersensitivity reaction that results from contact with an allergen to which the patient has **previously been exposed and sensitized.** Dermatitis develops when the patient is reexposed to the allergen or to a cross-reactive compound. More common in adults than in children.

HISTORY/PE

- Commonly presents with pruritus and rash, but can also present with edema, fever, and lymphadenopathy.
- Frequently implicated allergens include poison ivy, poison oak, nickel, soaps, detergents, cosmetics, and rubber products containing latex (e.g., gloves and elastic bands in clothing).
- Characteristic distributions involve areas where makeup, clothing, perfume, nickel jewelry, and plants come into contact with the skin.
- The dermatitis begins in the area of contact with the antigen, with its appearance varying with the acuity of the lesion.

Erythema toxicum of the newborn resembles eczema, presenting with red papules/ vesicles with surrounding erythema. ↑ eosinophils will be seen on biopsy. This typically benign rash rarely appears after five days of age and is usually gone in 7–14 days; treatment is typically observation.

- **Acute:** Approximately 24–48 hours after an allergic contact, the skin becomes erythematous, presenting with tiny blisters followed by scale and crusts. Lesions are intensely pruritic.
- **Subacute:** Results from episodic exposure or a weak allergen. Lesions are less "angry appearing" than those of an acute inflammatory rash, and some lichenification is seen.
- **Chronic:** Results from extended exposure to an allergen. Characterized by erythema and lichenification with fissuring, often with superimposed acute dermatitis.
- The overall shape of the rash often mimics that of the exposing object (see Figure 2.2-3), but it can also spread over the body via transfer of allergen by the hands or via circulating T lymphocytes. Patients are at ↑ risk of 2° infection.

The pathogenesis of contact dermatitis involves allergenic molecules that are passed through the epidermis and taken up by Langerhans cells, which carry them to the lymph nodes and expose them to T lymphocytes.

DIAGNOSIS

Diagnosed by clinical impression. A **patch test** can be used to establish the causative allergen after the acute-phase rash has been treated. The differential includes atopic dermatitis, seborrheic dermatitis, impetigo, HSV, herpes zoster, and fungal infection.

TREATMENT

- Prophylaxis consists of avoidance of the offending allergen.
- Treat with topical or systemic corticosteroids as needed and with cool, wet compresses to relieve and debride the skin.

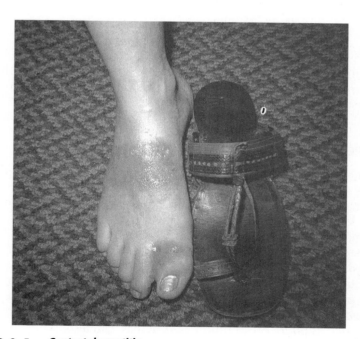

FIGURE 2.2-3. Contact dermatitis.

Shown above are erythematous papules and vesicles with serous weeping localized to areas of contact with the offending agent. (Reproduced, with permission, from Hurwitz RM. *Pathology of the Skin: Atlas of Clinical-Pathological Correlation*, 2nd ed. Stamford, CT: Appleton & Lange, 1998: 3.)

Seborrheic Dermatitis

A common disease that may be caused by *Pityrosporum ovale*, a generally harmless yeast found in sebum and hair follicles. It has a predilection for **areas with oily skin** such as the scalp, eyebrows, nasolabial folds, and midchest.

HISTORY/PE

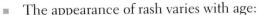

- The appearance of rash varies with age:
    - **Infants:** Presents as a severe, red diaper rash with yellow scale, erosions, and blisters. A thick crust ("cradle cap") may be seen on the scalp.
    - **Children/adults:** Red, scaly patches are seen around the ears, eyebrows, nasolabial fold, midchest, and scalp. The rash is more localized and less dramatic than that seen in infants.
- Patients with **HIV/AIDS can develop severe seborrheic dermatitis or an overlapping syndrome** of severe seborrheic dermatitis, psoriasis, psoriatic arthritis, and even Reiter's syndrome.

Suspect HIV in a young person with severe seborrheic dermatitis.

DIAGNOSIS

Diagnosed by clinical impression. Rule out contact dermatitis and psoriasis.

TREATMENT

Treatment consists of selenium sulfide or zinc pyrithione shampoos for the scalp, and topical antifungals and/or topical corticosteroids for other areas. Low-concentration coal tar shampoos are still available despite concerns about carcinogenicity.

Psoriasis

A T-cell-mediated inflammatory dermatosis characterized by **erythematous patches** and **silvery scales** due to dermal inflammation and epidermal hyperplasia. Five percent of patients also have a **seronegative arthritis.** The condition usually starts in puberty or young adulthood, and its incidence is 2–4%.

HISTORY/PE

- The typical lesion is a round, sharply bordered erythematous patch with silvery scales (see Figure 2.2-4A).
- Lesions are classically found on the **extensor surfaces,** including the elbows, knees, scalp, and lumbosacral regions.
- Lesions may initially appear very small (guttate) but may slowly enlarge and become confluent. Psoriatic nails feature pitting, "oil spots," and **onycholysis,** or lifting of the nail plate (see Figure 2.2-4B).
- Psoriatic lesions can be provoked by local irritation or by trauma (**Koebner's phenomenon**). Streptococcal infection can lead to cutaneous immune complex deposition, which triggers guttate psoriasis. Some medications, such as β-blockers, lithium, and ACEIs, can also induce psoriasis.
- **Psoriatic arthritis** usually begins in the hands with "**sausage digits,**" but the knees, wrists and ankles as well as the lumbosacral region may also be affected. Arthritic patients with spinal involvement are usually HLA-B27 ⊕.
- When pustular psoriasis, a less common form, is generalized, it can be life threatening, presenting with fever, electrolyte abnormalities, and loss of serum proteins.

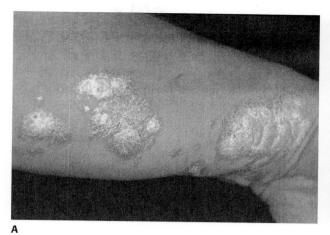
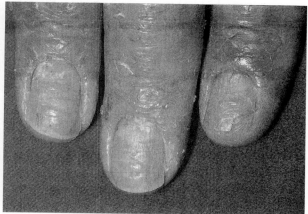

A

B

FIGURE 2.2-4.   Psoriasis.

(A) Skin changes. The classic sharply demarcated plaques with silvery scales are commonly located on the extensor surfaces (e.g., elbows, knees). (B) Nail changes. Note the pitting, onycholysis, and "oil spots." (Reproduced, with permission, from Hurwitz RM. *Pathology of the Skin: Atlas of Clinical-Pathological Correlation*, 2nd ed. Stamford, CT: Appleton & Lange, 1998: 15, 18.)

Diagnosis

- Clinical impression is usually sufficient for diagnosis.
- Classically presents with the **Auspitz sign** (bleeding when scale is scraped), but biopsy can be useful.
- Histology classically shows a thickened epidermis, elongated rete ridges, an absent granular cell layer, preservation of nuclei, and a sterile neutrophilic infiltrate (**Munro's microabscess**) in the stratum corneum.

Treatment

- Treat with topical steroids combined with keratolytic agents, tar, or anthralin along with UV therapy, including PUVA. Methotrexate may be used for severe cases. Retinoids (vitamin A derivatives) may also be used.
- Arthritis should be treated first with NSAIDs and then with methotrexate if necessary. Systemic corticosteroids should be avoided, as tapering can induce psoriatic flares.
- Recently, biologic agents such as TNF-α inhibitors have proven effective in severe psoriatic arthritis and psoriasis.

Urticaria (Hives)

Urticaria is characterized by superficial, intense edema in a localized area. It is usually acute but can also be chronic (lasting > 6 weeks). The condition results from the release of vasoactive substances (histamine, prostaglandins) from mast cells in a **type I hypersensitivity response.**

History/PE

- Hives can range in severity from a few itchy bumps to life-threatening anaphylaxis.

- The typical lesion is an elevated papule or plaque that is reddish or white and variable in size. Lesions are widespread and last a few hours.
- In severe allergic reactions, **extracutaneous manifestations** can include tongue swelling, angioedema (deeper, more diffuse swelling), asthma, GI symptoms, joint swelling, and fever.
- Acute urticaria is a response to a trigger that may be a food, drug, virus, insect bite, or physical stimulus. Chronic urticaria is usually idiopathic.

DIAGNOSIS

Diagnosed by clinical impression and patient report. Biopsy demonstrates perivascular edema. It can often be difficult to determine the cause.

TREATMENT

Treat with systemic antihistamines. Topical medications are of no benefit.

Drug Eruption

Maintain a high suspicion for a cutaneous drug reaction in patients who are hospitalized and develop rashes. Such reactions can take many forms, including urticarial, lupus-like, vasculitic, purpuric, lichenoid, and vesicular. Drugs can cause **all four types of hypersensitivity reactions,** and sometimes the same drug may cause different types of reactions in different patients.

HISTORY/PE

- Eruptions occur **7–14 days after exposure, so if a patient reacts within a day or two of starting a new drug (i.e., a drug they have never taken before), that drug is probably not the causative agent.**
- Eruptions are generally **widespread, relatively symmetrical,** and **pruritic.** Most are relatively short-lived, disappearing within 1–2 weeks following removal of the offending agent.
- The exception is **fixed drug eruption,** which consists of reddish macules or papules that develop in the same area (usually the genitalia, face, or extremities) each time the patient is exposed to the triggering agent. After these lesions resolve, there is often a persistent brown pigmentation.
- Extreme complications of drug eruptions include erythroderma and toxic epidermal necrolysis (TEN).

DIAGNOSIS

Diagnosed by clinical impression. Patients may have eosinophilia and eosinophils on histopathology.

TREATMENT

Discontinue the offending agent; treat symptoms with antihistamines.

Erythema Multiforme

A cutaneous reaction pattern with classic targetoid lesions that has many triggers and is often recurrent. Although some cases are idiopathic, many are triggered by recurrent HSV infection of the lip. Other common triggers are drugs (e.g., sulfa drugs, anticonvulsants, barbiturates, penicillin, NSAIDs) and mycoplasmal infections.

History/PE

- The characteristic lesion has a **target appearance** (see Figure 2.2-5), but other types of lesions may be seen as well.
- The disease can occur on mucous membranes, where erosions are seen. Typically, lesions start as erythematous macules that become centrally clear and then develop a blister. The **palms and soles** are often affected.
- May be associated with systemic symptoms, including fever, myalgias, headache, and arthralgias (these symptoms may precede eruption).
- In its minor form, the disease is uncomplicated and localized to the skin. However, severe erythema multiforme can lead to **TEN or Stevens-Johnson syndrome,** in which patients are very ill with involvement of at least two mucosal surfaces.

Diagnosis

Diagnosed by clinical impression. A **history of recurrent labial herpes** should be sought in all cases with multiple recurrences.

Treatment

- Symptomatic treatment is all that is necessary; systemic corticosteroids are of no benefit.
- Minor cases can be treated with antipruritics; major cases should be treated as burns. In patients with HSV, suppressive acyclovir may ↓ the frequency of rashes.

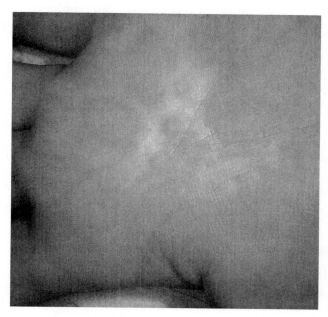

FIGURE 2.2-5.   Erythema multiforme.

Evolving erythematous plaques and papules are seen with a target appearance consisting of a dull red center, a pale zone, and a darker outer ring. (Reproduced, with permission, from Hurwitz RM. *Pathology of the Skin: Atlas of Clinical-Pathological Correlation*, 2nd ed. Stamford, CT: Appleton & Lange, 1998: 24.)

Stevens-Johnson Syndrome (SJS)/Toxic Epidermal Necrolysis (TEN)

SJS and TEN constitute two different points on the spectrum of life-threatening exfoliative mucocutaneous diseases that are often caused by a drug-induced immunologic reaction. The epidermal separation of SJS involves < 10% of body surface area (BSA), whereas TEN involves > 30% of BSA. Involvement of 10–30% of BSA is often considered SJS/TEN overlap.

HISTORY/PE

- May be preceded by erythema multiforme, a flulike prodrome, skin tenderness, a maculopapular drug rash, or painful mouth lesions.
- Often associated with a history of exposure to new drugs, such as penicillin, sulfonamides, seizure medications (e.g., phenytoin, carbamazepine), quinolones, cephalosporins, allopurinol, corticosteroids, or NSAIDs.
- Exam reveals severe mucosal erosions with widespread erythematous, cutaneous macules or atypical targetoid lesions. The epidermal lesions often become confluent and show a ⊕ Nikolsky's sign and epidermal detachment.
- Mucous membranes of the eyes, mouth, and genitals often become eroded and hemorrhagic as well.

DIAGNOSIS

- **SJS:** Biopsy shows **degeneration of the basal layer of the epidermis** and perivascular mononuclear infiltrate with some eosinophils in the papillary dermis. Subepidermal blisters may also be seen.
- **TEN:** Biopsy shows **full-thickness eosinophilic epidermal necrosis** with cell-poor infiltrate; there is a sparse perivascular lymphocytic infiltrate.
- **TEN vs. SSSS:** On biopsy, TEN demonstrates full-thickness epidermal damage, whereas SSSS shows only superficial damage.
- The differential also includes graft-versus-host reaction (usually after bone marrow transplant), radiation therapy, and burns.

TREATMENT

Patients have the **same complications as burn victims,** including thermoregulatory difficulties, electrolyte disturbances, and 2° infections. Treatment includes skin coverage and maintenance of fluid and electrolyte balance. Controversial treatments include systemic corticosteroids in the early stages of SJS/TEN or IVIG. There is a high risk of mortality.

Erythema Nodosum

A **panniculitis** whose triggers include **infection** (e.g., *Streptococcus, Coccidioides, Yersinia,* TB), **drug reactions** (e.g., sulfonamides, various antibiotics, OCPs), and **chronic inflammatory diseases** (e.g., sarcoidosis, Crohn's disease, ulcerative colitis, Behçet's disease).

HISTORY/PE

Painful, erythematous nodules appear on the patient's lower legs (see Figure 2.2-6) and slowly spread, turning brown or gray. Patients may present with **fever and joint pain.**

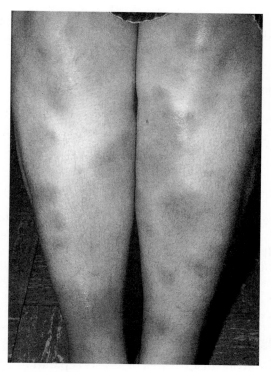

FIGURE 2.2-6.   Erythema nodosum.

Erythematous plaques and nodules are commonly located on pretibial areas. Lesions are painful and indurated but heal spontaneously without ulceration. (Reproduced, with permission, from Hurwitz RM. *Pathology of the Skin: Atlas of Clinical-Pathological Correlation*, 2nd ed. Stamford, CT: Appleton & Lange, 1998: 132.)

DIAGNOSIS

- Diagnosed by clinical impression. Histology shows nonspecific septal panniculitis.
- Workup should include an ASO titer, a PPD test in patients who are high risk, a CXR to rule out sarcoid, and a small bowel series to rule out IBD in patients with GI symptoms.

TREATMENT

Remove the triggering factor and treat the underlying disease where possible. NSAIDs can be used but may lead to erythema multiforme.

Pemphigus Vulgaris

A life-threatening autoimmune condition characterized by an **intraepidermal blister leading to widespread painful erosions** of the skin and mucous membranes. Antibodies are directed against desmoglein molecules responsible for keratinocyte adherence, leading to loss of cellular attachment. Patients are generally **middle-aged** (40–60).

HISTORY/PE

Initial presentation is with mucous membrane involvement, typically mouth ulcers, with progression to skin involvement. Rarely, an intact blister may be seen, but generally presents only with erosions, often accompanied by crusting, weeping, and 2° infections.

DIAGNOSIS

- Along with the clinical picture, a ⊕ **Nikolsky's sign** (the ability to produce a blister by rubbing skin adjacent to a natural blister) and skin biopsy with immunofluorescence confirm the diagnosis.
- Biopsy shows **acantholysis** (intraepidermal split with free-floating keratinocytes in the blister). Immunofluorescence and ELISA are confirmatory for antidesmoglein antibodies.

TREATMENT

- Long-term treatment is generally required. Initially, systemic corticosteroids are used at high doses in combination with steroid-sparing agents introduced early to ↓ corticosteroid side effects.
- Steroid-sparing agents include mycophenolate mofetil and azathioprine. Recently, rituximab and IVIG have been successfully used for recalcitrant disease.

Bullous Pemphigoid

An **acquired blistering disease** that leads to **separation at the epidermal basement membrane**. It is most commonly seen in patients **60–80 years of age**. Its pathogenesis involves **antibodies** that are developed against the bullous pemphigoid antigen, which lies superficially in the basement membrane zone (BMZ). Antigen-antibody complexes activate complement and eosinophil degranulation that provoke an inflammatory reaction and lead to

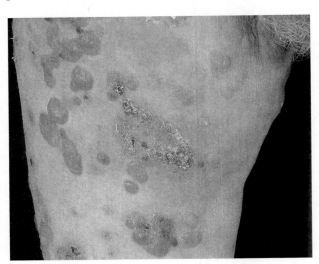

FIGURE 2.2-7. **Bullous pemphigoid.**

Multiple tense serous and partially hemorrhagic bullae can be seen. (Reproduced, with permission, from Fitzpatrick TB. *Color Atlas & Synopsis of Clinical Dermatology*, 4th ed. New York: McGraw-Hill, 2001: 100.)

separation at the BMZ. The **blisters are stable** because their roof consists of nearly normal epidermis.

HISTORY/PE

Presents with firm, stable blisters that arise on erythematous skin, often preceded by urticarial lesions. **Nikolsky's sign is** ⊖. The blisters form crusts and erosions (see Figure 2.2-7). Mucous membranes are less commonly involved than is the case in pemphigus.

DIAGNOSIS

Diagnosed according to the clinical picture. Skin biopsy shows a subepidermal blister, often with an eosinophil-rich infiltrate. Immunofluorescence demonstrates linear IgG and C3 immunoglobulin and complement at the dermal-epidermal junction.

TREATMENT

Systemic corticosteroids. Topical corticosteroids can help prevent blister formation when applied to early lesions.

▶ INFECTIOUS DISEASE MANIFESTATIONS

Viral Diseases

HERPES SIMPLEX

A painful, recurrent vesicular eruption of the mucocutaneous surfaces due to infection with HSV. **HSV-1 usually produces oral-labial lesions, whereas HSV-2 usually causes genital lesions.** The virus spreads through epidermal cells, causing them to fuse into **giant cells.** The local host inflammatory response leads to erythema and swelling.

HISTORY/PE

- The initial infection is passed by direct contact, after which the herpesvirus remains dormant in local nerve ganglia. **1° episodes** are generally longer and more severe than recurrences.
- Onset is preceded by prodromal tingling, burning, or pain but can also present with lymphadenopathy, fever, discomfort, malaise, and edema of involved tissue.
- **Recurrences** are limited to mucocutaneous areas innervated by the involved nerve.
  - **Recurrent oral herpes (HSV-1):** Typically consists of the common "cold sore," which presents as a cluster of crusted vesicles on an erythematous base (see Figure 2.2-8A). It is often triggered by sun and fever.
  - **Recurrent genital herpes (HSV-2):** Unilateral and characterized by a cluster of blisters on an erythematous base, but with less pain and systemic involvement than the 1° infection.

DIAGNOSIS

- Diagnosed primarily by the clinical picture. **Multinucleated giant cells** on **Tzanck smear** (see Figure 2.2-8B) yield a presumptive diagnosis.
- VZV has the same appearance on Tzanck, so culture or direct fluorescent antibody staining is needed for definitive diagnosis.

Dermatitis herpetiformis differs from HSV, consisting of pruritic papules and vesicles on the elbows, knees, buttocks, neck, and scalp. Granular IgA is seen on dermal papillae. The condition is associated with celiac disease (15–25% of celiac patients may have it). Treat with dapsone and a gluten-free diet.

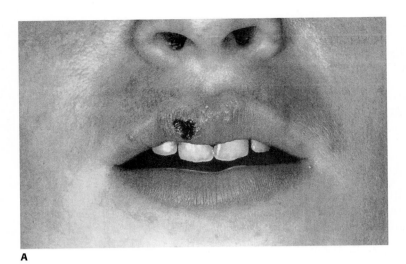
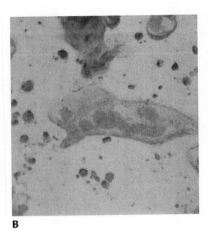

A

B

FIGURE 2.2-8. **Herpes simplex.**

(A) 1° infection. Grouped vesicles on an erythematous base on the patient's lips and oral mucosa may progress to pustules before resolving. (B) Tzanck smear. The multinucleated giant cells from vesicular fluid provide a presumptive diagnosis of HSV infection. The Tzanck smear cannot distinguish between HSV and VZV infection. (Reproduced, with permission, from Hurwitz RM. *Pathology of the Skin: Atlas of Clinical-Pathological Correlation*, 2nd ed. Stamford, CT: Appleton & Lange, 1998: 145.)

TREATMENT

- Oral or IV acyclovir (IV for severe cases or for immunocompromised patients) ↓ both the frequency and the severity of recurrences. Daily acyclovir, valacyclovir, or famciclovir suppressive therapy may be used in patients with > 6 outbreaks per year or for those with erythema multiforme.
- Acyclovir ointment is somewhat effective in reducing the duration of viral shedding but does not prevent recurrence.
- In AIDS patients, HSV can persist, with ulcers remaining resistant to antiviral therapy. Symptomatic HSV infection lasting > 1 month can be considered an AIDS-defining illness.

VARICELLA-ZOSTER VIRUS (VZV)

VZV causes two different diseases, **varicella and herpes zoster**—with transmission occurring via respiratory droplet or by direct contact. VZV has an incubation period of 10–20 days, with contagion beginning 24 hours before the eruption appears and lasting until lesions have crusted.

HISTORY/PE

- Varicella:
  - A prodrome consisting of malaise, fever, headache, and myalgia occurs 24 hours before the onset of the rash.
  - Pruritic lesions appear in crops over a period of 2–3 days, evolving from red macules to grouped central vesicles (**"dewdrop on a rose petal"**) and then crusting over.
  - At any given time, patients have **all stages of lesions over their entire body.** The trunk, face, scalp, and mucous membranes are involved, but the **palms and soles are spared.**
  - In adults, chickenpox is often more severe, with **systemic complications** such as **pneumonia** and **encephalitis.**

and even laryngeal mucosa. Laryngeal warts are transmitted to infants by mothers with genital HPV.

DIAGNOSIS

Diagnosed by the clinical picture. **Acetowhitening** can be helpful in visualizing mucosal lesions. There is a long latency period, with children sometimes acquiring HPV at birth and not manifesting any lesions until years later.

TREATMENT

Treatment centers on destruction of the tissue by curettage, cryotherapy, or acid keratolytics. Genital warts are treated locally with podophyllin, trichloroacetic acid, imiquimod, or 5-FU. HPV lesions on the cervix must be monitored cytologically and histologically for evidence of malignancy.

Bacterial Infections

IMPETIGO

A superficial, weeping local infection that primarily occurs in **children** and is caused by both **group A streptococcal and staphylococcal** organisms. It is transmitted by direct contact.

HISTORY/PE

- There are two types:
    - **Common type:** Characterized by pustules and **honey-colored crusts** on an erythematous base; generally appears on the face (see Figure 2.2-11).
    - **Bullous type:** Usually acral; characterized by large stable blisters.
- Bullous impetigo is almost always caused by *S. aureus* and can evolve into SSSS. Streptococcal impetigo can be complicated by acute streptococcal glomerulonephritis.

What is another skin condition caused by group A strep?
Erysipelas, *which presents as a small red patch on the cheek that turns into a painful raised, shiny red plaque. Patients often have a history of trauma or pharyngitis. Treat with penicillin.*

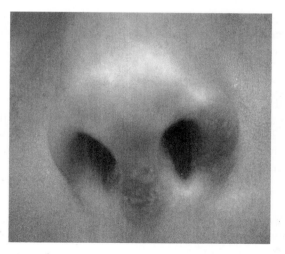

FIGURE 2.2-11. Impetigo.

Dried pustules with a superficial golden-brown crust are most commonly found around the nose and mouth. (Reproduced, with permission, from Hurwitz RM. *Pathology of the Skin: Atlas of Clinical-Pathological Correlation*, 2nd ed. Stamford, CT: Appleton & Lange, 1998: 165.)

- **Scarlet fever:** *"Sunburn with goosebumps" appearance; strawberry tongue. Caused by* S. pyogenes. *Treatment: Penicillin.*
- **Salmonella typhi:** *Small pink papules on the trunk ("rose spots") in groups of 10–20 plus gallbladder disease. Treatment: Cholecystectomy for chronic carrier state.*

Ludwig's angina is a bilateral cellulitis of the submaxillary/ sublingual spaces that usually results from an infected tooth. It presents with dysphagia, drooling, fever, and a red, warm mouth and can lead to death from asphyxiation.

DIAGNOSIS

Diagnosed by the clinical picture.

TREATMENT

Treat with antibiotics with antistaphylococcal activity. Topical antibiotics are often sufficient, but systemic agents can hasten recovery and prevent spread to other patients.

ERYTHRASMA

An infection caused by *Corynebacterium*, presenting as brownish-red patches with fine scales that characteristically appear along major skin folds. It is more common among diabetics.

DIAGNOSIS

Wood's light exam reveals coral-red fluorescence of lesions. Gram staining reveals gram-⊕, filamentous rods.

TREATMENT

Treat with erythromycin. (Remember: **erythr**asma is treated with **erythr**omycin.)

CELLULITIS

A **deep, local infection** involving the connective tissue, subcutaneous tissue, or muscle in addition to the skin. It is commonly caused by **staphylococci** or **group A streptococci** originating from an area of damaged skin or from a systemic source of infection. **Community-acquired MRSA** is an increasingly common cause. Risk factors include diabetes, IV drug use, venous stasis, and immune compromise.

HISTORY/PE

Presents with **red, hot, swollen, tender skin.** Fever and chills are also common.

DIAGNOSIS

Diagnosed by the clinical picture; wound culture may aid in diagnosis and help determine antibiotic sensitivities for treatment. Blood cultures should be obtained when bacteremia is suspected. Culture and sensitivities are important in case of MRSA. Rule out abscess, urticaria, contact dermatitis, osteomyelitis, and necrotizing fasciitis.

TREATMENT

Treat with 7–10 days of oral antibiotics for mild cases or with IV antibiotics if there is evidence of systemic toxicity, comorbid conditions, DM, extremes of age, hand or orbital involvement, or other concerns.

NECROTIZING FASCIITIS

Deep infection along a fascial plane causing severe pain followed by anesthesia. Infection is caused by *S. pyogenes* or *Clostridium perfringens*. A history of trauma or a recent surgery to the affected area is often but not always elicited.

HISTORY/PE

- Presents with sudden onset of pain and swelling at the site of trauma or recent surgery. Pain often progresses to anesthesia.
- An area of erythema quickly spreads over the course of hours to days. Margins move out into normal skin, and skin becomes dusky or purplish near the site of insult, ultimately leading to necrosis.
- Necrosis can initially have the appearance of undermining of the skin and subcutaneous layer; if the skin is open, gloved fingers can easily pass between the two layers to reveal yellow-green necrotic fascia (infection spreads quickly in deep fascia).
- The most important signs are tissue necrosis, a putrid discharge, bullae, severe pain, gas production, rapid burrowing through fascial planes, lack of classical tissue inflammatory signs, and intravascular volume loss.

Fournier gangrene is a form of necrotizing fasciitis that is localized to the scrotum and perineal area.

DIAGNOSIS

Local radiographs or CT scans show air in tissue. Biopsy from the edge of the lesion can be diagnostic.

TREATMENT

- A surgical emergency. Early and aggressive surgical debridement is critical.
- If *Streptococcus* is the principal organism involved, penicillin G is the drug of choice. Clindamycin is second line.
- For anaerobic coverage, give metronidazole or a third-generation cephalosporin.

FOLLICULITIS

Inflammation of the hair follicle. Although typically caused by infection with **Staphylococcus, Streptococcus,** and **gram-⊖ bacteria,** folliculitis may occasionally be caused by **yeast** such as *Candida albicans* or *Pityrosporum ovale.* It may also be **mechanical,** arising from ingrown hairs (most common in patients with curly hair).

HISTORY/PE

- Presents as a **tiny pustule** that appears at the opening of a hair follicle and usually has a hair penetrating it. When the infection is deeper, a **furuncle,** or hair follicle abscess, develops.
- Furuncles are larger and more painful than folliculitic lesions and may disseminate to adjacent follicles to form a **carbuncle.** Patients with diabetes or immunosuppression are at ↑ risk.
- Folliculitis can be a critical problem in AIDS patients, in whom the disease is intensely pruritic and resistant to therapy.

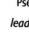

Pseudomonas aeruginosa leads to "hot tub folliculitis."

DIAGNOSIS

Diagnosed by the clinical picture.

TREATMENT

Topical antibiotics can be used to treat mild disease, but severe cases require systemic antibiotics. Large lesions must be incised, drained, and cultured to rule out MRSA. Patients who are prone to ingrown hairs should be advised not to shave.

ACNE VULGARIS

An endogenous skin disease that is common among adolescents. The pathogenesis involves hormonal activation of sebaceous glands, the development of the comedo or plugged sebaceous follicle, and involvement of *Propionibacterium acnes* in the follicle, causing inflammation. Comedones may be caused by medications (e.g., lithium, corticosteroids) or by topical occlusion (e.g., cosmetics).

HISTORY/PE

- There are three stages of acne lesions:
    - **Comedo:** May be open ("**blackheads**") or closed ("**whiteheads**"); present in large quantities but with little inflammation.
    - **Inflammatory:** The comedo ruptures, creating a pustule that can be large and nodular.
    - **Scar:** As the inflammation heals, scars may develop. Picking at papules exacerbates scarring.
- Two types of cysts can occur in acne: inflammatory cysts, which are large, fluctuant pustules, and epidermoid cysts, which develop along the eyebrows and behind the ears.
- Acne first develops at puberty and typically persists for several years. Males are more likely to have severe, cystic acne than are females. Women in their 20s tend to have a variant that flares cyclically with menstruation, featuring fewer comedones and more painful lesions on the chin. Androgenic stimulation may contribute to these lesions.

DIAGNOSIS

Diagnosed by the clinical picture.

*Ironically, erythromycin does **not** cause erythema with sun exposure. It is tetracycline and doxycycline that can cause serious photosensitivity!*

TREATMENT

- Treat comedones with topical **tretinoin** (Retin-A) and benzoyl peroxide.
- Inflammatory lesions should be treated with topical antibiotics (e.g., erythromycin, clindamycin) or systemic agents (e.g., tetracycline, erythromycin).
- Isotretinoin (**Accutane**) leads to marked improvement in > 90% of acne patients and has greatly improved the treatment of severe acne.
    - Isotretinoin is, however, a teratogen and may cause transient elevations in cholesterol, triglycerides, and LFTs, and it may also be associated with depression.
    - Patients on isotretinoin are thus carefully monitored and are required to get monthly blood tests to check quantitative serum β-hCG (to rule out pregnancy), LFTs, cholesterol, and triglycerides. Monthly refills are contingent on completion of blood testing and evaluation by a dermatologist.

PILONIDAL CYSTS

Abscesses in the sacrococcygeal region that usually occur near the top of the natal cleft. Their name may not be appropriate, as not all such cysts contain hair, and not all are true cysts. Repetitive trauma to the region plays a role. The condition is thought to start as a folliculitis that becomes an abscess complicated by perineal microbes, especially *Bacteroides*. It most commonly occurs between the ages of 20 and 40, affecting men more often than women.

HISTORY/PE

- Patients present with an abscess at the natal cleft that can be tender, fluctuant, warm, and indurated and is sometimes associated with purulent drainage or cellulitis. Systemic symptoms are uncommon, but cysts may develop into perianal fistulas.
- Risk factors include deep and hairy natal clefts, obesity, and a sedentary lifestyle.

DIAGNOSIS

Diagnosed by the clinical picture. Rule out perirectal and anal abscess.

TREATMENT

- Treatment consists of incision and drainage of the abscess under local anesthesia followed by sterile packing of the wound. Abscesses should be allowed to heal by 2° intention.
- Antibiotics are not needed unless cellulitis is present; if they are prescribed, both aerobic and anaerobic coverage is required.
- Good local hygiene and shaving of the sacrococcygeal skin can help prevent recurrence. Patients should follow up with a surgeon.

Fungal Infections

TINEA VERSICOLOR

Caused by *Malassezia furfur*, a yeast that is part of the normal skin flora (morphologic variants are *Pityrosporum ovale* and *Pityrosporum orbiculare*). It is unclear what leads the organism to overgrow on the skin surface and become a pathogen, but humid and sweaty conditions as well as host factors such as oily skin can contribute. Cushing's syndrome and immunosuppression are also risk factors.

HISTORY/PE

- Patients present with small, scaly patches of varying color, usually on the chest or back.
- Lesions may be hypopigmented as a result of interference with melanin production, or they may be hyperpigmented by virtue of thickened scale.

DIAGNOSIS

Diagnosed by clinical impression, and confirmed by potassium hydroxide **(KOH) preparation** of scale that reveals a **"spaghetti and meatballs"** pattern of hyphae and spores.

TREATMENT

Treat lesions with topical selenium sulfide daily for one week, followed by application once weekly for prophylaxis.

CANDIDIASIS

Commonly called "yeast infection" or "thrush," candidiasis can be caused by any *Candida* species but is most commonly caused by *C. albicans*. In immune-competent patients, it typically presents as a superficial infection of the skin or mucous membranes in moist areas such as skin folds, armpits, the vagina, and below the breasts. Oral thrush is not uncommon among children, but in adults it is often a sign of a weakened immune system.

HISTORY/PE

- Patients often have a history of antibiotic use, steroid use, or diabetes.
- Symptoms vary according to the site affected:
  - **Oral candidiasis:** Presents with painless white plaques that cannot easily be scraped off.
  - **Candidiasis of the skin:** Presents as pink, circular, erythematous macules that converge, with smaller satellite lesions seen nearby, often in skin folds.
- In infants, infection can often be seen in the diaper area and along the inguinal folds.

DIAGNOSIS

- Diagnosed by the clinical picture.
- Confirmed by KOH preparation of a scraping or swab of the affected area. KOH dissolves the skin cells but leaves the *Candida* untouched such that candidal hyphae and pseudospores become visible.

TREATMENT

- **Oral candidiasis:** Oral fluconazole; nystatin swish and swallow.
- **Superficial (skin) candidiasis:** Topical antifungals; keep skin clean and dry.
- **Diaper rash:** Topical nystatin.

DERMATOPHYTE INFECTIONS

Dermatophytes **live only in tissues with keratin** (i.e., the skin, nails, and hair) and are a common cause of infection. Causative organisms include *Microsporum*, *Trichophyton*, and *Epidermophyton*. The immune response to the dermatophyte, rather than the organism itself, is responsible for many of the symptoms. **Pets** are a reservoir for *Microsporum*. Other risk factors include diabetes, ↓ peripheral circulation, immune compromise, and chronic maceration of skin (e.g., from athletic activities).

HISTORY/PE

Presentation varies according to subtype:

- **Tinea corporis:** Presents as a scaly, pruritic eruption with a sharp, irregular border, often with central clearing. May be seen in immunocompromised patients or in children following contact with infected pets.

- **Tinea pedis/manuum:** Presents as chronic interdigital scaling with erosions between the toes (**"athlete's foot"**) or as a thickened, scaly skin on the soles. Asymmetric involvement of the hands is typical.
- **Tinea cruris ("jock itch"):** A chronic infection of the groin (typically sparing the scrotum) that is usually associated with tinea pedis.
- **Tinea capitis ("ringworm"):** A diffuse, scaly scalp eruption similar to seborrheic dermatitis.

DIAGNOSIS

Diagnosed by the clinical picture; confirmed by scales prepared in **KOH showing hyphae.**

TREATMENT

Patients can be treated with topical or systemic antifungals. Tinea capitis must be treated with systemic drugs.

Parasitic Infections

LICE

Lice live off blood and on specific parts of the body, depending on their species. The **head louse** lives on the scalp and lays its eggs as nits attached to hair; the **body louse** lives in clothing and bites only the body. The **pubic louse** lives on pubic hair. Lice are spread through body contact or by the sharing of bedclothes and other garments. They secrete local toxins that lead to pruritus.

HISTORY/PE

- Patients with lice often experience severe pruritus, and 2° bacterial infection of the excoriations is a risk. **Classroom epidemics** of head lice are common.
- Body lice are seen in people with inadequate hygiene or in those with crowded living conditions. Pubic lice (called "crabs" because of their squat, crablike body shape) contain anticoagulant in their saliva, so their bites often turn **blue.**

DIAGNOSIS

Lice can be seen on hairs or in clothes.

TREATMENT

- **Head lice:** Treat with OTC pyrethrin (RID) and mechanical removal of nits.
- **Body lice:** Wash body, clothes, and bedding thoroughly. Treating the body with topical permethrin or pyrethrin may also be required.
- **Pubic lice:** Treat with RID.

SCABIES

Caused by *Sarcoptes scabiei*, a tiny arthropod that mates on the skin surface, after which the female digs a passage into the stratum corneum and lays her eggs. The **burrowing** leads to **pruritus** that ↑ in intensity once an allergy to the mite or its products develops. Scabies mites are spread through close contact.

HISTORY/PE

- Patients present with intense pruritus, especially at **night and after hot showers.**
- The most commonly affected sites are the hands, axillae, and genitals.
- On exam, the mite's **track** can sometimes be seen along with **erythematous, excoriated papules.** 2° bacterial infection is common.

DIAGNOSIS

A history of pruritus in several family members is suggestive. The mite may be identifiable by scraping an intact tunnel and looking under the microscope, but this is often difficult.

TREATMENT

Patients should be treated overnight with 1–2 applications of 5% **permethrin from the neck down,** and their contacts should be treated as well. Oral **ivermectin** is also effective. Pruritus may persist for two weeks after treatment, so symptomatic treatment should be provided.

Other ulcers (all can be treated with specialized wound dressings):

- ***Venous stasis ulcers:** Found near the lateral or medial malleolus, often in association with lower extremity edema. Treat with compression (Unna boots or compression stockings) and elevation.*
- ***Arterial insufficiency ulcers:** Found on the heel and tips of toes. Typically very painful.*
- ***Neuropathic ulcers:** Found on the underside of the foot and toes, usually at pressure points. Typically painless.*

▶ **ISCHEMIC DISORDERS**

Decubitus Ulcers

Result from ischemic necrosis following continuous pressure on an area of skin that restricts microcirculation to the area. Ulcers are most commonly seen in **bedridden patients** who lie in one spot for too long. An underlying bony prominence or lack of fat ↑ the likelihood of ulcer formation. Patients who lack mobility or cutaneous sensation are also at ↑ risk. Incontinence of urine or stool may macerate the skin, facilitating ulceration.

HISTORY/PE

Ulcers are graded by degree of damage:

- **Grade I:** Characterized by persistent redness.
- **Grade II:** Marked by ulceration.
- **Grade III:** Involves destruction of structures beneath the skin such as muscle or fat.

DIAGNOSIS

Diagnosed by the history and clinical appearance.

TREATMENT

Prevention is key and involves routinely moving bedridden patients and using special beds that distribute pressure. Once an ulcer has developed, low-grade lesions can be treated with routine **wound care,** including hydrocolloid dressings. High-grade lesions require **surgical debridement.**

Gangrene

Defined as necrosis of body tissue. There are three subtypes: **dry, wet,** and **gas.** The presence of one subtype does not exclude the others. Etiologies are as follows:

- **Dry gangrene:** Due to insufficient blood flow to tissue, typically from atherosclerosis.
- **Wet gangrene:** Involves bacterial infection, usually with skin flora.
- **Gas gangrene:** Due to *Clostridium perfringens* infection.

HISTORY/PE

- **Dry gangrene:** Early signs are a dull ache, cold, and pallor of the flesh. As necrosis sets in, the tissue (usually a toe) becomes bluish-black, dry, and shriveled. Diabetes, vasculopathy, and smoking are risk factors.
- **Wet gangrene:** The tissue appears bruised, swollen, or blistered with pus.
- **Gas gangrene:** Typically occurs at a site of recent injury or surgery, presenting with swelling around the injury and with skin that turns pale and then dark red. Bacteria are rapidly destructive of tissue, producing gas that separates healthy tissue and exposes it to infection. **A medical emergency.**

DIAGNOSIS

Diagnosed by clinical impression.

TREATMENT

- Surgical **debridement,** with amputation if necessary, is the mainstay of treatment. **Antibiotics alone do not suffice** by virtue of inadequate blood flow, but they should be given as an adjuvant to surgery.
- **Gas gangrene can be treated with hyperbaric oxygen,** which is toxic to the anaerobic *C. perfringens.* Susceptible patients should maintain careful **foot care** and should avoid trauma.

▶ MISCELLANEOUS SKIN DISORDERS

Acanthosis Nigricans

- A condition in which the skin in the **intertriginous zones** (genital and axillary regions and especially the nape of the neck) is hyperkeratotic and hyperpigmented with a **velvety** appearance (see Figure 2.2-12).
- Associated with DM, Cushing's disease, HAIR-AN syndrome, and obesity. May also be a paraneoplastic sign of underlying adenocarcinoma (usually GI).
- **Dx:** Clinical appearance.
- **Tx:** May be treated with topical retinoids, but typically not treated. Patients should be encouraged to lose weight.

Lichen Planus

- A chronic inflammatory dermatosis involving the skin and mucous membranes. The condition is intensely pruritic, can be induced by drugs, and can be associated with HCV infection.
- Hx/PE:
  - Presents with **violaceous, flat-topped, polygonal papules.** Lesions may have **Wickham's striae** (white stripes), especially on the mucous mem-

*Lichen planus is the "P" disease: **P**lanar, **P**urple, **P**ruritic, **P**ersistent, **P**olygonal, **P**enile, **P**erioral, **P**uzzling, and Koebner's Phenomenon.*

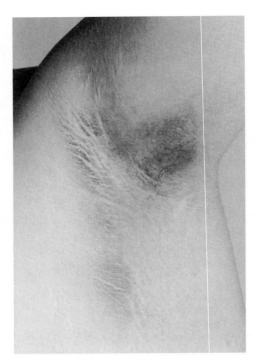

FIGURE 2.2-12. **Acanthosis nigricans.**

Velvety, dark brown epidermal thickening of the armpit is seen with prominent skin fold and feathered edges. (Reproduced, with permission, from Wolff K et al. *Fitzpatrick's Color Atlas & Synopsis of Clinical Dermatology*, 5th ed. New York: McGraw-Hill, 2005: 87.)

branes (see Figure 2.2-13), as well as prominent **Koebner's phenomena** (lesions that appear at the site of trauma). The initial lesions often appear on the genitalia, where they are ulcerated.
- Although most cases resolve spontaneously over 6–18 months, those with oral involvement have a more chronic course.
- **Dx:** Histology reveals a "lichenoid pattern"—i.e., a band of **T lymphocytes at the epidermal-dermal junction with damage to the basal layer.**
- **Tx:** Mild cases can be treated with topical corticosteroids. For severe disease, systemic corticosteroids may be used. Tretinoin gel may be helpful on oral mucosa.

Rosacea

A chronic disorder of pilosebaceous units. The disorder has a female predominance and is more common among those with fair skin. Its etiology is unclear.

HISTORY/PE

- Patients are generally **middle-aged** and often have an **abnormal flushing** response to various substances.
- Early in the disease, **central facial erythema** is seen with telangiectasias. Later, papules and pustules may develop.
- Associated findings include **ocular keratitis** and **rhinophyma** (sebaceous gland hyperplasia of the nose).

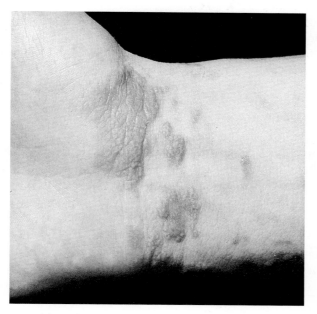

FIGURE 2.2-13.   Lichen planus.

Flat-topped, polygonal, sharply defined papules of violaceous color are grouped and confluent. The surface is shiny and reveals fine white lines (Wickham's striae). (Reproduced, with permission, from Wolff K et al. *Fitzpatrick's Color Atlas & Synopsis of Clinical Dermatology*, 5th ed. New York: McGraw-Hill, 2005: 125.)

DIAGNOSIS

- Diagnosed by the clinical picture. Rosacea can be confused with acne but is not follicular in origin and involves an older age group.
- In a high percentage of patients, ↑ numbers of *Demodex* mites (which normally live harmlessly in hair follicles, especially in the facial area) are found on the facial skin and can be seen by microscopic examination of skin scrapings.

TREATMENT

Treat with low-potency topical corticosteroids or topical metronidazole. In more severe disease, systemic antibiotics may be used. Extremely severe cases can be treated with short-term oral metronidazole.

Pityriasis Rosea

An acute dermatitis that is pink and scaly. Its etiology is unknown, but it has been hypothesized to represent a reaction to a **viral infection with human herpesvirus (HHV) 6** or **7** because it tends to occur in **mini-epidemics among young adults.**

HISTORY/PE

- The initial lesion is a **herald patch** that is several centimeters in diameter and erythematous with a peripheral scale.

- Days to weeks later, a 2° exanthem appears, presenting with multiple tiny, symmetric papules with a fine **"cigarette paper"** scale (see Figure 2.2-14). Papules are arranged along skin lines, giving a classic **"Christmas tree pattern"** on the patient's back.
- Patients are generally asymptomatic, although the disease may be more extensive, pruritic, and chronic among African-Americans.

DIAGNOSIS

Diagnosed by clinical impression and confirmed by KOH exam to rule out fungus (the herald patch may be mistaken for tinea corporis). The differential also includes 2° syphilis (RPR should be ordered), guttate psoriasis, and drug eruptions.

TREATMENT

Patients usually heal without treatment in 2–3 weeks, but skin lubrication, topical antipruritics, and systemic antihistamines may occasionally be necessary. Severe cases can be treated with a short course of systemic corticosteroids.

Vitiligo

A disease of **depigmentation** whose pathogenesis is unknown. The mechanism may be autoimmune, neurologic, or both.

HISTORY/PE

- Patients develop **small, sharply demarcated, depigmented macules or patches** on otherwise normal skin, often on the hands, face, or genitalia.

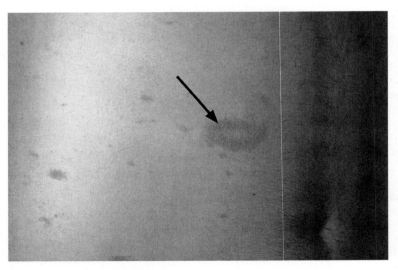

FIGURE 2.2-14. **Pityriasis rosea.**

The round to oval erythematous plaques are often covered with a fine white scale ("cigarette paper") and are often found on the trunk and proximal extremities. Plaques are often preceded by a larger herald patch (arrow). (Reproduced, with permission, from Hurwitz RM. *Pathology of the Skin: Atlas of Clinical-Pathological Correlation*, 2nd ed. Stamford, CT: Appleton & Lange, 1998: 13.)

These spots then expand, sometimes in dermatomal patterns, to include large segments of skin.

- The disease is usually **chronic and progressive,** with some patients becoming completely depigmented.
- Many patients have **serologic markers of autoimmune disease** (e.g., antithyroid antibodies, DM, pernicious anemia) but seldom present with these diseases. Patients with malignant melanoma may develop an **antimelanocyte immune response** that leads to vitiligo.

DIAGNOSIS

Diagnosed by the history and clinical picture, with **histology demonstrating total absence of melanocytes.** Conditions to rule out include postinflammatory hypopigmentation, scleroderma, piebaldism, and toxic exposure (phenolated cleansers are toxic to melanocytes).

TREATMENT

Topical or systemic psoralens and exposure to sunlight or PUVA may be helpful. Patients must wear **sunscreen** because depigmented skin lacks inherent sun protection. Dyes and makeup may be used to color the skin, or the skin may be chemically bleached to produce a uniformly white color.

▶ DYSPLASIAS

Seborrheic Keratosis

A very common skin tumor, appearing in almost all patients after age 40. The etiology is unknown. When many seborrheic keratoses erupt suddenly, they may be part of a **paraneoplastic syndrome** due to tumor production of epidermal growth factors. Lesions have no malignant potential but may be a cosmetic problem.

HISTORY/PE

- Present as **exophytic, waxy brown papules and plaques** with prominent follicle openings (see Figure 2.2-15). Lesions often appear in great numbers and **have a "stuck-on" appearance.**
- Lesions may become irritated either spontaneously or by external trauma, especially in the groin, breast, or axillae. Irritated lesions are smoother and redder.

"Seborrheic keratoses, or SKs, look StucK on."

DIAGNOSIS

Diagnosed by the clinical picture; can be confirmed by histology showing **hyperplasia of benign, basaloid epidermal cells** with **horn pseudocysts** (prominent follicular openings). Rule out actinic keratosis, lentigo (focal ↑ in melanocytes), squamous cell carcinoma (SCC), and basal cell carcinoma (BCC).

TREATMENT

Cryotherapy or curettage is curative.

Actinic Keratosis

A precursor of SCC in situ. Lesions are caused by exposure to **sunlight.**

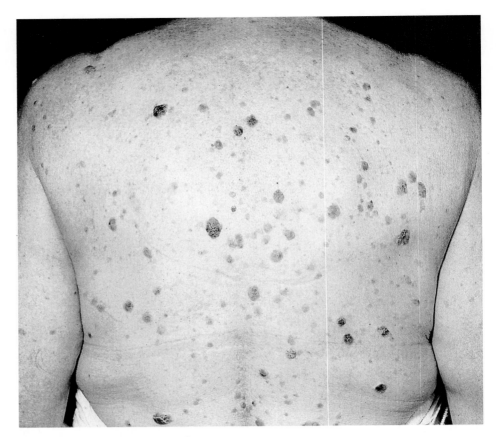

FIGURE 2.2-15. **Seborrheic keratoses.**

Multiple brown, warty papules and nodules are seen on the back, characterized by a "stuck-on" appearance. (Reproduced, with permission, from Fitzpatrick TB. *Color Atlas & Synopsis of Clinical Dermatology*, 4th ed. New York: McGraw-Hill, 2001: 195.)

HISTORY/PE

Lesions appear on sun-exposed areas (especially the face and arms) and primarily affect **older patients,** who rarely have a solitary lesion. They are erythematous with a light scale that can become thick and crusted (see Figure 2.2-16). Early lesions may be difficult to visualize and may be easier to find by palpation.

DIAGNOSIS

Diagnosed by clinical impression. Biopsy is seldom necessary but shows intraepidermal atypia over a sun-damaged dermis. The differential includes **Bowen's disease,** a form of squamous cell carcinoma in situ.

TREATMENT

Cryosurgery, topical 5-FU, or topical imiquimod can be used to destroy the lesion. If carcinoma is suspected, biopsy followed by excision or curettage is appropriate. Patients should be advised to use sun protection.

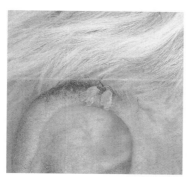

FIGURE 2.2-16. **Actinic keratosis.**

The discrete patch above has an erythematous base and a rough white scale. (Reproduced, with permission, from Hurwitz RM. *Pathology of the Skin: Atlas of Clinical-Pathological Correlation*, 2nd ed. Stamford, CT: Appleton & Lange, 1998: 359.)

Squamous Cell Carcinoma (SCC)

The second most common skin tumor, with locally destructive effects as well as the potential for **metastasis and death. UV light** is the most common causative factor, but exposure to **chemical carcinogens,** prior **radiation** therapy, and the presence of **chronically draining infectious sinuses** (as in osteomyelitis) also predispose patients to developing SCC. Most SCCs occur in older adults with sun-damaged skin, arising from actinic keratoses.

History/PE

- SCCs have a variety of forms, and a single patient will often have multiple variants (see Figure 2.2-17).

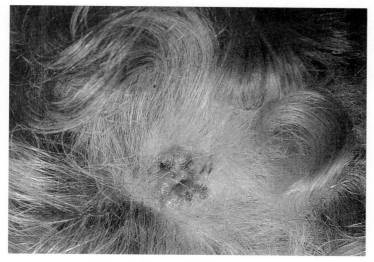

FIGURE 2.2-17. **Squamous cell carcinoma.**

Note the crusting and ulceration of this erythematous plaque. Most lesions are exophytic nodules with erosion or ulceration. (Reproduced, with permission, from Hurwitz RM. *Pathology of the Skin: Atlas of Clinical-Pathological Correlation*, 2nd ed. Stamford, CT: Appleton & Lange, 1998: 360.)

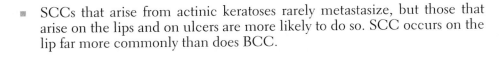

■ SCCs that arise from actinic keratoses rarely metastasize, but those that arise on the lips and on ulcers are more likely to do so. SCC occurs on the lip far more commonly than does BCC.

DIAGNOSIS

■ Diagnosed by clinical suspicion and confirmed by **biopsy,** which is necessary for accurate diagnosis and appropriate therapeutic planning.
■ Histology shows intraepidermal atypical keratinocytes, with penetration of the basement membrane by malignant epidermal cells growing into the dermis. SCCs are **graded histologically.**

TREATMENT

Surgical excision. Lesions with high metastatic potential may require additional radiation or chemotherapy.

Basal Cell Carcinoma (BCC)

The most common malignant skin tumor, BCC is slow growing and locally destructive but has **virtually no metastatic potential. Chronic UV light** exposure is the main risk factor. Multiple lesions on non-sun-exposed areas are suggestive of **arsenic exposure** or **inherited basal cell nevus syndrome.** Most lesions appear on the face and on other sun-exposed areas.

HISTORY/PE

There are many types of BCC with varying degrees of pigmentation, ulceration, and depth of growth (see Figure 2.2-18).

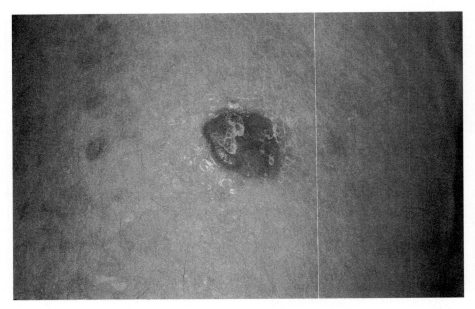

FIGURE 2.2-18.   Basal cell carcinoma.

Seen above is an erythematous, fleshy, telangiectatic nodule with a translucent surface. (Reproduced, with permission, from Hurwitz RM. *Pathology of the Skin: Atlas of Clinical-Pathological Correlation*, 2nd ed. Stamford, CT: Appleton & Lange, 1998: 362.)

Keratoacanthoma, a benign epithelial tumor, can look like SCC but develops more rapidly and may regress spontaneously. Treatment is usually similar to that of SCCs.

HIGH-YIELD FACTS

DERMATOLOGY

DIAGNOSIS

Diagnosed by clinical impression; confirmed by biopsy showing islands of proliferating epithelium resembling the basal layer of the epidermis. The differential includes benign tumors, hypopigmented melanocytic nevi, melanoma, dermatitis, psoriasis, and Paget's disease.

TREATMENT

Options include excision, curettage and electrodesiccation/cautery, deep cryotherapy, superficial radiation therapy, and Mohs' surgery. **Cure rates are > 95%.**

Melanoma

The **most common life-threatening dermatologic disease**; incidence has been increasing throughout the world. Risk factors include **short, intense bursts of sun exposure** (especially in childhood and with intermittent exposure) and the presence of **congenital melanocytic nevi, an ↑ number of nevi, or dysplastic nevi**. Immunosuppression also ↑ risk. Some patients inherit a predisposition to melanoma with the **familial atypical mole and melanoma (FAM-M) syndrome**. There are several subtypes (see Table 2.2-4).

HISTORY/PE

- Malignant melanomas usually begin in the epidermal basal layer, where melanocytes are normally found.
- The first growth phase is horizontal-intraepidermal, presenting with a lesion that is flat but increasing in diameter (typical of lentigo maligna or melanoma in situ). Later, there is a vertical growth phase with dermal invasion.
- Lesion characteristics that are suggestive of melanoma include **irregular pigment, irregular contour and border, nodule and ulcer formation, and changes in size/shape/color/contour/surface** noted by the patient (see Figure 2.2-19).

TABLE 2.2-4. Types of Melanoma

TYPE	PRESENTATION
Lentigo maligna	Arises in a lentigo. Usually found on sun-damaged skin of the face.
Superficial spreading	Typically affects younger adults, presenting on the trunk in men and on the legs in women. A relatively prolonged horizontal growth phase helps identify the disease early, when it is still confined to the epidermis.
Nodular	Lesions have a rapid vertical growth phase and appear as a rapidly growing reddish-brown nodule with ulceration or hemorrhage.
Acral lentiginous	Begins on the hands and feet as a slowly spreading, pigmented patch. Type most commonly seen in Asians and African-Americans.
Amelanotic	Presents as a lesion without clinical pigmentation. Extremely difficult to identify.

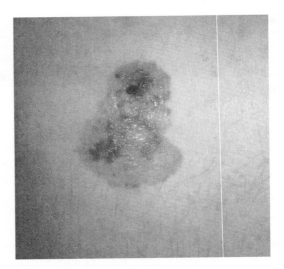

FIGURE 2.2-19. Melanoma.

Note the asymmetry, border irregularity, color variation, and large diameter of this plaque. (Reproduced, with permission, from Hurwitz RM. *Pathology of the Skin: Atlas of Clinical-Pathological Correlation*, 2nd ed. Stamford, CT: Appleton & Lange, 1998: 432.)

- Malignant melanoma may metastasize, and 10% of patients with metastatic melanoma have no known 1° lesion. Metastasis may be local (to nearby skin), regional (between the original lesion and its regional lymph nodes), or distant (via lymphatic or hematogenous spread to almost every organ in the body).

DIAGNOSIS

- Early recognition and treatment are essential. All adults should be examined for lesions that are suspicious for melanoma according to the **ABCDE criteria,** which identify dysplastic nevi and superficial spreading melanoma (see mnemonic).
- The onset of **pruritus** is also an early sign of malignant change. An **excisional biopsy** should be performed on any suspicious lesion. **Malignancy is determined histologically.**
- Malignant melanomas are staged by Breslow's thickness (depth of invasion measured in millimeters) and by tumor-node-metastasis (**TNM**) staging (see Table 2.2-5). **Clark's level is another classification system linking melanoma depth to prognosis** (see Table 2.2-6).

> **The ABCDEs of melanoma:**
>
> **A**symmetric
> Irregular **B**order
> Irregular **C**olor
> **D**iameter > 6 mm
> **E**volution: changing or new lesion

TABLE 2.2-5. TNM Staging of Melanoma

STAGE	EXTENT OF DISEASE	FIVE-YEAR SURVIVAL (%)
I	1° skin melanoma	70
II	Local or regional metastasis	30
III	Distant metastasis	0

TABLE 2.2-6. Characterization of Melanoma by Clark's Level

LEVEL	DEPTH OF LESION	FIVE-YEAR SURVIVAL (%)
I	Within the epidermis	99
II	Into the papillary dermis	95
III	Filling the papillary dermis	90
IV	Into the reticular dermis	65
V	To subcutaneous fat	25

TREATMENT

- Lesions confined to the skin are treated by **excision with margins.** Lymph node dissection is useful for staging but does not ↑ survival. Chemotherapy and radiation therapy may be used but are not likely to be successful.
- Malignant melanoma has the potential to **relapse after several years;** patients with early melanoma are at low risk for relapse but are at high risk for the development of **subsequent melanomas. Patient surveillance** is thus essential.

Kaposi's Sarcoma (KS)

A vascular proliferative disease that has been attributed to a herpesvirus, HHV-8, which is also called Kaposi's sarcoma–associated herpesvirus (KSHV).

HISTORY/PE

There are several types of KS:

- The **classic variant** is characterized by multicentric vascular macules and coalescent papules and plaques on the lower extremities. It usually occurs in the elderly, with a preponderance of cases in patients of Ashkenazi Jewish or Mediterranean descent.
- More disseminated cases occur in **African KS (endemic KS)** and in **immunocompromised** patients.
- **Epidemic HIV-associated KS** is an aggressive form of the disease, and although less common since the advent of HAART, it remains the **most common HIV-associated malignancy.**

DIAGNOSIS

Diagnosed by history and clinical impression, which are confirmed by biopsy showing spindle cells (elongated tumor cells) with ⊕ HHV-8 staining. The presence of the viral protein LANA in tumor cells can also be detected for diagnostic confirmation.

TREATMENT

Treatment is technically palliative. Local lesions may be treated with radiation or cryotherapy; surgery is not recommended. Widespread or internal disease is treated with systemic chemotherapy (anthracyclines, paclitaxil, or IFN-α).

Mycosis Fungoides (Cutaneous T-Cell Lymphoma)

Not a fungus, but rather a slow, progressive neoplastic proliferation of T cells. Its pathogenesis is thought to be related to chronic immunostimulation that leads **helper T cells to gather in the epidermis.** Industrial exposure to irritating chemicals appears to ↑ risk. The disease is chronic and is more common in men than in women.

HISTORY/PE

- The early lesion is a nonspecific, psoriatic-appearing plaque that is palpable and often pruritic.
- **Stage I** involves limited plaques, papules, and patches affecting < 10% BSA with no nodal involvement.
- **Stage II** is characterized by limited or generalized skin involvement with palpable lymph nodes or one or more skin tumors with multicentric, often confluent reddish-brown nodules (see Figure 2.2-20). Rarely, patients skip the plaque stage and present directly with tumors.
- **Stage III** is characterized by generalized erythroderma.

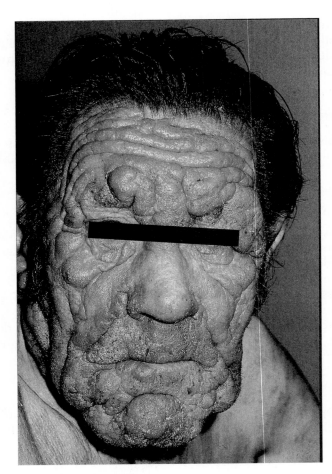

FIGURE 2.2-20. **Mycosis fungoides.**

Massive nodular infiltration of the face leads to a leonine facies. (Reproduced, with permission, from Fitzpatrick TB. *Color Atlas & Synopsis of Clinical Dermatology,* 4th ed. New York: McGraw-Hill, 2001: 541.)

- **Stage IV** is characterized by biopsy-⊕ lymph nodes or internal organ spread.
- Patients may have dermatopathic lymphadenopathy without actual tumor involvement of the node. However, the **internal organs can be involved,** including the nodes, liver, and spleen.
- **Sézary's syndrome** is the leukemic phase of cutaneous T-cell lymphoma and is characterized by circulating Sézary cells in the peripheral blood, erythroderma, and lymphadenopathy.

DIAGNOSIS

- Diagnosed by clinical features and histology, with immunologic characterization and electron microscopy showing the typical **Sézary or Lutzner cells** (cerebriform lymphocytes).
- The early lesion is clinically indistinguishable from dermatitis, so **histologic diagnosis is indicated for any dermatitis that is chronic and resistant to treatment.**
- Once clinical tumors have evolved, histology is useful for showing the type of cells present.

TREATMENT

- **Stage I disease:** Treat **topically** with steroids, retinoids, chemotherapy, or PUVA.
- **Stage II disease:** Treat **systemically** with retinoids, interferon, monoclonal antibodies, or chemotherapy.
- **Photopheresis** is the mainstay of treatment for many patients. For more extensive or advanced disease, **radiation therapy** is an effective option. Treatment modalities are often combined.

Endocrinology

Type 1 Diabetes Mellitus (Type 1 DM)

Due to autoimmune pancreatic β-cell destruction leading to insulin deficiency and abnormal fuel metabolism.

HISTORY/PE

- Classically presents with **polyuria** (especially nocturia), **polydipsia, polyphagia,** and rapid, unexplained weight loss. Patients may also present with **ketoacidosis.**
- Usually affects nonobese children or young adults.
- Associated with HLA-DR3 and -DR4.

DIAGNOSIS

At least one of the following is required to make the diagnosis:

- A fasting (> 8-hour) plasma glucose of ≥ 126 mg/dL on two separate occasions.
- A random plasma glucose of ≥ 200 mg/dL plus symptoms.
- A two-hour postprandial glucose of ≥ 200 mg/dL after a glucose tolerance test on two separate occasions if the results of initial testing are equivocal.

TREATMENT

- Insulin (see Table 2.3-1) and self-monitoring of blood glucose in the normal range (80–120 mg/dL). Higher blood glucose levels (≥ 200 mg/dL) can be tolerated, particularly in the very young, in light of the ↑ risk of hypoglycemia.
- Routine HbA_{1c} testing (with a goal HbA_{1c} < 8 in children), frequent BP checks, foot checks, annual dilated-eye exams, annual microalbuminuria screening, and a lipid profile every 2–5 years.

TABLE 2.3-1. Types of Insulin

INSULIN[a]	ONSET	PEAK EFFECT	DURATION
Regular	30–60 minutes	2–4 hours	5–8 hours
Humalog (lispro)	5–10 minutes	0.5–1.5 hours	6–8 hours
NovoLog (aspart)	10–20 minutes	1–3 hours	3–5 hours
Apidra (glulisine)	5–15 minutes	1.0–1.5 hours	1.0–2.5 hours
NPH	2–4 hours	6–10 hours	18–28 hours
Levemir (detemir)	2 hours	No discernible peak	20 hours
Lantus (glargine)	1–4 hours	No discernible peak	20–24 hours

[a] Combination preparations mix longer-acting and shorter-acting types of insulin together to provide immediate and extended coverage in the same injection (e.g., 70 NPH/30 regular = 70% NPH + 30% regular).

Table 2.3-2 outlines the acute, chronic, and treatment-related complications of DM.

Type 2 Diabetes Mellitus (Type 2 DM)

A dysfunction in glucose metabolism that is best characterized as varying degrees of insulin resistance that may lead to β-cell burnout and insulin dependence.

TABLE 2.3-2. Complications of DM

COMPLICATION	DESCRIPTION
Complications of treatment	
Dawn phenomenon	Early-morning hyperglycemia caused by ↓ effectiveness of insulin and ↑ secretion of growth hormone (GH) and other hormones overnight. **Move P.M. insulin closer to bedtime to treat.**
Acute complications	
Diabetic ketoacidosis (DKA)	Hyperglycemia-induced crisis that most commonly occurs in **type 1 DM.** Often precipitated by stress (including infections, MI, trauma, or alcohol) or by noncompliance with insulin therapy. May present with **abdominal pain, vomiting, Kussmaul respirations,** and a **fruity, acetone breath odor.** Patients are severely dehydrated with many electrolyte abnormalities and may also develop **mental status changes.** Treatment includes fluids, potassium, **insulin,** bicarbonate (if pH is < 7), and treatment of the initiating event or underlying disease process.
Hyperosmolar hyperglycemic state (HHS)	Presents as **profound dehydration,** mental status changes, hyperosmolarity, and extremely high plasma glucose (> 600 mg/dL) without acidosis and with small or absent ketones. Occurs in **type 2 DM;** precipitated by acute stress (dehydration, infections) and often can be fatal. Treatment includes **aggressive fluid and electrolyte replacement** and insulin. Treat the initiating event.
Chronic complications	
Retinopathy (nonproliferative, proliferative)	Appears when diabetes has been present for at least **3–5 years.** Preventive measures include control of hyperglycemia and hypertension, annual eye exams, and **laser photocoagulation therapy for retinal neovascularization.**
Diabetic nephropathy	Characterized by glomerular hyperfiltration followed by **microalbuminuria.** Preventive measures include **ACEIs** or ARBs and BP/glucose control.
Neuropathy	Peripheral, symmetric, sensorimotor neuropathy leading to burning pain, foot trauma, infections, and diabetic ulcers. Treat with preventive **foot care** and **analgesics.** Late complications due to autonomic dysfunction include delayed gastric emptying, esophageal dysmotility, impotence, and orthostatic hypotension.
Macrovascular complications	Cardiovascular, cerebrovascular, and peripheral vascular disease. Cardiovascular disease is the most common cause of death in diabetic patients. The goal BP is < 130/< 75; ↓ LDL to < 100 mg/dL; ↓ triglycerides to < 150 mg/dL. Patients should also be started on low-dose ASA.

HISTORY/PE

- Patients typically present with symptoms of hyperglycemia.
- Onset is more **insidious** than that of type 1 DM, and patients often present with complications.
- **Nonketotic hyperglycemia** may be seen in the setting of poor glycemic control.
- Usually occurs in older adults with obesity (often truncal); has a strong genetic predisposition.

DIAGNOSIS

- Diagnostic criteria are the **same as those for type 1 DM.**
- **Follow-up testing:**
  - **Patients with no risk factors: Test at 45 years of age; retest every three years.**
  - **Patients with impaired fasting glucose** (> 110 mg/dL but < 126 mg/dL): Follow up with frequent retesting.

TREATMENT

The goal of treatment is tight glucose control—i.e., blood glucose levels ranging from 80 to 120 mg/dL and HbA_{1c} levels < 7. Treatment measures include the following:

- Diet, weight loss, and exercise.
- **Oral agents** (monotherapy or combination if uncontrolled):
  - **Sulfonylureas (glipizide, glyburide, and glimepiride):** Insulin secretagogues. Hypoglycemia and weight gain are side effects.
  - **Meglitinides (repaglinide and nateglinide):** Short-acting agents whose mechanism of action is similar to that of sulfonylureas.
  - **Metformin:** Inhibits hepatic gluconeogenesis; ↑ peripheral sensitivity to insulin. Side effects include weight loss, GI upset, and, rarely, lactic acidosis. Contraindicated in the elderly (those > 80 years of age) and in patients with renal disease.
  - **Thiazolidinediones (the "glitazones"):** ↑ insulin sensitivity. Side effects include weight gain, edema, and potential hepatotoxicity.
  - **α-glucosidase inhibitors:** ↓ intestinal absorption of carbohydrates. Rarely used owing to the side effect of flatulence.
  - **DDP-4 inhibitors (sitagliptin):** Inhibit the degradation of the endogenous enzyme that breaks down glucagon-like peptide 1 (GLP-1).
- **Insulin** (alone or in conjunction with oral agents).
- **Incretins (exenatide):** GLP-1 agonists. Injected subcutaneously. Delay absorption of food; ↑ insulin secretion and ↓ glucagon secretion. Side effects include nausea and (rarely) pancreatitis.
- **Statins** for hypercholesterolemia (goal LDL < 100); glucose control and fibric acid derivatives for hypertriglyceridemia.
- **Strict BP control to < 130/80;** ACEIs/ARBs are usually first-line agents.
- **Antiplatelet agents** (ASA) for patients at risk of cardiovascular disease or for those > 40 years of age.
- Regular screening for cardiovascular disease, nephropathy, retinopathy, neuropathy, and smoking cessation.

COMPLICATIONS

See Table 2.3-2 for an outline of the complications of DM. Note that the **presence of diabetes is equivalent to the highest risk for cardiovascular disease** regardless of all other risk factors.

- **Somogyi effect:** Nocturnal hypoglycemia leading to a surge of counterregulatory hormones, leading in turn to hyperglycemia in the morning.
- **Dawn phenomenon:** Nocturnal secretion of GH leading to early-morning hyperglycemia.

Metabolic Syndrome

Also known as insulin resistance syndrome or syndrome X. Associated with an ↑ risk of CAD and mortality from a cardiovascular event.

HISTORY/PE

Presents with **abdominal obesity, high BP, impaired glycemic control,** and **dyslipidemia.**

DIAGNOSIS

Three out of five of the following criteria must be met:

- Abdominal obesity (↑ waist girth): > 40 inches in men and > 35 inches in women.
- Triglycerides ≥ 150 mg/dL.
- HDL < 40 mg/dL in men and < 50 mg/dL in women.
- BP ≥ 130/85 mmHg or administration of antihypertensive drugs.
- Fasting glucose ≥ 100 mg/dL.

TREATMENT

Intensive weight loss, aggressive cholesterol lowering, and BP control. Metformin has been shown to slow the onset of diabetes in this high-risk population.

▶ THYROID DISORDERS

Testing of Thyroid Function

TFTs include the following (see also Table 2.3-3):

- **TSH measurement: The single best test for assessing thyroid function.** High TSH levels lead to 1° hypothyroidism; low TSH levels lead to thyrotoxicosis.
- **Radioactive iodine uptake (RAIU) and scan:** Determines the level of iodine uptake by the thyroid. Useful in differentiating thyrotoxic states, but has a limited role in determining malignancy.

In 1° endocrine disturbances, the gland itself is abnormal. In 2° endocrine disturbances, the HPA malfunctions.

TABLE 2.3-3. Common Thyroid Function Abnormalities

DIAGNOSIS	TSH	T₄	T₃	CAUSES
1° hyperthyroidism	↓	↑	↑	Graves' disease, toxic multinodular goiter, toxic adenoma, amiodarone, molar pregnancy, postpartum thyrotoxicosis, postviral thyroiditis.
1° hypothyroidism	↑	↓	↓	Hashimoto's thyroiditis, hypothyroid phase of thyroiditis, iatrogenic factors (radioactive iodine thyroid ablation, excision with inadequate supplementation, external radiation, lithium, or amiodarone), iodine deficiency, infiltrative disease.

- **Total T_4 measurement:** Not an adequate screening test. Ninety-nine percent of circulating T_4 is bound to thyroxine-binding globulin (TBG). Total T_4 levels can be altered by changes in levels of binding proteins.
- **T_3 resin uptake (T3RU):** Used with total T_4 or T_3 to correct for changes in TBG levels (e.g., the free thyroxine index = total $T_4 \times$ T3RU).
- **Free T_4 measurement:** The preferred screening test for thyroid hormone levels; more useful for unstable thyroid states.

Hyperthyroidism

Refers to causes of thyrotoxicosis ($\uparrow$ levels of T_3/T_4 due to any cause) in which the thyroid overproduces thyroid hormone, including **Graves' disease,** toxic multinodular goiter (also called Plummer's disease), and toxic adenomas.

HISTORY/PE

- Presents with **weight loss, heat intolerance, nervousness, palpitations,** $\uparrow$ **bowel frequency,** insomnia, and menstrual abnormalities.
- Exam reveals warm, moist skin, goiter, sinus **tachycardia** or **atrial fibrillation,** fine **tremor, lid lag,** and hyperactive reflexes. **Exophthalmos,** pretibial myxedema, and thyroid bruits are seen only in Graves' disease (see Figure 2.3-1).

DIAGNOSIS

The initial test of choice is serum TSH level, followed by T_4 levels and, rarely, T_3 (unless TSH is low and free T_4 is not elevated). See Table 2.3-3.

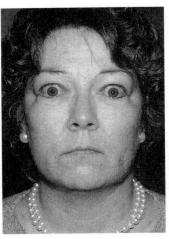
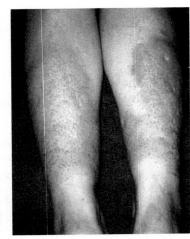

A

B

FIGURE 2.3-1. Physical signs of Graves' disease.

(A) Graves' ophthalmopathy. (B) Pretibial myxedema. (Figure 2.3-1A reproduced, with permission, from the Pathology Education Instructional Resource [PEIR] digital library [http://peir.net] at the University of Alabama, Birmingham. Figure 2.3-1B reproduced, with permission, from Greenspan FS, Strewler GJ. *Basic and Clinical Endocrinology,* 5th ed. Stamford, CT: Appleton & Lange, 1997.)

TREATMENT

- 1° therapy is **radioactive ^{131}I thyroid ablation;** antithyroid drugs (methimazole or propylthiouracil) may also be used if radioactive iodine is not indicated. Thyroidectomy is rarely indicated.
- Give **propranolol** for adrenergic symptoms while awaiting the resolution of hyperthyroidism.
- Administer levothyroxine to prevent hypothyroidism in patients who have undergone ablation or surgery.

TSH receptor antibodies are seen in patients with Graves' disease.

Hypothyroidism

Hashimoto's thyroiditis is the most common cause of hypothyroidism (see Table 2.3-3). Anti-TPO antibodies are ⊕. The second most common cause is iatrogenic. **Myxedema coma** refers to severe hypothyroidism with ↓ mental status, hypothermia, and other parasympathetic symptoms. Mortality is 30–60%.

HISTORY/PE

Presents with weakness, fatigue, **cold intolerance, constipation,** weight gain, **depression,** menstrual irregularities, and **hoarseness.** Exam may reveal **dry, cold, puffy skin** accompanied by edema, **bradycardia,** and delayed relaxation of DTRs.

DIAGNOSIS

See Table 2.3-3.

TREATMENT

- **Uncomplicated hypothyroidism (e.g., Hashimoto's disease):** Administer levothyroxine.
- **Myxedema coma:** Treat with IV levothyroxine and IV hydrocortisone (if adrenal insufficiency has not been excluded).

Thyroiditis

Inflammation of the thyroid gland. Common subtypes include subacute granulomatous, radiation-induced, autoimmune (lymphocytic, chronic, or Hashimoto's), postpartum, and drug-induced (e.g., amiodarone) thyroiditis.

HISTORY/PE

The **subacute** form presents with a **tender thyroid** accompanied by malaise and URI symptoms. Other forms are associated with painless goiter.

DIAGNOSIS

Thyroid dysfunction (typically thyrotoxicosis followed by hypothyroidism), with ↓ uptake on RAIU during the thyrotoxic phase.

TREATMENT

- β-blockers for hyperthyroidism; levothyroxine for hypothyroidism.
- Subacute thyroiditis is usually self-limited; treat with **NSAIDs** or with oral **corticosteroids** for severe cases.

Thyroid Neoplasms

Thyroid nodules are very common and show an ↑ incidence with age. Most are benign.

Check calcitonin levels if medullary cancer is suspected.

HISTORY/PE

- Usually **asymptomatic** on initial presentation.
- **Hyperfunctioning nodules** present with hyperthyroidism and local symptoms (dysphagia, dyspnea, cough, choking sensation) and are associated with a ⊕ family history (especially **medullary thyroid cancer**).
- An ↑ risk of malignancy is associated with a **history of neck irradiation, "cold" nodules** on radionuclide scan, male sex, age < 20 or > 70, firm and fixed solitary nodules, a ⊕ family history (especially medullary thyroid cancer), and **rapidly growing nodules with hoarseness.**
- Check for anterior cervical lymphadenopathy. Carcinoma (see Table 2.3-4) may be **firm and fixed.**
- Medullary thyroid carcinoma is associated with multiple endocrine neoplasia (MEN) type 2 and familial medullary thyroid cancer.

DIAGNOSIS

- The best method of assessing a nodule for malignancy is **fine-needle aspiration** (FNA), which has high sensitivity and moderate specificity.
- **TFTs** (TSH to exclude hyperfunction).
- **Ultrasound** determines if the nodule is solid or cystic; a radioactive scan determines whether it is hot or cold (cancers are usually cold and solid). Hot nodules are never cancerous and should not be biopsied.

TABLE 2.3-4. Types of Thyroid Carcinoma

TYPE[a]	CHARACTERISTICS	PROGNOSIS
Papillary	Represents 75–80% of thyroid cancers. The female-to-male ratio is 3:1. Slow growing; found in thyroid hormone–producing cells.	Ninety percent of patients survive 10 years or more after diagnosis; the prognosis is worse in elderly patients or those with large tumors.
Follicular	Accounts for 17% of thyroid cancers; found in thyroid hormone–producing cells.	Ninety percent of patients survive 10 years or longer after diagnosis; the prognosis is worse in elderly patients or those with large tumors.
Medullary	Responsible for 6–8% of thyroid cancers; found in calcitonin-producing C cells; the prognosis is related to degree of vascular invasion.	Eighty percent of patients survive at least 10 years after surgery.
Anaplastic	Accounts for < 2% of thyroid cancers; rapidly enlarges and metastasizes.	Ten percent of patients survive for > 3 years.

[a] Tumors may contain mixed papillary and follicular pathologies.

- **Benign FNA:** Follow with physical exam/ultrasound or a trial of levothyroxine suppression treatment.
- **Malignant FNA:** Surgical resection is first-line treatment; adjunctive radioiodine ablation following excision is appropriate for follicular lesions.
- **Indeterminate FNA:** Remove the nodule by surgical excision and wait for final pathology.
- Medullary thyroid cancer has a poorer prognosis than papillary and follicular types. Anaplastic thyroid cancer has an extremely poor prognosis.

Multiple Endocrine Neoplasia (MEN)

Associated with autosomal-dominant inheritance. Subtypes are as follows:

- **MEN type 1 (Wermer's syndrome):** Pancreatic islet cell tumors (e.g., Zollinger-Ellison syndrome, insulinomas, VIPomas), parathyroid hyperplasia, and pituitary adenomas.
- **MEN type 2A (Sipple's syndrome):** Medullary carcinoma of the thyroid, pheochromocytoma or adrenal hyperplasia, parathyroid gland hyperplasia.
- **MEN type 2B:** Medullary carcinoma of the thyroid, pheochromocytoma, oral and intestinal ganglioneuromatosis (mucosal neuromas), marfanoid habitus.

> **MEN 1 affects "P" organs:**
>
> **P**ancreas
> **P**ituitary
> **P**arathyroid

▶ BONE AND MINERAL DISORDERS

Osteoporosis

A common metabolic bone disease characterized by low bone mass and microarchitectural disruption, with bone mineral density > 2.5 SDs below normal peak bone mass. Most often affects thin, postmenopausal women (17%), especially Caucasians and Asians, with risk doubling (30%) after age 65.

HISTORY/PE

- Commonly asymptomatic even in the presence of a vertebral fracture.
- Exam may reveal **hip fractures, vertebral compression fractures** (loss of height and progressive thoracic kyphosis), and/or distal radius fractures following minimal trauma (see Figure 2.3-2).
- Bone pain unrelated to fracture is most likely osteomalacia rather than osteoporosis.
- **Smoking,** excessive caffeine or alcohol intake, a history of estrogen-depleting conditions (e.g., amenorrhea, eating disorders), thyroid dysfunction, and **steroid use** are all associated with an ↑ risk.

DIAGNOSIS

- **DEXA:** The gold standard; reveals significant osteopenia (bone mineral density < 2.5 SDs from normal peak level), most commonly in the vertebral bodies, proximal femur, and distal radius.
- **Labs:** Markers of bone turnover (↑ urinary N-telopeptides and deoxypyridinoline) can facilitate diagnosis in equivocal cases but are not routinely used; rule out 2° causes with TFTs, CMP, serum 25-hydroxyvitamin D, CBC, and testosterone (in men).
- **X-rays:** Global demineralization is apparent only after > 30% of bone density is lost.

Osteoporosis is the most common cause of pathologic fractures in elderly, thin women.

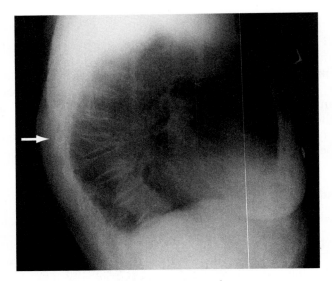

FIGURE 2.3-2.   Radiographic findings in osteoporosis.

Lateral spine x-ray shows severe osteopenia and a severe wedge-type deformity (severe anterior compression). (Reproduced, with permission, from Kasper DL et al. *Harrison's Principles of Internal Medicine*, 16th ed. New York: McGraw-Hill, 2005: 2269.)

TREATMENT

- Prevention with **calcium supplementation** and vitamin D.
- Smoking cessation and weight-bearing exercises help maintain bone density.
- Bisphosphonates (e.g., alendronate, risedronate, ibandronate, zoledronic acid), selective estrogen receptor modulators (e.g., raloxifene), and intranasal calcitonin may be used to prevent resorption and stabilize bone mineral density.
- Estrogen replacement therapy may be indicated for short-term treatment in the symptomatic perimenopausal period.
- Recombinant PTH may be used in patients with the highest level of risk.

Paget's Disease

Characterized by an ↑ rate of bone turnover. Causes both excessive resorption and excessive formation of bone, leading to a "mosaic" lamellar bone pattern. Suspected to be due to latent viral infection in genetically susceptible individuals. Found in roughly 4% of men and women > 40 years of age, and associated with 1° hyperparathyroidism in up to one-fifth of patients.

HISTORY/PE

Usually asymptomatic, but may present with **aching bone or joint pain,** headaches, skull deformities, fractures, or nerve entrapment (leads to loss of hearing in 30–40% of cases).

DIAGNOSIS

Based on clinical history, characteristic radiographic changes (see Figure 2.3-3), and lab findings.

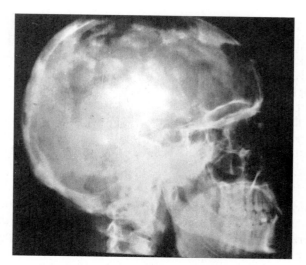

FIGURE 2.3-3.   Radiographic findings in Paget's disease.

Skull of a 58-year-old woman with Paget's disease of bone. (Reproduced, with permission, from Kasper DL et al. *Harrison's Principles of Internal Medicine*, 16th ed. New York: McGraw-Hill, 2005: 2280.)

- **Imaging:** Radionuclide bone scan is the most sensitive test.
- **Labs:** Abnormalities include ↑ serum alkaline phosphatase with normal calcium and phosphate levels; urinary pyridinolines may be helpful. Must be differentiated from metastatic bone disease.

TREATMENT

- **The majority of patients are asymptomatic and require no treatment.**
- There is no cure for Paget's disease. Bisphosphonates and calcitonin are used to slow osteoclastic bone resorption; NSAIDs and acetaminophen can be given for arthritis pain.

COMPLICATIONS

Pathologic fractures, cardiac complications, osteosarcoma (up to 1%).

Hyperparathyroidism

Eighty percent of 1° cases are due to a single **adenoma** and 15% to parathyroid hyperplasia. The most common 2° cause is phosphate retention in chronic kidney disease, which leads to renal osteodystrophy. **3° hyperparathyroidism** occurs when chronic 2° hyperparathyroidism progresses to an unregulated state, resulting in hypercalcemia.

HISTORY/PE

- Most cases are **asymptomatic,** but signs and symptoms may be mild and include **stones** (nephrolithiasis), **bones** (bone pain, myalgias, arthralgias, fractures), abdominal **groans** (abdominal pain, nausea, vomiting, PUD, pancreatitis), and **psychiatric overtones** (fatigue, depression, anxiety, sleep disturbances).
- Chronic renal insufficiency and gout are also associated with 1° hyperparathyroidism.

DIAGNOSIS

- Labs reveal **hypercalcemia, hypophosphatemia,** and hypercalciuria. Intact PTH is inappropriately ↑ relative to ionized calcium (see Table 2.3-5). Vitamin D deficiency may obscure mild cases.
- A radionuclide parathyroid scan may help with localization of an adenoma, although localization is not always necessary.
- Cancer is the most likely alternative diagnosis and must be ruled out, but with carcinoma PTH is usually < 25 pg/mL unless hyperparathyroidism is also present. Lithium and thiazides may exacerbate hyperparathyroidism.

TREATMENT

Relative surgical criteria for hyperparathyroidism include age < 50, markedly ↓ bone mass, nephrolithiasis/renal insufficiency, profoundly elevated serum calcium or life-threatening hypercalcemia, and urine calcium > 400 mg in 24 hours.

- **Parathyroidectomy** if the patient is **symptomatic** or if certain criteria are met. For acute hypercalcemia, give **IV fluids (with a loop diuretic in the setting of renal or heart failure), IV bisphosphonate,** and **calcitonin.**
- Oral phosphate binders (aluminum hydroxide, calcium salts, sevelamer hydrochloride, and lanthanum carbonate) and dietary phosphate restriction are used in patients with 2° hyperparathyroidism regardless of dialysis status.
- Cinacalcet ↓ PTH as well as calcium and phosphate and may be a helpful adjunct in end-stage renal disease.

COMPLICATIONS

Hypercalcemia is the most severe complication, presenting acutely with coma or altered mental status, bone disease, nephrolithiasis, and abdominal pain with nausea and vomiting.

> ► **PITUITARY AND HYPOTHALAMIC DISORDERS**

Cushing's Syndrome

The most common endogenous cause of Cushing's syndrome is hypersecretion of ACTH from a pituitary adenoma (known as Cushing's disease, or **central** hypercortisolism). Other endogenous causes include ectopic ACTH secretion from neoplasia (e.g., carcinoid tumor, small cell lung cancer) and excess adrenal secretion of cortisol (e.g., bilateral adrenal hyperplasia, adenoma, adrenal cancer). The condition is most commonly iatrogenic, resulting from treatment with exogenous corticosteroids.

TABLE 2.3-5. Functions and Mechanisms of PTH

SOURCE	FUNCTIONS	MECHANISMS	REGULATION
Chief cells of parathyroid	↑ bone resorption of calcium and phosphate. ↑ kidney resorption of calcium in the distal convoluted tubule. ↓ kidney resorption of phosphate. ↑ 1,25-$(OH)_2$ vitamin D (cholecalciferol) production by stimulating kidney 1α-hydroxylase.	PTH ↑ serum Ca^{2+}, ↓ serum $(PO_4)^{3-}$, and ↑ urine $(PO_4)^{3-}$. PTH stimulates both osteoclasts and osteoblasts.	↓ in free serum Ca^{2+} ↑ PTH secretion.

HISTORY/PE

- Presents with **hypertension, central obesity,** muscle wasting, thin skin with purple **striae,** psychological disturbances, **hirsutism, moon facies,** and **"buffalo hump."**
- Exam reveals **depression,** oligomenorrhea, growth retardation, proximal weakness, acne, **excessive hair growth,** symptoms of **diabetes** (2° to glucose intolerance), and ↑ susceptibility to infection. **Headache** or cranial nerve deficits are also seen with increasing size of the pituitary mass.

DIAGNOSIS

Diagnosis is as follows (see also Table 2.3-6):

- **Begin with a screen:** An elevated 24-hour free urine cortisol or evening salivary cortisol or a ⊕ overnight low-dose dexamethasone suppression test is considered **abnormal if A.M. cortisol is persistently elevated following overnight suppression.**
- **Distinguish ACTH-dependent from ACTH-independent causes:** If late-afternoon ACTH levels are elevated, Cushing's disease or ectopic ACTH is likely.
- Hyperglycemia, glycosuria, and **hypokalemia** may also be present.

TREATMENT

- **Surgical resection** of the hypersecretory source (pituitary, adrenal).
- Pituitary radiotherapy may also be considered.
- Blockers of adrenal steroidogenesis (e.g., **ketoconazole, aminoglutethimide**) may be of benefit.
- Permanent hormone replacement therapy to correct deficiencies after treatment of the 1° lesion.

Acromegaly

An adult condition due to a benign pituitary GH adenoma. Children with excess GH production present with **gigantism.**

HISTORY/PE

- Presents with **enlargement of the jaw, hands, and feet and coarsening of facial features.** May lead to carpal tunnel syndrome, diastolic dysfunction, hypertension, and arthritis.

TABLE 2.3-6. **Laboratory Findings in Cushing's Syndrome**

	CUSHING'S DISEASE (PITUITARY HYPERSECRETION)	EXOGENOUS STEROID USE	ECTOPIC ACTH SECRETION	ADRENAL CORTISOL HYPERSECRETION
ACTH	↑	↓	↑	↓
Urinary free cortisol	↑	↑	↑	↑

- **Bitemporal hemianopia** may result from compression of the optic chiasm by a pituitary adenoma.
- Excess GH may also lead to **glucose intolerance** or **diabetes.**

DIAGNOSIS

- **Imaging:** MRI of the pituitary shows a sellar lesion.
- **Labs:** Screen by measuring insulin-like growth factor 1 (IGF-1) levels ($\uparrow$ with acromegaly); confirm the diagnosis with an oral glucose suppression test (GH levels will remain elevated despite glucose suppression; baseline GH is not a reliable test).

TREATMENT

- Transsphenoidal surgical resection or external beam radiation of the tumor.
- Octreotide can be used to suppress GH secretion.
- Pegvisomant can be used to block GH receptors in refractory cases.

Hyperprolactinemia

- Prolactinoma is the **most common functioning pituitary tumor.**
- Other pathologic causes include craniopharyngioma, irradiation, drugs (e.g., dopamine), and cirrhosis.
- **Hx/PE:** Hypogonadism is manifested by infertility, oligomenorrhea, or amenorrhea. Galactorrhea, gynecomastia, or bitemporal hemianopia may be prominent.
- **Dx:** The serum prolactin level is typically > 200 mg/mL.
- **Tx:**
  - **Dopamine agonists (first-line therapy):** Cabergoline or bromocriptine.
  - **Surgery:** Should be considered when medical treatment has failed, when the patient desires future pregnancies, or in the setting of visual field defects.

Diabetes Insipidus (DI)

Failure to concentrate urine as a result of central or nephrogenic ADH dysfunction. Subtypes are as follows:

- **Central DI:** The posterior pituitary fails to secrete ADH. Causes include **tumor,** ischemia (Sheehan's syndrome), traumatic cerebral injury, infection, and autoimmune disorders.
- **Nephrogenic DI:** The kidneys fail to respond to circulating ADH. Causes include renal diseases and drugs (e.g., **lithium,** demeclocycline).

For unknown reasons, patients with DI prefer ice-cold beverages.

HISTORY/PE

- Presents with **polydipsia, polyuria,** and **persistent thirst** with dilute urine.
- Patients may present with hypernatremia and dehydration, but if given unlimited access to water, they are typically normonatremic.

DIAGNOSIS

- During a **water deprivation test,** patients excrete a high volume of dilute urine.

- Desmopressin acetate (DDAVP), a synthetic analog of ADH, can be used to distinguish central from nephrogenic DI.
  - **Central DI:** DDAVP challenge will ↓ **urine output and** ↑ **urine osmolarity.**
  - **Nephrogenic DI:** DDAVP challenge will not significantly ↓ urine output.
- MRI may show a pituitary or hypothalamic mass in central DI.

TREATMENT

- Treat the underlying cause.
- **Central DI:** Administer DDAVP intranasally or orally.
- **Nephrogenic DI:** Salt restriction and water intake are the 1° treatment. Thiazide diuretics are used to promote mild volume depletion and to stimulate proximal reabsorption of salt and water.

SIADH

A common cause of euvolemic hyponatremia that results from **stimulated ADH release independent of serum osmolality.**

HISTORY/PE

Associated with **CNS disease** (e.g., head injury, tumor), **pulmonary disease** (e.g., sarcoid, pneumonia), ectopic tumor production/paraneoplastic syndrome (e.g., small cell carcinoma), drugs (e.g., antipsychotics, antidepressants), or surgery.

DIAGNOSIS

- Diagnose on the basis of a urine osmolality > 50–100 mOsm/kg with concurrent serum hyposmolarity in the absence of a physiologic reason for ↑ ADH (e.g., CHF, cirrhosis, hypovolemia).
- **Urinary sodium ≥ 20 mEq/L** demonstrates that the patient is not hypovolemic.

TREATMENT

- **Restrict fluid** and address the underlying cause.
- If hyponatremia is severe (< 110 mEq/L) or if the patient is significantly symptomatic (e.g., comatose, seizing), cautiously give hypertonic saline.
- **Demeclocycline** can help normalize serum sodium by antagonizing the action of ADH in the collecting duct.
- Chronic correction depends on treatment of the underlying disorder.
- **Tolvaptan** (a vasopressin agonist) can be used to treat refractory chronic cases.

Fluid restriction is the cornerstone of SIADH treatment.

▶ ADRENAL GLAND DISORDERS

Adrenal Insufficiency (AI)

May be 1° or 2°. Etiologies are as follows:
- **1°:**
  - Most commonly caused by autoimmune adrenal cortical destruction (**Addison's disease**), leading to deficiencies of mineralocorticoids and glucocorticoids. **Autoimmune destruction** may occur as part of a

polyglandular autoimmune syndrome (hypothyroidism, type 1 DM, vitiligo, premature ovarian failure, testicular failure, pernicious anemia).
- Other causes of 1° AI include congenital enzyme deficiencies, adrenal hemorrhage, TB, and other infections.
- 2°: Caused by ↓ ACTH production by the pituitary; most often due to **cessation of long-term glucocorticoid treatment.**

History/PE
- Most symptoms are nonspecific.
- **Weakness, fatigue,** and **anorexia with weight loss** are common. GI manifestations, hypotension, and salt craving are also seen.
- **Hyperpigmentation** (due to ↑ ACTH secretion) is seen in Addison's disease, especially in areas of sun exposure or friction.

Diagnosis
- Labs show **hyponatremia** and **eosinophilia** (1° or 2°).
- **Hyperkalemia** is specific to 1° AI.
- Hypercalcemia is seen in up to one-third of cases.
- Diagnosis is confirmed with plasma **cortisol levels:**
    - Low plasma cortisol levels (< 20 μg/dL) during a period of high physiologic stress is confirmatory.
    - A random plasma cortisol level > 20 μg/dL excludes the diagnosis.
- **Confirmatory test with synthetic ACTH stimulation test:** A plasma cortisol level > 20 μg/dL excludes the diagnosis.

Treatment
- **Glucocorticoid replacement, with mineralocorticoid** replacement if 1°.
- In adrenal crisis, correct electrolyte abnormalities as needed; provide 50% dextrose to correct hypoglycemia; and initiate volume resuscitation.
- ↑ steroids during periods of stress (e.g., major surgery, trauma, infection). Avoid 2° AI by tapering steroids slowly.

Pheochromocytoma
- A tumor of chromaffin tissue found either in the adrenal medulla or in extra-adrenal sites that secrete catecholamines. May be associated with von Hippel–Lindau syndrome, neurofibromatosis, or MEN 2 syndromes.
- **Hx/PE:** Presents with intermittent tachycardia, palpitations, chest pain, diaphoresis, hypertension, headache, tremor, and anxiety. Crises may be precipitated by anesthesia.
- **Dx:** CT or MRI often demonstrates a suprarenal mass. Screen with plasma-free metanephrines (metanephrine and normetanephrine) or 24-hour urine metanephrines. MIBG scan is sometimes helpful.
- **Tx:** Surgical resection. Preoperatively, **use α-adrenergic blockade first** to control hypertension, followed by β-blockade to control tachycardia. Never give β-blockade first; otherwise, unopposed α-adrenergic stimulation will lead to refractory hypertension.

Hyperaldosteronism
Results from excessive secretion of aldosterone from the zona glomerulosa of the adrenal cortex. It is usually due to adrenocortical hyperplasia (70%) but can also result from unilateral adrenal adenoma (**Conn's syndrome**).

The 4 S's of adrenal crisis management:

Salt: 0.9% saline
Steroids: IV hydrocortisone 100 mg q 8 h
Support
Search for the underlying illness

Do not delay in giving steroids when diagnosing a patient with AI.

Pheochromocytoma rule of 10's:

10% extra-adrenal
10% bilateral
10% malignant
10% occur in children
10% familial

The 5 P's of pheochromocytoma:

Pressure (BP)
Pain (headache)
Perspiration
Palpitations
Pallor/diaphoresis

HISTORY/PE

- Presents with **hypertension, headache, polyuria,** and **muscle weakness.**
- Tetany, paresthesias, and peripheral edema are seen in severe cases.

DIAGNOSIS

- Patients have diastolic hypertension without edema.
- Labs show **hypokalemia, mild hypernatremia,** metabolic alkalosis, hypomagnesemia, and an ↑ **aldosterone/plasma renin activity ratio** (from hyposecretion of renin that fails to ↑ appropriately with volume depletion as well as from hypersecretion that does not suppress with volume expansion).
- CT or MRI may reveal an adrenal mass.

TREATMENT

- Laparoscopic or open **adrenalectomy** for adrenal tumors (after correcting BP and potassium).
- Treat bilateral hyperplasia with **spironolactone,** an aldosterone receptor antagonist.

Congenital Adrenal Hyperplasia

A family of inherited disorders that lead to **cortisol deficiency.** Most cases are due to **21-hydroxylase deficiency (autosomal recessive)** that leads to ↓ cortisol production with elevated cortisol precursors (e.g., 17-OH progesterone). In severe cases, mineralocorticoid deficiency with salt wasting may develop. Other causes include 11- and 17-hydroxylase deficiencies. Cortisol deficiency stimulates ACTH synthesis, leading to overproduction of adrenal androgens.

HISTORY/PE

- Presents with **ambiguous genitalia** in female infants and **virilization** when manifested later in life.
- Also characterized by **macrogenitosomia** in male infants; precocious puberty (if manifested later in life); and hypertension (with 11- and 17-hydroxylase deficiencies).

DIAGNOSIS

Diagnosed by high levels of cortisol precursors and androgens found in blood and urine.

TREATMENT

- **Medical: Immediate fluid resuscitation and salt repletion.** Administer cortisol to ↓ ACTH and adrenal androgens. Fludrocortisone is appropriate for severe 21-hydroxylase deficiency.
- **Surgical:** May be required in the case of ambiguous genitalia in female infants.
- Refer to the Gynecology chapter for information on the diagnosis and treatment of late-onset congenital adrenal hyperplasia.

Epidemiology

▶ ASSESSMENT OF DISEASE FREQUENCY

- The **prevalence** of a disease is the number of existing cases in the population at a specific moment in time.
- The **incidence** of a disease is the number of new cases in the disease-free population that develop over a period of time.
- Prevalent cases are incident cases that have persisted in a population for various reasons:

$$\text{Prevalence} = \text{Incidence} \times \text{Average duration of disease}$$

Prevalence Studies

A **prevalence study** is one in which people in a population are examined for the presence of a disease of interest at a given point in time.

- The **advantages** of prevalence studies are as follows:
    - They provide an efficient means of examining a population, allowing cases and noncases to be assessed all at once.
    - They can be used as a basis for diagnostic testing.
    - They can be used to plan which health services to offer and where.
- Their **disadvantages** include the following:
    - One cannot determine causal relationships because information is obtained only at a single point in time.
    - The risk or incidence of disease cannot be directly measured.

▶ ASSESSMENT OF DIAGNOSTIC STUDIES

Sensitivity and Specificity

Physicians often use tests to try to ascertain a diagnosis, but because no test is perfect, a given result may be falsely ⊕ or ⊖ (see Figure 2.4-1). When deciding whether to administer a test, one should thus consider both its sensitivity and its specificity.

- **Sensitivity** is the probability that a patient with a disease will have a ⊕ test result. **A sensitive test will rarely miss people with the disease and is therefore good at ruling people out.**

$$\text{False-}\ominus \text{ ratio} = 1 - \text{sensitivity}$$

	Disease Present	**No Disease**	
Positive test	a	b	$PPV = a/(a + b)$
Negative test	c	d	$NPV = d/(c + d)$
	Sensitivity = $a/(a + c)$ Specificity = $d/(b + d)$		

FIGURE 2.4-1.   **Sensitivity, specificity, PPV, and NPV.**

- **Specificity** is the probability that a patient without a disease will have a ⊖ test result. **A specific test will rarely determine that someone has the disease when in fact they do not and is therefore good at ruling people in.**

$$\text{False-} \oplus \text{ ratio} = 1 - \text{specificity}$$

- The ideal test is both sensitive and specific, but a trade-off must often be made between sensitivity and specificity.
  - **High sensitivity** is particularly desirable when there is a significant penalty for missing a disease. It is also desirable early in a diagnostic workup, when it is necessary to reduce a broad differential. **Example:** An initial ELISA test for HIV infection.
  - **High specificity** is useful for confirming a likely diagnosis or for situations in which false-⊕ results may prove harmful. **Example:** A Western blot confirmatory HIV test.
- **Example:** You search for your physician, Mary Adel, MD, in the local phone book.
  - Identifying all individuals named "Mary" would be a sensitive test, as anyone named Mary Adel would likely be included in the results. However, it is not specific, as numerous other physicians would also be included. Remember the mnemonic **"Snout"**: High **SEN**sitivity would allow one to rule **out** physicians not listed with this first name.
  - Identifying only individuals with the full name "Mary Lucy Adel IV" is very specific, since individuals not named Mary Adel are especially likely to be declined. However, it is not sensitive, as she may be overlooked if she is not listed by her complete name. Remember the mnemonic **"SPin"**: High **SP**ecificity would allow one to rule **in** physicians listed with this full name.

Positive and Negative Predictive Values

Once a test has been administered and a patient's result has been made available, that result must be interpreted through use of predictive values (or post-test probabilities):

- The **positive predictive value (PPV)** is the probability that a patient with a ⊕ test result truly has the disease. The more specific a test, the higher its PPV. The higher the disease prevalence, the higher the PPV of the test for that disease.
- The **negative predictive value (NPV)** is the probability that a patient with a ⊖ test result truly does not have the disease. The more sensitive a test, the higher its NPV. The lower the disease prevalence, the higher the NPV of the test for that disease.

Likelihood Ratio

Another way to describe the performance of a diagnostic test involves the use of **likelihood ratios (LRs)**, which express how much more or less likely a given test result is in diseased as opposed to nondiseased people:

$$\oplus \text{LR} = \frac{\text{Diseased people with a } \oplus \text{ test result}}{\text{Nondiseased people with a } \oplus \text{ test result}} = \frac{\text{Sensitivity}}{1 - \text{specificity}}$$

$$\ominus \text{LR} = \frac{\text{Diseased people with a } \ominus \text{ test result}}{\text{Nondiseased people with a } \ominus \text{ test result}} = \frac{1 - \text{sensitivity}}{\text{Specificity}}$$

SnOUT: Sensitive tests rule **OUT** disease.
SpIN: Specific tests rule **IN** disease.

Because the predictive value of a test is affected by disease prevalence, it is advantageous to apply diagnostic tests to patients with an ↑ likelihood of having the disease being sought (i.e., an at-risk population).

If a test has an LR of 1, it does not change the pretest probability of disease. If the LR is 10, it makes disease 45% more likely. If the LR is 0.1, disease is 45% less likely.

Knowledge of risk factors may be used to predict future disease in a given patient. Risk factors may be causal (immediate or distant causes of disease) or disease markers (in which removing the risk factor does not necessarily ↓ the likelihood of disease). Risk factors can be difficult to discover for a variety of reasons, including the following:

- A disease may have a long **latency period,** with risky exposures remote and forgotten.
- A risky exposure may be so common that its impact is hard to discern.
- Disease incidence may be low, and it is hard to draw conclusions from infrequent events.
- Risk associated with any individual exposure is small and hard to parse out.
- There is seldom a close, constant relationship between a risk factor and a disease.

The best way to determine whether an exposure actually ↑ disease risk is with a prospective study. The ideal study for risk factor assessment would be an experiment in which the researcher controls risk exposure and then relates it to disease incidence. Doing so, however, may be unethical as well as prohibitively intrusive, time consuming, and expensive. Instead, observational studies such as cohort or case-control studies are used to determine risk.

Cohort Studies

If you see a set of COworkers being followed over time, think COhort study.

In a **cohort study,** a group of people is assembled, **none of whom have the outcome of interest** (i.e., the disease), but **all of whom could potentially experience that outcome.** For each possible risk factor, the members of the cohort are classified as either exposed or unexposed. All the cohort members are then followed over time, and **rates of outcome events are compared in the two exposure groups.**

- **Advantages** of cohort studies are as follows:
  - They follow the same logic as the clinical question (if people are exposed, will they get the disease?).
  - They are the only way to directly determine incidence.
  - They can be used to assess the relationship of a given exposure to many diseases.
  - In prospective studies, exposure is elicited without bias from a known outcome.
- The **disadvantages** of such studies include the following:
  - They can be time consuming and expensive.
  - Studies assess only the relationship of the disease to the few exposure factors recorded at the start of the study.
  - They require many subjects and are thus inefficient and cannot be used to study rare diseases.

Cohort studies are also known as longitudinal studies or incidence studies.

Cohort studies may be prospective—in which a cohort is assembled in the present and followed into the future—or they may be retrospective, in which a cohort is identified from past records and followed to the present.

Case-Control Studies

Case-control studies are essentially cohort studies in reverse. In such studies, a researcher selects **two groups—one with disease (cases) and one without (controls)—and then looks back in time to measure the comparative frequency of exposure to a possible risk factor** in the two groups.

- The validity of a case-control study depends on **appropriate selection of cases and controls, the manner in which exposure is measured, and the manner in which extraneous variables (confounders) are dealt with.**
  - Cases and controls should be comparable in terms of opportunity for exposure (i.e., they should be members of the same base population with an equal opportunity of risk factor exposure).
  - Cases should be newly diagnosed using explicit criteria for diagnosis.
  - Exposures should be assessed in as unbiased a fashion as possible.
  - Confounding may be ↓ by matching subjects or through the stratification of subjects. Multivariable analysis may be helpful in this context.
- **Advantages** of such studies are as follows:
  - Studies use small groups, thereby reducing expense.
  - They can be used to study rare diseases and can easily examine multiple risk factors.
- **Disadvantages** include the following:
  - Studies cannot calculate disease prevalence, incidence, or relative risk, because the numbers of subjects with and without a disease are determined artificially by the investigator rather than by nature (an odds ratio can be used to estimate relative risk).
  - Retrospective data may be inaccurate owing to recall or survivorship biases.

If alcohol intake among individuals with breast cancer is compared with that of individuals without breast cancer, think case-control study.

Absolute risk: The number of finger injuries among hospital staff this week.

▶ MEASURES OF EFFECT

There are several ways to express and compare risk. These include the following:

- **Absolute risk:** Defined as the incidence of disease.
- **Attributable risk (or risk difference):** The additional incidence of disease that is due to a risky exposure, on top of the background incidence from other causes.

Attributable risk = Incidence of disease in exposed − Incidence in unexposed

- **Relative risk (or risk ratio):** Expresses how much more likely an exposed person is to get disease in comparison to an unexposed person. This indicates the **strength of the association between exposure and disease**, making it useful when one is considering disease etiology.

$$\text{Relative risk} = \frac{\text{Incidence in exposed}}{\text{Incidence in unexposed}}$$

- **Odds ratio:** An estimate of relative risk that is used in case-control studies. The odds ratio tells how much more likely it is that a person with a disease has been exposed to a risk factor than someone without the disease. The

Attributable risk: (number of injuries among staff who used scissors) − (number of injuries among staff who did not use scissors).

Relative risk: (number of injuries among staff who used scissors) ÷ (number of injuries among staff who did not use scissors).

	Disease Develops	No Disease	
Exposure	a	b	$RR = \dfrac{a\,/\,(a+b)}{c\,/\,(c+d)}$
No exposure	c	d	$OR = ad/bc$

FIGURE 2.4-2. Relative risk (RR) vs. odds ratio (OR).

lower the disease incidence, the more closely it approximates relative risk (see Figure 2.4-2).

$$\text{Odds ratio} = \frac{\text{Odds that a diseased person is exposed}}{\text{Odds that a nondiseased person is exposed}}$$

Odds ratio: (odds that injured staff used scissors) ÷ (odds that uninjured staff used scissors).

$$Odds = \frac{Probability\ of\ event}{1 - probability\ of\ event}$$

$$Probability = \frac{Odds}{1 + odds}$$

► SURVIVAL CURVES

Once a diagnosis has been established, it is important to be able to describe the associated prognosis. **Survival analysis is used to summarize the average time from one event (e.g., presentation, diagnosis, or start of treatment) to any outcome that can occur only once during follow-up (e.g., death or recurrence of cancer).** The usual method is with a Kaplan-Meier curve (see Figure 2.4-3) describing the survival (or time-to-event if the measured outcome is not death) in a cohort of patients, with the probability of survival decreasing over time as patients die or drop out (are censored) from the study.

► TREATMENT

Studies are typically used to judge the best treatment for a disease. Although the gold standard for such evaluation is a randomized, double-masked controlled trial, other types of studies may be used as well (e.g., an observational

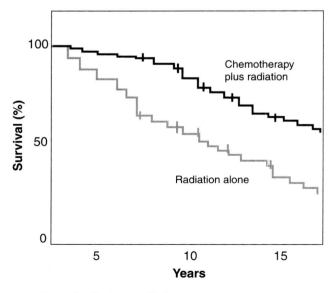

FIGURE 2.4-3. Example of a Kaplan-Meier curve.

study, in which the exposure in question is a therapeutic intervention). In descending order of quality, published studies regarding treatment options include meta-analyses, randomized controlled trials, and case series/case reports.

Randomized Controlled Trials

A randomized controlled trial is **an experimental, prospective study in which subjects are randomly assigned to a treatment or control group.** Random assignment helps ensure that the two groups are truly comparable. The control group may be treated with a placebo or with the accepted standard of care. The study may be masked in **one of two ways:** single-masked, in which patients do not know which treatment group they are in, or double-masked, in which neither the patients nor their physicians know who is in which group. Double-masked studies are the gold standard for studying treatment effects.

Randomization minimizes bias and confounding; double-blinded studies prevent observation bias.

- **Advantages** of randomized controlled trials are as follows:
  - They involve minimal bias.
  - They have the potential to demonstrate causal relationships.
- **Disadvantages** include the following:
  - They are costly and time intensive.
  - Informed consent may be difficult to obtain.
  - Some interventions (e.g., surgery) are not amenable to masking.
  - Ethical standards cannot allow all variables to be controlled.

Bias

Defined as **any process that causes results to systematically differ from the truth.** Good studies and data analyses seek to minimize potential bias. Types of bias include the following:

- **Selection bias:** Occurs when samples or participants are selected that differ from other groups in additional determinants of outcome. **Examples:** A surgeon may select patients without significant comorbid conditions to receive surgery, resulting in unexpectedly positive outcomes compared to previous studies. Similarly, individuals concerned about a family history of breast cancer may be more likely to self-select in entering a mammography program, giving the impression of a prevalence that is higher than reality.
- **Measurement bias:** Occurs when measurement or data-gathering methods differ between groups. **Example:** One group is assessed by CT while another group is assessed by MRI.
- **Confounding bias:** Occurs when a third variable is associated with both the dependent variable and the independent variable (either positively or negatively), inducing a false-$\oplus$ association (type I bias). **Example:** Fishermen in an area may experience a higher incidence of cataracts than the general population. However, becoming a fisherman will not in itself give you cataracts; rather, it is the sunlight to which those fishermen are exposed in their outdoor work.
- **Recall bias:** Results from a difference between two groups in the retrospective recall of past factors or outcomes. **Example:** A patient with cancer may be more motivated than a healthy individual to recall past episodes of chemical exposure.
- **Lead-time bias:** Results from earlier detection of disease, giving an appearance of prolonged survival when in fact the natural course is not altered. **Example:** A new and widely used screening test that detects cancer five

Studies that are masked and randomized are better protected from the effects of bias, whereas observational studies are particularly susceptible to bias.

years earlier may give the impression that patients are living longer with the disease.

- **Length bias:** Occurs when screening tests detect a disproportionate number of slowly progressive diseases but miss rapidly progressive ones, leading to overestimation of the benefit of the screen. **Example:** A better prognosis for patients with cancer is celebrated after implementation of a new screening program. However, this test disproportionally detects slow-growing tumors, which generally tend to be less aggressive.

Confounding variables reduce the internal validity of a study.

Chance

Even with bias reduction, unsystematic random error is unavoidable owing to chance variation in studied data. Types of errors are as follows:

- **Type I (α) error:**
    - Defined as the probability of saying that there is a difference in treatment effects between groups when in fact there is not (i.e., a false-$\oplus$ conclusion).
    - The **p-value** is an estimate of the probability that differences in treatment effects in a study could have happened by chance alone. Classically, differences associated with a $p < 0.05$ are statistically significant.
- **Type II (β) error:**
    - Defined as the probability of saying that there is no difference in treatment effects (i.e., a false-$\ominus$ conclusion) when in fact a difference exists.
    - **Power** is the probability that a study will find a statistically significant difference when one is truly there. It relates directly to the number of subjects. Power (β) = 1 − type II error.
- The **confidence interval (CI)** is a way of expressing statistical significance (p-value) that shows the size of the effect and the statistical power. CIs are interpreted as follows:
    - If one is using a 95% CI, there is a 95% chance that the interval contains the true effect size, which is likely to be closest to the point estimate near the center of the interval.
    - **Example:** You would like to estimate the percentage of women with a specific disease. A 10% result from a sample of 3000 women would provide a 95% CI of 9%–11%, whereas a 10% finding from a sample of 30 women would yield a CI of −1% of 21%. The first case has more power because the sample size is larger, producing a narrow interval. In the latter case, you cannot state with 95% certainty that women in general even have the disease!
- If the CI includes the value corresponding to a relative risk of 1.0 (i.e., zero treatment difference), the results are not statistically significant.
- If the CI is wide, power is low.

▶ PREVENTION

- There are three levels of prevention:
    - **1° prevention:** Includes measures to ↓ the incidence of disease.
    - **2° prevention:** Focuses on identifying the disease early, when it is asymptomatic or mild, and implementing measures that can halt or slow disease progression.
    - **3° prevention:** Includes measures that ↓ morbidity or mortality resulting from the presence of disease.

TABLE 2.4-1. Types of Vaccinations

Vaccine Type	Targeted Diseases
Live attenuated	Measles, mumps, rubella, polio (Sabin), yellow fever, influenza (nasal spray).
Inactivated (killed)	Cholera, influenza, HAV, polio (Salk), rabies, influenza (injection).
Toxoid	Diphtheria, tetanus.
Subunit	HBV, pertussis, *Streptococcus pneumoniae*, HPV, meningococcus.
Conjugate	Hib, *S. pneumoniae*.

■ Prevention may be accomplished by a **combination of immunization, chemoprevention, behavioral counseling, and screening.** A good screening test has the following characteristics:
  ■ It has high sensitivity and specificity.
  ■ It has a high PPV.
  ■ It is inexpensive, easy to administer, and safe.
  ■ Treatment after screening is more effective than subsequent treatment without screening.

Vaccination

■ Vaccines work by mimicking infections and triggering an immune response in which memory cells are formed to recognize and fight any future infection. There are several different vaccine formulations, as indicated in Table 2.4-1.
■ Recommended vaccination schedules for children and adults are outlined in Figures 2.4-4 through 2.4-6.

> ■ **1° prevention:** A woman reduces dietary intake of fat or alcohol to reduce her risk of developing breast cancer.
> ■ **2° prevention:** A woman obtains a mammogram to screen for breast cancer.
> ■ **3° prevention:** A woman undergoes surgical intervention for breast cancer.

Vaccine ▼ Age ►	Birth	1 month	2 months	4 months	6 months	12 months	15 months	18 months	19–23 months	2–3 years	4–6 years
Hepatitis B	HepB	HepB				HepB					
Rotavirus			RV	RV	RV						
Diphtheria, Tetanus, Pertussis			DTaP	DTaP	DTaP		DTaP				DTaP
Haemophilus influenzae type b			Hib	Hib	Hib	Hib					
Pneumococcal			PCV	PCV	PCV	PCV				PPSV	
Inactivated Poliovirus			IPV	IPV		IPV					IPV
Influenza						Influenza (Yearly)					
Measles, Mumps, Rubella						MMR					MMR
Varicella						Varicella					Varicella
Hepatitis A						HepA (2 doses)				HepA Series	
Meningococcal										MCV	

Range of recommended ages

Certain high-risk groups

FIGURE 2.4-4. Recommended vaccinations for children 0–6 years of age.

(Reproduced from the Centers for Disease Control and Prevention, Atlanta, Georgia.)

Vaccine ▼ Age ►	7–10 years	11–12 years	13–18 years
Tetanus, Diphtheria, Pertussis		Tdap	Tdap
Human Papillomavirus		HPV (3 doses)	HPV Series
Meningococcal	MCV	MCV	MCV
Influenza		Influenza (Yearly)	
Pneumococcal		PPSV	
Hepatitis A		HepA Series	
Hepatitis B		HepB Series	
Inactivated Poliovirus		IPV Series	
Measles, Mumps, Rubella		MMR Series	
Varicella		Varicella Series	

Range of recommended ages

Catch-up immunization

Certain high-risk groups

FIGURE 2.4-5.   Recommended vaccinations for children 7–18 years of age.

(Reproduced from the Centers for Disease Control and Prevention, Atlanta, Georgia.)

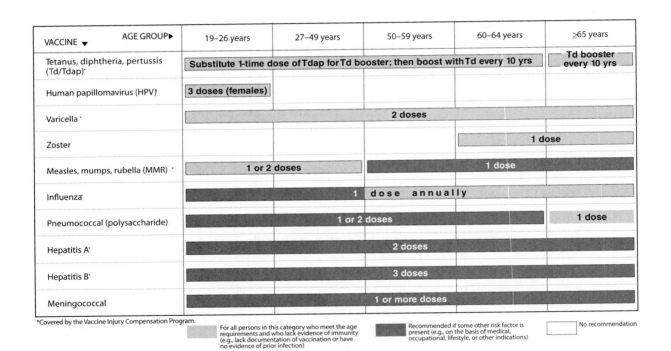

VACCINE ▼ AGE GROUP ►	19–26 years	27–49 years	50–59 years	60–64 years	≥65 years
Tetanus, diphtheria, pertussis (Td/Tdap)*	Substitute 1-time dose of Tdap for Td booster; then boost with Td every 10 yrs				Td booster every 10 yrs
Human papillomavirus (HPV)	3 doses (females)				
Varicella *	2 doses				
Zoster				1 dose	
Measles, mumps, rubella (MMR) *	1 or 2 doses		1 dose		
Influenza	1 dose annually				
Pneumococcal (polysaccharide)	1 or 2 doses				1 dose
Hepatitis A*	2 doses				
Hepatitis B*	3 doses				
Meningococcal	1 or more doses				

*Covered by the Vaccine Injury Compensation Program.

For all persons in this category who meet the age requirements and who lack evidence of immunity (e.g., lack documentation of vaccination or have no evidence of prior infection)

Recommended if some other risk factor is present (e.g., on the basis of medical, occupational, lifestyle, or other indications)

No recommendation

FIGURE 2.4-6.   Recommended vaccinations for adults.

(Reproduced from the Centers for Disease Control and Prevention, Atlanta, Georgia.)

TABLE 2.4-2. Stages of Change in Behavioral Counseling

STAGE OF CHANGE	CHARACTERIZATION	EXAMPLE
Precontemplation	Denial or ignorance of the problem.	A 51-year-old smoker has not even thought about cessation.
Contemplation	Ambivalence or conflicted emotions; assessing benefits and barriers to change.	A 43-year-old crack cocaine addict considers treatment for her addiction.
Preparation	Experimenting with small changes; collecting information about change.	A 28-year-old heroin addict visits his doctor to ask questions about quitting.
Action	Taking direct action toward achieving a goal.	A 33-year-old enters a rehabilitation facility for treatment of addiction to prescription narcotics.
Maintenance	Maintaining a new behavior; avoiding temptation.	A 41-year-old continues to visit Alcoholics Anonymous meetings to gain support and reinforcement against relapse.

- **Live vaccines should not be administered to immunosuppressed patients.** Such vaccines are also **contraindicated in pregnant women** owing to a theoretical risk of maternal-fetal transmission.

Chemoprevention

Defined as the use of drugs to prevent disease. Examples include supplementation of water and food with healthful vitamins and minerals; aspirin prophylaxis for heart disease; statin treatment for hypercholesterolemia; and perioperative β-blockade.

Behavioral Counseling

In offering counsel, physicians should tailor their education and suggestions to the individual patient as well as to his or her **stage of change** (see Table 2.4-2). Counseling is most likely to be successful when it accommodates the patient's willingness to change or lack thereof.

► SCREENING RECOMMENDATIONS

Tables 2.4-3 and 2.4-4 outline recommended health care screening measures by age group and modality.

TABLE 2.4-3. Health Screening Methods by Age

AGE GROUP	MEASURES
Birth–10 years	Height and weight, BP, vision and hearing screening, hemoglobinopathy screen (at birth), phenylalanine level (at birth), TSH and/or T$_4$ (at birth), lead level (at least one time before six years of age).
11–24 years	Height and weight, BP, Pap test, gonorrhea and chlamydia (GC) screen (if sexually active), rubella serology or vaccination (women only); screen for risky behaviors, including substance abuse.
25–64 years	Height and weight, BP (every two years), cholesterol (every five years), Pap test and bimanual pelvic exam, fecal occult blood test (FOBT) or fecal immunochemical test (FIT), sigmoidoscopy or colonoscopy, mammography, rubella serology or vaccination (women only); screen for alcohol abuse and depression.
≥ 65 years	Height and weight, BP, FOBT or FIT, sigmoidoscopy or colonoscopy, Pap test, vision and hearing screening, osteoporosis (DEXA) scans for women; screen for alcohol abuse and depression.

TABLE 2.4-4. Health Screening Methods by Modality

MODALITY	RECOMMENDATION[a]
Colonoscopy	Once every 10 years in patients ≥ 50 years of age (or ≥ 40 years of age for high-risk patients). The preferred modality if there is a known history of dysplasia. CT virtual colonoscopy is comparable to standard colonoscopy and can be used every five years as an initial screening exam.
Flexible sigmoidoscopy	Once every five years in patients ≥ 50 years of age (or ≥ 40 years of age for high-risk patients).
FOBT or FIT	Once every year in patients ≥ 50 years of age (or ≥ 40 years of age for high-risk patients).
Bimanual pelvic exam	Once every 1–3 years in patients 20–40 years of age; once yearly in patients ≥ 40 years of age.
Pap test	Once every year within three years after onset of vaginal intercourse, but no later than age 21 up to age 30; once every two years with liquid-based Pap test. The interval can be ↑ to once every 2–3 years for women > 30 years of age with three ⊖ cytology tests.
Mammography	Once every 1–2 years in patients ≥ 40 years of age; once yearly in patients ≥ 50 years of age (controversial).
Endometrial tissue sampling	Not recommended as a screening test; indicated for postmenopausal bleeding.
CXR	Not recommended as a screening test.
Skin exam	Insufficient evidence.
DRE	Offer every year to high-risk patients at 40 years and to others at 50 years of age (controversial).
PSA	Offer every year to high-risk patients at 40 years and to others at 50 years of age (controversial).
Clinical breast exam	Offer every three years to female patients in 20s and 30s, and every year to females 40 or more years of age (controversial).

[a] Different medical societies have various recommendations regarding cancer screening. Refer to the National Cancer Institute's Web site for a recent summary of recommendations: www.nci.nih.gov/cancer_information/testing.

The leading cause of cancer mortality in the United States is lung cancer. Prostate and breast cancers are the most prevalent cancers in men and women, respectively, with lung and colorectal cancers ranking second and third most common in both sexes. Table 2.4-5 lists the principal causes of death in the United States by age group.

TABLE 2.4-5. Leading Causes of Death by Age Group

AGE GROUP	VARIABLE
All ages	Heart disease, cancer, stroke, chronic lower respiratory disease, injuries, diabetes.
< 1 year	Congenital anomalies, disorders related to low birth weight, SIDS, maternal complications.
1–4 years	Injuries, congenital anomalies, cancer, homicide, heart disease.
5–14 years	Injuries, cancer, congenital anomalies, homicide, suicide, heart disease.
15–24 years	Injuries, homicide, suicide, cancer, heart disease.
25–44 years	Injuries, cancer, heart disease, suicide, **HIV**, homicide.
45–64 years	Cancer, heart disease, injuries, stroke, diabetes, chronic lower respiratory disease.
≥ 65 years	Heart disease, cancer, stroke, chronic lower respiratory disease, Alzheimer's disease, diabetes.

Adapted, with permission, from the National Center for Health Statistics, Department of Health and Human Services, www.cdc.gov/nchs.

HIGH-YIELD FACTS

EPIDEMIOLOGY

By law, disease reporting is mandated at the state level, and the list of diseases that must be reported to public health authorities varies slightly by state. The CDC has a list of nationally notifiable diseases that states voluntarily report to the CDC. These diseases include but are not limited to those listed in Table 2.4-6.

TABLE 2.4-6. Common Reportable Diseases

DISEASE CATEGORY	EXAMPLES
STDs	HIV, AIDS, syphilis, gonorrhea, chlamydia, chancroid, HCV.
Tick-borne disease	Lyme disease, ehrlichiosis, Rocky Mountain spotted fever.
Potential bioweapons	Anthrax, smallpox, plague.
Vaccine-preventable disease	Diphtheria, tetanus, pertussis, measles, mumps, rubella, polio, varicella, HAV, HBV, *H. influenzae* (invasive), meningococcal disease.
Water-/food-borne disease	Cholera, giardiasis, legionella, listeriosis, botulism, shigellosis, shiga toxin–producing *E. coli*, salmonellosis, trichinellosis, typhoid.
Zoonoses	Tularemia, psittacosis, brucellosis, rabies.
Miscellaneous	TB, leprosy, toxic shock syndrome, SARS, West Nile virus, VRSA, coccidioidomycosis, cryptosporidiosis.

Ethics and Legal Issues

- **Respect for autonomy:** Clinicians are obligated to respect patients as individuals and to honor their preferences in medical care. **Example:** A surgeon presents the risks and benefits of tumor resection to her patient before consent is given to proceed with the procedure.
- **Beneficence:** Physicians have a responsibility to act in the patient's best interest. As a fiduciary, the physician stands in a special relationship of trust and responsibility to patients. Respect for patient autonomy may conflict with beneficence. **Example:** An elderly woman is adamant that she does not want to go to a rehabilitation facility and thus refuses amputation of a potentially gangrenous foot. The procedure is necessary to prevent life-threatening complications. The physician has a responsibility to act in the patient's best interest.
- **Nonmaleficence:** "Do no harm." The responsibility to avert avoidable harms is a strong duty. However, if the potential benefits of an intervention outweigh the risks, an autonomous patient may make an informed decision to consent and proceed. **Example:** A patient may choose to undergo dialysis, accepting that his discomfort would be outweighed by the greater good of sustaining life.
- **Justice:** With regard to individual patients, fairness is expressed as the notion that equal persons should be treated equally. Health care is an important resource, and access to quality health care gives individuals a greater chance for a healthy and productive life. Fair distribution of this resource is an ongoing challenge for health policy and in the clinical arena.

▶ **INFORMED CONSENT**

BRAIN of informed consent:

Benefits
Risks
Alternatives
Indications
Nature

- Defined as willing acceptance (without coercion) of a medical intervention by a patient after adequate discussion with a physician about the **nature** of the intervention along with its **indications, risks, benefits,** and potential **alternatives** (including no treatment).
- **Patients may change their minds at any time.**
- Informed consent is required for significant procedures unless:
  - Emergency treatment is required. **Examples:** An unconscious patient presents with cerebral edema after a motor vehicle collision, or a patient without previously indicated DNR/DNI status undergoes cardiac arrest.
  - Patients lack decision-making capacity (consent can be obtained from a surrogate decision maker). **Examples:** Patients may present with dementia or significant psychiatric disturbances. Minors generally require surrogate decision makers until they demonstrate adequate decision-making capacity or are of legal age.

▶ **MINORS**

- **Consent for treatment** is implied in life-threatening situations when parents cannot be contacted.
- Emancipated minors do not require parental consent for medical care. Minors are emancipated if they are married, in the armed services, or are financially independent of their parents and have sought legal emancipation.
- Minors may consent to care for **sexually transmitted infections** without parental consent or knowledge. Rules concerning contraception, preg-

nancy, and abortion services and treatment for drug and alcohol dependency vary across the United States. (Some states leave the decision of informing parents about adolescent use of confidential services to the physician, based on the best interest of the patient. Other states limit disclosure.)

- **Refusal of treatment:** A parent has the right to refuse treatment for his/her child as long as those decisions do not pose a serious threat to the child's well-being (e.g., refusing immunizations is not considered a serious threat). If a decision is not in the best interest of the child, a physician may seek a court order to provide treatment against parental wishes. In emergent situations, if withholding treatment jeopardizes the child's safety, treatment can be initiated on the basis of legal precedent. **Example:** A physician provides blood transfusion to save the life of a six-year-old child seriously injured in a motor vehicle collision despite parental requests to withhold such a measure.

Minors may consent to care for sexually transmitted infections without parental consent or knowledge.

▶ COMPETENCE AND DECISION-MAKING CAPACITY

- **Competence:** Refers to a person's **legal capacity to make decisions** and be held accountable in a court of law. Competence is assessed by the courts and is often used interchangeably with the term *decision-making capacity* (see below).
- **Decision-making capacity:** A medical term that refers to the ability of a patient to understand relevant information, appreciate the severity of the medical situation and its consequences, communicate a choice, and deliberate rationally about one's values in relation to the decision being made. This can be assessed by the physician.
- Decision-making capacity is best understood as varying with the complexity of the decision involved. **Example:** The level of capacity needed for a decision about liver transplantation is different from that needed to choose between two types of pain medication for fracture-related pain.
- Incompetent patients, as assessed by the courts, or temporarily incapacitated patients cannot decide to accept or refuse treatment. **Example:** An intoxicated patient with altered mental status cannot refuse thiamine supplementation.
- In general, patients who have decision-making capacity have the right to refuse or discontinue treatment. **Example:** Jehovah's Witnesses can refuse blood products.

▶ END-OF-LIFE ISSUES

Written Advance Directives

- **Living will:** Addresses a patient's wishes to maintain, withhold, or withdraw life-sustaining treatment in the event of terminal disease or a persistent vegetative state. Examples include **DNR** (do not resuscitate) and **DNI** (do not intubate) orders.
- **Durable power of attorney for health care (DPOAHC):** Legally designates a surrogate health care decision maker if a patient lacks decision-making capacity. **More flexible** than a living will. Surrogates should make decisions consistent with the person's stated wishes.
- If no living will or DPOAHC exists, decisions should be made by close family members (spouse, adult children, parents, and adult siblings), friends, or personal physicians, in that order.

*In the absence of a living will or DPOA, the **Spouse CHIPS** in For the **Person**: **Spouse**, **CHI**ldren, Parent, Sibling, Friend, **Person**al physician.*

*DNR/DNI orders do **not** mean "do not treat."*

Withdrawal of Care

- Patients and their decision makers have the right to forgo or withdraw life-sustaining treatment.
- **No ethical distinction is considered to exist between withdrawing a treatment that offers no benefit and withholding one that is not indicated.** This may include ventilation, fluids, nutrition, and medications such as antibiotics.
- If the intent is to relieve suffering and medications administered are titrated for that purpose, then it is considered ethical to provide palliative treatment to relieve pain and suffering, even if it may hasten a patient's death. **Example:** A physician prescribes midazolam to a patient who is expected to die within a day in order to offer relief from the acute distress of grand mal seizures and pain.

Euthanasia and Physician-Assisted Suicide

- **Euthanasia** is the administration of a lethal agent with the intent to end life.
- It is opposed by the AMA Code of Medical Ethics and is **illegal in all states.**
- Patients who request euthanasia should be evaluated for inadequate pain control and comorbid depression.
- **Physician-assisted suicide** is prescribing a lethal agent to a patient who will self-administer it to end his/her own life. This is currently illegal except in the state of Oregon.

Futility

Physicians are not ethically obligated to provide treatment and may refuse a family member's request for further intervention on the grounds of futility under the following circumstances:

Patients cannot demand futile treatment from their physicians.

- There is no pathophysiologic rationale for treatment.
- A given intervention has already failed.
- Maximal intervention is currently failing.
- Treatment will not achieve the goals of care.

▶ DISCLOSURE

Full Disclosure

A patient's family cannot require that a doctor withhold information from the patient.

- Patients have a right to know about their medical status, prognosis, and treatment options (full disclosure).
- A patient's family cannot require that a doctor withhold information from the patient.
- A doctor may withhold information only if the patient requests not to be told or in the rare case when a physician determines that disclosure would severely harm the patient or undermine their informed decision-making capacity (**therapeutic privilege**).

Medical Errors

- **Physicians are obligated to inform patients of mistakes made in their medical treatment.**
- If the specific error or series of errors is not known, the physician should communicate this with the family promptly and maintain contact with the patient as investigations reveal more facts.

Clinical Research

- Physicians are obligated to inform patients considering involvement in a clinical research protocol about the purpose of the research study and the entire study design as it will affect the patient's treatment. This includes the possible risks, benefits, and alternatives to the research protocol.
- An informed consent form approved by the overseeing research institutional review board (IRB) must be completed for participation in any clinical research protocol, describing the possible risks and benefits of involvement in the research study.

► CONFIDENTIALITY

- Information disclosed by a patient to his/her physician and information about a patient's medical condition are confidential and cannot be divulged without expressed patient consent.
- A patient may waive the right to confidentiality (e.g., with insurance companies).
- It is ethically and legally necessary to override confidentiality in the following situations:
    - **Patient intent to commit a violent crime (Tarasoff decision):** Physicians have a **duty to protect** the intended victim through reasonable means (e.g., warn the victim, notify police).
    - Suicidal patients.
    - Child and elder abuse.
    - Reportable infectious diseases (duty to warn public officials and identifiable people at risk).
    - Gunshot and knife wounds (duty to notify the police).
    - Impaired automobile drivers. **Example:** A patient begins to drive one week after hospitalization for seizures, although the department of motor vehicles in his state requires that licensed drivers be seizure free for at least three months.

► CONFLICT OF INTEREST

- Occurs when physicians find themselves having two interests in a given situation and their professional obligations are influenced by personal interest in another matter. **Example:** A physician may own stock in a pharmaceutical company (financial interest) that produces a drug he is prescribing to his patient (patient care interest).
- Physicians should disclose existing conflicts of interest to affected parties (e.g., patients, institutions, audiences of journal articles or scientific meetings).

Overriding confidentiallty—

WAIT a SEC before letting a dangerous patient go!

Wounds
Automobile-driving impairment
Infectious diseases
Tarasoff— Violent crimes
Suicide
Elder abuse
Child abuse

The 4 D's of malpractice:

Duty
Dereliction
Damage
Direct cause

- The essential elements of a civil suit under negligence include the **four D's:**
  - The physician has a **D**uty to the patient.
  - **D**ereliction of duty occurs.
  - There is **D**amage to the patient.
  - Dereliction is the **D**irect cause of damage.
- Unlike a criminal suit, in which the burden of proof is "beyond a reasonable doubt," the burden of proof in a malpractice suit is "a preponderance of the evidence."

Gastrointestinal

Dysphagia/Odynophagia

Difficulty swallowing (dysphagia) or pain with swallowing (odynophagia) due to abnormalities of the oropharynx or esophagus.

HISTORY/PE

- Presentation varies according to the location:
  - **Oropharyngeal dysphagia:** Presents with difficulty passing material from the oropharynx to the esophagus. Usually involves **liquids** more than solids. Causes can be **neurologic** or **muscular** and include stroke, Parkinson's disease, myasthenia gravis, prolonged intubation, and Zenker's diverticula.
  - **Esophageal dysphagia:** Usually involves **solids** more than liquids for most **obstructive** causes (strictures, Schatzki rings, webs, carcinoma) and is generally progressive. **Motility** disorders (achalasia, scleroderma, esophageal spasm) present with **both** liquid and solid dysphagia.
- Examine for masses (e.g., goiter, tumor) and anatomic defects.

DIAGNOSIS

- **Oropharyngeal dysphagia:** Cine-esophagram.
- **Esophageal dysphagia:** Barium swallow followed by endoscopy, manometry, and/or pH monitoring. If an obstructive lesion is suspected, proceed directly to endoscopy with biopsy.
- **Odynophagia:** Upper endoscopy.

TREATMENT

Etiology dependent.

Esophageal webs are associated with iron deficiency anemia and glossitis (Plummer-Vinson syndrome).

Infectious Esophagitis

Table 2.6-1 outlines the etiology, diagnosis, and treatment of infectious esophagitis.

Diffuse Esophageal Spasm

- A motility disorder in which normal peristalsis is periodically interrupted by high-amplitude **nonperistaltic** contractions of unknown etiology. Also known as **nutcracker esophagus.**

Candidal esophagitis is an AIDS-defining illness.

TABLE 2.6-1. Causes of Infectious Esophagitis

ETIOLOGIC AGENT	EXAM FINDINGS	UPPER ENDOSCOPY	TREATMENT
Candida albicans	Oral thrush	Yellow-white plaques adherent to the mucosa.	Fluconazole PO
HSV	Oral ulcers	Small, deep ulcerations; multinucleated giant cells with nuclear inclusions on biopsy.	Acyclovir IV
CMV	Retinitis, colitis	Large, superficial ulcerations; intranuclear inclusions on biopsy.	Ganciclovir IV

The musculature of the upper one-third of the esophagus is skeletal, whereas that of the lower two-thirds is smooth muscle.

Malignancy may mimic achalasia (pseudoachalasia).

- **Hx/PE:** Presents with **chest pain,** dysphagia, and odynophagia. Often precipitated by ingestion of hot or cold liquids; relieved by nitroglycerin.
- **Dx:** Barium swallow may show a **corkscrew**-shaped esophagus. **Esophageal manometry** reveals high-amplitude, simultaneous contractions.
- **Tx:** Nitrates and calcium channel blockers (CCBs) for symptomatic relief; surgery (esophageal myotomy) for severe, incapacitating symptoms.

Achalasia

- A motor disorder of the esophagus characterized by **impaired relaxation of the lower esophageal sphincter (LES)** and loss of peristalsis in the distal two-thirds of the esophagus. Thought to result from the loss or absence of inhibitory ganglion cells in the myenteric (Auerbach's) plexus.
- **Hx/PE:** Progressive dysphagia, chest pain, regurgitation of undigested food, weight loss, and nocturnal cough are common symptoms.
- **Dx:**
    - **Barium swallow** reveals esophageal **dilation** with a **"bird's beak" tapering** of the distal esophagus (see Figure 2.6-1).
    - **Manometry** shows ↑ **resting LES pressure, incomplete LES relaxation** upon swallowing, and ↓ **peristalsis** in the body of the esophagus.
    - Mechanical causes of obstruction must be ruled out by endoscopy.
- **Tx:** Nitrates, CCBs, or endoscopic injection of botulinum toxin into the LES may provide short-term relief of symptoms. Pneumatic balloon dilation or surgical (Heller) myotomy are definitive treatment options.

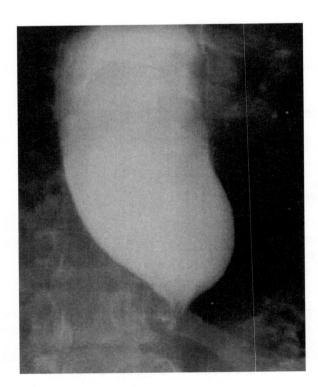

FIGURE 2.6-1.   Achalasia.

Barium esophagram reveals esophageal dilation with a "bird's beak" tapering of the distal esophagus. (Reproduced from Waters PF, DeMeester TR. Foregut motor disorders and their surgical management. *Med Clin North Am* 65: 1235, © 1981, with permission from Elsevier.)

Esophageal Diverticula

- The second most common esophageal motility disorder (after achalasia).
- Cervical outpouching through the cricopharyngeal muscle is called Zenker's diverticulum. Diverticula can also occur in the middle and distal third of the esophagus.
- **Hx/PE:** Patients complain of chest pain, dysphagia, halitosis, and regurgitation of undigested food.
- **Dx: Barium swallow** will demonstrate outpouchings.
- **Tx:** If symptomatic, treat with surgical excision of the diverticulum. For Zenker's diverticulum, **myotomy** of the cricopharyngeus is required to relieve the high-pressure zone.

Esophageal Cancer

- **Squamous cell carcinoma** (SCC) is the most common type of esophageal cancer worldwide, while **adenocarcinoma** is most prevalent in the United States, Europe, and Australia. The latter is associated with Barrett's esophagus (columnar metaplasia of the distal esophagus 2° to chronic GERD).
- Alcohol use and smoking have been identified as major risk factors for SCC.
- **Hx/PE:** Progressive dysphagia, initially to solids and later to liquids, is common. Weight loss, odynophagia, GERD, GI bleeding, and vomiting are also seen.
- **Dx:** Barium study shows narrowing of the esophagus with an irregular border protruding into the lumen. EGD and biopsy confirm the diagnosis. CT and endoscopic ultrasound are used for staging.
- **Tx:** Chemoradiation and surgical resection is the definitive treatment, but the prognosis is poor. Surgery is also offered for high-grade Barrett's dysplasia. Patients who are not candidates for surgery may require an endoscopically placed esophageal stent for palliation and improved quality of life.

Gastroesophageal Reflux Disease (GERD)

Symptomatic reflux of gastric contents into the esophagus, most commonly as a result of **transient LES relaxation.** Can be due to an incompetent LES, gastroparesis, or hiatal hernia.

HISTORY/PE

- Patients present with **heartburn** that commonly occurs 30–90 minutes **after a meal, worsens with reclining,** and often improves with antacids, sitting, or standing. Substernal chest pain can be difficult to distinguish from other causes.
- Sour taste ("water brash"), globus, unexplained cough, and morning hoarseness can be clues.
- Exam is usually **normal** unless a systemic disease (e.g., scleroderma) is present.

DIAGNOSIS

- The history and clinical impression are important.
- An empiric trial of lifestyle modification and medical treatment is often attempted first. Studies may include barium swallow (to look for hiatal hernia), esophageal manometry, and 24-hour pH monitoring.

Squamous cell esophageal cancer is associated with tobacco and alcohol use.

Esophageal cancer metastasizes early because the esophagus lacks a serosa.

Risk factors for GERD include hiatal hernia and ↑ intra-abdominal pressure (e.g., obesity, pregnancy).

GERD can mimic cough-variant asthma.

- **EGD** with biopsies should be performed in patients whose symptoms are unresponsive to initial empiric therapy, long-standing (to rule out Barrett's esophagus and adenocarcinoma), or suggestive of complicated disease (e.g., anorexia, weight loss, dysphagia/odynophagia).

TREATMENT

- **Lifestyle:** Weight loss, head-of-bed elevation, reduction of meal size, and avoidance of nocturnal meals and substances that ↓ LES tone.
- **Pharmacologic:** Start with **antacids** in patients with mild, intermittent symptoms; use **H₂ receptor antagonists** (cimetidine, ranitidine) or **PPIs** (omeprazole, lansoprazole) in patients with chronic and frequent symptoms. PPIs are preferred for severe or erosive disease.
- **Surgical:** For refractory or severe disease, **Nissen fundoplication** may offer significant relief.

COMPLICATIONS

Esophagitis, esophageal stricture, aspiration of gastric contents, upper GI bleeding, **Barrett's esophagus.**

Hiatal Hernia

- Herniation of a portion of the stomach upward into the chest through a diaphragmatic opening. There are two common types:
    - **Sliding hiatal hernias (95%):** The gastroesophageal junction and a portion of the stomach are displaced above the diaphragm.
    - **Paraesophageal hiatal hernias (5%):** The gastroesophageal junction remains below the diaphragm, while a neighboring portion of the fundus herniates into the mediastinum.
- **Hx/PE:** May be asymptomatic. Those with sliding hernias may present with GERD.
- **Dx:** Commonly an incidental finding on CXR; also frequently diagnosed by barium swallow or EGD.
- **Tx:**
    - **Sliding hernias:** Medical therapy and lifestyle modifications to ↓ GERD symptoms.
    - **Paraesophageal hernias:** Surgical gastropexy (attachment of the stomach to the rectus sheath and closure of the hiatus) is recommended to prevent gastric volvulus.

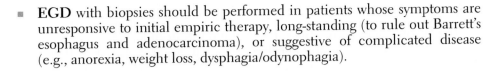

▶ **DISORDERS OF THE STOMACH AND DUODENUM**

Gastritis

Inflammation of the stomach lining. Subtypes are as follows:

- **Acute gastritis:** Rapidly developing, superficial lesions that are often due to **NSAID** use, alcohol, *H. pylori* infection, and stress from severe illness (e.g., burns, CNS injury).
- **Chronic gastritis:**
    - **Type A (10%):** Occurs in the fundus and is due to **autoantibodies to parietal cells.** Causes **pernicious anemia** and is associated with other autoimmune disorders, such as thyroiditis. Also ↑ the risk of gastric adenocarcinoma.

Patients with GERD should avoid caffeine, alcohol, chocolate, garlic, onions, mints, and nicotine.

BARRett's—

Becomes
Adenocarcinoma
Results from
Reflux

Type A gastritis is associated with pernicious anemia due to the lack of intrinsic factor necessary for the absorption of vitamin B₁₂.

- **Type B (90%):** Occurs in the antrum and may be caused by NSAID use or *H. pylori* infection. Often asymptomatic, but associated with ↑ risk of PUD and gastric cancer.

HISTORY/PE

Patients may be asymptomatic or may complain of epigastric pain, nausea, vomiting, hematemesis, or melena.

DIAGNOSIS

- Upper endoscopy can visualize the gastric lining.
- *H. pylori* infection can be detected by **urease breath test**, serum IgG antibodies (which indicate exposure, not current infection), *H. pylori* stool antigen, or endoscopic biopsy.

TREATMENT

- ↓ intake of offending agents. Antacids, sucralfate, H₂ blockers, and/or PPIs may help.
- Triple therapy (amoxicillin, clarithromycin, omeprazole) to treat *H. pylori* infection.
- Give prophylactic H₂ blockers or PPIs to patients at risk for stress ulcers (e.g., ICU patients).

Gastric Cancer

- This malignant tumor is the second most common cause of cancer-related death worldwide and is particularly common in Korea and Japan. Tumors are generally adenocarcinomas, which exhibit two morphologic types:
  - **Intestinal type:** Thought to arise from intestinal metaplasia of **gastric mucosal cells.** Risk factors include a diet high in nitrites and salt and low in fresh vegetables (antioxidants), *H. pylori* colonization, and chronic gastritis.
  - **Diffuse type:** Tends to be poorly differentiated and not associated with *H. pylori* infection or chronic gastritis. Risk factors are largely unknown; signet ring cells are seen on pathology.
- **Hx/PE:** Early signs are indigestion and loss of appetite. Advanced cases generally present with abdominal pain, weight loss, or upper GI bleeding.
- **Dx:** Early gastric carcinoma is largely asymptomatic and is discovered serendipitously with endoscopic examination of high-risk individuals.
- **Tx:** Successful treatment rests entirely on early detection and surgical removal of the tumor. Five-year survival is < 10% for advanced disease.

Gastric adenocarcinoma that metastasizes to the ovary is called a Krukenberg tumor.

*Gastric cancer may present with **Virchow's node** (an enlarged left supraclavicular lymph node).*

Peptic Ulcer Disease (PUD)

Damage to the gastric or duodenal mucosa caused by impaired mucosal defense and/or ↑ acidic gastric contents. *H. pylori* plays a causative role in > 90% of duodenal ulcers and 70% of gastric ulcers. Other risk factors include **corticosteroid, NSAID, alcohol,** and **tobacco** use. Males are affected more often than females.

HISTORY/PE

- Classically presents with chronic or periodic **dull, burning epigastric pain** that **improves with meals** (especially duodenal ulcers), worsens 2–3 hours after eating, and can radiate to the back.

After a meal, pain from a Gastric ulcer is Greater, whereas Duodenal pain Decreases.

Roughly 5–7% of lower GI bleeds are from an upper GI source.

Rule out Zollinger-Ellison syndrome with serum gastrin levels in cases of GERD and PUD that are refractory to medical management.

Misoprostol can help patients with PUD who require NSAID therapy (e.g., for arthritis).

- Patients may also complain of nausea, hematemesis ("coffee-ground" emesis), or blood in the stool (melena or hematochezia).
- Exam may reveal varying degrees of **epigastric tenderness** and, if there is active bleeding, a ⊕ stool guaiac.
- An acute perforation can present with a rigid abdomen, rebound tenderness, guarding, or other signs of peritoneal irritation.

DIAGNOSIS

- **AXR to rule out perforation** (free air under the diaphragm); CBC to assess for GI bleeding (low or ↓ hematocrit).
- **Upper endoscopy** with biopsy to confirm PUD and to rule out active bleeding or gastric adenocarcinoma (10% of gastric ulcers); barium swallow is an alternative.
- *H. pylori* testing.
- In recurrent or refractory cases, serum gastrin can be used to screen for Zollinger-Ellison syndrome (patients must discontinue PPI use prior to testing).

TREATMENT

- **Acute:**
  - Rule out active bleeding with serial hematocrits, a rectal exam with stool guaiac, and NG lavage.
  - Monitor the patient's hematocrit and BP and treat with IV hydration, transfusion, IV PPIs, endoscopy, and surgery as needed for complications.
  - If perforation is likely, **emergent surgery** is indicated.
- **Pharmacologic:**
  - Involves protecting the mucosa, decreasing acid production, and eradicating *H. pylori* infection.
  - Treat mild disease with antacids or with sucralfate, bismuth, and misoprostol (a prostaglandin analog) for mucosal protection. PPIs or H₂ receptor antagonists may be used to ↓ acid secretion.
  - Patients with confirmed *H. pylori* infection should receive triple therapy (amoxicillin, clarithromycin, and omeprazole).
  - Discontinue use of exacerbating agents. Patients with recurrent or severe disease may require chronic symptomatic therapy.
- **Endoscopy and surgery:**
  - Patients with symptomatic gastric ulcers for > **2 months** that are **refractory** to medical therapy should have either endoscopy or an upper GI series with barium to rule out gastric adenocarcinoma.
  - Refractory cases may require a surgical procedure such as **parietal cell vagotomy** (the most selective and preferred surgical approach).

COMPLICATIONS

Hemorrhage (posterior ulcers that erode into the gastroduodenal artery), gastric outlet obstruction, perforation (usually anterior ulcers), intractable pain.

Zollinger-Ellison Syndrome

- A rare condition characterized by **gastrin-producing tumors** in the duodenum and/or pancreas that lead to oversecretion of gastrin.
- ↑ gastrin results in the production of high levels of **gastric acid** by the gastric mucosa, leading to recurrent/intractable **ulcers** in the stomach and duodenum (may occur more distally).

Complications of PUD—

HOPI

Hemorrhage
Obstruction
Perforation
Intractable pain

- In 20% of cases, gastrinomas are associated with MEN 1 (pancreas, pituitary, and parathyroid tumors).
- **Hx/PE:** Patients may present with unresponsive, recurrent **gnawing, burning abdominal pain** as well as with **diarrhea**, nausea, vomiting, fatigue, weakness, weight loss, and **GI bleeding.**
- **Dx:** ↑ fasting serum gastrin levels are characteristic, as is ↑ gastrin following a secretin stimulation test. Octreotide scan can localize the tumor.
- **Tx:**
  - Requires ↓ **acid production.** H₂ blockers are typically ineffective, but a moderate- to high-dose PPI often controls symptoms.
  - In light of the malignant potential of the tumor, surgical resection should be attempted where possible.

Zollinger-Ellison syndrome is associated with MEN 1 syndrome in roughly 20% of cases.

▶ DISORDERS OF THE SMALL BOWEL

Diarrhea

Defined as the production of **> 200 g of feces per day along with ↑ frequency or ↓ consistency of stool.** Broadly, the four etiologic mechanisms are ↑ motility, ↑ secretion, ↑ luminal osmolarity, and inflammation (see also Table 2.6-2).

HISTORY/PE

- **Acute diarrhea:**
  - Acute onset with < 2 weeks of symptoms; usually infectious and self-limited.
  - Causes include bacteria with preformed toxins (e.g., *S. aureus, Bacillus cereus*), noninvasive bacteria (e.g., enterotoxigenic *E. coli, Vibrio cholerae, C. difficile*), invasive bacteria (e.g., enteroinvasive *E. coli, Salmonella, Shigella, Campylobacter, Yersinia*), parasites (e.g., *Giardia, Entamoeba histolytica*), and opportunistic organisms (e.g., *Cryptosporidium, Isospora, Microsporidium,* CMV).
  - One of the most common causes of **pediatric diarrhea** is **rotavirus infection** (most common during **winter**).
- **Chronic diarrhea:**
  - Insidious onset with > 4 weeks of symptoms.
  - Can be due to ↑ intestinal **secretion** (e.g., carcinoid, VIPomas), **malabsorption/osmotic** diarrhea (e.g., bacterial overgrowth, pancreatic insufficiency, mucosal abnormalities, lactose intolerance), **inflammatory bowel disease (IBD),** or altered **motility** (e.g., IBS). ↑ stool osmotic gap and resolution of diarrhea with fasting suggest osmotic diarrhea. See Figure 2.6-2 for a diagnostic algorithm.

Acute diarrhea is generally infectious and self-limited.

DIAGNOSIS

- Acute diarrhea usually does not require laboratory investigation unless the patient has a high fever, bloody diarrhea, or diarrhea lasting > 4–5 days.
- Send stool for fecal leukocytes, bacterial culture, *C. difficile* toxin, and O&P.
- Consider sigmoidoscopy in patients with bloody diarrhea.

Organisms that cause bloody diarrhea include Salmonella, Shigella, E. coli, and Campylobacter.

TREATMENT

- **Acute diarrhea:**
  - When bacterial infection is **not** suspected, treat with antidiarrheals (e.g., loperamide, bismuth salicylate) and oral rehydration solutions.

Diarrhea after ingestion of raw eggs or dairy: think Salmonella.

TABLE 2.6-2. Causes of Infectious Diarrhea

INFECTIOUS AGENT	HISTORY	EXAM	COMMENTS	TREATMENT
Campylobacter	**The most common etiology of infectious diarrhea.** Ingestion of contaminated food or water. Affects young children and young adults. Generally lasts 7–10 days.	Fecal RBCs and WBCs. Frequently bloody diarrhea.	Rule out appendicitis and IBD.	Erythromycin.
Clostridium difficile	Recent treatment with antibiotics (penicillins, cephalosporins, **clindamycin**). Affects hospitalized adult patients. **Watch for toxic megacolon.**	Fever, abdominal pain, possible systemic toxicity. Fecal RBCs and WBCs.	Most commonly causes colitis, but can involve the small bowel. Identify C. difficile toxin in the stool. Sigmoidoscopy shows pseudomembranes.	**Cessation of the inciting antibiotic.** PO metronidazole or vancomycin; IV metronidazole if the patient cannot tolerate PO.
Entamoeba histolytica	Ingestion of contaminated food or water; history of travel in developing countries. Incubation period can last up to three months.	Severe abdominal pain, fever. Fecal RBCs and WBCs.	Chronic amebic colitis mimics IBD.	Steroids can lead to fatal perforation. Treat with metronidazole.
E. coli O157:H7	Ingestion of contaminated food (raw meat). Affects children and the elderly. Generally lasts 5–10 days.	Severe abdominal pain, low-grade fever, vomiting. Fecal RBCs and WBCs.	It is important to rule out GI bleed and ischemic colitis. HUS is a possible complication.	Avoid antibiotic or antidiarrheal therapy, which ↑ HUS risk.
Salmonella	Ingestion of contaminated poultry or eggs. Affects young children and elderly patients. Generally lasts 2–5 days.	Prodromal headache, fever, myalgia, abdominal pain. Fecal WBCs.	Sepsis is a concern, as 5–10% of patients become bacteremic. Sickle cell patients are susceptible to invasive disease leading to osteomyelitis.	Treat bacteremia or at-risk patients (e.g., sickle cell patients) with oral quinolone or TMP-SMX.
Shigella	Extremely contagious; transmitted between people by the fecal-oral route. Affects young children and institutionalized patients.	Fecal RBCs and WBCs.	May lead to severe dehydration. Can also cause febrile seizures in the very young.	Treat with TMP-SMX to ↓ person-to-person spread.

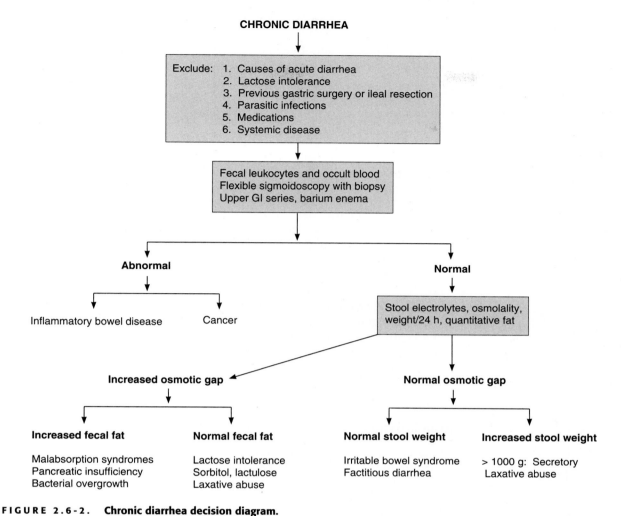

CHRONIC DIARRHEA

Exclude:
1. Causes of acute diarrhea
2. Lactose intolerance
3. Previous gastric surgery or ileal resection
4. Parasitic infections
5. Medications
6. Systemic disease

Fecal leukocytes and occult blood
Flexible sigmoidoscopy with biopsy
Upper GI series, barium enema

Abnormal

Inflammatory bowel disease   Cancer

Normal

Stool electrolytes, osmolality, weight/24 h, quantitative fat

Increased osmotic gap

Increased fecal fat

Malabsorption syndromes
Pancreatic insufficiency
Bacterial overgrowth

Normal fecal fat

Lactose intolerance
Sorbitol, lactulose
Laxative abuse

Normal osmotic gap

Normal stool weight

Irritable bowel syndrome
Factitious diarrhea

Increased stool weight

> 1000 g: Secretory
Laxative abuse

FIGURE 2.6-2. Chronic diarrhea decision diagram.

(Reproduced, with permission, from McPhee SJ et al. *Current Medical Diagnosis & Treatment*, 48th ed. New York: McGraw-Hill, 2009: Fig. 15-2.)

- If the patient has evidence of systemic infection (e.g., fever, chills, malaise), avoid antimotility agents and consider antibiotics after stool studies have been sent.
- **Chronic diarrhea:** Identify the underlying cause and treat symptoms with loperamide, opioids, octreotide, or cholestyramine.
- **Pediatric diarrhea:** For children who cannot take medication or PO fluids—hospitalize, give IV fluids, replete electrolytes, and treat the underlying cause.

Malabsorption

- Inability to absorb nutrients as a result of an underlying condition such as **bile salt deficiency** (e.g., bacterial overgrowth, ileal disease), **short bowel syndrome, mucosal abnormalities** (e.g., celiac disease, Whipple's disease, tropical sprue), and **pancreatic insufficiency.** The small bowel is most commonly involved.

- May result in ↓ absorption of protein, fat, carbohydrates, and micronutrients (folate/B$_{12}$/iron).
- **Hx/PE:** Presents with **frequent, loose, watery stools** and/or **pale, foul-smelling, bulky stools** associated with abdominal pain, **flatus, bloating,** weight loss, **nutritional deficiencies,** and fatigue.
- **Tx:** Etiology dependent. Institute a gluten-free diet for patients with celiac sprue. Severely affected patients may receive TPN, immunosuppressants, and anti-inflammatory medications.

Lactose Intolerance

- Results from a **deficiency of lactase,** a brush-border enzyme that hydrolyzes the disaccharide lactose into glucose and galactose.
- Lactase deficiency is common among populations of African, Asian, and Native American descent. It may also occur transiently 2° to an acute episode of gastroenteritis or other disorders affecting the proximal small intestinal mucosa.
- **Hx/PE:** Presents with **abdominal bloating, flatulence, cramping,** and **watery diarrhea following milk ingestion.**
- **Dx: Hydrogen breath test** reveals ↑ breath hydrogen following ingestion of a lactose load (indicates metabolism of lactose by colonic bacteria). An empiric lactose-free diet that results in symptom resolution is highly suggestive of the diagnosis.
- **Tx:** Avoidance of dairy products; lactase enzyme replacement.

Carcinoid Syndrome

Cutaneous flushing, diarrhea, wheezing, and cardiac valvular lesions are the most common manifestations of carcinoid tumors.

- Due to liver metastasis of **carcinoid tumors** (hormone-producing enterochromaffin cells) that most commonly arise from the ileum and appendix and produce vasoactive substances such as serotonin and substance P. Prior to metastasis, most secreted hormones undergo first-pass metabolism by the liver and do not reach systemic circulation.
- **Hx/PE: Cutaneous flushing, diarrhea, abdominal cramps, wheezing,** and right-sided **cardiac valvular lesions** are the most common manifestations. Symptoms usually follow eating, exertion, or excitement.
- **Dx:** High urine levels of the serotonin metabolite 5-HIAA are diagnostic. Octreotide scan can localize the tumor.
- **Tx:** Treatment includes **octreotide** (for symptoms) and debulking of tumor mass.

Irritable Bowel Syndrome (IBS)

Half of all patients with IBS have comorbid psychiatric disturbances.

An idiopathic **functional disorder** that is characterized by changes in bowel habits that ↑ with stress as well as by abdominal pain that is **relieved by bowel movements.** It is most common in the second and third decades, but since the syndrome is chronic, patients may present at any age. Half of all IBS patients who seek medical care have comorbid psychiatric disorders (e.g., depression, anxiety, fibromyalgia).

HISTORY/PE

- Patients present with abdominal pain, a change in bowel habits (diarrhea and/or constipation), abdominal distention, mucous stools, and relief of pain with a bowel movement.

- IBS rarely awakens patients from sleep; vomiting, significant weight loss, and constitutional symptoms are also uncommon.
- Exam is usually unremarkable except for mild abdominal tenderness.

DIAGNOSIS

- A **diagnosis of exclusion** based on clinical history.
- Tests to rule out other GI causes include CBC, TSH, electrolytes, stool cultures, abdominal films, and barium contrast studies.
- Manometry can assess sphincter function.

IBS is a diagnosis of exclusion.

TREATMENT

- **Psychological:** Patients need **reassurance** from their physicians. They should not be told that their symptoms are "all in their head."
- **Dietary:** Fiber supplements (psyllium) may help.
- **Pharmacologic:** Treat with TCAs, **antidiarrheals** (loperamide), and **antispasmodics** (anticholinergics such as dicyclomine).

Small Bowel Obstruction (SBO)

Defined as blocked passage of bowel contents through the small bowel. Fluid and gas can build up proximal to the obstruction, leading to fluid and electrolyte imbalances and significant abdominal discomfort. The obstruction can be complete or partial, and ischemia or necrosis of the bowel may occur. SBO may arise from **adhesions** from a prior abdominal surgery (60% of cases), **hernias** (10–20%), neoplasms (10–20%), intussusception, gallstone ileus, stricture due to IBD, or volvulus.

The leading cause of SBO in children is hernias. The leading cause of SBO in adults is adhesions.

HISTORY/PE

- Patients typically experience cramping abdominal pain with a recurrent **crescendo-decrescendo pattern** at 5- to 10-minute intervals.
- **Vomiting** typically follows the pain; early emesis is bilious and nonfeculent if the obstruction is proximal but **feculent** if it is distal.
- In partial obstruction, there is continued passage of flatus but no stool, whereas in complete obstruction, no flatus or stool is passed (**obstipation**).
- Abdominal exam often reveals distention, tenderness, prior surgical scars, or hernias.
- Bowel sounds are characterized by **high-pitched tinkles** and **peristaltic rushes.**
- Peristalsis may disappear later in disease progression. Fever, hypotension, rebound tenderness, and tachycardia suggest **peritonitis,** a surgical emergency.

DIAGNOSIS

- CBC may demonstrate **leukocytosis** if there is ischemia or necrosis of bowel.
- Labs often reflect **dehydration** and **metabolic alkalosis** due to vomiting. Lactic acidosis is particularly worrisome, as it suggests necrotic bowel and the need for emergent surgical intervention.
- Abdominal films often demonstrate a **stepladder pattern of dilated small-bowel loops, air-fluid levels** (see Figure 2.6-3), and a paucity of gas in the colon. The presence of radiopaque material at the cecum is suggestive of gallstone ileus.

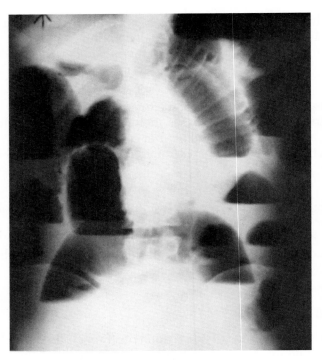

FIGURE 2.6-3. **Acute mechanical obstruction of the small intestine (upright film).**

Note the air-fluid levels, marked distention of bowel loops, and absence of colonic gas. (Reproduced, with permission, from Kasper DL et al. *Harrison's Principles of Internal Medicine*, 16th ed. New York: McGraw-Hill, 2005: 1804.)

TREATMENT

- For partial obstruction, supportive care may be sufficient and should include NPO status, NG suction, IV hydration, correction of electrolyte abnormalities, and Foley catheterization to monitor fluid status.
- Surgery is required in cases of complete SBO, vascular compromise (necrotic bowel), or symptoms lasting > 3 days without resolution.
- Exploratory laparotomy may be performed with lysis of adhesions, resection of necrotic bowel, and evaluation for stricture, IBD, and hernias.
- There is a 2% mortality risk for a nonstrangulated SBO; strangulated SBO is associated with up to a 25% mortality rate depending on the time between diagnosis and treatment.
- A second-look laparotomy or laparoscopy may be performed 18–36 hours after initial surgical treatment to reevaluate bowel viability if ischemia is a concern.

Never let the sun rise or set on a complete SBO.

Anticholinergics, opioids, and hypokalemia slow GI motility.

Ileus

Loss of peristalsis without structural obstruction. Risk factors include recent surgery/GI procedures, severe medical illness, immobility, hypokalemia or other electrolyte imbalances, hypothyroidism, DM, and medications that slow GI motility (e.g., anticholinergics, opioids).

- Presenting symptoms include diffuse, constant, moderate abdominal discomfort; **nausea and vomiting** (especially with eating); and an **absence of flatulence or bowel movements.**
- Exam may reveal diffuse tenderness and **abdominal distention, no peritoneal signs,** and ↓ **or absent bowel sounds.**
- A **rectal exam is required** to rule out fecal impaction in elderly patients.

DIAGNOSIS

- Diffusely **distended loops of small and large bowel** are seen on **supine AXR** with air-fluid levels on upright view.
- A Gastrografin study can rule out partial obstruction; CT can rule out neoplasms.

TREATMENT

- ↓ or discontinue the use of narcotics and any other drugs that reduce **bowel motility.**
- Temporarily ↓ or discontinue oral feeds.
- Initiate **NG suction/parenteral feeds** as necessary.
- Replete electrolytes as needed.

In diagnosing ileus, look for air throughout the small and large bowel on AXR.

Mesenteric Ischemia

↓ mesenteric blood supply leading to insufficient perfusion to intestinal tissue and ischemic injury. Causes include **acute arterial occlusion** (usually involving the SMA) from **thrombosis** (due to atherosclerosis) or **embolism** (due to atrial fibrillation or ↓ ejection fraction); nonocclusive arterial disease (low cardiac output, arteriolar vasospasm); and venous thrombosis (due to hypercoagulable states).

HISTORY/PE

- Patients present with sudden onset of **severe abdominal pain out of proportion to the exam.**
- A history of prior episodes of similar abdominal pain after eating ("intestinal angina") may be present.
- Other symptoms may include nausea, vomiting, diarrhea, and bloody stools.
- Early abdominal exam is often unremarkable; later findings may include peritoneal signs (suggest bowel infarction).

DIAGNOSIS

- Lab tests may show **leukocytosis, metabolic acidosis** with ↑ lactate, ↑ amylase, ↑ LDH, and ↑ CK.
- AXR and CT may reveal bowel wall edema ("thumbprinting") and air within the bowel wall (pneumatosis intestinalis).
- Mesenteric **angiography** is the gold standard for arterial occlusive disease.

TREATMENT

- Volume resuscitation, broad-spectrum antibiotics, optimization of hemodynamics, and avoidance of vasoconstrictors.
- Anticoagulation for arterial or venous thrombosis or embolism.

- **Early laparotomy** for acute arterial occlusive disease or if evidence of peritonitis or clinical deterioration is present.
- Angioplasty and thrombectomy +/– endovascular stenting for acute arterial thrombosis.
- Embolectomy for acute arterial embolism.
- Resection of infarcted bowel.

COMPLICATIONS

Sepsis/septic shock, multisystem organ failure, death.

The mortality rate for acute mesenteric ischemia is > 50%.

Appendicitis

See the Emergency Medicine chapter.

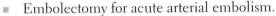
► **DISORDERS OF THE LARGE BOWEL**

Diverticular Disease

Outpouchings of mucosa and submucosa (false diverticula) that herniate through the colonic muscle layers in areas of high intraluminal pressure; most commonly found in the sigmoid colon. Diverticulosis is the **most common cause of acute lower GI bleeding** in patients > 40 years of age. Risk factors include a **low-fiber and high-fat diet,** advanced age (65% occur in those > 80 years of age), and connective tissue disorders (e.g., Ehlers-Danlos syndrome). **Diverticulitis** is due to inflammation and, potentially, perforation of a diverticulum 2° to fecalith impaction.

Diverticulosis is the most common cause of acute lower GI bleeding in patients > 40 years of age.

HISTORY/PE

- Diverticulosis is often **asymptomatic.**
- Bleeding is painless and sudden, generally presenting as hematochezia with symptoms of anemia (fatigue, lightheadedness, dyspnea on exertion).
- **Diverticulitis** presents with **LLQ abdominal pain, fever,** nausea, vomiting, and constipation. Perforation is a serious complication that leads to peritonitis and shock.

DIAGNOSIS

- CBC may show **leukocytosis.**
- Diagnosis is based on AXR (to rule out free air, ileus, or obstruction), colonoscopy, or barium enema. Sigmoidoscopy/colonoscopy must be avoided in those with early diverticulitis due to the risk of perforation.
- In patients with severe disease or in those who show lack of improvement, abdominal CT may reveal abscess or free air.

Diverticular disease must be distinguished from colon cancer with perforation.

Avoid flexible sigmoidoscopy and barium enemas in the initial stages of diverticulitis because of perforation risk.

TREATMENT

- **Uncomplicated diverticulosis:** Patients can be followed and placed on a **high-fiber diet** or fiber supplements.
- **Diverticular bleeding:** Bleeding usually stops spontaneously; transfuse and hydrate as needed. If bleeding does not stop, angiography with embolization or **surgery** is indicated.
- **Diverticulitis:** Treat with **bowel rest** (NPO), NG tube placement, and **broad-spectrum antibiotics** (metronidazole and a fluoroquinolone or a second- or third-generation cephalosporin) if the patient is stable. Avoid barium enema and flexible sigmoidoscopy if diverticulitis is suspected.

- For perforation, perform immediate surgical resection of diseased bowel via a Hartmann's procedure with a temporary colostomy.

Large Bowel Obstruction (LBO)

Table 2.6-3 describes features that distinguish SBO from LBO. Figure 2.6-4 demonstrates the classic radiographic findings of LBO.

Colon and Rectal Cancer

The second leading cause of cancer mortality in the United States after lung cancer. There is an ↑ incidence with age, with a peak incidence at 70–80 years. There has also been an observed association between colon cancer

TABLE 2.6-3. **Characteristics of Small and Large Bowel Obstruction**

	SBO	LBO
History	Moderate to severe acute abdominal pain; **copious emesis.** Cramping pain with distal SBO. Fever, signs of dehydration, and hypotension may be seen.	Constipation/obstipation, deep and cramping abdominal pain (less intense than SBO), nausea/vomiting (less than SBO but more commonly **feculent**).
PE	**Abdominal distention** (distal SBO), abdominal tenderness, visible peristaltic waves, fever, hypovolemia. Look for **surgical scars/hernias;** perform a rectal exam. **High-pitched "tinkly" bowel sounds;** later, absence of bowel sounds.	Significant **distention,** tympany, and tenderness; examine for peritoneal irritation or mass; fever or signs of shock suggest perforation/peritonitis or ischemia/necrosis. **High-pitched "tinkly" bowel sounds;** later, absence of bowel sounds.
Etiologies	**Adhesions** (postsurgery), **hernias,** neoplasm, volvulus, intussusception, gallstone ileus, foreign body, Crohn's disease, CF, stricture, hematoma.	**Colon cancer,** diverticulitis, volvulus, fecal impaction, benign tumors. **Assume colon cancer until proven otherwise.**
Differential	LBO, paralytic ileus, gastroenteritis.	SBO, paralytic ileus, appendicitis, IBD, Ogilvie's syndrome (pseudo-obstruction).
Diagnosis	CBC, electrolytes, lactic acid, AXR (see Figure 2.6-3); contrast studies (determine if it is partial or complete), CT scan.	CBC, electrolytes, lactic acid, AXR (see Figure 2.6-4), CT scan; water contrast enema (if perforation is suspected); sigmoidoscopy/colonoscopy if stable.
Treatment	Hospitalize. Partial SBO can be treated conservatively with **NG decompression** and NPO status. Patients with complete SBO should be managed aggressively with NPO status, NG decompression, IV fluids, electrolyte replacement, and **surgical correction.**	Hospitalize. Obstruction can be relieved with a Gastrografin enema, colonoscopy, or a **rectal tube;** however, **surgery** is usually required. Ischemic colon usually requires partial colectomy with a diverting colostomy. Treat the underlying cause (e.g., neoplasm).

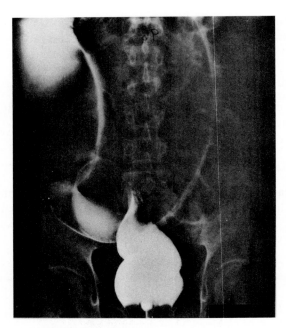

FIGURE 2.6-4. **Large bowel obstruction.**

Barium study shows the "bird-beak" sign, with juxtaposed adjacent bowel walls in the dilated loop pointing toward the site of obstruction. (Reproduced, with permission, from Way LW. *Current Surgical Diagnosis & Treatment*, 10th ed. Stamford, CT: Appleton & Lange, 1994: 676.)

and *Streptococcus bovis* bacteremia. Risk factors and screening protocols are summarized in Table 2.6-4.

HISTORY/PE

- In the absence of screening, colon and rectal cancer typically present with symptoms only after a prolonged period of silent growth.

TABLE 2.6-4. **Risk Factors and Screening for Colorectal Cancer**

RISK FACTORS	SCREENING
Age.	A DRE should be performed yearly for patients ≥ 50 years of age. Up to 10% of all lesions are palpable with DRE.
Hereditary syndromes—familial adenomatous polyposis (100% risk by age 40), Gardner's disease, hereditary nonpolyposis colorectal cancer (HNPCC).	Stool guaiac should be performed every year for patients ≥ 50 years of age. Up to 50% of ⊕ guaiac tests are due to colorectal cancer.
Family history.	
IBD—ulcerative colitis carries a higher risk than does Crohn's disease.	Colonoscopy every 10 years in those ≥ 50 years of age **OR** yearly FOBT with sigmoidoscopy every 5 years.
Adenomatous polyps—villous polyps progress more often than tubular polyps and sessile more than pedunculated polyps. Lesions > 2 cm carry an ↑ risk.	Colonoscopy should be performed every 10 years in patients ≥ 40 years of age who have a first-degree relative with colorectal cancer or adenomatous polyps, or 10 years prior to the age at diagnosis of the youngest family member.
Past history of colorectal cancer.	
High-fat, low-fiber diet.	

- Although often asymptomatic, patients may present with unexplained anemia or vague abdominal pain. Other features depend on location:
    - **Right-sided lesions:** Often bulky, ulcerating masses that lead to **anemia from chronic occult blood loss.** Patients may complain of weight loss, anorexia, diarrhea, weakness, or vague abdominal pain. Obstruction is rare.
    - **Left-sided lesions:** Typically **"apple-core"** obstructing masses (see Figure 2.6-5). Patients complain of a **change in bowel habits** (e.g., ↓ stool caliber, constipation, obstipation), colicky abdominal pain, and/or blood-streaked stools. Obstruction is common.
    - **Rectal lesions:** Usually present with bright red blood per rectum, often with tenesmus and/or rectal pain. Can coexist with hemorrhoids, so rectal cancer must be ruled out in all patients with rectal bleeding.

Iron deficiency anemia in an elderly male is colorectal cancer until proven otherwise.

DIAGNOSIS

- Order a CBC (often shows microcytic anemia) and stool occult blood.
- Perform sigmoidoscopy to evaluate rectal bleeding and all suspicious left-sided lesions.
- Rule out synchronous right-sided lesions with colonoscopy. If colonoscopy is incomplete, rule out additional lesions with an air-contrast barium enema.
- Determine the degree of invasion in **rectal cancer** with endorectal ultrasound.
- Order a CXR, LFTs, and an abdominal/pelvic CT for metastatic workup. Metastases may arise from direct extension to local viscera, hematogenous spread (40–50% go to the liver, but spread may also occur to bone, lungs, and brain), or lymphatic spread (to pelvic lymph nodes).

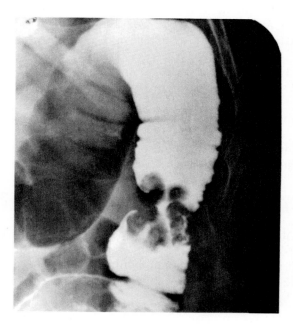

FIGURE 2.6-5.   Colon carcinoma.

The encircling carcinoma appears as an "apple-core" filling defect in the descending colon on barium enema x-ray. (Reproduced, with permission, from Way LW. *Current Surgical Diagnosis & Treatment*, 10th ed. Stamford, CT: Appleton & Lange, 1994: 658.)

- Staging is based on the depth of tumor penetration into the bowel wall and the presence of lymph node involvement and distant metastases.

TREATMENT

- Surgical resection of the 1° cancer is the treatment of choice. Regional lymph node dissection should be performed for staging purposes.
- For **rectal lesions,** the resection technique depends on the proximity of the lesion to the anal verge (the junction between the anal canal and the anal skin).
  - **Abdominoperineal resection:** For distal lesions < 10 cm from the anal verge, when the sphincter cannot be preserved, the rectum and anus are resected and a permanent colostomy is placed.
  - **Low anterior resection:** For proximal lesions > 10 cm from the anal verge, a 1° anastomosis is created between the colon and rectum.
  - **Wide local excision:** For small, low-grade, well-differentiated tumors in the lower third of the rectum.
- **Adjuvant chemotherapy:** Used in cases of colon cancer with ⊕ lymph nodes. Can be considered for rectal cancers.
- Follow with serial CEA levels (diagnostically nonspecific, but useful for monitoring recurrence), colonoscopy, LFTs, CXR, and abdominal CT (for metastasis).

Ischemic Colitis

- Due to lack of arterial blood supply to the colon. Severity ranges from superficial mucosal involvement to full-thickness necrosis.
- The most commonly affected site is the left colon, particularly the "watershed area" at the splenic flexure. Incidence ↑ with age.
- **Hx/PE:** Presents with crampy **lower abdominal pain** associated with **bloody diarrhea.** Fever and peritoneal signs suggest infarction.
- **Dx:**
  - CBC may reveal **leukocytosis.**
  - Flexible sigmoidoscopy or **colonoscopy** to assess colonic mucosa.
- **Tx:**
  - Supportive therapy with bowel rest, IV fluids, and broad-spectrum antibiotics.
  - Surgery with resection is indicated for infarction, fulminant colitis, or obstruction 2° to ischemic stricture.

Ischemic colitis is a known complication of AAA repair due to sacrifice of the inferior mesenteric artery.

▶ GASTROINTESTINAL BLEEDING

Bleeding from the GI tract may present as hematemesis, hematochezia, and/or melena. Upper GI tract bleeding is defined as bleeding from lesions proximal to the ligament of Treitz (the anatomic boundary between the duodenum and jejunum). Table 2.6-5 presents the features of upper and lower GI bleeding.

One unit of PRBCs should ↑ hemoglobin by 1 unit and hematocrit by 3–4 units.

▶ INFLAMMATORY BOWEL DISEASE (IBD)

Comprises **Crohn's disease and ulcerative colitis** (see Figure 2.6-6). Most common in Caucasians and **Ashkenazi Jews,** appearing most frequently during the teens to early 30s or in the 50s. Table 2.6-6 summarizes the features of IBD.

TABLE 2.6-5. Features of Upper and Lower GI Bleeding

VARIABLE	UPPER GI BLEEDING	LOWER GI BLEEDING
History/PE	Hematemesis ("coffee-ground" emesis), melena > hematochezia, depleted volume status (e.g., tachycardia, lightheadedness, hypotension).	Hematochezia > melena, but can be either.
Diagnosis	NG tube and NG lavage; endoscopy if stable.	Rule out upper GI bleed with NG lavage. Anoscopy/sigmoidoscopy for patients < 45 years of age with small-volume bleeding. Colonoscopy if stable; arteriography or exploratory laparotomy if unstable.
Etiologies	**PUD,** esophagitis/gastritis, Mallory-Weiss tear, esophageal varices.	**Diverticulosis** (60%), IBD, hemorrhoids/fissures, neoplasm, AVM.
Initial management	Protect the airway (may need intubation). Stabilize the patient with IV fluids and PRBCs (hematocrit may be normal early in acute blood loss).	Similar to upper GI bleed.
Long-term management	Endoscopy followed by therapy directed at the underlying cause (e.g., high-dose PPIs for PUD; octreotide and/or banding for varices).	Depends on the underlying etiology. Endoscopic therapy (e.g., epinephrine injection), intra-arterial vasopressin infusion or embolization, or surgery for diverticular disease or angiodysplasia.

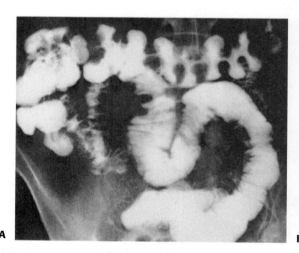
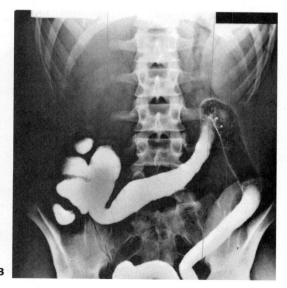

A   B

FIGURE 2.6-6. **Inflammatory bowel disease.**

(A) Crohn's disease. Barium enema x-ray reveals deep transverse fissures, ulcers, and edema of the bowel. (B) Ulcerative colitis. Barium enema x-ray demonstrates shortening of the colon, loss of haustra ("lead pipe" appearance), and fine serrations of the bowel edges from small ulcers. (Reproduced, with permission, from Stobo J et al. *The Principles and Practice of Medicine,* 23rd ed. Stamford, CT: Appleton & Lange, 1996: 135.)

TABLE 2.6-6. Features of Ulcerative Colitis and Crohn's Disease

VARIABLE	ULCERATIVE COLITIS	CROHN'S DISEASE
Site of involvement	The **rectum** is always involved. May extend proximally in a **continuous fashion.** Inflammation and ulceration are **limited to the mucosa and submucosa.**	May involve **any portion** of the GI tract, particularly the **ileocecal region,** in a **discontinuous pattern** ("skip lesions"). The rectum is often spared. **Transmural inflammation** is seen.
History/PE	**Bloody diarrhea,** lower abdominal cramps, tenesmus, urgency. Exam may reveal orthostatic hypotension, tachycardia, abdominal tenderness, frank blood on rectal exam, and extraintestinal manifestations.	Abdominal pain, abdominal mass, low-grade fever, weight loss, watery diarrhea. Exam may reveal fever, abdominal tenderness or mass, **perianal fissures, fistulas,** and extraintestinal manifestations.
Extraintestinal manifestations	Aphthous stomatitis, episcleritis/uveitis, arthritis, **primary sclerosing cholangitis,** erythema nodosum, and pyoderma gangrenosum.	The same as ulcerative colitis, as well as gallstones, nephrolithiasis, and fistulas to the skin, bladder, or between bowel loops.
Diagnosis	CBC, AXR, stool cultures, O&P, stool assay for *C. difficile.* Colonoscopy can show diffuse and continuous rectal involvement, friability, edema, and **pseudopolyps.** Definitive diagnosis can be made with biopsy.	The same lab workup as ulcerative colitis. Upper GI series with small bowel follow-through. Colonoscopy may show aphthoid, linear, or stellate ulcers, strictures, **"cobblestoning,"** and **"skip lesions."** "Creeping fat" may also be present during laparotomy. Definitive diagnosis can be made with biopsy.
Treatment	**5-ASA agents** (e.g., sulfasalazine, mesalamine), topical or oral; corticosteroids and immunomodulating agents (e.g., azathioprine) for refractory disease. **Total proctocolectomy is curative** for long-standing or fulminant colitis or **toxic megacolon;** it also ↓ cancer risk.	**5-ASA agents;** corticosteroids and immunomodulating agents (e.g., azathioprine, infliximab) are indicated if no improvement is seen. Surgical resection may be necessary for suspected perforation, stricture, fistula, or abscess; **may recur** anywhere in the GI tract.
Incidence of cancer	**Markedly ↑ risk of colorectal cancer** in long-standing cases (monitor with frequent fecal occult blood screening and yearly colonoscopy with multiple biopsies after eight years of disease).	Incidence of 2° malignancy is lower than in ulcerative colitis, but greater than the general population.

▶ **INGUINAL HERNIAS**

Abnormal **protrusions of abdominal contents** (usually the small intestine) into the inguinal region through a weakness or defect in the abdominal wall. Defined as **direct or indirect** on the basis of their relationship to the inguinal canal.

- **Indirect:** Herniation of abdominal contents through the internal and then **external inguinal rings** and eventually into the scrotum (in males).
    - The **most common hernia in both genders.**
    - Due to a **congenital patent processus vaginalis.**

- Protrudes **lateral** to the inferior epigastric vessels.
- **Direct:** Herniation of abdominal contents through the floor of **Hessel-bach's triangle.**
  - Protrudes **medial** to the epigastric vessels.
  - Hernial sac contents do not traverse the internal **inguinal ring;** they herniate directly through the abdominal wall and are contained within the **aponeurosis** of the **external oblique muscle.**
  - Most often due to an acquired defect in the **transversalis fascia** from mechanical breakdown that ↑ with age.

TREATMENT

- Because of the risk of **incarceration** and **strangulation,** surgical management (open or laparoscopic) is indicated unless specific contraindications are present.
- Repair of a direct inguinal hernia involves correcting the defect in the transversalis fascia.
- Indirect inguinal hernias are repaired by isolating and ligating the hernial sac and reducing the size of the internal inguinal ring to allow only the spermatic cord structures in males to pass through.

Hesselbach's triangle is an area bounded by the inguinal ligament, the inferior epigastric artery, and the rectus abdominis.

► BILIARY DISEASE

Cholelithiasis and Biliary Colic

Colic results from transient cystic duct blockage from impacted stones. Although risk factors include the **4 F's—Female, Fat, Fertile, and Forty**—the disorder is common and can occur in any patient. Flatulence can be thought of as a "5th F." Other risk factors include OCP use, rapid weight loss, a ⊕ family history, chronic hemolysis (pigment stones in sickle cell disease), small bowel resection, and TPN.

HISTORY/PE

- Patients present with **postprandial abdominal pain** (usually in the **RUQ**) that radiates to the right subscapular area or the epigastrium.
- Pain is abrupt; is followed by gradual relief; and is often associated with **nausea and vomiting,** fatty food intolerance, dyspepsia, and flatulence.
- Gallstones may be asymptomatic in up to 80% of patients. Exam may reveal RUQ tenderness and a palpable gallbladder.

Pigmented gallstones result from hemolysis (black) or infection (brown).

DIAGNOSIS

- Plain x-rays are rarely diagnostic; only 10–15% of stones are radiopaque.
- **RUQ ultrasound** is the imaging modality of choice (85–90% sensitive).
- Table 2.6-7 contrasts lab findings with those of other forms of biliary disease.

TREATMENT

- **Cholecystectomy** is curative and can be performed electively for symptomatic gallstones. It is generally performed laparoscopically. Asymptomatic gallstones do not require any intervention.
- Patients may require preoperative endoscopic retrograde cholangiopancreatography (ERCP) for common bile duct stones.
- Treat nonsurgical candidates with **dietary modification** (avoid triggers such as fatty foods).

Most gallstones are precipitations of cholesterol and are not radiopaque.

TABLE 2.6-7.   Differential Diagnosis of Biliary Disease

	FEVER/ELEVATED WBC COUNT	ELEVATED TOTAL BILIRUBIN/ ALKALINE PHOSPHATASE	ELEVATED SERUM AMYLASE
Cholelithiasis (colic)	–	–	–
Acute cholecystitis	+	–	–
Choledocholithiasis/ ascending cholangitis	+	+	–
Gallstone pancreatitis	+	+	+

COMPLICATIONS

Recurrent biliary colic, acute cholecystitis, choledocholithiasis, ascending cholangitis, gallstone ileus, gallstone pancreatitis.

Acute Cholecystitis

Prolonged blockage of the cystic duct, usually by an impacted stone, that leads to obstructive distention, inflammation, superinfection, and possibly gangrene of the gallbladder (acute gangrenous cholecystitis). **Acalculous cholecystitis** occurs in the absence of cholelithiasis in patients who are chronically debilitated, those who are critically ill in the ICU or on TPN, and trauma or burn victims.

HISTORY/PE

- Patients present with **RUQ pain, nausea, vomiting, and fever.** Symptoms are typically more severe and of longer duration than those of biliary colic.
- RUQ tenderness, inspiratory arrest during deep palpation of the RUQ (**Murphy's sign**), low-grade fever, mild icterus, and possibly guarding or rebound tenderness may be present on exam.

DIAGNOSIS

- Fever is often present, and CBC shows leukocytosis (see Table 2.6-7).
- Ultrasound may demonstrate stones, bile sludge, pericholecystic fluid, a thickened gallbladder wall, gas in the gallbladder, and an ultrasonic Murphy's sign (see Figure 2.6-7).
- Obtain a **HIDA scan** when ultrasound is equivocal (see Figure 2.6-8); nonvisualization of the gallbladder on HIDA scan suggests acute cholecystitis.

TREATMENT

- Hospitalize patients, administer broad-spectrum **IV antibiotics** and **IV fluids,** and replete electrolytes.
- If diagnosed soon after onset, **early cholecystectomy** is indicated.
- For stable patients or those with significant medical problems, surgery can be delayed for 4–6 weeks.

The cystic artery usually passes through the anatomic triangle of Calot, comprising the common hepatic duct, the cystic duct, and the inferior border of the liver.

In patients with significant medical problems (including DM), delay cholecystectomy until acute inflammation resolves.

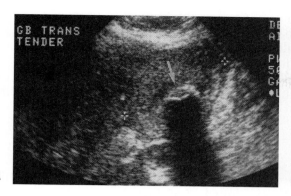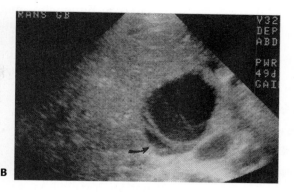

FIGURE 2.6-7. Acute cholecystitis, ultrasound.

(A) Note the sludge-filled, thick-walled gallbladder with a hyperechoic stone and acoustic shadow (arrow). (B) This patient exhibits sludge and pericholecystic fluid (arrow) but no gallstones. (Reproduced, with permission, from Grendell J. *Current Diagnosis & Treatment in Gastroenterology*, 1st ed. Stamford, CT: Appleton & Lange, 1996: 212.)

COMPLICATIONS

Gangrene, empyema, perforation, emphysematous gallbladder (due to infection by gas-forming organisms), fistulization, gallstone ileus, sepsis, abscess formation.

Choledocholithiasis

- Gallstones in the common bile duct. Symptoms vary according to the degree of obstruction, the duration of the obstruction, and the extent of bacterial infection.

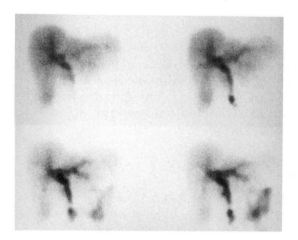

FIGURE 2.6-8. Acute cholecystitis, HIDA scan.

IV dye is taken up by hepatocytes and is conjugated and excreted into the common bile duct. The gallbladder is not visualized, although activity is present in the liver, common duct, and small bowel, suggesting cystic duct obstruction due to acute cholecystitis. (Reproduced, with permission, from Grendell J. *Current Diagnosis & Treatment in Gastroenterology*, 1st ed. Stamford, CT: Appleton & Lange, 1996: 217.)

Gallstone pancreatitis occurs when stones in the ampulla also obstruct the pancreatic duct.

- **Hx/PE:** Although sometimes asymptomatic, it often presents with biliary colic, jaundice, fever, and pancreatitis.
- **Dx:** The hallmark is ↑ **alkaline phosphatase** and **total bilirubin,** which may be the only abnormal lab values (see Table 2.6-7).
- **Tx:** Management generally consists of ERCP with sphincterotomy followed by semielective cholecystectomy. Common bile duct exploration may be necessary.

Ascending Cholangitis

An acute bacterial infection of the biliary tree that commonly occurs 2° to **obstruction,** usually from **gallstones (choledocholithiasis)** or primary sclerosing cholangitis (progressive inflammation of the biliary tree associated with ulcerative colitis). Other etiologies include bile duct stricture and malignancy (biliary or pancreatic). Gram-⊖ enterics (e.g., *E. coli, Enterobacter, Pseudomonas*) are commonly identified pathogens.

Charcot's triad consists of RUQ pain, jaundice, and fever/chills. Reynolds' pentad consists of RUQ pain, jaundice, fever/chills, shock, and altered mental status.

HISTORY/PE

- **Charcot's triad**—RUQ pain, jaundice, and **fever/chills**—is classic and seen in 50–70% of cases.
- **Reynolds' pentad**—Charcot's triad plus septic **shock** and **altered mental status**—may be present in acute suppurative cholangitis and suggests sepsis.

DIAGNOSIS

- Look for **leukocytosis,** ↑ **bilirubin,** and ↑ **alkaline phosphatase** (see Table 2.6-7).
- Obtain blood cultures to rule out sepsis. **Ultrasound** or CT may be a useful adjunct, but diagnosis is often clinical. Magnetic resonance cholangiopancreatography (MRCP) is a noninvasive test that may also be useful.
- **ERCP** is both diagnostic and therapeutic (biliary drainage).

TREATMENT

- Patients often require **ICU admission** for monitoring, hydration, BP support, and broad-spectrum **IV antibiotic treatment.**
- Patients with acute suppurative cholangitis require **emergent bile duct decompression** via ERCP/sphincterotomy, percutaneous transhepatic drainage, or open decompression.

Gallstone Ileus

- A mechanical obstruction resulting from the passage of a large (> 2.5-cm) stone into the bowel through a cholecystoduodenal fistula. Obstruction is often at the terminal ileum (TI)/ileocecal valve.
- **Hx/PE:** Many patients have no previous history of biliary symptoms and present as an SBO. The classic presentation is that of a subacute SBO in an elderly woman.
- **Dx:** Pneumobilia (gas in the biliary tree) seen on imaging can confirm, in addition to an upper GI series with small bowel follow-through showing a TI obstruction.
- **Tx:** Laparotomy with stone extraction (enterolithotomy) or manipulation into the colon.

Primary Sclerosing Cholangitis

- An idiopathic disorder characterized by inflammation, fibrosis, and strictures of extra- and intrahepatic bile ducts. The disease usually presents in **young men with IBD** (most often ulcerative colitis).
- **Hx/PE:** Presents with progressive **jaundice, pruritus,** and **fatigue.**
- **Dx:**
  - Laboratory findings include ↑ **alkaline phosphatase** and ↑ bilirubin.
  - MRCP/ERCP show **multiple bile duct strictures** with dilatations between strictures.
  - Liver biopsy reveals periductal sclerosis ("onion skinning").
- **Tx:** High-dose ursodeoxycholic acid; endoscopic dilation and short-term stenting of bile duct strictures; liver transplantation. Patients are at ↑ risk for **cholangiocarcinoma.**

Primary sclerosing cholangitis is significantly associated with ulcerative colitis.

▶ LIVER DISEASE

Abnormal Liver Function Tests

Liver diseases can be divided into distinct patterns based on LFT results:

- **Hepatocellular injury:** ↑ AST and ALT.
- **Cholestasis:** ↑ alkaline phosphatase and bilirubin.
- **Isolated hyperbilirubinemia:** ↑ bilirubin; normal aminotransferases and alkaline phosphatase.

Jaundice, which can be seen in any of the patterns outlined above, is a clinical sign that arises when excess bilirubin (> 2.5 mg/dL) is circulating in the blood. Figures 2.6-9 and 2.6-10 summarize the clinical approaches toward cholestasis and isolated hyperbilirubinemia. Hepatocellular injury is described in the section that follows.

Hepatitis

Inflammation of the liver leading to liver cell injury and necrosis. The causes of **acute** hepatitis include **viruses** (e.g., HAV, HBV, HCV, HDV, HEV) and **drug-induced** disease (e.g., alcohol, acetaminophen, INH, methyldopa). The

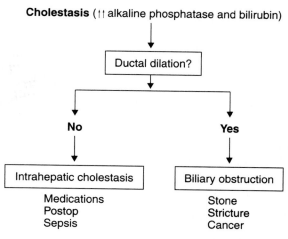

FIGURE 2.6-9. **Approach to cholestasis.**

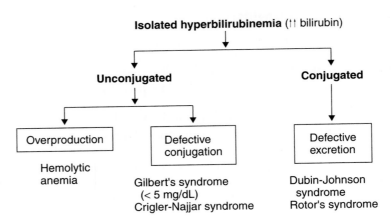

Isolated hyperbilirubinemia ($\uparrow\uparrow$ bilirubin)

Unconjugated → Overproduction (Hemolytic anemia), Defective conjugation (Gilbert's syndrome (< 5 mg/dL), Crigler-Najjar syndrome)

Conjugated → Defective excretion (Dubin-Johnson syndrome, Rotor's syndrome)

FIGURE 2.6-10. **Approach to isolated hyperbilirubinemia.**

HCV is Chronic. Eighty percent of patients with HCV infection will develop chronic hepatitis.

causes of **chronic** hepatitis include viruses (e.g., HBV, HCV, HDV), **alcoholic** hepatitis, **autoimmune** hepatitis, ischemic hepatitis, and **hereditary** etiologies (e.g., Wilson's disease, hemochromatosis, α_1-antitrypsin deficiency).

- HAV and HEV are transmitted by the fecal-oral route.
- HBV and HCV are transmitted by bodily fluids, although the risk of acquiring HCV sexually is very low.

HISTORY/PE

- Acute hepatitis often starts with a viral prodrome of nonspecific symptoms (e.g., **malaise,** fever, joint pain, fatigue, URI symptoms, **nausea, vomiting,** changes in bowel habits) followed by **jaundice** and RUQ tenderness.
- Exam often reveals **jaundice,** scleral icterus, **tender hepatomegaly,** possible splenomegaly, and lymphadenopathy.
- Chronic hepatitis usually gives rise to symptoms indicative of chronic liver disease (jaundice, fatigue, hepatosplenomegaly). At least 80% of those infected with HCV and 10% of those with HBV will develop chronic hepatitis.

DIAGNOSIS

- Dramatically $\uparrow$ **ALT and AST** and $\uparrow$ bilirubin/alkaline phosphatase are present in the acute form.
- In chronic hepatitis, ALT and AST are $\uparrow$ for > 6 months with a concurrent $\uparrow$ in alkaline phosphatase/bilirubin and hypoalbuminemia. In severe cases, PT will be prolonged, as all clotting factors except factor VIII are produced by the liver.
- The diagnosis of viral hepatitis is made by **hepatitis serology** (see Table 2.6-8 and Figure 2.6-11 for a description and timing of serologic markers) and by liver biopsy in chronic or severe cases.
- ANA, anti–smooth muscle antibody, and antimitochondrial antibody point to autoimmune hepatitis. Iron saturation (hemochromatosis) and ceruloplasmin (Wilson's disease) can identify other causes.

An AST/ALT ratio > 2 suggests alcoholic hepatitis–you're toASTed.

TREATMENT

Treatment is etiology specific; monitor for resolution of symptoms over time.

- Steroids for severe alcoholic hepatitis.
- **Immunosuppression** with steroids and other agents (azathioprine) for autoimmune hepatitis.

TABLE 2.6-8. Key Hepatitis Serologic Markers

SEROLOGIC MARKER	DESCRIPTION
IgM HAVAb	IgM antibody to HAV; the best test to detect active hepatitis A.
HBsAg	Antigen found on the surface of HBV; continued presence indicates carrier state.
HBsAb	Antibody to HBsAg; **provides immunity** to HBV.
HBcAg	Antigen associated with core of HBV.
HBcAb	Antibody to HBcAg; ⊕ during the **window period.** IgM HBcAb is an indicator of recent disease.
HBeAg	A second, different antigenic determinant in the HBV core. An important indicator of transmissibility (**BE**ware!).
HBeAb	Antibody to e antigen; indicates low transmissibility.

- **IFN-α, lamivudine (3TC),** or **adefovir** for chronic HBV infection; **peginterferon** and **ribavirin** for chronic HCV infection.
- **Liver transplantation** is the treatment of choice for patients with end-stage liver failure.
- ICU management and emergent transplant for fulminant hepatic failure.

The sequelae of chronic hepatitis include cirrhosis, liver failure, and hepatocellular carcinoma.

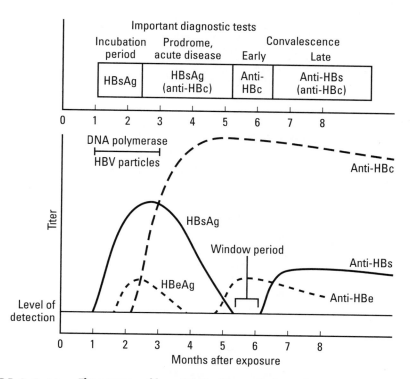

FIGURE 2.6-11.   Time course of hepatitis B with serologic markers.

Cirrhosis, liver failure, hepatocellular carcinoma (3–5%).

Cirrhosis

Defined as **fibrosis** and **nodular regeneration** resulting from hepatocellular injury. Etiologies include causes of chronic hepatitis, biliary tract disease (e.g., primary biliary cirrhosis, primary sclerosing cholangitis), right-sided heart failure, constrictive pericarditis, and Budd-Chiari syndrome (hepatic vein thrombosis 2° to hypercoagulability).

Alcoholism, chronic hepatitis, and other chronic liver diseases lead to cirrhosis.

HISTORY/PE

- Presents with **jaundice, ascites, spontaneous bacterial peritonitis, hepatic encephalopathy** (e.g., asterixis, altered mental status), **gastroesophageal varices,** coagulopathy, and renal dysfunction. Weakness, anorexia, and weight loss are also seen in advanced disease.
- Exam may reveal an enlarged, palpable, or firm liver. Stigmata of portal hypertension and signs of liver failure may be present (see Figures 2.6-12 and 2.6-13).

DIAGNOSIS

Gut, butt, and caput–the three anastomoses commonly seen in cirrhosis.

- Lab studies show ↓ **albumin**, ↑ **PT/PTT**, and ↑ **bilirubin**. Anemia or thrombocytopenia (2° to hypersplenism) may also be seen.
- Abdominal ultrasound with Doppler can assess liver size, the presence of ascites, and the patency of splenic and hepatic veins. The etiology of ascites can be established through measurement of the **serum-ascites albumin gradient** (**SAAG** = serum albumin – ascites albumin); see Table 2.6-9.
- Obtain hepatitis serologies and autoimmune hepatitis studies.
- Serum ferritin, ceruloplasmin, and α_1-antitrypsin may help identify additional causes, such as hemochromatosis, Wilson's disease, and α_1-antitrypsin deficiency, respectively.
- Liver biopsy showing bridging fibrosis and nodular regeneration.

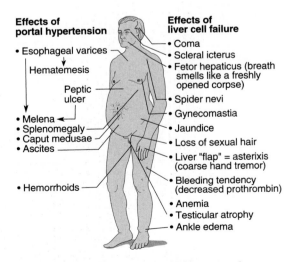

FIGURE 2.6-12. Presentation of cirrhosis/portal hypertension.

(Adapted, with permission, from Chandrasoma P, Taylor CE. *Concise Pathology*, 3rd ed. Stamford, CT: Appleton & Lange, 1998: 654.)

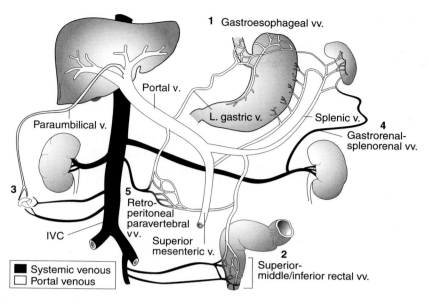

FIGURE 2.6-13.   Portosystemic anastomoses.

1. Left gastric–azygos → esophageal varices. 2. Superior–middle/inferior rectal → hemorrhoids.
3. Paraumbilical–inferior epigastric → caput medusae (navel). 4. Gastrorenal-splenorenal.
5. Retroperitoneal paravertebral.

TREATMENT

Aimed at ameliorating the complications of cirrhosis/portal hypertension.

- **Ascites:**
    - Sodium restriction and diuretics (furosemide and spironolactone).
    - Rule out infectious and neoplastic causes; perform paracentesis to obtain SAAG, cell count with differential, and cultures.
    - If possible, treat underlying liver disease.
- **Spontaneous bacterial peritonitis:**
    - Presents with fever, abdominal pain, and altered mental status.
    - Check peritoneal fluid if there is a possibility of infection. The fluid is ⊕ if there are > 250 PMNs/mL or > 500 WBCs.
    - Treat with **IV antibiotics** (e.g., third-generation cephalosporin) to cover both gram-⊕ (*Enterococcus*) and gram-⊖ (*E. coli, Klebsiella*) organisms until a causative organism is identified.

Noncirrhotic causes of portal hypertension include right heart failure, splenic vein thrombosis, and schistosomiasis.

TABLE 2.6-9.   Serum-Ascites Albumin Gradient

SAAG > 1.1	SAAG < 1.1
Ascites is related to portal hypertension:	Ascites is due to protein leakage:
■ **Presinusoidal:** Splenic or portal vein thrombosis, schistosomiasis	■ Nephrotic syndrome
■ **Sinusoidal:** Cirrhosis, massive hepatic metastases	■ Tuberculosis
■ **Postsinusoidal:** Right heart failure, constrictive pericarditis, Budd-Chiari syndrome	■ Malignancy (e.g., ovarian cancer)

Spontaneous bacterial peritonitis is diagnosed by > 250 PMNs/mL or > 500 WBCs in the ascitic fluid.

- **Hepatorenal syndrome:** A diagnosis of exclusion; difficult to treat and often requires dialysis.
- **Hepatic encephalopathy:**
  - Due to ↓ clearance of ammonia.
  - Often precipitated by dehydration, infection, electrolyte abnormalities, and GI bleeding.
  - Treat with dietary protein restriction, **lactulose,** and **rifaximin.**
- **Esophageal varices:**
  - Monitor for GI bleeding; treat medically (β-blockers, octreotide), endoscopically (band ligation), or surgically (portocaval shunt).
  - Consider **liver transplantation** for patients with advanced disease.

Primary Biliary Cirrhosis

Primary biliary cirrhosis is an autoimmune disease that presents with jaundice and pruritus in middle-aged women.

- An **autoimmune** disorder characterized by **destruction of intrahepatic bile ducts.** The disease most commonly presents in **middle-aged women** with other autoimmune conditions.
- **Hx/PE:** Presents with progressive **jaundice, pruritus,** and **malabsorption** of the fat-soluble vitamins (A, D, E, K).
- **Dx:** Laboratory findings include ↑ **alkaline phosphatase,** ↑ bilirubin, ⊕ **antimitochondrial antibody,** and ↑ cholesterol.
- **Tx:** Ursodeoxycholic acid (slows progression of disease); cholestyramine for pruritus; liver transplantation.

Hepatocellular Carcinoma

One of the most common cancers worldwide despite its relatively low incidence in the United States. 1° risk factors for the development of hepatocellular carcinoma in the United States are **cirrhosis** and **chronic hepatitis** (HCV). In developing countries, **aflatoxins** (in various food sources) and **HBV infection** are also major risk factors.

HISTORY/PE

- Patients commonly present with **RUQ tenderness, abdominal distention,** and signs of chronic liver disease such as **jaundice, easy bruisability,** and **coagulopathy.** Cachexia and weakness may be present.
- Exam may reveal tender **enlargement** of the liver.

DIAGNOSIS

- Often suggested by the presence of a mass on **ultrasound** or **CT** as well as by abnormal LFTs and significantly elevated α-fetoprotein (AFP) levels.
- Liver biopsy for definitive diagnosis.

TREATMENT

Complications of hepatocellular carcinoma include GI bleeding, liver failure, and metastasis.

- For small tumors that are detected early, aggressive tumor resection or **orthotopic liver transplantation** may be successful.
- Chemotherapy and radiation are generally not effective, although they may be used to shrink large tumors prior to surgery (**neoadjuvant therapy**).
- Monitor tumor recurrence with serial AFP levels. Prevent exposure to hepatic carcinogens and vaccinate against hepatitis in high-risk individuals.

Hemochromatosis

Caused by hyperabsorption of iron with parenchymal hemosiderin accumulation in the liver, pancreas, heart, adrenals, testes, pituitary, and kidneys. It is an **autosomal-recessive** disease that usually occurs in males of northern European descent and is rarely recognized before the fifth decade. 2° hemochromatosis may occur with iron overload and is common in patients receiving **chronic transfusion therapy** (e.g., for α-thalassemia) as well as in **alcoholics** (alcohol ↑ iron absorption).

HISTORY/PE

- Patients may present with abdominal pain or **symptoms of DM, hypogonadism, arthropathy of the MCP joints, heart failure,** or cirrhosis.
- Exam may reveal **bronze skin pigmentation,** pancreatic dysfunction, **cardiac dysfunction** (CHF), hepatomegaly, and testicular atrophy.

DIAGNOSIS

- ↑ **serum iron,** percent saturation of iron, and ferritin with ↓ serum transferrin.
- Fasting transferrin saturation (serum iron divided by transferrin level) > 45% is the most sensitive diagnostic test.
- **Glucose intolerance** and mildly elevated AST and alkaline phosphatase can be present.
- Perform a **liver biopsy** (to determine hepatic iron index), hepatic MRI, or *HFE* gene mutation screen.

TREATMENT

- **Weekly phlebotomy;** when serum iron levels ↓, perform maintenance phlebotomy every 2–4 months.
- **Deferoxamine** can be used for maintenance therapy.

COMPLICATIONS

Cirrhosis, hepatocellular carcinoma, cardiomegaly leading to CHF and/or conduction defects, DM, impotence, arthropathy, hypopituitarism.

Wilson's Disease (Hepatolenticular Degeneration)

- ↓ ceruloplasmin and **excessive deposition of copper** in the liver and brain due to a deficient copper-transporting protein. Linked to an autosomal-recessive defect on chromosome 13. Usually occurs in patients < 30 years of age; 50% of patients are symptomatic by age 15.
- Hx: Patients with present hemolytic anemia, **liver abnormalities** (jaundice 2° to hepatitis/cirrhosis), and neurologic (loss of coordination, **tremor,** dysphagia) as well as **psychiatric** (psychosis, anxiety, mania, depression) **abnormalities.**
- PE: May reveal **Kayser-Fleischer rings** in the cornea (green-to-brown deposits of copper in Descemet's membrane) as well as jaundice, hepatomegaly, asterixis, choreiform movements, and rigidity.
- Dx: ↓ serum ceruloplasmin, ↑ urinary copper excretion, ↑ hepatic copper.
- Tx: **Dietary copper restriction** (avoid shellfish, liver, legumes), **penicillamine** (a copper chelator that ↑ urinary copper excretion; administer with pyridoxine), and possibly oral zinc (↑ fecal excretion).

Wilson's disease—

ABCD

Asterixis
Basal ganglia deterioration
Ceruloplasmin ↓, **C**irrhosis, **C**opper ↑, **C**arcinoma (hepatocellular), **C**horeiform movements
Dementia

Pancreatitis

Table 2.6-10 outlines the important features of acute and chronic pancreatitis. Table 2.6-11 lists Ranson's criteria for predicting mortality associated with acute pancreatitis.

TABLE 2.6-10. **Features of Acute and Chronic Pancreatitis**

VARIABLE	ACUTE PANCREATITIS	CHRONIC PANCREATITIS
Pathophysiology	Leakage of pancreatic enzymes into pancreatic and peripancreatic tissue, often 2° to gallstone disease or alcoholism.	Irreversible parenchymal destruction leading to pancreatic dysfunction.
Time course	Abrupt onset of severe pain.	Persistent, recurrent episodes of severe pain.
Risk factors	**Gallstones, alcoholism,** hypercalcemia, hypertriglyceridemia, trauma, drug side effects (thiazide diuretics), viral infections, post-ERCP, scorpion bites.	**Alcoholism** (90%), gallstones, hyperparathyroidism, hypercholesterolemia, cystic fibrosis. May also be idiopathic.
History/PE	**Severe epigastric pain (radiating to the back);** nausea, vomiting, weakness, fever, shock. Flank discoloration (**Grey Turner's sign**) and periumbilical discoloration (**Cullen's sign**) may be evident on exam.	Recurrent episodes of **persistent epigastric pain;** anorexia, nausea, constipation, flatulence, **steatorrhea,** weight loss, DM.
Diagnosis	↑ **amylase,** ↑ **lipase,** ↓ **calcium** if severe; **"sentinel loop"** or **"colon cutoff sign"** on AXR. Abdominal ultrasound or CT may show an enlarged pancreas with stranding, abscess, hemorrhage, necrosis, or pseudocyst.	↑ or normal amylase and lipase, ↓ stool elastase, glycosuria, **pancreatic calcifications,** and mild ileus on AXR and CT (**"chain of lakes"**).
Treatment	Removal of the offending agent if possible. Standard supportive measures: IV fluids/electrolyte replacement, analgesia, bowel rest, NG suction, nutritional support, O_2, "tincture of time." IV antibiotics, respiratory support, and surgical debridement if necrotizing pancreatitis is present.	Analgesia, exogenous lipase/trypsin and medium-chain fatty-acid diet, avoidance of causative agents (EtOH), celiac nerve block, surgery for intractable pain or structural causes.
Prognosis	Roughly 85–90% are mild and self-limited; 10–15% are severe, requiring ICU admission. Mortality may approach 50% in severe cases.	Can have chronic pain and pancreatic exocrine and endocrine dysfunction.
Complications	**Pancreatic pseudocyst, fistula formation,** hypocalcemia, renal failure, pleural effusion, chronic pancreatitis, sepsis. Mortality 2° to acute pancreatitis can be predicted with Ranson's criteria (see Table 2.6-11).	**Chronic pain,** malnutrition/weight loss, pancreatic cancer.

TABLE 2.6-11. Ranson's Criteria for Acute Pancreatitis[a]

On Admission	After 48 Hours
"GA LAW":	**"C HOBBS":**
Glucose > 200 mg/dL	Ca^{2+} < 8.0 mg/dL
Age > 55 years	Hematocrit ↓ by > 10%
LDH > 350 IU/L	PaO_2 < 60 mmHg
AST > 250 IU/dL	Base excess > 4 mEq/L
WBC > 16,000/mL	BUN ↑ by > 5 mg/dL
	Sequestered fluid > 6 L

[a] The risk of mortality is 20% with 3–4 signs, 40% with 5–6 signs, and 100% with ≥ 7 signs.

Pancreatic Cancer

Roughly 75% are adenocarcinomas in the head of the pancreas. Risk factors include smoking, chronic pancreatitis, a first-degree relative with pancreatic cancer, and a high-fat diet. Incidence rises after age 45; slightly more common in men.

HISTORY/PE

- Presents with **abdominal pain** radiating toward the back, as well as with **obstructive jaundice,** loss of appetite, nausea, vomiting, **weight loss,** weakness, fatigue, and indigestion.
- Often asymptomatic, and thus presents late in the disease course.
- Exam may reveal a palpable, nontender gallbladder (**Courvoisier's sign**) or migratory thrombophlebitis (**Trousseau's sign**).

DIAGNOSIS

- Use **CT** to detect a pancreatic mass, dilated pancreatic and bile ducts, the extent of vascular involvement (particularly the SMA, SMV, and portal vein), and metastases (hepatic).
- If a mass is not visualized, use ERCP or endoscopic ultrasound for better visualization.
- CA-19-9 is often elevated, but this measure lacks sensitivity and specificity.

TREATMENT

- Most patients present with metastatic disease, and treatment is palliative.
- Some 10–20% of pancreatic head tumors have no evidence of metastasis or major vessel involvement and may be resected using the Whipple procedure (pancreaticoduodenectomy).
- Chemotherapy with 5-FU and gemcitabine may improve short-term survival, but long-term prognosis is poor (5–10% five-year survival).

The classic presentation of pancreatic cancer is painless, progressive obstructive jaundice.

HIGH-YIELD FACTS

GASTROINTESTINAL

Hematology/Oncology

Bleeding disorders due to platelet dysfunction usually manifest as petechiae, whereas disorders of coagulation factors cause other symptoms, such as hemarthroses.

Coagulation Cascade

Hemostasis requires the interaction of blood vessels, platelets, monocytes, and coagulation factors. This activates the clotting cascade, as shown in Figure 2.7-1.

- **Heparin:** ↑ PTT, activates antithrombin III and affects the **intrinsic pathway,** and ↓ fibrinogen levels; **protamine sulfate** is the antidote.
- **Warfarin:** ↑ PT, inhibits vitamin K and affects the **extrinsic pathway,** and is teratogenic, since its small size allows it to cross the placenta. **Vitamin K** is the antidote. **Goal INR of 2.0–3.0** (2.5–3.5 in patients with mechanical valves).
- **Enoxaparin** (low-molecular-weight heparin [LMWH]): Inhibits factor Xa and does not have to be monitored; dosing is once or twice daily.

Heparin-to-warfarin conversion is necessary because warfarin inhibits proteins C and S before other vitamin K–dependent factors (II, VII, IX, and X), leading to a transient period of **paradoxical hypercoagulability** before proper anticoagulation.

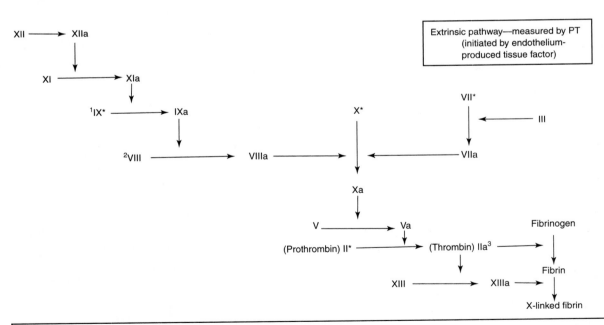

FIGURE 2.7-1. **Coagulation cascade.**

Hemophilia

A deficiency of a clotting factor that leads to a bleeding diathesis. Subtypes are distinguished on the basis of which factor is lacking (see Table 2.7-1). The condition is usually hereditary but may be **acquired** through the development of an antibody to a clotting factor. This may occur in patients with autoimmune or lymphoproliferative disease, postpartum, or following a blood transfusion. Patients are nearly always male and may have a ⊕ family history.

HISTORY/PE

- Presents with spontaneous hemorrhage into the tissues and joints that, if left untreated, can lead to **arthropathy and joint destruction.**
- Spontaneous intracerebral hemorrhages, renal and retroperitoneal bleeding, and GI bleeding may also be seen.
- **Mild cases** may have major hemorrhage after surgery or trauma but are otherwise asymptomatic.

DIAGNOSIS

- **Evaluate for suspected clotting factor deficiency:**
  - **PT:** Usually normal, but isolated elevations are seen in congenital factor VII deficiency.
  - **aPTT:** Prolonged (the more prolonged, the more severe the hemophilia).
  - **Thrombin time, fibrinogen, bleeding time:** Usually normal.
- **Conduct a mixing study:** Mix the patient's plasma with normal plasma; if this corrects the aPTT, a factor deficiency is likely. If the aPTT does not correct, the patient may have a clotting factor inhibitor.
- **Obtain factor assays:** Specific factor assays should then be performed for factors VII, VIII, IX, XI, and XII. Hemophilia is characterized according to factor level as follows:
  - **Mild:** > 5% of normal.
  - **Moderate:** 1–3% of normal.
  - **Severe:** ≤ 1% of normal.

TREATMENT

- Treat bleeding episodes with immediate **transfusion of clotting factors (or cryoprecipitate) to at least 40% of normal concentration.** Factor VIII has a half-life of 12 hours, so patients should be dosed BID to maintain ad-

*The classic case of hemophilia is the **boy** (**X**-linked) from the Imperial **R**ussian family (**R**ecessive) who presents with hemarthroses following minimal or no trauma.*

Cryoprecipitate consists of factors VIII and XIII, vWF, fibrinogen, and fibronectin.

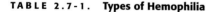

TABLE 2.7-1. Types of Hemophilia

SUBTYPE	PATHOGENESIS
Hemophilia A (factor VIII deficiency) (90%)	X-linked inheritance; the most common severe congenital clotting deficiency.
Hemophilia B (factor IX deficiency) (9%)	X-linked inheritance.
Hemophilia C (factor XI deficiency) (< 1%)	Most common in Ashkenazi Jews.
Factor VII deficiency (< 1%)	Presents in a milder, likely heterozygous form.

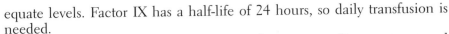

DDAVP helps the body release extra factor VIII.

equate levels. Factor IX has a half-life of 24 hours, so daily transfusion is needed.

- The length of treatment varies with the lesion, extending up to several weeks after orthopedic surgery.
- Mild hemophiliacs may be treated with desmopressin (**DDAVP**); if so, they should be **fluid restricted** to prevent the side effect of **hyponatremia.**
- It may be necessary to transfuse RBCs, depending on the degree of blood loss.
- Fifteen percent of patients who are treated for hemophilia A develop neutralizing IgG antibodies to factor VIII, which precludes further treatment with replacement factor.

von Willebrand's Disease (vWD)

An **autosomal-dominant** condition in which patients have deficient or defective von Willebrand's factor (vWF) with low levels of factor VIII, which is carried by vWF. Symptoms are due to platelet dysfunction and to deficient factor VIII. The disease is milder than hemophilia. vWD is the **most common inherited bleeding disorder** (1% of the population is affected).

ASA ↑ the risk of bleeding in patients with von Willebrand's disease.

HISTORY/PE

Presents with easy bruising, mucosal bleeding (e.g., epistaxis, oral bleeding), menorrhagia, and postincisional bleeding. Platelet dysfunction is not severe enough to produce petechiae. Symptoms worsen with ASA use.

DIAGNOSIS

- Look for a family history of bleeding disorders.
- Platelet count and **PT** are **normal,** but a **prolonged aPTT** may be seen as a result of factor VIII deficiency.
- A **ristocetin cofactor assay** of patient plasma can measure the capacity of vWF to agglutinate platelets.

Ristocetin cofactor assay measures the ability of vWF to agglutinate platelets in vitro in the presence of ristocetin.

TREATMENT

- Bleeding episodes can be treated with **DDAVP**; menorrhagia can be controlled with **OCPs.**
- Avoid ASA and other inhibitors of platelet function.

Hypercoagulable States

Also called **thrombophilias** or **prothrombotic states,** *hypercoagulable states* is an all-inclusive term describing conditions that ↑ a patient's risk of developing thromboembolic disease. Causes are multiple and may be **genetic, acquired, or physiologic** (see Table 2.7-2). Acquired causes are usually 2° to an underlying clinical condition, disease process, or lifestyle. Inherited causes are collectively called *hereditary thrombotic disease,* of which **factor V Leiden** (a polymorphism in factor V, rendering it resistant to inactivity by activated protein C, or APC) is the most common.

Suspect pulmonary embolism in a patient with rapid onset of hypoxia, hypercapnia, tachycardia, and an ↑ alveolar-arterial oxygen gradient without another obvious explanation.

HISTORY/PE

- Presents with **recurrent** thrombotic complications, including **DVT, pulmonary embolism, arterial thrombosis, MI, and stroke.** Women may have recurrent miscarriages.

TABLE 2.7-2. Causes of Hypercoagulable States

Genetic	Acquired	Physiologic
Antithrombin III deficiency	Surgery	Age
Protein C deficiency	Trauma	Pregnancy
Protein S deficiency	Malignancy	
Factor V Leiden	Immobilization	
Hyperhomocysteinemia	Smoking	
Dysfibrinogenemia	Obesity	
Plasminogen deficiency	Antiphospholipid syndrome	
Prothrombin G20210A	Nephrotic syndrome	
mutation	OCPs/HRT	
MTHFR gene mutation		

- Although patients may have no recognizable predisposing factors, they usually have one or more of the causative factors outlined in Table 2.7-2. They may also have a ⊕ family history.

DIAGNOSIS

- Under ideal circumstances, patients should be diagnosed before they are symptomatic, but this rarely occurs.
- Prior to workup for hereditary causes, acquired causes of abnormal coagulation values should be ruled out. **Confirmation of a hereditary abnormality requires two abnormal values that are obtained while the patient is asymptomatic and untreated, with similar values obtained in two other family members.**
- Workup for hypercoagulability includes lupus antigen/antiphospholipid syndrome, antithrombin III deficiency, protein C and S deficiencies, APC resistance, homocysteine elevation, and prothrombin G20210A mutation.

TREATMENT

- Treatment should address the type of thrombotic event as well as the area of thrombosis.
- Treat DVT and pulmonary embolism with heparin (unfractionated or LMWH) followed by 3–6 months of oral warfarin anticoagulation for the first event, 6–12 months for the second, and lifelong anticoagulation for subsequent events.
- Heparin-to-warfarin conversion is necessary (see the "Coagulation Cascade" discussion above).

Disseminated Intravascular Coagulation (DIC)

A common disorder among hospitalized patients, second only to liver disease as a cause of acquired coagulopathy. It is caused by **deposition of fibrin in small blood vessels,** leading to thrombosis and end-organ damage. **Depletion of clotting factors and platelets** leads to a bleeding diathesis. May be associated with almost any severe illness.

HISTORY/PE

- Disorders commonly associated with DIC include obstetric complications, infections with septicemia, neoplasms, acute promyelocytic leukemia, pan-

DIC is characterized by both thrombosis and hemorrhage.

Petechiae suggest Platelet deficiency.

Bleeding into body Cavities or joints suggests Clotting factor deficiency.

creatitis, intravascular hemolysis, vascular disorders (e.g., aortic aneurysm), massive tissue injury and trauma, drug reactions, acidosis, and ARDS.

- Presentation varies according to whether the disease is acute or chronic:
    - **Acute:** Presents with generalized bleeding out of venipuncture sites into organs, with ecchymoses and petechiae. Patients who are in shock may have acral cyanosis.
    - **Chronic:** Presents with bruising and mucosal bleeding, thrombophlebitis, renal dysfunction, and transient neurologic syndromes.

DIAGNOSIS

- Diagnosed as outlined in Table 2.7-3.
- DIC may be confused with severe liver disease, but **unlike liver disease, factor VIII is depressed.**

TREATMENT

Treatment of the underlying illness often results in spontaneous reversal. Patients often require RBC transfusion and shock management. Platelets should be transfused in the event of hemorrhage with a platelet count < 20,000.

Thrombotic Thrombocytopenic Purpura (TTP)

Part of a spectrum of diseases that includes hemolytic-uremic syndrome (HUS) and HELLP syndrome (see the Obstetrics chapter); thought to be due to **platelet microthrombi** that block off small blood vessels, leading to end-organ ischemia and dysfunction. **RBCs are fragmented** by contact with the microthrombi, leading to hemolysis (microangiopathic hemolytic anemia). The cause of initial microthrombus formation is unknown but may be infectious (bacterial toxins), drug related, autoimmune, or idiopathic.

HISTORY/PE

A **clinical syndrome** characterized by **five signs/symptoms:** low platelet count, microangiopathic hemolytic anemia, neurologic changes (delirium, seizure, stroke), impaired renal function, and fever.

DIAGNOSIS

- Diagnosis is largely clinical.
- It is rare for all signs to be present, but the presence of schistocytes (broken RBCs) on peripheral smear with low platelets and rising creatinine is highly suggestive. Nucleated RBCs are also often seen in the peripheral smear.
- Hemolytic anemia labs include elevated indirect bilirubin, LDH, and AST along with low haptoglobin. **Coagulation factors are normal.**

The three causes of microangiopathic hemolytic anemia are HUS, TTP, and DIC.

TABLE 2.7-3. Laboratory Values in DIC

	PT	aPTT	THROMBIN TIME	PLATELETS	FDPs + D-DIMER	CLOTTING FACTORS
Acute	↑	↑	↑	↓	↑	↓
Chronic	↑	↑	↑	Normal	↑	Normal

- Overlapping conditions are HUS, HELLP syndrome, and DIC.
  - **HUS:** Characterized by renal failure, hemolytic anemia, and low platelets. **Severe elevations in creatinine are more typical of HUS than of TTP.**
  - **HELLP syndrome:** Affects pregnant women, often occurring in conjunction with preeclampsia (see the Obstetrics chapter).
  - **DIC:** Distinguished from TTP by prolonged PT and aPTT.

TREATMENT

Treat with **corticosteroids** to ↓ the formation of microthrombi along with plasma replacement and plasmapheresis (the mainstay of severe cases). Rarely, splenectomy is performed with mixed results. Platelet transfusions are contraindicated.

Idiopathic Thrombocytopenic Purpura (ITP)

A relatively common cause of thrombocytopenia. **IgG antibodies** are formed against the patient's platelets. Bone marrow production of platelets is ↑, with ↑ megakaryocytes in the marrow. The **most common immunologic disorder in women of childbearing age.** May be acute or chronic.

HISTORY/PE

- Patients often feel well and present with no systemic symptoms. They may have minor bleeding, easy bruising, petechiae, hematuria, hematemesis, or melena. Bleeding is mucocutaneous. Usually there is no splenomegaly.
- ITP is associated with a range of conditions, including lymphoma, leukemia, SLE, HIV, and HCV.
- The clinical presentation is as follows:
  - **Acute:** Abrupt onset of hemorrhagic complications following a viral illness. Commonly affects children 2–6 years of age, with males and females affected equally.
  - **Chronic:** Insidious onset that is unrelated to infection. Most often affects adults 20–40 years of age; women are three times more likely to be affected than men.

DIAGNOSIS

- A **diagnosis of exclusion,** as the test for platelet-associated antibodies is a poor one.
- Once other causes of thrombocytopenia have been ruled out, a diagnosis can be made on the basis of the history and physical, a CBC, and a peripheral blood smear showing normal RBC morphology. Most patients do not require bone marrow biopsy, which would show ↑ megakaryocytes as the only abnormality.

TREATMENT

- Most patients with acute childhood ITP spontaneously remit, but this is rarely the case in chronic ITP.
- Treatment is reserved for patients with symptomatic bleeding. Those with platelet counts > 20,000 are generally asymptomatic.
- Platelet transfusions are of no benefit, as patients' IgG levels will also lead to destruction of platelets.
- The main therapies are **corticosteroids, high-dose gamma globulin (IVIG), and splenectomy.** Most patients respond to corticosteroids, but if

Anti-D (Rh) immunoglobulin and rituximab are emerging therapies for ITP.

Anti-D (Rh) immunoglobulin and IVIG act as "decoys" so that WBCs will recognize them instead of IgG on platelets.

they cannot be tapered after 3–6 months, splenectomy should be considered.

■ An emerging therapy is anti-D (Rh) immunoglobulin, which binds to RBCs so that they are destroyed instead of the patient's platelets. Patients will have a drop in their hematocrit. Rh-⊖ and splenectomized patients should not receive this treatment.

■ In **pregnant patients, severe thrombocytopenia may occur in the fetus.**

▶ **BLOOD CELL DIFFERENTIATION**

Figure 2.7-2 illustrates the various blood cell categories and lineages.

▶ **RED BLOOD CELL DISORDERS**

Anemias

Anemia is a disorder of **low hematocrit and hemoglobin.** There are several subtypes, which are classified according to red cell morphology (MCV, RDW, color, shape) and reticulocyte count (see Figure 2.7-3). Once anemia has been diagnosed by a low hemoglobin/hematocrit, the approach starts with the MCV. An MCV < 80 fL indicates **microcytic** anemia; between 80 fL and 100 fL is **normocytic;** and > 100 fL is **macrocytic.**

IRON DEFICIENCY ANEMIA (A MICROCYTIC ANEMIA)

A condition in which iron loss exceeds intake. May occur when **dietary intake is insufficient** for the patient's needs (e.g., when needs are ↑ by growth or pregnancy) or in the setting of **chronic blood loss,** usually 2° to menstruation or GI bleeding. **Toddlers, adolescent girls,** and **women of childbearing age** are most commonly affected.

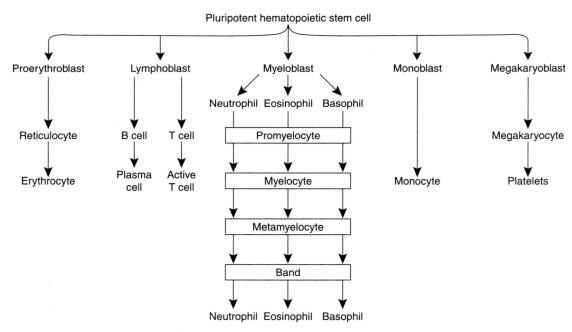

FIGURE 2.7-2. Blood cell differentiation.

194

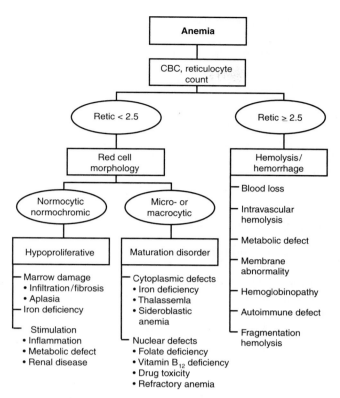

FIGURE 2.7-3. **Anemia algorithm.**

HISTORY/PE

- Symptoms include **fatigue, weakness, brittle nails,** and **pica.** If the anemia develops slowly, patients are generally asymptomatic.
- Physical findings include **glossitis, angular cheilitis,** and **koilonychia ("spoon nails").**

DIAGNOSIS

- Bone marrow biopsy looking for evidence of iron stores is the gold standard but is seldom performed.
- Iron deficiency is often confused with **anemia of chronic disease,** in which iron use by the body is impaired. Labs can help differentiate the two conditions (see Table 2.7-4).
- Peripheral blood smear shows **hypochromic and microcytic RBCs** with a **low reticulocyte count.**
- Low serum ferritin reflects low body stores of iron and confirms the diagnosis. However, ferritin is also an acute-phase reactant and may thus obscure evidence of iron deficiency.

TREATMENT

- Treat with **replacement iron for 4–6 months.** Oral iron sulfate may lead to nausea, constipation, diarrhea, and abdominal pain. Antacids may interfere with iron absorption.
- If necessary, IV iron dextran can be administered but is associated with a 10% risk of serious side effects, including anaphylaxis. Hence, this is usually done only by a hematologist.

Iron deficiency anemia in an elderly patient could be due to colorectal cancer and needs to be evaluated to rule out malignancy.

Iron deficiency anemia can be due to a hookworm infection.

Causes of microcytic anemia—

TICS

Thalassemia
Iron deficiency
Chronic disease
Sideroblastic anemia

TABLE 2.7-4. Iron Deficiency Anemia vs. Anemia of Chronic Disease

	IRON DEFICIENCY	CHRONIC DISEASE	BOTH
Serum iron	↓	↓	↓
TIBC or transferrin	↑	↓	Normal/↑
Ferritin	↓	↑	Normal/↓
Serum transferrin receptor	↑	Normal	Normal/↑

Most macrocytic anemias are caused by processes that interfere with normal DNA synthesis and replication.

B_{12} deficiency can be due to infection by a tapeworm, Diphyllobothrium latum.

Causes of oxidative stress in G6PD deficiency include infection, metabolic acidosis, fava beans, antimalarials, dapsone, sulfonamides, and nitrofurantoin.

MEGALOBLASTIC ANEMIA (A MACROCYTIC ANEMIA)

Vitamin B_{12} (cobalamin) and **folate deficiency** interfere with DNA synthesis, leading to a delay in blood cell maturation. Cobalamin deficiency is due to malabsorption, usually from **pernicious anemia** (destruction of parietal cells, which produce the intrinsic factor needed for cobalamin absorption). Folate deficiency results from insufficient dietary folate, malabsorption, alcoholism, or use of certain drugs. **Drugs that interfere with DNA synthesis,** including many chemotherapeutic agents, may lead to megaloblastic anemia.

HISTORY/PE

- Presents with **fatigue, pallor, diarrhea, loss of appetite, headaches,** and **tingling/numbness of the hands and feet.**
- Cobalamin deficiency affects the nervous system, so patients lacking that vitamin may develop a **demyelinating disorder** and may present with symptoms of motor, sensory, autonomic, and/or neuropsychiatric dysfunction, known as **subacute combined degeneration of the cord.**

DIAGNOSIS

- Peripheral smear shows RBCs with an **elevated MCV.** Hypersegmented (> 5) granulocytes can also be seen.
- Bone marrow sample reveals **giant neutrophils** and **hypersegmented mature granulocytes.**
- The **Schilling test** (ingestion of radiolabeled cobalamin both with and without added intrinsic factor) is classic for measuring absorption of cobalamin but is rarely performed.
- Serum vitamin levels are poorly diagnostic of deficiencies and are thus used with adjunctive tests, including methylmalonic acid (MMA) and homocysteine levels:
  - **B_{12} deficiency:** Elevated MMA and homocysteine.
  - **Folate deficiency:** Normal MMA; elevated homocysteine.

TREATMENT

Address the cause of the anemia, and correct the underlying cause.

HEMOLYTIC ANEMIA (A NORMOCYTIC ANEMIA)

Occurs when bone marrow production is unable to compensate for ↑ destruction of circulating blood cells. Etiologies include the following:

196

- **G6PD deficiency:** An X-linked recessive disease that ↑ RBC sensitivity to oxidative stress.
- **Paroxysmal nocturnal hemoglobinuria:** A disorder in which blood cell sensitivity to complement activation is ↑.
- **Hereditary spherocytosis:** An abnormality of the RBC membrane.
- **Autoimmune RBC destruction:** Occurs 2° to EBV infection, mycoplasmal infection, CLL, rheumatoid disease, or medications.
- **Sickle cell disease:** A recessive β-globin mutation (see the following section).
- **Microangiopathic hemolytic anemia:** TTP, HUS, DIC.
- **Mechanical hemolysis:** Associated with mechanical heart valves.
- **Other:** Malaria, hypersplenism.

HISTORY/PE

- Presents with **pallor, fatigue, tachycardia,** and **tachypnea.**
- Patients are typically **jaundiced,** with low haptoglobin and elevated indirect bilirubin and LDH. Urine is dark with **hemoglobinuria,** and there is ↑ excretion of urinary and fecal urobilinogen. **Reticulocyte count is elevated.**

The classic case of G6PD deficiency is an African-American male soldier in Vietnam who took quinine.

DIAGNOSIS

Diagnosed by the history and clinical presentation. High LDH, elevated indirect bilirubin, and ↓ haptoglobin levels are consistent with a diagnosis of hemolytic anemia. Also obtain a reticulocyte count. A **Coombs' test** is used to detect autoimmune hemolysis.

TREATMENT

Treatment varies with the cause of hemolysis but typically includes **corticosteroids** to address immunologic causes and **iron supplementation** to replace urinary losses. Splenectomy may be helpful, and transfusion may be necessary to treat severe anemia.

Indirect Coombs' tests detect antibodies to RBCs in the patient's serum. Direct Coombs' tests detect sensitized erythrocytes.

APLASTIC ANEMIA

A rare condition caused by failure of blood cell production due to **destruction of bone marrow cells.** It may be hereditary, as in **Fanconi's anemia;** may have an **autoimmune** or a **viral** etiology (e.g., HIV, parvovirus B19); or may result from exposure to **toxins** (e.g., drugs, cleaning solvents) or **radiation.**

HISTORY/PE

- Patients are typically **pancytopenic,** with symptoms resulting from a lack of RBCs, WBCs, and platelets—e.g., **pallor, weakness, a tendency to infection, petechiae, bruising, and bleeding.**
- The disease may be of sudden or sustained onset and may be of variable severity, depending on the patient's blood counts.

DIAGNOSIS

- Diagnosed by clinical presentation and CBC; **verified by a bone marrow biopsy** revealing hypocellularity and space occupied by fat.
- The differential includes megaloblastic anemia, as both diseases feature an elevated MCV.

Patients with Fanconi's anemia may be identified on physical exam by café au lait spots, short stature, and radial/thumb hypoplasia/aplasia.

TREATMENT

Blood transfusion and stem cell transplantation to replace absent cells; immunosuppression with cyclosporin A and antithymocyte globulin to prevent autoimmune destruction of marrow. **Infections** are a major cause of mortality and should be treated aggressively.

SICKLE CELL DISEASE (SCD)

SCD represents a qualitative defect in the β-globin chain.

An **autosomal-recessive** disorder most commonly caused by a mutation of adult hemoglobin (the β chain has glu replaced by val). Signs and symptoms are due to ↓ **red cell survival** and a tendency of sickled cells to lead to **vaso-occlusion.**

HISTORY/PE

- Asymptomatic during the first year or two of life; may first present with dactylitis in childhood. Later, hemolysis results in **anemia, jaundice, cholelithiasis,** ↑ **cardiac output (murmur and cardiomegaly),** and **delayed growth.**
- Vaso-occlusion leads to ischemic organ damage, especially **splenic infarction,** which predisposes to pneumococcal sepsis, and acute chest syndrome (pneumonia and/or pulmonary infarction). Patients also experience painful crises of unknown etiology. Common triggers for a vaso-occlusive crisis (VOC) include cold temperatures, dehydration, and infection.
- Other potential complications include splenic sequestration, which occurs in patients who have not infarcted their spleens, and aplastic crisis, which is usually 2° to infection with parvovirus B19.

DIAGNOSIS

Patients with SCD classically get osteomyelitis with Salmonella. They are also at ↑ risk of avascular necrosis of the hip.

The sickle cell screen is based on a blood smear with sickle cells and target cells. The gold standard is quantitative hemoglobin electrophoresis.

TREATMENT

- Treat with **hydroxyurea,** which stimulates the production of fetal hemoglobin (hydroxyurea is teratogenic, so it is contraindicated in pregnancy).
- If hydroxyurea does not prove effective, chronic transfusion therapy, which carries the risk of iron overload, can be tried.
- Treat cholelithiasis with cholecystectomy.
- VOCs must be treated with adequate pain management, O_2 therapy, IV fluid rehydration, and antibiotics (if infection is suspected to be the trigger).
- To prevent VOCs from progressing to acute chest syndrome, initiate aggressive hydration and incentive spirometry, and keep the sickle variant < 40%. This can be done with simple transfusions or, if necessary, exchange transfusion in an ICU setting.

Thalassemias

Hereditary disorders involving ↓ or absent production of normal globin chains of hemoglobin. α-**thalassemia** is caused by a mutation of one or more of the four genes for α-hemoglobin; β-**thalassemia** results from a mutation of one or both of the two genes for β-hemoglobin.

Thalassemia is most common among people of **African, Middle Eastern,** and **Asian descent.** Disease presentation and prognosis vary with the number of genes missing (see Table 2.7-5).

DIAGNOSIS

Diagnosed by hemoglobin electrophoresis evaluation (but note that this is normal in α-thalassemia) and DNA studies.

TREATMENT

Most patients do not require treatment, but those with β-thalassemia major and hemoglobin H disease are commonly transfusion dependent and should be given iron chelators (deferoxamine) to prevent overload.

Polycythemias

Erythrocytosis (an abnormal elevation of hematocrit) may be either 1° (due to ↑ RBC production) or 2° (due to ↓ plasma volume and hemoconcentration).

TABLE 2.7-5. Differential Diagnosis of Thalassemias

SUBTYPE	NUMBER OF GENES PRESENT	CLINICAL FEATURES
β-thalassemia major	0/2 β	Patients develop severe microcytic anemia in the first year of life and need chronic transfusions or marrow transplant to survive.
β-thalassemia minor	1/2 β	Patients are asymptomatic, but their cells are microcytic and hypochromic on peripheral smear.
Hydrops fetalis	0/4 α	Patients die in utero.
Hemoglobin H disease	1/4 α	Patients have severe hypochromic, microcytic anemia with chronic hemolysis, splenomegaly, jaundice, and cholelithiasis. The reticulocyte count elevates to compensate, and one-third of patients have skeletal changes due to expanded erythropoiesis.
α-thalassemia trait	2/4 α	Patients have low MCV but are usually asymptomatic.
Silent carrier	3/4 α	Patients have no signs or symptoms of disease.

HISTORY/PE

- Characterized by ↑ hematocrit, ↓ tissue blood flow and oxygenation, and ↑ cardiac work.
- Patients present with **"hyperviscosity syndrome,"** which consists of easy bleeding/bruising, blurred vision, neurologic abnormalities, plethora, pruritus (especially after a warm bath), hepatomegaly, splenomegaly, and CHF.
- 1° erythrocytosis is associated with hypoxia (from lung disease, smoking, high altitudes, or a poor intrauterine environment), neoplasia (erythropoietin-producing tumors), or **polycythemia vera (PCV)**, in which there is clonal proliferation of a pluripotent marrow stem cell.
- 2° erythrocytosis is associated with excessive diuresis, severe gastroenteritis, and burns.

DIAGNOSIS

- Erythrocytosis is diagnosed clinically and by cell counts, with ABGs used to assess hypoxia or imaging to demonstrate neoplasia.
- Patients with PCV have excess RBCs, WBCs, and platelets. **Levels of erythropoietin** may be useful in distinguishing PCV, in which levels are low, from other causes of polycythemia.

TREATMENT

- **Phlebotomy** relieves symptoms of erythrocytosis, but treatment should also address the underlying cause.
- PCV can be treated with **cytoreductive drugs** such as hydroxyurea or interferon. Because PCV is prothrombotic, **ASA** should also be used. With treatment, survival is 7–10 years.

Transfusion Reactions

Blood transfusion is generally safe but may result in a variety of adverse reactions. Nonhemolytic febrile reactions and minor allergic reactions are the most common, each occurring in 3–4% of all transfusions. Etiologies are as follows:

- **Nonhemolytic febrile reactions:** Involve cytokine formation during the storage of blood, and WBC antibodies.
- **Minor allergic reactions:** Involve antibody formation (usually IgA) against donor proteins. Usually occur following transfusion of plasma-containing product.
- **Hemolytic transfusion reactions:** Entail the development of antibodies against donor erythrocytes. Usually result from ABO incompatibility or from antibody against minor antigens.

HISTORY/PE

- **Nonhemolytic febrile reactions:** Present with fever, chills, rigors, and malaise. Symptom onset is 1–6 hours following transfusion.
- **Minor allergic reactions:** Characterized by urticaria.
- **Hemolytic transfusion reactions:** Present with fever, chills, nausea, flushing, apprehension, back pain, burning at the IV site, tachycardia, tachypnea, and hypotension. Symptoms begin following the transfusion of only a small amount of blood.

True polycythemia vera is characterized by a high red cell mass.

Premedication with acetaminophen and diphenhydramine is sometimes used to prevent transfusion reactions.

Hemoglobinuria in hemolytic transfusion reaction may lead to acute tubular necrosis and subsequent renal failure.

DIAGNOSIS

Diagnosed by clinical impression.

TREATMENT

- **Nonhemolytic febrile reactions:** Stop the transfusion and control fever with acetaminophen. Rule out infection.
- **Minor allergic reactions:** Administer antihistamines. In the setting of a severe reaction, stop the transfusion and give epinephrine +/– steroids.
- **Hemolytic transfusion reactions:** Stop the transfusion immediately. Replace donor blood with normal saline; administer vigorous IV fluids; and maintain good urine output (diuretics and pressors may be used to ↑ renal blood flow).

Porphyria

The porphyrias are a group of inherited disorders that include acute intermittent porphyria, porphyria cutanea tarda, and erythropoietic porphyria. Some porphyrias are **autosomal dominant** (e.g., acute intermittent porphyria) and others **autosomal recessive** (e.g., erythropoietic porphyria). All involve **abnormalities of heme production** that lead to an accumulation of porphyrins.

Heme is necessary for the production of hemoglobin, myoglobin, and cytochrome molecules.

HISTORY/PE

- Signs and symptoms vary with the type of porphyria. In general, however, porphyrias are characterized by a combination of **photodermatitis, neuropsychiatric complaints,** and **visceral complaints** that typically take the form of a **colicky abdominal pain and seizures.**
- Physical exam reveals **tachycardia, skin erythema and blisters, areflexia,** and a **nonspecific abdominal exam.**
- Patients with the erythropoietic form present with **hemolytic anemia.** Acute attacks are associated with stimulants of ↑ heme synthesis such as fasting or chemical exposures; well-known triggers are alcohol, barbiturates, and OCPs. Urine may appear red or brown after an acute attack. Patients may have a ⊕ family history.

The telltale sign of porphyria is pink urine.

DIAGNOSIS

Diagnosed by a combination of the history and physical along with labs showing elevated blood, urine, and stool porphyrins. Enzyme assays may also be helpful.

TREATMENT

- Avoidance of triggers of acute attacks; symptomatic treatment during acute episodes.
- High doses of **glucose** may be administered to ↓ heme synthesis during mild attacks, and **IV hematin** can be given for severe attacks (provides ⊖ feedback to the heme synthetic pathway).

The classic case of porphyria involves a college student who consumes alcohol and barbiturates at a party, and then has an acute episode of abdominal pain and brown urine the next day.

▶ WHITE BLOOD CELL DISORDERS

Leukemias

Malignant proliferations of hematopoietic cells, categorized by the type of cell involved and their level of differentiation. Leukemias may be acute or chronic, lymphocytic or myelogenous.

HIGH-YIELD FACTS

HEMATOLOGY/ONCOLOGY

ACUTE LEUKEMIAS

Acute myelogenous and lymphocytic leukemias are clonal disorders of early hematopoietic stem cells. They are characterized by rapid growth of immature blood cells (blasts), which overwhelms the ability of bone marrow to produce normal cells.

HISTORY/PE

- Acute myelogenous leukemia (AML) and acute lymphocytic leukemia (ALL) affect children as well as adults. ALL is the **most common childhood malignancy.**
- Disease onset and progression are rapid; patients present with signs and symptoms of anemia (pallor, fatigue) and thrombocytopenia (**petechiae, purpura, bleeding**). Medullary expansion and periosteal involvement may lead to **bone pain** (common in ALL).
- On exam, patients may have **hepatosplenomegaly** and **swollen/bleeding gums** from leukemic infiltration and ↓ platelets. Leukemic cells also infiltrate the skin and CNS.

DIAGNOSIS

- Based on examination of the patient's bone marrow, obtained by **biopsy and aspiration,** or **peripheral blood** if circulating blasts are present. Marrow that is infiltrated with blast cells (> 20–30%) is consistent with a leukemic process. **In AML, the leukemic cells are myeloblasts; in ALL they are lymphoblasts.** These cells may be distinguished by examination of morphology, cytogenetics, cytochemistry, and immunophenotyping (see Table 2.7-6).
- The WBC count is usually elevated, but the cells are dysfunctional, and patients may be neutropenic with a **history of frequent infection.** If the WBC is very high (> 100,000), there is a risk of **leukostasis** (blasts occluding the microcirculation, leading to pulmonary edema, CNS symptoms, ischemic injury, and DIC).
- The type of acute leukemia is further classified according to the **FAB system** (ALL: L1–L3; AML: M0–M7) and karyotype analysis. Prognosis varies with leukemic cytogenetics.

TABLE 2.7-6. Myeloblasts vs. Lymphoblasts

	MYELOBLAST	LYMPHOBLAST
Size	Larger (2–4 times RBC)	Smaller (1.5–3.0 times RBC)
Amount of cytoplasm	More	Less
Nucleoli	Conspicuous	Inconspicuous
Granules	Common, fine	Uncommon, coarse
Auer rods	Present in 50% of cases	Absent
Myeloperoxidase	⊕	⊖

TREATMENT

- ALL and AML are treated primarily with chemotherapeutic agents, although transfusions, antibiotics, and colony-stimulating factors are also used. Patients with unfavorable genetics or those who do not achieve remission may be candidates for bone marrow transplantation.
- Prior to therapy, patients should be well hydrated, and if their WBC counts are high, they may be started on **allopurinol** to prevent hyperuricemia and renal insufficiency resulting from blast lysis (**tumor lysis syndrome**).
- Leukostasis syndrome may be treated with hydroxyurea +/– leukapheresis to rapidly ↓ WBC count.
- Indicators of a poor prognosis are as follows:
  - **ALL:** Age < 1 year or > 10 years; an ↑ in WBC count to > 50,000; the presence of the Philadelphia chromosome t(9,22) (associated with B-cell cancer); CNS involvement at diagnosis; and L3 morphology (associated with Burkitt's lymphoma).
  - **AML:** Age > 60 years, CD34+ or MDR1+ phenotype, elevated LDH, mutations in chromosomes 5 or 7, t(6,9), trisomy 8 or a more complex karyotype, *FLT3* gene mutation, and FAB M7 (acute megakaryocytic variant).
- AML type (FAB) **M3—acute promyelocytic leukemia (APL)**—has a good prognosis because it is responsive to **all-*trans*-retinoic acid (ATRA) therapy.** The mutation that causes this form of AML contains the retinoic acid receptor. ATRA is less toxic than conventional chemotherapy.

*A characteristic sign for AML type M3 (APL) is the **Auer rod**.*

Eighty-five percent of children with ALL achieve complete remission with chemotherapy.

CHRONIC LYMPHOCYTIC LEUKEMIA (CLL)

A malignant, clonal proliferation of functionally incompetent lymphocytes that accumulate in the bone marrow, peripheral blood, lymph nodes, spleen, and liver. The most common type of leukemia. A rare form of T-cell CLL exists, but almost all cases involve **well-differentiated B lymphocytes.** The etiology is unknown, although there is some genetic contribution, as first-degree relatives of patients with CLL are three times more likely than others to develop a lymphoid malignancy. Primarily affects **older adults** (median age 65); the male-to-female ratio is 2:1.

HISTORY/PE

Often asymptomatic, but many patients present with **fatigue, malaise, and infection.** Common physical findings are **lymphadenopathy and splenomegaly.**

DIAGNOSIS

- Diagnosed by the clinical picture; may be confirmed by **flow cytometry** demonstrating the presence of CD5—normally found only on T cells—on leukemic cells with the characteristic B-cell antigens CD20 and CD21.
- CBC shows lymphocytosis (lymphocyte count > 5000) with an abundance of small, normal-appearing lymphocytes and ruptured **smudge cells** on peripheral smear. **Granulocytopenia, anemia, and thrombocytopenia** are common owing to marrow infiltration with leukemic cells. Abnormal function by the leukemic cells leads to **hypogammaglobulinemia.**
- Bone marrow biopsy is rarely required for diagnosis or staging but may provide prognostic information and may help assess response to therapy.

CLL may be complicated by autoimmune hemolytic anemia.

The lymphoid equivalent of CLL is small lymphocytic lymphoma.

TREATMENT

- The clinical stage correlates with expected survival (see Table 2.7-7).
- Treatment is palliative. The degree of peripheral lymphocytosis does not correlate with prognosis, nor does it dictate when treatment should be initiated. **Treatment is often withheld until patients are symptomatic**—e.g., when they present with recurrent infection, severe lymphadenopathy or splenomegaly, anemia, and thrombocytopenia.
- Treatment consists primarily of **chemotherapy,** especially with alkylating agents, although radiation may be useful for localized lymphadenopathy.
- Although CLL is **not curable**, long disease-free intervals may be achieved with adequate treatment of symptoms.

CHRONIC MYELOGENOUS LEUKEMIA (CML)

Involves clonal expansion of myeloid progenitor cells, leading to leukocytosis with excess granulocytes and basophils and sometimes ↑ erythrocytes and platelets as well. To truly be CML, the BCR-ABL translocation must be present. In > 90% of patients, this is reflected by the **Philadelphia chromosome t(9,22).** CML primarily affects **middle-aged** patients.

HISTORY/PE

- With routine blood testing, many patients are diagnosed while asymptomatic. However, typical signs and symptoms are those of **anemia.**
- Patients frequently have **splenomegaly** with LUQ pain and early satiety. Hepatomegaly may be present as well. **Constitutional symptoms** of weight loss, anorexia, fever, and chills may also be seen.
- Patients with CML go through three disease phases:
    - **Chronic:** Without treatment, typically lasts 3.5–5.0 years. Signs and symptoms are as described above. Infection and bleeding complications are rare.
    - **Accelerated:** A transition toward blast crisis, with an ↑ in peripheral and bone marrow blood counts. Should be suspected when the differential shows an abrupt ↑ in basophils and thrombocytopenia < 100,000.
    - **Blast:** Resembles acute leukemia; survival is 3–6 months.

DIAGNOSIS

- Diagnosed by the clinical picture, including labs; cytogenetic analysis usually reveals the Philadelphia chromosome.

TABLE 2.7-7. Clinical Staging of CLL (Rai Staging)

STAGE	FINDINGS	MEDIAN SURVIVAL
0	Lymphocytosis ($> 15 \times 10^9$)	> 150 months
I	Lymphocytosis + lymphadenopathy	101 months
II	Lymphocytosis + splenomegaly	71 months
III	Lymphocytosis + anemia	19 months
IV	Lymphocytosis + thrombocytopenia	19 months

- CBwC shows a **very high WBC**—often > 100,000 at diagnosis, and sometimes reaching > 500,000. Differential shows granulocytes in all stages of maturation. Rarely, the WBC count will be so elevated as to cause a **hyperviscosity syndrome.**
- **Leukocyte alkaline phosphatase is low; LDH, uric acid, and B$_{12}$ levels are elevated.**

TREATMENT

Varies with disease phase and is undergoing rapid change, particularly since the introduction of targeted therapies:

- **Chronic:** Imatinib. Younger patients can be treated with allogeneic stem cell transplantation if a suitable matched sibling donor is available.
- **Blast:** Therapy as for acute leukemia or dasatinib plus hematopoietic stem cell transplant or clinical trial.

Imatinib (Gleevec) is a selective inhibitor of the BCR-ABL tyrosine kinase.

HAIRY CELL LEUKEMIA (HCL)

A malignant disorder of well-differentiated B lymphocytes with an unclear cause. HCL is a **rare** disease that accounts for 2% of adult leukemia cases and most commonly affects **older males.**

HISTORY/PE

- Typically presents with pancytopenia, bone marrow infiltration, and splenomegaly.
- Patients complain of weakness, fatigue, petechiae and bruising, infection (especially with atypical mycobacteria such as *Mycobacterium avium–intracellulare*), abdominal pain, early satiety, and weight loss. Symptoms are similar to those of CLL except that patients rarely have lymphadenopathy.

DIAGNOSIS

- Diagnosed by the history, physical exam, and labs; confirmed through the identification of hairy cells in the blood, marrow, or spleen.
- **Tartrate-resistant acid phosphatase (TRAP) staining of hairy cells,** electron microscopy, and **flow cytometry** (quantification of fluorescence on cells with fluorescent-labeled monoclonal antibodies bound to cell-specific antigens) are helpful in distinguishing the pathognomonic hairy cells.
- CBC usually demonstrates **leukopenia** (making the name *leukemia* a misnomer); roughly 85% of the time, a peripheral smear shows **hairy cells,** or **mononuclear cells with abundant pale cytoplasm and cytoplasmic projections.**

TREATMENT

- Ten percent of patients have a benign course and never require therapy, but the remainder develop progressive pancytopenia and splenomegaly. The median survival without treatment is five years.
- Treatment begins when patients are symptomatic or extremely cytopenic. **Nucleoside analogs** are currently the initial treatment of choice, and effectively induce remission. Other treatment options include splenectomy, which may improve blood counts, and IFN-α.

Lymphomas

Malignant transformations of lymphoid cells residing primarily in lymphoid tissues, especially the lymph nodes. Classically organized into Hodgkin's and non-Hodgkin's varieties.

Non-Hodgkin's Lymphoma (NHL)

NHL represents a progressive clonal expansion of B cells, T cells, and/or natural killer (NK) cells stimulated by chromosomal translocations, most commonly t(14,18); by the inactivation of tumor suppressor genes; or by the introduction of exogenous genes by oncogenic viruses (e.g., EBV, HTLV-1, HCV). There is a strong association between *H. pylori* infection and MALT gastric lymphoma. **Most NHLs (almost 85%) are of B-cell origin.** NHL is the **most common hematopoietic neoplasm** and is five times more common than Hodgkin's lymphoma.

History/PE

The median patient age is > **50 years,** but NHL may also be found in children, who tend to have more aggressive, higher-grade disease. Patient presentation varies with disease grade (see Table 2.7-8).

Diagnosis

- **Excisional lymph node biopsy** is necessary for diagnosis; the disease may first present at an extranodal site, which should be biopsied for diagnosis as well.
- A CSF exam should be done in patients with HIV, neurologic signs or symptoms, or 1° CNS lymphoma. **Disease staging (Ann Arbor classification) is based on the number of nodes and on whether the disease crosses the diaphragm.**

Treatment

- Treatment is based on histopathologic classification rather than on stage. Symptomatic patients are treated with radiation and chemotherapy

The treatment of high-grade NHL may be complicated by tumor lysis syndrome, in which rapid cell death releases intracellular contents and leads to hyperkalemia, hyperphosphatemia, hyperuricemia, and hypocalcemia.

TABLE 2.7-8. Presentation of Non-Hodgkin's Lymphoma

GRADE	HISTORY	PHYSICAL
Low	Painless peripheral adenopathy. Cytopenia from bone marrow involvement. Fatigue and weakness.	Peripheral adenopathy, splenomegaly, hepatomegaly.
Intermediate to high	Adenopathy. Extranodal disease (GI, GU, skin, thyroid, CNS). B symptoms (temperature > 38.5°C, night sweats, weight loss). Mass formation (e.g., abdominal mass with bowel obstruction in Burkitt's lymphoma; mediastinal mass and SVC syndrome in lymphoblastic lymphoma).	Bulky adenopathy, splenomegaly, hepatomegaly. Masses (abdominal, testicular, mediastinal). Skin findings.

(CHOP: cyclophosphamide [Cytoxan], Adriamycin, Oncovin [vincristine], and prednisone).

- The rule of thumb is for **low-grade, indolent NHL** to be treated with a **palliative approach** in symptomatic patients, and for **high-grade, aggressive NHL** to be treated **aggressively** with a **curative approach.**

HODGKIN'S DISEASE (HD)

A **predominantly B-cell malignancy** with an unclear etiology. There is a possible association with EBV. HD has a **bimodal age distribution,** peaking first in the third decade (primarily the nodular sclerosing type) and then in the elderly at around age 60 (mainly the lymphocyte-depleted type). It has a male predominance in childhood.

HISTORY/PE

- HD commonly presents as **cervical adenopathy,** although it may also present as a mediastinal mass; it is **usually found above the diaphragm,** with infradiaphragmatic involvement suggesting more widely disseminated disease.
- Patients also have **systemic B symptoms, pruritus, and hepatosplenomegaly. Pel-Ebstein fevers** (1–2 weeks of high fever alternating with 1–2 afebrile weeks) and **alcohol-induced pain** at nodal sites are rare signs that are specific for HD.

DIAGNOSIS

- Fine-needle biopsy is usually nondiagnostic, so diagnosis is usually made by **excisional lymph node biopsy,** which is examined for the classic **Reed-Sternberg (RS) cells** (giant abnormal B cells with bilobar nuclei and huge, eosinophilic nucleoli, which create an "owl's-eye" appearance) and for abnormal nodal morphology.
- Histologic types, in descending order of frequency, include nodular sclerosing, mixed cellularity, lymphocyte predominant, and lymphocyte depleted. Staging is based on the **number of nodes, the presence of B symptoms, and whether the disease crosses the diaphragm;** staging laparotomy is not recommended.

TREATMENT

- Treatment is stage dependent, involving chemotherapy and/or radiation. **Radiation is directed toward the involved lymph node area** plus the next contiguous region. Chemotherapy regimens used include ABVD (Adriamycin, bleomycin, vinblastine, dacarbazine) and MOPP (mechlorethamine, Oncovin [vincristine], procarbazine, and prednisone).
- **Five-year survival rates are very good** and are 90% for stage I and II disease (nodal disease limited to one side of the diaphragm), 84% for stage III, and 65% for stage IV.

Chemotherapy and radiation can lead to 2° neoplasms such as AML, NHL, breast cancer, and thyroid cancer.

► PLASMA CELL DISORDERS

Multiple Myeloma

Clonal proliferation of malignant plasma cells at varying stages of differentiation, with **excessive production of monoclonal immunoglobulins or immunoglobulin fragments** (kappa/lambda light chains). It is commonly believed to be a disease of the elderly, with a peak incidence in the seventh decade. Risk factors for disease development include radiation; monoclonal gammopathy of undetermined significance (MGUS); and, possibly, petroleum, pesticides, and other chemicals.

HISTORY/PE

Patients present with **anemia, plasmacytosis of the bone marrow, lytic bone lesions, hypercalcemia,** and **renal abnormalities.** They are prone to **infection** and have **elevated monoclonal (M) proteins** in the serum and/or urine.

DIAGNOSIS

- The classic triad of diagnostic criteria are > 10% plasma cells in the bone marrow and/or histologically proven plasma cell infiltration, M protein in serum or urine, and evidence of lytic bone lesions.
- The **presence of M proteins alone is insufficient for the diagnosis of multiple myeloma;** MGUS is relatively common. Other lymphoproliferative diseases may also result in M proteins, including CLL, lymphoma, Waldenström's macroglobulinemia, and amyloidosis.
- Patients should be evaluated with a skeletal survey, a bone marrow biopsy, serum and urine protein electrophoresis, and CBC.

TREATMENT

- Treat with **chemotherapy.**
- **Common initial treatment** involves a combination of melphalan (an oral alkylating agent) and prednisone and other agents. Myeloma cells tend to become resistant to drugs by an **MDR gene** mechanism, and autologous stem cell transplantation may be used to support more intensive doses of chemotherapy.

Waldenström's Macroglobulinemia

A clonal disorder of B cells that leads to a malignant monoclonal gammopathy. **Elevated levels of IgM** result in hyperviscosity syndrome, coagulation abnormalities, cryoglobulinemia, cold agglutinin disease (leading to autoimmune hemolytic anemia), and amyloidosis. Tissue is infiltrated by IgM and neoplastic plasma cells. A **chronic, indolent disease of the elderly.**

HISTORY/PE

- Presents with nonspecific symptoms of lethargy and weight loss along with **Raynaud's phenomenon** from cryoglobulinemia. Patients complain of **neurologic problems** ranging from mental status changes to sensorimotor peripheral neuropathy and blurry vision. Organomegaly and organ dysfunction affecting the skin, GI tract, kidneys, and lungs are also seen.
- As with multiple myeloma, **MGUS is a precursor** to disease.

DIAGNOSIS

- Labs show elevated ESR, uric acid, LDH, and alkaline phosphatase.
- **Bone marrow biopsy and aspirate** are required to establish the diagnosis. Marrow shows abnormal plasma cells, classically with **Dutcher bodies** (PAS-⊕ IgM deposits around the nucleus). Serum and urine protein electrophoresis and immunofixation are also used.

The combination of anemia and bone pain must always raise suspicion of multiple myeloma.

*Bone pain **at rest** should raise concern for malignancy.*

Hypercalcemia manifests in symptoms of polyuria, constipation, confusion, nausea, vomiting, and lethargy.

Because multiple myeloma is an osteoclastic process, a bone scan, which detects osteoblastic activity, may be ⊖.

TREATMENT

Excess immunoglobulin is removed with plasmapheresis; underlying lymphoma is treated with chemotherapy.

Amyloidosis

A generic term referring to extracellular deposition of protein fibrils. There are many different kinds of amyloidosis, involving different types of deposited fibrils with varying etiologies (see Table 2.7-9). Classically a disease of the **elderly.**

HISTORY/PE

- The clinical presentation depends on the type of precursor protein, tissue distribution, and the amount of amyloid deposition. In the two most common forms of systemic amyloidosis, 1° (AL) and 2° (AA), the major sites of clinically important amyloid deposition are in the kidneys, heart, and liver.
- In some disorders, clinically important amyloid deposition is limited to one organ (e.g., the brain in **Alzheimer's disease**).

DIAGNOSIS

Diagnosed by the clinical picture; confirmed by tissue biopsy with **Congo red staining** showing apple-green birefringence under polarized light.

TREATMENT

1° amyloidosis is treated with experimental chemotherapy to reduce protein burden; in 2° amyloidosis, the underlying condition should be addressed. Transplantation is also used; kidney transplantation may cure dialysis-related amyloid, and liver transplantation may cure heritable amyloid.

TABLE 2.7-9. Types of Amyloidosis

AMYLOID	CAUSE
AL	A plasma cell dyscrasia, with deposition of monoclonal light-chain fragments. Associated with multiple myeloma and Waldenström's macroglobulinemia.
AA	Deposition of the acute-phase reactant serum amyloid A. Associated with chronic inflammatory diseases (e.g., rheumatoid arthritis), infections, and neoplasms.
Dialysis-related	Deposition of β_2 microglobulin, which accumulates in patients on long-term dialysis.
Heritable	Deposition of abnormal gene products (e.g., transthyretin, aka prealbumin). A heterogeneous group of disorders.
Senile-systemic	Deposition of otherwise normal transthyretin.

An **absolute neutrophil count (ANC) < 1500,** where ANC = (WBC count) (% bands + % segmented neutrophils) (0.01). Neutropenia may be due to a combination of ↓ production, sequestration to marginated or tissue pools, and ↑ destruction or utilization. It may be acquired or intrinsic (see Table 2.7-10).

HISTORY/PE

Patients are at ↑ **risk of infection,** which varies inversely with neutrophil count.

- **Acute neutropenia:** Associated with **S. aureus, Pseudomonas, E. coli, Proteus,** and **Klebsiella** sepsis.
- **Chronic and autoimmune neutropenia:** Presents with **recurrent sinusitis, stomatitis, gingivitis,** and **perirectal infections** rather than sepsis. Some chronic neutropenias are accompanied by splenomegaly (e.g., Felty's syndrome, Gaucher's disease, sarcoidosis).

DIAGNOSIS

- The history and physical exam are the cornerstones of diagnosis.
- CBC with ANC may be used to follow neutropenia. If thrombocytopenia or anemia is present, bone marrow biopsy and aspirate should be performed.
- Serum immunologic evaluation, ANA levels, and a workup for collagen vascular disease may be merited.

TABLE 2.7-10. Acquired vs. Intrinsic Neutropenia

TYPE	CAUSE
Acquired	Drug induced (e.g., **chemotherapy,** ethanol, antibiotics, NSAIDs), usually by marrow suppression. Marrow-infiltrating disorders.
	Postinfectious.
	HIV infection.
	Benign familial leukopenia (seen in Yemenite Jews, West Indians, and people of African descent; due to genetic variation).
	Chronic idiopathic neutropenia (occurs in infancy and childhood; thought to be due to production of antineutrophil IgG).
	Autoimmune neutropenia (isolated or 2° to rheumatoid arthritis or SLE).
	Nutritional deficiency (B_{12}/folate or thiamine deficiency).
	Metabolic disease (ketoacidosis, hyperglycinuria, orotic aciduria, MMA, hypothyroidism, Gaucher's disease).
Intrinsic	Dyskeratosis congenita (X-linked, with integument abnormalities and hypocellular marrow).
	Kostmann's syndrome (aka infantile agranulocytosis).
	Shwachman-Diamond-Oski syndrome (neutropenia, metaphyseal dysplasia, and pancreatic insufficiency).
	Chédiak-Higashi syndrome (oculocutaneous albinism, neurologic impairment, and giant granules in cells).
	Fanconi's anemia.

TREATMENT

- Infection management is most important; patients may not be able to mount an inflammatory response to infection owing to their lack of neutrophils.
- Fever in the context of neutropenia should be treated immediately with **broad-spectrum antibiotics.** Suspected fungal infections should be treated appropriately as well.
- Hematopoietic stem cell factors such as **G-CSF** can be used to shorten the duration of neutropenia. In some instances, **IVIG and allogeneic bone marrow transplantation** may be used.

Hypothermia can be caused by fungemia.

► EOSINOPHILIA

Absolute eosinophil count = (WBC) (% eosinophils) (0.01). **Normal levels do not exceed 350.** Eosinophilia can be triggered by the overproduction of one or more of three eosinophilopoietic cytokines (IL-3, IL-5, and GM-CSF) or by chemokines that stimulate the migration of eosinophils into peripheral blood and tissues. Eosinophilia may be a 1° disorder, but it **usually occurs 2° to another cause** (see Table 2.7-11).

HISTORY/PE

- A **travel, medication, atopic, and diet history** should be elicited along with a history of symptoms relating to lymphoma/leukemia.
- Physical exam findings vary. Patients with hypereosinophilic syndrome (HES) may present with fever, anemia, and prominent cardiac findings (emboli from mural thrombi, abnormal ECGs, CHF, murmurs). Other affected organs include the lung, liver, spleen, skin, and nervous system (due to eosinophilic infiltration).

DIAGNOSIS

- In addition to a history and physical, a CBC and differential should be obtained, and **CSF should be analyzed for eosinophilia,** which is suggestive

Causes of 2° eosinophilia—

NAACP

Neoplasm
Allergies
Asthma
Collagen vascular disease
Parasites

TABLE 2.7-11. Etiologies of Eosinophilia

TYPE	CAUSES
1°	**Hypereosinophilic syndrome:** Unknown etiology.
	Hereditary eosinophilia: Autosomal-dominant inheritance; rare.
	Eosinophilia-myalgia syndrome: Results from abnormal tryptophan metabolism.
2°	**Allergic states with elevated serum IgE:** The most common cause in the United States.
	Parasitic diseases: The most common cause worldwide.
	Other:
	Coccidioidomycosis.
	Vasculitis (e.g., Churg-Strauss syndrome).
	Benign or malignant hematologic disorders; also solid tumors.
	Collagen vascular diseases (e.g., dermatomyositis, PAN).
	Drug induced (e.g., sulfonamides, iodides, ASA, phenytoin).

of a drug reaction or infection with a coccidioidomycosis or a helminth. Hematuria with eosinophilia may be a sign of schistosomiasis.

- **Imaging of the lungs, abdomen, pelvis, and brain** may demonstrate a focal defect that may be helpful in narrowing down the potential causes.

TREATMENT

Medication should be tailored to the cause of the eosinophilia. HES is treated with corticosteroid and cytotoxic agents to ↓ the eosinophilia.

▶ TRANSPLANT MEDICINE

- Tissue transplantation is increasingly used to treat a variety of diseases. Types of transplantation include the following:
    - **Autologous:** Transplantation from the patient to him/herself.
    - **Allogeneic:** Transplantation from a donor to a genetically different patient.
    - **Syngeneic:** Transplantation between identical twins (i.e., from a donor to a genetically identical patient).
- With allogeneic donation, efforts are made to ABO and HLA match the donor and recipient. Even with antigenic matching and immunosuppression, however, transplants may be rejected. There are three types of rejection: hyperacute, acute, and chronic (see Table 2.7-12).
- **Graft-versus-host disease** (GVHD) is a complication specific to allogeneic bone marrow transplantation in which donated T cells attack host tissues. It may be acute (occurring < 100 days post-transplant) or chronic (occurring > 100 days afterward).
    - **Minor histocompatibility antigens are thought to be responsible for GVHD,** which typically presents with **skin changes, cholestatic liver dysfunction, obstructive lung disease,** or **GI problems.**
    - Patients are treated with **high-dose corticosteroids.**

TABLE 2.7-12.   Types of Transplant Rejection

	HYPERACUTE	ACUTE	CHRONIC
Timing after transplant	Within minutes.	Five days to three months.	Months to years.
Pathomechanism	Preformed antibodies.	T-cell mediated.	Chronic immune reaction causing fibrosis.
Tissue findings	Vascular thrombi; tissue ischemia.	Laboratory evidence of tissue destruction such as ↑ GGT, alkaline phosphatase, LDH, BUN, or creatinine.	Gradual loss of organ function.
Prevention	Check ABO compatibility.	N/A	N/A
Treatment	Cytotoxic agents.	Confirm with sampling of transplanted tissue; treat with corticosteroids, antilymphocyte antibodies (OKT3), tacrolimus, or mycophenolate mofetil (MMF).	No treatment; biopsy to rule out treatable acute reaction.

- The typical regimen after transplant can include these commonly used drugs: prednisone, MMF, FK506 (tacrolimus), TMP-SMX, ganciclovir, and ketoconazole.
- A variant of GVHD is the **graft-versus-leukemia effect,** in which leukemia patients who are treated with an allogeneic bone marrow transplant have significantly lower relapse rates than those treated with an autologous transplant. This difference is thought to be due to a reaction of donated T cells against leukemic cells.

▶ **DISEASES ASSOCIATED WITH NEOPLASMS**

Table 2.7-13 outlines conditions that are commonly associated with neoplasms.

TABLE 2.7-13. Disorders Associated with Neoplasms

CONDITION	NEOPLASM
Down syndrome	ALL ("We will **ALL** go **Down** together").
Xeroderma pigmentosum	Squamous cell and basal cell carcinomas of the skin.
Chronic atrophic gastritis, pernicious anemia, postsurgical gastric remnants	Gastric adenocarcinoma.
Tuberous sclerosis (facial angiofibroma, seizures, mental retardation)	Astrocytoma and cardiac rhabdomyoma.
Actinic keratosis	Squamous cell carcinoma of the skin.
Barrett's esophagus (chronic GI reflux)	Esophageal adenocarcinoma.
Plummer-Vinson syndrome (atrophic glossitis, esophageal webs, anemia; all due to iron deficiency)	Squamous cell carcinoma of the esophagus.
Cirrhosis (alcoholic, HBV or HCV)	Hepatocellular carcinoma.
Ulcerative colitis	Colonic adenocarcinoma.
Paget's disease of bone	2° osteosarcoma and fibrosarcoma.
Immunodeficiency states	Malignant lymphomas.
AIDS	Aggressive malignant NHLs and Kaposi's sarcoma.
Autoimmune diseases (e.g., myasthenia gravis)	Benign and malignant thymomas.
Acanthosis nigricans (hyperpigmentation and epidermal thickening)	Visceral malignancy (stomach, lung, breast, uterus).
Dysplastic nevus	Malignant melanoma.

Infectious Disease

Pneumonia

Some common causes of pneumonia are outlined in Table 2.8-1.

HISTORY/PE

- **May present classically or atypically.**
  - **Classic symptoms:** Sudden onset, fever, productive cough (purulent yellow-green sputum or hemoptysis), dyspnea, night sweats, pleuritic chest pain.
  - **Atypical symptoms:** Gradual onset, dry cough, headaches, myalgias, sore throat.
- Lung exam may show ↓ or bronchial breath sounds, rales, wheezing, dullness to percussion, egophony, and tactile fremitus.
- Elderly patients as well as those with COPD, diabetes, or immunocompromised status may have minimal or atypical signs on physical exam.

DIAGNOSIS

- Workup includes physical exam, **CXR**, CBC, sputum Gram stain and culture (see Figures 2.8-1 and 2.8-2), nasopharyngeal aspirate, blood culture, and ABG.
- Tests for specific pathogens include the following:
  - **Legionella:** Urine *Legionella* antigen test (detects only serogroup 1), sputum staining with direct fluorescent antibody (DFA), culture.
  - **Chlamydia pneumoniae:** Serologic testing, culture, PCR.

TABLE 2.8-1. Common Causes of Pneumonia

CHILDREN (6 WKS–18 YRS)	ADULTS (18–40 YRS)	ADULTS (40–65 YRS)	ELDERLY
Viruses (RSV)	*Mycoplasma*	*S. pneumoniae*	*S. pneumoniae*
Mycoplasma	*C. pneumoniae*	*H. influenzae*	Viruses
Chlamydia pneumoniae	*S. pneumoniae*	Anaerobes	Anaerobes
Streptococcus pneumoniae		Viruses	*H. influenzae*
		Mycoplasma	Gram-⊕ rods

Special groups:	
Atypical	*Mycoplasma, Legionella, Chlamydia*
Nosocomial (hospital acquired)	Gram-⊖ rods (GNRs), *Staphylococcus,* anaerobes
Immunocompromised	*Staphylococcus,* gram-⊕ rods, fungi, viruses, *Pneumocystis jiroveci* (with HIV), mycobacteria
Aspiration	Anaerobes
Alcoholics/IV drug users	*S. pneumoniae, Klebsiella, Staphylococcus*
Cystic fibrosis (CF)	*Pseudomonas, Burkholderia, S. aureus,* mycobacteria
COPD	*H. influenzae, Moraxella catarrhalis, S. pneumoniae*
Postviral	*Staphylococcus, H. influenzae*
Neonate	Group B streptococci (GBS), *E. coli*
Recurrent	Obstruction, bronchogenic carcinoma, lymphoma, Wegener's granulomatosis, immunodeficiency, unusual organisms (e.g., *Nocardia, Coxiella burnetii, Aspergillus, Pseudomonas*)

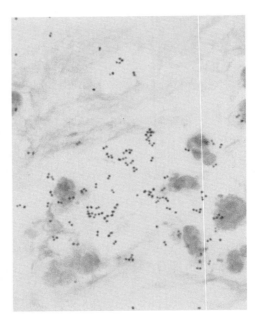

FIGURE 2.8-1. *S. aureus.*

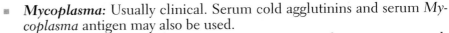

These clusters of gram-⊕ cocci were isolated from the sputum of a patient who developed pneumonia while hospitalized.

An adequate sputum Gram stain sample has many PMNs (> 25 cells/hpf) and few epithelial cells (< 25 cells/hpf).

- ■ *Mycoplasma:* Usually clinical. Serum cold agglutinins and serum *Mycoplasma* antigen may also be used.
- ■ *Streptococcus pneumoniae:* Urine pneumococcal antigen test, culture.
- ■ **Viral:** Nasopharyngeal aspirate, rapid tests for pathogens (e.g., influenza, RSV), DFA, viral culture.

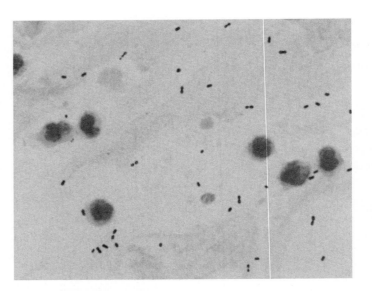

FIGURE 2.8-2. *S. pneumoniae.*

Sputum sample from a patient with pneumonia. Note the characteristic lancet-shaped gram-⊕ diplococci.

- Table 2.8-2 summarizes the recommended initial treatment for pneumonia.
- Outpatient treatment with oral antibiotics is recommended only in uncomplicated cases.
- **In-hospital treatment with IV antibiotics** is recommended for patients > 65 years of age and in those with comorbidity (alcoholism, COPD, diabetes, malnutrition), immunosuppression, unstable vitals or signs of respiratory failure, altered mental status, and/or multilobar involvement.
- For patients with obstructive diseases (e.g., CF or bronchiectasis), consider adding pseudomonal, staphylococcal, or anaerobic coverage.

The PORT criteria (i.e., pneumonia severity index) risk-stratifies patients with pneumonia on the basis of age, comorbidity, and presentation. Note: The PORT criteria do not apply to AIDS patients.

Tuberculosis (TB)

Infection due to *Mycobacterium tuberculosis*. Initial infection usually leads to latent TB infection (LTBI) that is asymptomatic. Most symptomatic cases (i.e., cases of active disease) are due to reactivation of latent infection rather

TABLE 2.8-2. Treatment of Pneumonia

PATIENT TYPE	SUSPECTED PATHOGENS	EMPIRIC COVERAGE
Outpatient community-acquired pneumonia, patients ≤ 65 years of age, otherwise healthy	*S. pneumoniae, Mycoplasma pneumoniae, C. pneumoniae, H. influenzae,* viral.	Macrolide (azithromycin), doxycycline, or fluoroquinolone.
Patients > 65 years of age or with comorbidity (COPD, heart failure, renal failure, diabetes, liver disease, EtOH abuse)	*S. pneumoniae, H. influenzae,* aerobic GNRs (*E. coli, Enterobacter, Klebsiella*), *S. aureus, Legionella,* viruses.	Macrolide or fluoroquinolone. Consider adding a second-generation cephalosporin or β-lactam to the macrolide.
Community-acquired pneumonia requiring hospitalization	*S. pneumoniae, H. influenzae,* anaerobes, aerobic GNRs, *Legionella, Chlamydia.*	Extended-spectrum cephalosporin, β-lactam/β-lactamase inhibitor, or fluoroquinolone. Add a macrolide if atypical organisms are suspected.
Community-acquired pneumonia requiring ICU care	*S. pneumoniae, H. influenzae,* anaerobes, aerobic GNRs, *Mycoplasma, Legionella, Pseudomonas.*	Fluoroquinolone or extended-spectrum cephalosporin or β-lactam/β-lactamase inhibitor + macrolide.
Institution-/hospital-acquired pneumonia—patients hospitalized > 48 hours or in a long-term care facility > 14 days	GNRs (including *Pseudomonas and Acinetobacter*), *S. aureus, Legionella,* mixed flora.	Extended-spectrum cephalosporin or β-lactam with antipseudomonal activity or carbapenem. Consider adding an aminoglycoside or a fluoroquinolone for coverage of resistant organisms (*Pseudomonas*) until lab sensitivities identify the best single agent.
Patients who are critically ill or worsening over 24–48 hours on initial antibiotic therapy	Methicillin-resistant *S. aureus* (MRSA).	Add vancomycin or linezolid; broader gram-⊖ coverage.

than to 1° exposure. Pulmonary TB is most common, but disseminated or extrapulmonary TB should be considered as well.

- TB can infect almost any organ system, including the lungs, CNS, GU tract, bone, and GI tract.
- Risk factors for active disease (i.e., reactivation) include immunosuppression (HIV), alcoholism, preexisting lung disease, diabetes, and advancing age. Risk factors for TB exposure include **homelessness** and crowded living conditions (e.g., **prison**), immigration/travel from developing nations, working in an allied health profession, and interacting with known TB contacts.

TB almost always presents with an extended duration (> 3 weeks) of symptoms.

HISTORY/PE

Presents with cough, **hemoptysis**, dyspnea, **weight loss, fatigue, night sweats, fever,** cachexia, hypoxia, tachycardia, lymphadenopathy, an abnormal lung exam, and a prolonged (> 3-week) symptom duration. TB is a common cause of fever of unknown origin (FUO). HIV patients can present with atypical signs and symptoms and have higher rates of extrapulmonary TB.

DIAGNOSIS

- **Active disease:** Mycobacterial culture of sputum (or blood/tissue for extrapulmonary disease) is the gold standard but can take weeks to obtain. A sputum **acid-fast stain** (see Figure 2.8-3) can yield rapid preliminary results but lacks sensitivity.
  - Three A.M. sputum samples for AFB stain and a mycobacterial culture are advised. If the results of the stain are ⊖ but there is a high degree of clinical suspicion, proceed to bronchoscopy with bronchoalveolar lavage or biopsy. HIV patients have a high rate of ⊖ sputum stains (i.e., a ⊖ AFB smear accompanied by a ⊕ culture).
  - The most common finding among typical hosts is a cavitary infiltrate in the upper lobe on CXR. HIV patients or those with 1° TB may show lower lobe infiltrates with or without cavitation. Multiple fine nodular

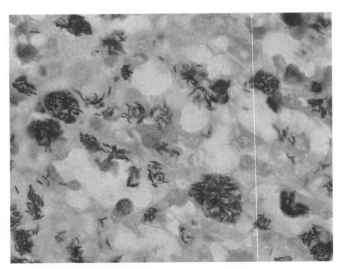

FIGURE 2.8-3. **TB organisms are identified by their red color ("red snappers") on acid-fast staining.**

(Reproduced, with permission, from the Pathology Education Instructional Resource Digital Library [http://peir.net] at the University of Alabama, Birmingham.)

densities distributed throughout both lungs are typical of miliary TB, which represents hematologic or lymphatic dissemination.

- **LTBI (i.e., previous exposure):** Diagnose with a ⊕ PPD test (see Figure 2.8-4). Immunocompromised individuals with LTBI may not mount a ⊕ PPD (anergy). Interferon-gamma release assays are now available to diagnose LTBI as well. All cases of LTBI should be evaluated (e.g., with a CXR) to rule out active disease.

TREATMENT

All cases should be reported to local and state health departments. Respiratory isolation should be instituted if TB is suspected. Treatment is as follows:

- **Active TB:** Directly observed multidrug therapy with a four-drug regimen (**INH, pyrazinamide, rifampin, ethambutol**) × 2 months, followed by four months with INH and rifampin.
- Administer **vitamin B$_6$** (pyridoxine) with **INH** to prevent peripheral neuritis.
- **Latent TB:** For conversion of PPD without signs/symptoms of active disease, initiate therapy with INH × 9 months. Alternative regimens include INH × 6 months or rifampin × 4 months.

Rifampin turns body fluids orange. Ethambutol can cause optic neuritis. INH causes peripheral neuritis and hepatitis.

Acute Pharyngitis

Viral causes are more common (90% in adults), but it is important to identify streptococcal pharyngitis (**group A β-hemolytic *Streptococcus pyogenes***). Etiologies are as follows:

- **Bacterial:** Group A streptococci (GAS), *Neisseria gonorrhoeae, Corynebacterium diphtheriae, M. pneumoniae.*
- **Viral:** Rhinovirus, coronavirus, adenovirus, HSV, EBV, CMV, influenza virus, coxsackievirus, acute HIV infection.

HISTORY/PE

- **Typical of streptococcal pharyngitis:** Fever, sore throat, pharyngeal erythema, tonsillar exudate, cervical lymphadenopathy, soft palate petechiae, headache, vomiting, scarlatiniform rash (indicates scarlet fever).
- **Atypical of streptococcal pharyngitis:** Coryza, hoarseness, rhinorrhea, cough, conjunctivitis, anterior stomatitis, ulcerative lesions, GI symptoms.

PPD is injected intradermally on the volar surface of the forearm. The diameter of induration is measured at 48–72 hours. BCG vaccination typically renders a patient PPD ⊕ but should not preclude prophylaxis as recommended for unvaccinated individuals. The size of induration that indicates a ⊕ test is interpreted as follows:

- **≥ 5 mm:** HIV or risk factors, close TB contacts, CXR evidence of TB.
- **≥ 10 mm:** Indigent/homeless, residents of developing nations, IV drug use, chronic illness, residents of health and correctional institutions, and health care workers.
- **≥ 15 mm:** Everyone else, including those with no known risk factors.

A ⊖ reaction with ⊖ controls implies anergy from immunosuppression, old age, or malnutrition and thus does not rule out TB.

FIGURE 2.8-4.   PPD interpretation.

DIAGNOSIS

Diagnosed by clinical evaluation, rapid GAS antigen detection, and throat culture. With three out of four of the Centor criteria, the sensitivity of rapid antigen testing is > 90%.

TREATMENT

If GAS is suspected, begin empiric antibiotic therapy with penicillin × 10 days. Cephalosporins, amoxicillin, and azithromycin are alternative options. Symptom relief can be attained with fluids, rest, antipyretics, and salt-water gargles.

COMPLICATIONS

- **Nonsuppurative:** Acute rheumatic fever (see the Cardiovascular chapter), poststreptococcal glomerulonephritis.
- **Suppurative:** Cervical lymphadenitis, mastoiditis, sinusitis, otitis media, retropharyngeal or peritonsillar abscess, and, rarely, thrombophlebitis of the jugular vein (**Lemierre's syndrome**) due to *Fusobacterium*, an oral anaerobe.
- **Peritonsillar abscess** may present with odynophagia, trismus ("lockjaw"), a muffled voice, unilateral tonsillar enlargement, and erythema, with the uvula and soft palate deviated away from the affected side. Culture abscess fluid and localize the abscess via intraoral ultrasound or CT. Treat with antibiotics and **surgical drainage.**

Sinusitis

Refers to inflammation of the paranasal sinuses. The maxillary sinuses are most commonly affected. Can be classified by site, organism, or chronicity. Subtypes include the following:

- **Acute sinusitis (symptoms lasting < 1 month):** Most commonly associated with viruses, *S. pneumoniae*, *H. influenzae*, and *M. catarrhalis*. Bacterial causes are rare and are characterized by symptoms lasting < 1 week.
- **Chronic sinusitis (symptoms persisting > 3 months):** Represents a chronic inflammatory process. Often due to obstruction of sinus drainage and ongoing low-grade anaerobic infections. In diabetic patients, mucormycosis should be considered.

HISTORY/PE

- Presents with **fever, facial pain/pressure, headache,** nasal congestion, and discharge. Exam may reveal tenderness, erythema, and swelling over the affected area.
- High fever, leukocytosis, and a purulent nasal discharge are suggestive of acute bacterial sinusitis.

DIAGNOSIS

- A clinical diagnosis. Culture and radiography are generally not required for acute sinusitis but may guide the management of chronic cases.
- Transillumination shows opacification of the sinuses (low sensitivity).
- CT is the test of choice for sinus imaging (see Figure 2.8-5) but is usually necessary only if symptoms persist after treatment. MRI is useful for differentiating soft tissue (as in a tumor) from mucus.

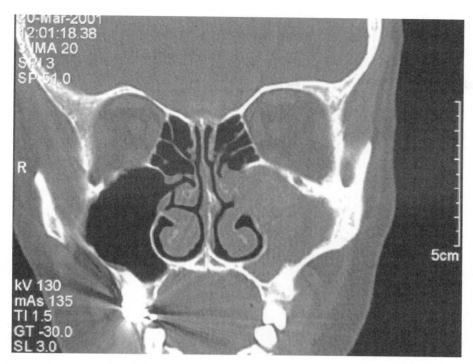

FIGURE 2.8-5. Sinusitis.

Compare the opacified left maxillary sinus and normal air-filled right sinus on this coronal CT scan. (Reproduced, with permission, from Lalwani AK. *Current Diagnosis & Treatment in Otolaryngology: Head and Neck Surgery*, 2nd ed. New York: McGraw-Hill, 2008: Fig. 14-2.)

- Bacterial culture by sinus tap is the gold standard for diagnosis but is not routinely performed because of discomfort. Endoscopically guided cultures from the middle meatus are gaining popularity.

TREATMENT

- Most cases of acute sinusitis are viral and/or self-limited and can thus be treated with symptomatic therapy (decongestants, antihistamines, pain relief).
- **Acute bacterial sinusitis (usually < 7 days):** Consider amoxicillin/clavulanate 500 mg PO TID × 10 days or, alternatively, clarithromycin, azithromycin, TMP-SMX, fluoroquinolone, or a second-generation cephalosporin × 10 days.
- **Chronic sinusitis (4–12 weeks): Adjuvant** therapy with intranasal corticosteroids, decongestants, and antihistamines may be useful in combating the allergic/inflammatory component of the disease. Antibiotics given are similar to those used for acute disease, although a **longer course** (3–6 weeks) may be necessary. **Surgical** intervention may also be required.

Coccidioidomycosis

A pulmonary fungal infection endemic to the **southwestern United States** (e.g., San Joaquin Valley, California). Can present as an acute or subacute pneumonia or as a flulike illness, and may involve extrapulmonary sites, including bone, CNS, and skin. The incubation period is 1–4 weeks after exposure. Filipino, African-American, pregnant, and HIV-⊕ patients are at ↑ risk.

Potential complications of sinusitis include meningitis, frontal bone osteomyelitis, cavernous sinus thrombosis, and abscess formation.

Consider coccidioidomycosis in the HIV-⊕, Filipino, African-American, or pregnant patient from the southwestern United States with respiratory infection.

HISTORY/PE

Patients present with **fever,** anorexia, headache, chest pain, **cough,** dyspnea, arthralgias, and **night sweats.** Disseminated infection can present with meningitis, bone lesions, and soft tissue abscesses.

DIAGNOSIS

- Obtain bronchoalveolar lavage along with fungal cultures of sputum, wound exudate, or other affected tissue.
- Identify *Coccidioides immitis* spherules on H&E or other special stains of sputum or tissue.
- Precipitin antibodies (IgM) ↑ within two weeks and disappear after two months; complement fixation antibodies (IgG) ↑ at 1–3 months. Titers > 1:16 indicate disseminated infection.
- CXR findings may be normal or may show infiltrates, nodules, cavity, mediastinal or hilar adenopathy, or pleural effusion.
- Consider bronchoscopy, fine-needle biopsy, open lung biopsy, or pleural biopsy if serology is indeterminate.

TREATMENT

- **Acute:** IV therapy is rarely necessary; however, consider **IV amphotericin B** for severe or protracted 1° pulmonary infection and disseminated disease. PO fluconazole or itraconazole may be used for mild infection or continuation therapy once the patient is stable.
- **Chronic:** No treatment is needed for asymptomatic chronic pulmonary nodules or cavities. Progressive cavitary or symptomatic disease usually requires surgery plus long-term azole therapy for 8–12 months.

Influenza

A highly contagious orthomyxovirus transmitted by droplet nuclei. There are three types of influenza: A, B, and C. Subtypes of influenza A (e.g., H5N1, H1N1) are classified on the basis of glycoproteins (hemagglutinin and neuraminidase). Relevant terms are as follows:

- **Antigenic drift:** Refers to small, gradual changes in surface proteins through point mutations. These small changes are sufficient to allow the virus to escape immune recognition, accounting for the fact that individuals can be infected with influenza multiple times.
- **Antigenic shift:** Refers to an acute, major change in the influenza A subtype (significant genetic reassortment) circulating among humans; leads to pandemics.

In the United States, the typical influenza season begins in November and lasts until March. Vaccination with inactivated influenza virus is recommended for patients > 50 years of age, children 6 months to 19 years of age, patients of any age with chronic medical problems (e.g., diabetes, heart disease, renal failure, HIV), pregnant women, nursing home residents, and contacts of high-risk groups (e.g., health care workers).

HISTORY/PE

Patients typically present with abrupt onset of fevers, myalgias, chills, cough, coryza, and weakness. Elderly patients may have atypical presentations characterized only by confusion.

DIAGNOSIS

Leukopenia is a common finding. Rapid influenza tests of viral antigens from nasopharyngeal swabs are available. More definitive diagnosis can be made with DFA tests or viral culture.

TREATMENT

Symptomatic care with analgesics and cough medicine. Antivirals such as oseltamivir or zanamivir are most effective when used within two days of onset and may shorten the course of infection by 1–2 days.

COMPLICATIONS

- Severe 1° viral pneumonia, 2° bacterial pneumonia, sinusitis, bronchitis, and exacerbation of COPD and asthma can occur.
- Reye's syndrome, or fatty liver encephalopathy, has been associated with ASA use in children with viral infections, including influenza.

A live attenuated, nasally delivered influenza vaccine is available for healthy people 2–49 years of age who are not pregnant or severely immunocompromised.

▶ CNS INFECTIONS

Meningitis

Risk factors for meningitis include recent ear infection, sinusitis, immunodeficiencies, recent neurosurgical procedures, and sick contacts. Causes are listed in Table 2.8-3.

HISTORY/PE

Patients present with **fever,** malaise, **headache, neck stiffness, photophobia,** altered mental status, **nausea/vomiting,** seizures, or signs of meningeal irritation (⊕ Kernig's and Brudzinski's signs).

DIAGNOSIS

- Obtain **blood cultures.**
- **LP** for **CSF Gram stain and culture;** obtain glucose, protein, WBC count plus differential, RBC count, and opening pressure (in the absence of papilledema or focal neurologic deficits).
- **Viral PCRs** (e.g., HSV); **cryptococcal antigen** (for HIV patients).
- **CT or MRI** to rule out other diagnoses. CBC may reveal leukocytosis; CSF findings vary (see Table 2.8-4).

TABLE 2.8-3. **Causes of Meningitis**[a,b]

| | CHILDREN | | |
NEWBORN (0–6 MOS)	(6 MOS–6 YRS)	6–60 YRS	60 YRS +
GBS	S. pneumoniae	N. meningitidis	S. pneumoniae
E. coli/GNRs	Neisseria meningitidis	Enteroviruses	GNRs
Listeria	H. influenzae type b	S. pneumoniae	Listeria
	Enteroviruses	HSV	N. meningitidis

[a] Causes in HIV include *Cryptococcus,* CMV, HSV, VZV, TB, toxoplasmosis (brain abscess), and JC virus (PML).

[b] Note: The incidence of *H. influenzae* meningitis has ↓ greatly with the introduction of the *H. influenzae* vaccine in the last 10–15 years.

TABLE 2.8-4. CSF Profiles

	RBCs (per mm³)	WBCs (per mm³)	GLUCOSE (mg/dL)	PROTEIN (mg/dL)	OPENING PRESSURE (cm H₂O)	APPEARANCE	GAMMA GLOBULIN (% PROTEIN)
Normal	< 10	< 5	~2/3 of serum	15–45	10–20	Clear	3–12
Bacterial meningitis	↔	↑ (> 1000 PMNs)	↓	↑	↑	Cloudy	↔ or ↑
Viral meningitis	↔	↑ (monos/ lymphs)	↔	↔ or ↑	↔ or ↑	Most often clear	↔ or ↑
Aseptic meningitis	↔	↑	↔	↔ or ↑	↔	Clear	↔
SAH	↑↑	↑	↔	↑	↔ or ↑	Yellow/red	↔ or ↑
Guillain-Barré syndrome	↔	↔	↔ or ↑	↑↑	↔	Clear or yellow (high protein)	↔
MS	↔	↔ or ↑	↔	↔	↔	Clear	↑↑
Pseudotumor cerebri	↔	↔	↔	↔	↑↑↑	Clear	↔

TREATMENT

- Antibiotics should be administered rapidly (see Table 2.8-5) and may be given empirically up to two hours before an LP is performed.
- Some cases of viral meningitis can be treated with supportive care and close follow-up.
- Close contacts of patients with meningococcal meningitis should receive **rifampin,** ciprofloxacin, or ceftriaxone prophylaxis.

TABLE 2.8-5. Empiric Treatment of Bacterial Meningitis

AGE	CAUSATIVE ORGANISM	TREATMENT
< 1 month	GBS, *E. coli*/GNRs, *Listeria*.	Ampicillin + cefotaxime or gentamicin.
1–3 months	Pneumococci, meningococci, *H. influenzae*.	Vancomycin IV + ceftriaxone or cefotaxime.
3 months – adulthood	Pneumococci, meningococci.	Vancomycin IV + ceftriaxone or cefotaxime.
> 60 years/alcoholism/ chronic illness	Pneumococci, gram-⊖ bacilli, *Listeria*, meningococci.	Ampicillin + vancomycin + cefotaxime or ceftriaxone.

- **Dexamethasone** may be beneficial in bacterial meningitis, especially S. *pneumoniae*, if given 15–20 minutes before antibiotics.

COMPLICATIONS

- **Cerebral edema:** Visible on CT/MRI. Presents with loss of oculocephalic reflex. Treat with IV mannitol.
- **Subdural effusions:** May be seen on CT scan. Occur in 50% of infants with *H. influenzae* meningitis. No treatment is necessary.
- **Ventriculitis/hydrocephalus:** Presents as a worsening clinical picture with improved CSF findings. Requires ventriculostomy and possibly intraventricular antibiotics.
- **Seizures:** Treat with benzodiazepines and phenytoin.
- **Hyponatremia:** Administer fluids and monitor sodium concentration.
- **Subdural empyema:** Presents with intractable seizures. Requires surgical evacuation.
- **Other:** Cranial nerve palsies, sensorineural hearing loss, coma, death.

Although other medications may be used, rifampin is the frequently tested prophylaxis of choice for close contacts of patients with meningococcal meningitis.

Encephalitis

HSV and **arboviruses** are the most common causes of encephalitis. Rarer etiologies include CMV, toxoplasmosis, West Nile virus, VZV, *Borrelia*, *Rickettsia*, *Legionella*, enterovirus, *Mycoplasma*, and cerebral malaria. Children and the elderly are the most vulnerable.

HISTORY/PE

- Presents with **altered consciousness, headache, fever, and seizures.** Lethargy, confusion, coma, and focal neurologic deficits (cranial nerve deficits, accentuated DTRs) may also be present.
- The differential includes brain abscess or malignancy, toxic-metabolic encephalopathy, subdural hematoma, and SAH.

DIAGNOSIS

- CSF shows lymphocytic pleocytosis and moderately ↑ protein. RBCs without evidence of trauma suggest HSV encephalitis. The glucose level is low in tuberculous, fungal, bacterial, and amebic infections.
- Obtain a CSF Gram stain (bacteria), acid-fast stain (mycobacteria), India ink (*Cryptococcus*), wet preparation (free-living amebae), and Giemsa stain (trypanosomes). **PCR** for HSV, CMV, EBV, VZV, and enterovirus.
- **MRI** may demonstrate a **contrast-enhancing lesion** in the **temporal** lobe (in HSV).

The presence of RBCs in CSF without a history of trauma indicates HSV encephalitis.

TREATMENT

HSV encephalitis requires immediate IV acyclovir. CMV encephalitis is treated with IV ganciclovir +/− foscarnet. Give doxycycline for suspected Rocky Mountain spotted fever, Lyme disease, or ehrlichiosis.

HSV encephalitis is associated with high morbidity. PCR is highly sensitive and specific. A full course of IV acyclovir is mandatory.

Brain Abscess

A focal, suppurative infection of the brain parenchyma, usually with a **"ring-enhancing"** appearance due to fibrous capsule. The most common infective organisms are **streptococci, staphylococci,** and **anaerobes; multiple** organisms are often implicated (80–90% of cases are polymicrobial). Nonbacterial

When fever is absent, 1° and metastatic brain tumors become the major differential diagnoses.

In general, do not LP a patient with a mass lesion in the brain.

Some commonly tested AIDS-defining illnesses:

- Oropharyngeal/ esophageal candidiasis
- CMV retinitis
- Kaposi's sarcoma
- CNS lymphoma, toxoplasmosis, or PML
- P. jiroveci pneumonia or recurrent bacterial pneumonia
- HIV encephalopathy
- Disseminated mycobacterial or fungal infection
- Invasive cervical cancer

causes include *Toxoplasma*, *Aspergillus*, and *Candida*; zygomycosis should be contemplated in immunocompromised hosts, and neurocysticercosis should be considered in relevant epidemiologic settings. Modes of transmission include the following:

- **Direct spread:** Due to paranasal sinusitis (10% of cases; frequently affects young males; often due to *Streptococcus milleri*), **otitis media** or **mastoiditis** (33%), or **dental infection** (2%).
- **Direct inoculation:** Affects patients with a history of head trauma or neurosurgical procedures.
- **Hematogenous spread** (25% of cases): Often shows an **MCA distribution** with **multiple abscesses** that are poorly encapsulated and located at the **gray-white junction.**

HISTORY/PE

- **Headache,** drowsiness, inattention, confusion, and **seizures** are early symptoms, followed by signs of **increasing ICP** and then **a focal neurologic deficit.**
- **Headache is the most common symptom** and is **often dull, constant, and refractory to treatment.** ↑ ICP leads to **CN III** and **CN VI deficits.**

DIAGNOSIS

- **CT scan** will show a **ring-enhancing lesion** with a low-density core. MRI has higher sensitivity for early abscesses and posterior fossa lesions.
- **CSF analysis** is not necessary and **may precipitate a herniation syndrome.**
- Lab values may show peripheral leukocytosis, ↑ **ESR,** and ↑ **CRP.**

TREATMENT

- **Initiate broad-spectrum IV antibiotics** and **surgical drainage** (aspiration or excision) if necessary for diagnostic and/or therapeutic purposes. Lesions < 2 cm can often be treated medically.
- Administer a third-generation cephalosporin + metronidazole +/– vancomycin; give IV therapy for 6–8 weeks followed by 2–3 weeks PO. Obtain serial CT/MRIs to follow resolution.
- **Dexamethasone** with taper may be used in severe cases to ↓ cerebral edema; **IV mannitol** may be used to ↓ ICP.

▶ HUMAN IMMUNODEFICIENCY VIRUS (HIV)

A retrovirus that targets and destroys CD4+ T lymphocytes. Infection is characterized by a progressively high rate of viral replication that leads to a progressive decline in CD4+ count (see Figure 2.8-6).

- **CD4+ count:** Indicates the **degree of immunosuppression;** guides therapy and prophylaxis and helps determine prognosis.
- **Viral load:** May predict the **rate** of disease progression; provides indications for treatment and gauges response to antiretroviral therapy.

HISTORY/PE

- In acute HIV (acute infection/seroconversion, acute retroviral syndrome), the initial infection is often **asymptomatic,** but patients may also present with **mononucleosis-like or flulike symptoms** (e.g., fever, lymphadenop-

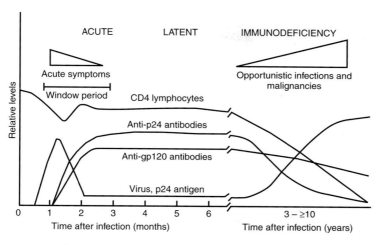

FIGURE 2.8-6. **Time course of HIV infection.**

(Adapted, with permission, from Levinson W, Jawetz E. *Medical Microbiology and Immunology: Examination & Board Review*, 6th ed. New York: McGraw-Hill, 2000: 276.)

athy, maculopapular rash, pharyngitis, diarrhea, nausea/vomiting, weight loss, headache).
■ HIV may later present as night sweats, weight loss, thrush, recurrent infections, or opportunistic infections. Complications are inversely correlated with CD4+ count (see Figure 2.8-7).

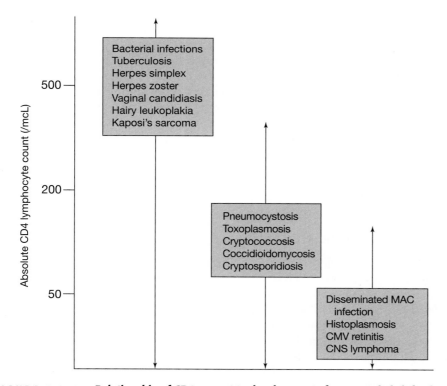

FIGURE 2.8-7. **Relationship of CD4+ count to development of opportunistic infections.**

(Reproduced, with permission, from McPhee SJ et al. *Current Medical Diagnosis & Treatment*, 48th ed. New York: McGraw-Hill, 2009: Fig. 31-1.)

AIDS pathogens—

**The Major Pathogens
Concerning Complete
T-Cell Collapse**

Toxoplasma gondii
Mycobacterium avium-
intracellulare
Pneumocystis jiroveci
Candida albicans
Cryptococcus
neoformans
Tuberculosis
CMV
Cryptosporidium
parvum

DIAGNOSIS

- **ELISA test** (high sensitivity, moderate specificity): Detects anti-HIV antibodies in the bloodstream (can take up to six months to appear after exposure).
- **Western blot** (low sensitivity, high specificity): Confirmatory.
- **Rapid HIV tests** are now available.
- Baseline evaluation should include HIV RNA PCR (viral load), CD4+ cell count, CXR, PPD skin testing, Pap smear, VDRL/RPR, and serologies for CMV, hepatitis, toxoplasmosis, and VZV.
- Evaluation for acute retroviral syndrome (acute HIV) should include **HIV RNA PCR** (viral load); ELISA may be ⊖.

TREATMENT

- Initiate antiretroviral therapy for the following: (1) symptomatic patients (i.e., those with AIDS-defining illness) regardless of CD4+ count or viral load; (2) asymptomatic patients with a CD4+ count < 350; (3) pregnant patients; and (4) those with specific HIV-related conditions (e.g., HIV-associated nephropathy).
- The **initial regimen** should generally consist of some combination of **two nucleoside/nucleotide reverse transcriptase inhibitors (RTIs) plus either one non-nucleoside RTI (NNRTI) or one protease inhibitor.** The most important principle is to select multiple medications (usually at least three) in order to achieve durable treatment response and limit the emergence of resistance.
    - The choice of regimen depends on drug-drug interactions, drug tolerance, patient adherence, and comorbid conditions (e.g., hyperlipidemia, reflux). Monotherapy/dual therapy should not be used.
    - The goal of therapy is viral suppression (< 50 copies), which usually occurs more rapidly than immune reconstitution. CD4+ count and viral load should thus be carefully monitored.
    - An HIV genotype should be obtained before the initiation of therapy and when resistance is suspected, as such testing can provide mutation information and identify resistance to specific antiretrovirals.
- Table 2.8-6 outlines prophylactic measures against opportunistic infections.

▶ OPPORTUNISTIC INFECTIONS

Figure 2.8-8 illustrates the microscopic appearance of some common opportunistic organisms.

Oropharyngeal Candidiasis (Thrush)

- Risk factors include xerostomia, antibiotic use, denture use, and immunosuppressed states (e.g., HIV, leukemias, lymphomas, cancer, diabetes, corticosteroid inhaler use, immunosuppressive treatment).
- **Hx/PE:** Presents with **soft white plaques that can be rubbed off,** with an erythematous base and possible mucosal burning. The differential includes oral hairy leukoplakia (lateral borders of the tongue; not easily rubbed off). Odynophagia is characteristic of candidal esophagitis.
- **Dx:** Usually clinical. KOH or Gram stain shows **budding yeast and/or pseudohyphae.**
- **Tx:** Treat thrush with local therapy (e.g., nystatin suspension or clotrimazole tablets, or a PO azole such as fluconazole). Treat candidal esophagitis with PO azole therapy.

TABLE 2.8-6. Prophylaxis for HIV-Related Opportunistic Infections

PATHOGEN	INDICATION FOR PROPHYLAXIS	TREATMENT	NOTES
P. jiroveci pneumonia	CD4+ < 200/mm³, prior *P. jiroveci* infection, unexplained fever × 2 weeks, or HIV-related oral candidiasis.	Single-strength TMP-SMX or dapsone +/− pyrimethamine.	Discontinue prophylaxis when CD4+ is > 200 for ≥ 3 months.
Mycobacterium avium complex (MAC)	CD4+ < 50–100/mm³.	Weekly azithromycin or daily clarithromycin.	Discontinue prophylaxis when CD4+ is > 100/mm³ for > 6 months.
Toxoplasma gondii	CD4+ < 100/mm³ + ⊕ IgG serologies.	Double-strength TMP-SMX.	—
M. tuberculosis	PPD > 5 mm or "high risk" (see TB section).	**Sensitive:** INH × 9 months (+ pyridoxine) or rifampin +/− pyrazinamide × 2 months.	Include pyridoxine with INH-containing regimens.
Candida	Multiple recurrences.	**Esophagitis:** Fluconazole. **Oral:** Nystatin swish and swallow.	—
HSV	Multiple recurrences.	Acyclovir, famciclovir, or valacyclovir.	—
S. pneumoniae	All patients.	Pneumovax.	Give every five years or when CD4+ is < 200.
Influenza	All patients.	Influenza vaccine annually.	—

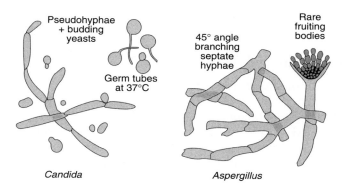
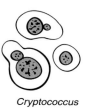
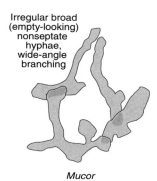

Pseudohyphae + budding yeasts

Germ tubes at 37°C

Candida

45° angle branching septate hyphae

Aspergillus

Rare fruiting bodies

5–10 μm yeasts with wide capsular halo

Narrow-based unequal budding

Cryptococcus

Irregular broad (empty-looking) nonseptate hyphae, wide-angle branching

Mucor

FIGURE 2.8-8. Common opportunistic organisms.

Cryptococcal Meningitis

- Risk factors include AIDS and exposure to **pigeon droppings.**
- Hx/PE: Presents with headache, fever, impaired mentation, and **absent meningismus.** The differential includes toxoplasmosis, lymphoma, TB meningitis, AIDS dementia complex, PML, HSV encephalitis, and other fungal disease.
- **Dx: LP** ($\downarrow$ CSF glucose; $\uparrow$ protein; $\uparrow$ leukocyte count with monocytic predominance, $\uparrow\uparrow$ opening pressure); $\oplus$ **CSF cryptococcal antigen test, India ink stain,** and fungal culture.
- **Tx:**
  - **IV amphotericin B** + flucytosine × 2 weeks; then give fluconazole 400 mg × 8 weeks. Lifelong **maintenance therapy** should be administered with fluconazole 200 mg QD, or until CD4+ is > 200 for > 6 months.
  - $\uparrow$ opening pressure may require serial LPs or VP shunt for management.

The CSF antigen test for cryptococcal meningitis is highly sensitive and specific.

Histoplasmosis

Risk factors include AIDS, spelunking, and exposure to bird or bat excrement, especially in the **Ohio** and **Mississippi** river valleys.

HISTORY/PE

- 1° exposure is often asymptomatic or causes a flulike illness.
- Presentation may range from no symptoms to fulminant disease with pulmonary or extrapulmonary manifestations.
- Fever, weight loss, hepatosplenomegaly, lymphadenopathy, nonproductive cough, and pancytopenia indicate disseminated infection (most often within 14 days).
- The differential includes atypical bacterial pneumonias, blastomycosis, coccidioidomycosis, TB, sarcoidosis, pneumoconiosis, and lymphoma.

DIAGNOSIS

- **CXR** shows diffuse nodular densities, focal infiltrate, cavity, or hilar lymphadenopathy (chronic infection is usually cavitary).
- The **urine and serum polysaccharide antigen test** is the most sensitive test for making the initial diagnosis, monitoring response to therapy, and diagnosing relapse. Culture is also diagnostic (blood, sputum, bone marrow, CSF).
- The yeast form is seen with **silver stain** on biopsy (bone marrow, lymph node, liver) or bronchoalveolar lavage.

TREATMENT

Depends on the severity of disease and the host:

- **Mild pulmonary disease or stable nodules:** Treat supportively in the immunocompromised host.
- **Chronic cavitary lesions:** Give itraconazole for > 1 year.
- **Severe acute pulmonary disease or disseminated disease:** Amphotericin **B** or amphotericin B liposomal × 3–10 days followed by itraconazole × 12 weeks or longer. Maintenance therapy with daily itraconazole.

Pneumocystis jiroveci Pneumonia

Formerly known as *Pneumocystis carinii* pneumonia, or PCP. Risk factors include impaired cellular immunity and AIDS.

HISTORY/PE

- Presents with **dyspnea on exertion**, fever, **nonproductive cough**, tachypnea, weight loss, fatigue, and **impaired oxygenation**.
- Can also present as disseminated disease or as local disease in other organ systems.
- The differential includes TB, histoplasmosis, and coccidioidomycosis.

DIAGNOSIS

- Diagnosed by cytology of induced sputum or bronchoscopy specimen with silver stain and immunofluorescence. Obtain an ABG to check PaO_2.
- CXR may show diffuse, bilateral interstitial infiltrates with a ground-glass appearance, but any presentation is possible.

TREATMENT

- Treat with **high-dose** TMP-SMX × 21 days. Clindamycin and primaquine constitute an alternative regimen for patients with sulfa allergy.
- A prednisone taper should be used in patients with moderate to severe hypoxemia ($PaO_2 < 70$ mm or an arterial-alveolar oxygen gradient > 35).

Suspect P. jiroveci *pneumonia in any HIV patient who presents with nonproductive cough and dyspnea.*

Cytomegalovirus (CMV)

Most 1° CMV infections are asymptomatic; serious reactivation generally occurs only in immunocompromised patients. Seventy percent of adults in the United States have been infected. Transmission occurs via **sexual contact**, in **breast milk**, via **respiratory droplets** in nursery or day care facilities, and through **blood transfusions**. Risk factors for reactivation include the first 100 days status post tissue or bone marrow transplant and HIV positivity with a CD4+ < 100 or a viral load > 10,000.

HISTORY/PE

- Systemic infection may resemble EBV mononucleosis (see the discussion of infectious mononucleosis).
- Specific manifestations are as follows:
  - **CMV retinitis:** Has a high rate of retinal detachment ("pizza pie" retinopathy), and presents with floaters and visual field changes (CD4+ < 50).
  - **GI and hepatobiliary involvement:** Can present with multiple nonspecific GI symptoms, including bloody diarrhea. CMV, microsporidia, and cryptosporidia have been implicated in the development of **AIDS cholangiopathy.**
  - **CMV pneumonitis:** Presents with cough, fever, and sparse sputum production; associated with a high mortality rate. Much more common in patients with hematologic malignancies and transplant patients than in those with AIDS.
  - **CNS involvement:** Can include **polyradiculopathy, transverse myelitis,** and subacute **encephalitis** (CD4+ < 50; periventricular calcifications).

HIGH-YIELD FACTS

INFECTIOUS DISEASE

233

Virus isolation, culture, **tissue examination, serum PCR**.

TREATMENT

Treat CMV infection with ganciclovir.

Treat with **ganciclovir** or foscarnet. Treat underlying disease if the patient is immunocompromised.

Mycobacterium avium Complex (MAC)

Ubiquitous organisms causing **pulmonary** and **disseminated** infection in several demographic groups. The 1° form occurs in **apparently healthy non-smokers (Lady Windermere syndrome);** a 2° pulmonary form affects patients with **preexisting pulmonary disease** such as COPD, TB, or CF. Disseminated infection occurs in AIDS patients with a **CD4+ < 50.** There is no evidence that behavioral change affects exposure.

HISTORY/PE

- Disseminated *M. avium* infection in AIDS is associated with **fever, weakness, and weight loss in patients who are not on HAART or chemoprophylaxis for MAC.**
- Hepatosplenomegaly and lymphadenopathy are occasionally seen.
- Adrenal insufficiency is possible in the setting of infiltration into the adrenals.

DIAGNOSIS

- Obtain mycobacterial **blood cultures** ($\oplus$ in 2–3 weeks).
- Labs show anemia, hypoalbuminemia, and ↑ **serum alkaline phosphatase and LDH.**
- Biopsy of bone marrow, intestine, or liver reveals **foamy macrophages** with **acid-fast bacilli.** Typical granulomas may be absent in immunocompromised patients.

TREATMENT

Treat with **clarithromycin** and **ethambutol +/– rifabutin** and **HAART.** Continue for > 12 months and until CD4+ is > 100 for > 6 months.

PREVENTION

Weekly azithromycin for those with a CD4+ < 50 or AIDS-defining opportunistic infection.

Toxoplasmosis

Risk factors include ingesting **raw or undercooked meat** and **changing cat litter.** Worldwide, exposure is highest in **France.**

HISTORY/PE

- 1° infection is usually asymptomatic.
- Reactivated toxoplasmosis occurs in immunosuppressed patients and may present in specific organs (brain, lung, and eye > heart, skin, GI tract, and liver).

- Encephalitis is common in seropositive AIDS patients. Classically, CNS lesions present with fever, headache, altered mental status, seizures, and focal neurologic deficits.

DIAGNOSIS

- **Serology, PCR** (indicates exposure and risk for reactivation); tissue examination for histology, isolation of the organism in mice, or tissue culture.
- In the setting of CNS involvement, obtain a **CT scan** (can show **multiple isodense or hypodense, ring-enhancing** mass lesions) or an **MRI** (predilection for **basal ganglia;** more sensitive).

TREATMENT

- Induction with high-dose PO pyrimethamine + sulfadiazine and leukovorin × 4–8 weeks; maintenance with low-dose pyrimethamine + sulfadiazine and leukovorin until the disease has resolved clinically and radiographically.
- TMP-SMX (Bactrim DS) or pyrimethamine + dapsone can be used for prophylaxis in patients with a CD4+ < 100 and a ⊕ toxoplasmosis IgG.

The two most likely differential diagnoses of ring-enhancing lesions in AIDS patients are toxoplasmosis and CNS lymphoma.

► SEXUALLY TRANSMITTED DISEASES (STDs)

Chlamydia

The most common bacterial STD in the United States. Caused by *Chlamydia trachomatis*, which can infect the genital tract, urethra, anus, and eye. Risk factors include **unprotected sexual intercourse, new or multiple partners, and frequent douching.** Often coexists with or mimics N. *gonorrhoeae* infection (known as nongonococcal urethritis when gonorrhea is absent). LGV serovars of *Chlamydia* cause lymphogranuloma venereum, an emerging cause of proctocolitis.

Chlamydia infection is a common cause of nongonococcal urethritis in men.

HISTORY/PE

- Infection is often asymptomatic but may present with **urethritis, mucopurulent cervicitis,** or **PID.**
- Exam may reveal cervical/adnexal tenderness in women or penile discharge and testicular tenderness in men.
- The differential includes gonorrhea, endometriosis, PID, orchitis, vaginitis, and UTI.
- Lymphogranuloma venereum presents in its 1° form as a painless, transient papule or shallow ulcer. In its 2° form, it presents as painful swelling of the inguinal nodes, and in its 3° form it can present as an "anogenital syndrome" (anal pruritus with discharge, rectal strictures, rectovaginal fistula, and elephantiasis).

Chlamydia species cause arthritis, neonatal conjunctivitis, pneumonia, nongonococcal urethritis/ PID, and lymphogranuloma venereum.

DIAGNOSIS

- Diagnosis is usually clinical.
- Culture is the **gold standard.**
- Urine tests (PCR or ligase chain reaction) are a rapid means of detection, while DNA probes and immunofluorescence (for gonorrhea/chlamydia) take 48–72 hours.
- **Gram stain** of urethral or genital discharge may show **PMNs but no bacteria (intracellular).**

TREATMENT

Doxycycline 100 mg PO BID × 7 days or azithromycin 1 g PO × 1 day. Use erythromycin in pregnant patients. **Treat sexual partners,** and maintain a low threshold to treat for *N. gonorrhoeae*. LGV serovars require prolonged therapy for 21 days.

COMPLICATIONS

- Chronic infection and pelvic pain, Reiter's syndrome (urethritis, conjunctivitis, arthritis), Fitz-Hugh–Curtis syndrome (perihepatic inflammation and fibrosis).
- Ectopic pregnancy/infertility can result from PID (in women) and epididymitis (in men).

Gonorrhea

A gram-$\ominus$ intracellular diplococcus that can infect almost any site in the female reproductive tract. Infection in men tends to be limited to the urethra.

HISTORY/PE

- Presents with a **greenish-yellow discharge,** pelvic or **adnexal pain,** and swollen Bartholin's glands. Men experience a **purulent urethral discharge,** dysuria, and erythema of the urethral meatus.
- The differential includes chlamydia, endometriosis, pharyngitis, PID, vaginitis, UTI, salpingitis, and tubo-ovarian abscess.

DIAGNOSIS

- **Gram stain and culture** is the gold standard for any site (i.e., pharynx, cervix, urethra, or anus). **Nucleic acid amplification tests** can be sent on penile/vaginal tissue or from urine.
- Disseminated disease may present with **monoarticular septic arthritis,** rash, and/or **tenosynovitis.**

Treat for gonorrhea and chlamydia in light of the high prevalence of coinfection.

TREATMENT

- **Ceftriaxone IM or cefepime PO × 1 dose.** Also treat for presumptive chlamydia coinfection (doxycycline × 7 days or macrolide × 1 dose). Condoms are effective prophylaxis. Treat the sexual partner or partners if possible. Fluoroquinolones should not be used because of emerging resistance.
- Disseminated disease requires IV ceftriaxone for at least 24 hours.

COMPLICATIONS

Persistent infection with pain; infertility; tubo-ovarian abscess with rupture; disseminated gonococcal infection (see Figure 2.8-9).

Syphilis

Caused by *Treponema pallidum*, a spirochete. AIDS can accelerate the course of disease progression.

Syphilis is the "great imitator" because its dermatologic findings resemble those of many other diseases.

HISTORY/PE

- 1° **(10–90 days after infection):** Presents with a **painless ulcer (chancre;** see Figure 2.8-10).

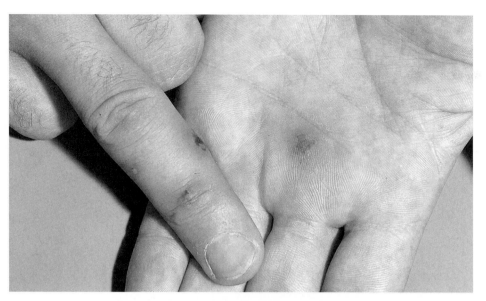

FIGURE 2.8-9. **Disseminated gonococcal infection.**

Hemorrhagic, painful pustules on erythematous bases. (Reproduced, with permission, from Wolff K et al. *Fitzpatrick's Color Atlas & Synopsis of Clinical Dermatology*, 5th ed. New York: McGraw-Hill, 2005: Fig. 27-17.)

- **2° (4–8 weeks after chancre):** Presents with low-grade fever, headache, malaise, and generalized lymphadenopathy with a diffuse, symmetric, asymptomatic (nonpruritic) **maculopapular rash on the soles and palms.** Highly infective 2° eruptions include mucous patches or **condylomata lata** (see Figure 2.8-11). Meningitis, hepatitis, nephropathy, and eye involvement may also be seen.
    - **Early latent** (period from resolution of 1° or 2° syphilis to end of **first year** of infection): No symptoms; ⊕ serology.
    - **Late latent** (period of asymptomatic infection **beyond the first year**): No symptoms; ⊕ or ⊖ serology. One-third progress to 3° syphilis.

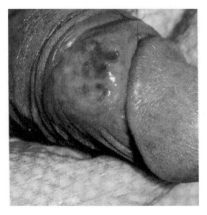

FIGURE 2.8-10. **1° syphilis.**

The chancre is an ulcerated papule with a smooth, clean base; raised, indurated borders; and scant discharge. (Reproduced, with permission, from Bondi EE. *Dermatology: Diagnosis and Therapy*, 1st ed. Stamford, CT: Appleton & Lange, 1991: 394.)

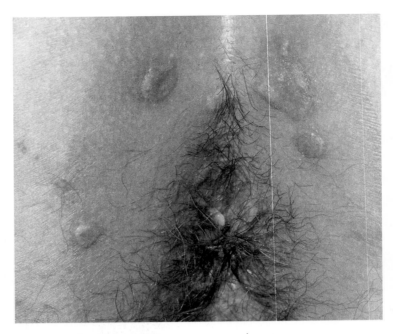

FIGURE 2.8-11. **Condylomata lata.**

Typical appearance of the verrucous heaped-up lesions of condylomata lata. (Reproduced, with permission, from Wolff K et al. *Fitzpatrick's Color Atlas & Synopsis of Clinical Dermatology,* 5th ed. New York: McGraw-Hill, 2005: Fig. 27-27.)

- **3°** (late manifestations appearing 1–20 years after initial infection): Presents with destructive, granulomatous **gummas. Neurosyphilis** includes **tabes dorsalis** (posterior column degeneration), meningitis, and **Argyll Robertson pupil** (constricts with accommodation but not reactive to light). **Cardiovascular** findings include dilated aortic root, aortitis, **aortic root aneurysms,** and aortic regurgitation.

DIAGNOSIS

- See Table 2.8-7. **VDRL false positives** are seen with **V**iruses (mononucleosis, HSV, HIV, hepatitis), **D**rugs/IV drug use, **R**heumatic fever/**R**heumatoid arthritis, and **S**LE/**L**eprosy.

TABLE 2.8-7. **Diagnostic Tests for Syphilis**

TEST	COMMENTS
Dark-field microscopy	Identifies motile spirochetes (only 1° and 2° lesions).
VDRL/RPR	Rapid and cheap, but sensitivity is only 60–75% in 1° disease. Many false positives.
FTA-ABS	Sensitive and specific. Used as a 2° diagnostic test.
TPPA[a]	Sensitivity and specificity similar to FTA-ABS but easier to use. Becoming the 2° test of choice.

[a] TPPA = *T. pallidum* particle agglutination test.

- Neurosyphilis should be suspected and ruled out in any AIDS patient with neurologic symptoms and a ⊕ **RPR**.

TREATMENT

- **1°/2°: Benzathine penicillin IM × 1 day.** Tetracycline or doxycycline × 14 days may be used for patients with penicillin allergies.
- **Latent infection:** Treat with benzathine penicillin once weekly × 3 weeks.
- **Neurosyphilis:** Treat with penicillin IV; penicillin-allergic patients should be desensitized prior to therapy.

Genital Lesions

See Table 2.8-8 for a description of common sexually transmitted genital lesions along with an outline of their diagnosis and treatment.

Remember that treatment of syphilis can result in an acute flulike illness known as the Jarisch-Herxheimer reaction.

▶ GENITOURINARY INFECTIONS

Urinary Tract Infections (UTIs)

Affect females more frequently than males, and ⊕ *E. coli* cultures are obtained in 80% of cases. See the mnemonic **SEEKS PP** for other pathogens. Risk factors include the presence of catheters or other urologic instrumentation, anatomic abnormalities (e.g., BPH, vesicoureteral reflux), previous UTIs or pyelonephritis, diabetes mellitus (DM), recent antibiotic use, immunosuppression, and pregnancy.

Common UTI bugs—
SEEKS PP

Serratia
E. coli
Enterobacter
Klebsiella pneumoniae
S. saprophyticus
Pseudomonas
Proteus mirabilis

HISTORY/PE

Present with **dysuria, urgency, frequency,** suprapubic pain, and possibly hematuria. Children may present with **bed-wetting,** poor feeding, recurrent fevers, and foul-smelling urine. The differential includes vaginitis, STDs, urethritis or acute urethral syndrome, and prostatitis.

DIAGNOSIS

- Diagnosed by **clinical symptoms.** In the absence of symptoms, treatment is warranted only for children, those with anatomical GU tract anomalies, pregnant women, those with instrumented urinary tracts, patients scheduled for GU surgery, and renal transplant patients.
- **Urine dipstick/UA:** ↑ **leukocyte esterase** (a marker of WBCs) is 75% sensitive and up to 95% specific. ↑ **nitrites** (a marker of bacteria), ↑ urine pH (*Proteus* infections), and hematuria (seen with cystitis) are also commonly seen.
- **Microscopic analysis:** Pyuria (> 5 WBCs/hpf) and **bacteriuria** (1 organism/hpf = 10^6 organisms/mL) are suggestive.
- **Urine culture:** The gold standard is > 10^5 **CFU/mL.**

TREATMENT

- **Uncomplicated UTI:** Treat on an outpatient basis with PO **TMP-SMX** or a **fluoroquinolone** × 3 days, or nitrofurantoin × 7 days. Note that resistance to TMP-SMX and fluoroquinolones has been increasing.
- **Complicated UTI** (urinary obstruction, men, renal transplant, catheters, instrumentation): Administer the same antibiotics as above, but for 7–14 days.

TABLE 2.8-8. **Sexually Transmitted Genital Lesions**

	KLEBSIELLA GRANULOMATIS[a] (GRANULOMA INGUINALE-DONOVANOSIS)	*HAEMOPHILUS DUCREYI* (CHANCROID)	HSV-1 OR HSV-2[b]	HPV[c]	*TREPONEMA PALLIDUM*
Lesion	Papule becomes a **beefy-red ulcer** with a characteristic rolled edge of granulation tissue	Papule or pustule (chancroid; see Figure 2.8-12)	Vesicle (3–7 days postexposure)	Papule (condylomata acuminata; warts)	Papule (chancre)
Appearance	Raised red lesions with a white border	Irregular, deep, well demarcated, necrotic	Regular, red, shallow ulcer	Irregular, pink or white, raised; cauliflower	Regular, red, round, raised
Number	1 or multiple	1–3	Multiple	Multiple	Single
Size	5–10 mm	10–20 mm	1–3 mm	1–5 mm	1 cm
Pain	No	**Yes**	**Yes**	No	No
Concurrent signs and symptoms	Granulomatous ulcers	Inguinal lymphadenopathy	Malaise, myalgias, and fever with vulvar burning and pruritus	Pruritus	Regional adenopathy
Diagnosis	Clinical exam, biopsy (Donovan bodies)	Difficult to culture; diagnosis is made on clinical grounds	Tzanck smear shows multinucleated giant cells; viral cultures; DFA or serology	Clinical exam; biopsy for confirmation	Spirochetes seen under dark-field microscopy; *T. pallidum* identified by serum antibody test
Treatment[d]	Doxycycline (100 mg BID) or azithromycin (1 g weekly) × 3 weeks	Doxycycline (100 mg BID) or azithromycin (1 g weekly) × 3 weeks	Acyclovir or valacyclovir for 1° infection	Cryotherapy; topical agents such as podophyllin, trichloroacetic acid, or 5-FU cream	Penicillin IM

[a] Previously known as *Calymmatobacterium granulomatis.*

[b] Some 85% of genital herpes lesions are caused by HSV-2.

[c] HPV serotypes 6 and 11 are associated with genital warts; types 16, 18, and 31 are associated with cervical cancer.

[d] For all, treat sexual partners.

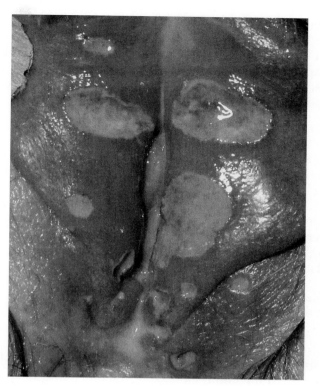

FIGURE 2.8-12.   Chancroid.

Multiple, painful ulcers. (Reproduced, with permission, from Wolff K et al. *Fitzpatrick's Color Atlas & Synopsis of Clinical Dermatology*, 5th ed. New York: McGraw-Hill, 2005: Fig. 27-31.)

- **Pregnant patients:** Treat asymptomatic bacteruria or symptomatic UTI with nitrofurantoin or cephalosporin × 3–7 days. Avoid fluoroquinolones. Confirm clearance with a repeat culture post-treatment.
- Patients with urosepsis should be hospitalized and initially treated with **IV antibiotics.** Consider broader coverage to include resistant GNRs or enterococcus.
- Prophylactic antibiotics may be given to women with uncomplicated recurrent UTIs. Check for prostatitis in men.

Pyelonephritis

Nearly 85% of community-acquired cases of pyelonephritis result from the same pathogens that cause cystitis. Cystitis and pyelonephritis have similar risk factors.

HISTORY/PE

- Signs and symptoms are similar to those of cystitis but show evidence of **upper urinary tract disease.**
- Symptoms include **flank pain, fever/chills,** and nausea/vomiting. Dysuria, frequency, and urgency are also possible.

DIAGNOSIS

- **UA and culture:** Results are similar to those of cystitis, but with **WBC casts.** Send blood cultures to rule out urosepsis.

Pyelonephritis is the most common serious medical complication of pregnancy. Twenty to thirty percent of patients with untreated bacteriuria will develop pyelonephritis.

- **CBC:** Reveals leukocytosis.
- **Imaging:** In general, imaging is not necessary. **Ultrasound** can be used to rule out obstruction and calculi and can often confirm the diagnosis non-invasively, but **CT** is becoming the **test of choice** in patients with adequate renal function who are not responding to therapy. In recurrent cases, IVP may demonstrate renal scarring.

TREATMENT

- For mild cases, patients may be treated on an outpatient basis for 10–14 days. **Fluoroquinolones** are first-line therapy. Encourage ↑ PO fluids and monitor closely.
- Admit and administer IV antibiotics to patients who have serious medical complications or systemic symptoms, are **pregnant,** present with severe **nausea and vomiting,** or have suspected bacteremia. Fluoroquinolones, third- or fourth-generation cephalosporins, β-lactam/β-lactamase inhibitors, and carbapenem may be used depending on disease severity.

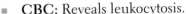

▶ **HEMATOLOGIC INFECTIONS**

Sepsis

Defined as the presence of systemic inflammatory response syndrome (**SIRS**) with a **documented infection,** induced by microbial invasion or toxins in the bloodstream. **Severe sepsis** refers to sepsis with end-organ dysfunction due to poor perfusion. **Septic shock** refers to sepsis with hypotension and organ dysfunction from vasodilation. Examples include the following:

- **Gram-⊕ shock** (e.g., staphylococci and streptococci) 2° to fluid loss caused by exotoxins.
- **Gram-⊖ shock** (e.g., *E. coli, Klebsiella, Proteus,* and *Pseudomonas*) 2° to vasodilation caused by endotoxins (lipopolysaccharide).
- **Neonates:** GBS, *E. coli, Listeria monocytogenes, H. influenzae.*
- **Children:** *H. influenzae,* pneumococcus, meningococcus.
- **Adults:** Gram-⊕ cocci, aerobic gram-⊖ bacilli, anaerobes (dependent on the presumed site of infection).
- **IV drug users/indwelling lines:** *S. aureus,* coagulase-⊖ *Staphylococcus* species.
- **Asplenic patients:** Pneumococcus, *H. influenzae,* meningococcus (encapsulated organisms).

HISTORY/PE

- Presents with abrupt onset of fever and chills, altered mental status, tachycardia, and tachypnea. Severe sepsis is seen in end-organ dysfunction. **Hypotension** occurs in cases of septic shock.
- Septic shock is typically a warm shock with **warm skin and extremities.** This contrasts with cardiogenic shock, which typically presents with **cool skin and extremities.**
- Petechiae, ecchymoses, or abnormal coagulation tests suggest DIC (2–3% of cases).

DIAGNOSIS

- A clinical diagnosis.
- Labs show leukocytosis or leukopenia with ↑ bands, thrombocytopenia

When in doubt, admit a patient with pyelonephritis and administer IV antibiotics.

Urosepsis must be considered in any elderly patient with altered mental status.

SIRS = two or more of the following:

1. *Temperature: Either < 36°C or > 38°C (i.e., hypothermia or fever).*

2. *Tachypnea: > 20 breaths per minute or $Paco_2 < 32$ mmHg on ABG.*

3. *Tachycardia: HR > 90 bpm.*

4. *Leukocytosis/leukopenia: WBC < 4000 cells/mm³ or > 12,000 cells/mm³.*

(50% of cases), evidence of ↓ tissue perfusion (↑ creatinine, ↑ LFTs), and abnormal coagulation studies (↑ INR).

- It is critical to obtain cultures of all appropriate sites (e.g., blood, sputum, CSF, wound, urine).
- Imaging (CXR, CT) may aid in establishing the etiology or site of infection.

TREATMENT

- ICU admission may be required. Treat aggressively with IV fluids, pressors, and empiric antibiotics (based on the likely source of infection).
- Treat underlying factors (e.g., remove Foley catheter or infected lines).
- The 1° goal is to **maintain BP and perfusion** to end organs.

Malaria

A protozoal disease caused by four strains of the genus **Plasmodium** (*P. falciparum, P. vivax, P. ovale,* and *P. malariae*) and transmitted by the bite of an infected female **Anopheles** mosquito. **P. falciparum** has the highest morbidity and causes the largest number of deaths, occasionally within 24 hours of symptom onset. Recent outbreaks have occurred in parts of the southern and eastern United States and in Europe, mainly through the arrival of infected travelers and immigrants from endemic areas. Travelers to endemic areas should take chemoprophylaxis and use mosquito repellent and bed nets to minimize exposure.

Malaria should be considered in the differential for any patient who has emigrated from or recently traveled to tropical locations and presents with fever.

HISTORY/PE

- Patients have a history of exposure in a malaria-endemic area, with **periodic** attacks of sequential **chills, fever (> 41°C),** and **diaphoresis** occurring over 4–6 hours. **Splenomegaly** often appears four or more days after onset of symptoms. Patients are often asymptomatic between attacks, which recur every 2–3 days, depending on the *Plasmodium* strain.
- Severely ill patients may present with hyperpyrexia, prostration, impaired consciousness, agitation, hyperventilation, and bleeding. The presence of rash, lymphadenopathy, neck stiffness, or photophobia suggests a different or additional diagnosis.

P. vivax, P. ovale, and P. malariae can all cause symptoms months to years after initial infection.

DIAGNOSIS

- Timely diagnosis of the correct strain is essential because *P. falciparum* can be fatal and is often resistant to standard chloroquine treatment.
- **Giemsa- or Wright-stained thick and thin blood films** should be sent for expert microscopic evaluation to determine the strain as well as the degree of parasitemia. Specimens should be obtained at eight-hour intervals for three days, including during and between febrile periods.
- CBC usually demonstrates normochromic, normocytic anemia with reticulocytosis.
- If resources allow, more sensitive serologic tests are available, including rapid antigen detection methods, fluorescent antibody methods, and PCR.

Obtain a finger stick in a patient with malaria and mental status changes to rule out hypoglycemia.

TREATMENT

- Uncomplicated malarial infection can be treated orally, with the choice of medication determined by the *Plasmodium* strain. **Chloroquine** has been the standard antimalarial medication, but increasing resistance has led to the use of other medications, including quinine with clindamycin or doxy-cycline, atovaquone, mefloquine, artesunate, and halofantrine.

- The life cycles of *P. vivax* and *P. ovale* strains include dormant liver hyp-nozoite forms, which are resistant to treatment with **chloroquine.** Thus, in cases of *P. vivax, P. ovale,* or an unknown strain, **primaquine** is added to eradicate the hypnozoites in the liver.
- Severe infections can be treated with parenteral antimalarial medications **(IV quinidine)** with transition to oral regimens as tolerated. Newer combi-nations such as **proguanil/atovaquone (Malarone)** eliminate the need for multiple medications. Symptoms can be treated with supportive care.

COMPLICATIONS

- **Cerebral malaria:** Headache, change in mental status, neurologic signs, retinal hemorrhages, convulsions, delirium, **coma.**
- **Severe hemolytic anemia:** Usually associated with *P. falciparum* infection.
- **Acute tubular necrosis and renal failure:** Associated with **blackwater fe-ver** (dark urine due to hemoglobinuria).
- **Noncardiogenic pulmonary edema:** Often precipitated by overly rapid re-hydration.
- **Other:** Additional complications include gram-$\ominus$ bacteremia, acute he-patopathy, hypoglycemia, cardiac dysrhythmias, secretory diarrhea, lactic acidosis, DIC, and a low birth rate in children of infected mothers.

Infectious Mononucleosis

Most commonly occurs in **young adult** patients; usually due to acute EBV infection. Transmission most often occurs through exchange of body fluids, including saliva.

HISTORY/PE

*A young adult who presents with the triad of **fever, sore throat,** and **lymphadenopathy** may have infectious mononucleosis.*

- Presents with **fever** and **pharyngitis. Fatigue** invariably accompanies ini-tial illness and may persist for 3–6 months. Exam may reveal low-grade fe-ver, generalized lymphadenopathy (especially **posterior cervical**), tonsillar exudate and enlargement, palatal petechiae, a generalized maculopapular rash, splenomegaly, and **bilateral upper eyelid edema.**
- Patients who present with pharyngitis as their 1° symptom may be misdiag-nosed as having streptococcal pharyngitis (30% of patients with infectious mononucleosis are asymptomatic carriers of group A strep in their orophar-ynx).
- **Treatment of patients with ampicillin (for streptococcal pharyngitis) during acute EBV infection can cause a prolonged, pruritic, drug-related maculopapular rash.** This rash does not portend future sensitivity to β-lactams and will remit with discontinuation of ampicillin.
- The differential also includes CMV, toxoplasmosis, HIV, HHV-6, other causes of viral hepatitis, and lymphoma.

DIAGNOSIS

The lymphocytosis in EBV infection is predominantly due to B-cell proliferation, but the atypical cells are T lymphocytes.

- Diagnosed by the **heterophil antibody (Monospot) test** (may be $\ominus$ in the first few weeks after symptoms begin). The EBV-infected proliferating B cells produce a characteristic antibody that agglutinates the horse and sheep RBCs that are the basis for the Monospot test.
- **EBV-specific antibodies** can be ordered in patients with suspected mono-

nucleosis and a ⊖ Monospot test. Infectious mononucleosis syndromes that are Monospot ⊖ and EBV-antibody ⊖ are most often due to CMV infection. Acute HIV and other viral etiologies should be considered.

- CBC with differential often reveals mild **thrombocytopenia** with relative **lymphocytosis** and > 10% **atypical T lymphocytes.**
- CMP usually reveals mildly elevated transaminases, alkaline phosphatase, and total bilirubin.

TREATMENT

Treatment is mostly supportive, as there is no effective antiviral therapy. Corticosteroids are indicated for airway compromise due to tonsillar enlargement, severe thrombocytopenia, or severe autoimmune hemolytic anemia.

COMPLICATIONS

- **CNS infection:** Can present as aseptic meningitis, encephalitis, meningoencephalitis, cranial nerve palsies (particularly CN VII), optic and peripheral neuritis, transverse myelitis, or Guillain-Barré syndrome.
- **Splenic rupture:** Occurs in < 0.5% of cases. More common in males, and presents with abdominal pain, referred shoulder pain, or hemodynamic compromise.
- **Upper airway obstruction:** Treat with steroids.
- **Bacterial superinfection:** Ten percent of patients develop streptococcal pharyngitis secondarily.
- **Fulminant hepatic necrosis:** More common in males; the most common cause of death in affected males.
- **Autoimmune hemolytic anemia:** Occurs in 2% of patients during the first two weeks. Coombs ⊕. Mild anemia lasts 1–2 months. Treat with corticosteroids if severe.
- **Other:** Rare complications associated with acute EBV infection include hepatitis (which can be fulminant), myocarditis or pericarditis with electrocardiographic changes, pneumonia with pleural effusion, interstitial nephritis, genital ulcerations, and vasculitis.

About one-third of patients with infectious mononucleosis have coexisting streptococcal pharyngitis that requires treatment.

▶ **FEVER**

Fever of Unknown Origin (FUO)

A temperature of > 38.3°C of at least three weeks' duration that remains undiagnosed following three outpatient visits or three days of hospitalization.

HISTORY/PE

Presents with fever, headache, myalgia, and malaise. The differential includes the following:

- **Infectious:** TB, endocarditis (e.g., HACEK organisms; see the discussion of infective endocarditis), occult abscess, osteomyelitis, catheter infections. In HIV patients, consider MAC, histoplasmosis, CMV, or lymphoma.
- **Neoplastic:** Lymphomas, leukemias, hepatic and renal cell carcinomas.
- **Autoimmune:** Still's disease, SLE, cryoglobulinemia, polyarteritis nodosa, connective tissue disease, granulomatous disease (including sarcoidosis).
- **Miscellaneous:** Pulmonary emboli, alcoholic hepatitis, drug fever, familial Mediterranean fever, factitious fever.
- Undiagnosed (10–15%).

Overall, infections and cancer account for the majority of cases of FUO (> 60%). Autoimmune diseases account for ~15%. In the elderly, rheumatic diseases account for one-third of cases.

DIAGNOSIS

- **Labs:** Confirm the presence of fever and take a detailed history (including family, social, sexual, occupational, dietary, exposures [pets/animals], and travel); obtain a CXR, CBC with differential, ESR, multiple blood cultures, sputum Gram stain and culture, UA and culture, and PPD. Specific tests (ANA, RF, viral cultures, viral serologies/antigen tests) can be obtained if an infectious or autoimmune etiology is suspected.
- **Imaging:** CT of the chest and abdomen should be done early in the workup of a true FUO. Rule out drug fever. Invasive testing (marrow/liver biopsy) is generally low yield. Laparoscopy and colonoscopy are higher yield as second-line tests (after CT).

TREATMENT

Stop unnecessary medications. Give empiric antibiotics to severely ill patients until the etiology has been determined. Stop antibiotics if there is no response.

FUO patients without other symptoms do not require empiric antibiotic therapy.

Neutropenic Fever

- Defined as a single oral temperature of $\geq 38.3°C$ (101°F) or a temperature of $\geq 38.0°C$ (100.4°F) for ≥ 1 hour in a neutropenic patient (i.e., an absolute neutrophil count of < 500 cells/mm³).
- **Hx/PE:** Common in cancer patients undergoing chemotherapy (neutropenic nadir 7–10 days postchemotherapy). Inflammation may be minimal or absent.
- **Dx:**
  - Send appropriate cultures, including blood, urine, sputum, and wound. Consider testing for viruses, fungi, and mycobacteria.
  - Conduct a thorough physical exam, but **avoid a rectal exam** in light of the bleeding risk if the patient is thrombocytopenic.
  - Obtain a CBC with differential, serum creatinine, BUN, and transaminases; order blood, urine, lesion, and stool cultures.
  - CXR for patients with respiratory symptoms; CT scan to evaluate for abscesses or other occult infection.
- **Tx:** Empiric antibiotic therapy (see Figure 2.8-13). Routine use of colony-stimulating factors is not indicated. If fevers persist after 72 hours despite antibiotic therapy, start antifungal treatment.

> **TICK-BORNE INFECTIONS**

Lyme Disease

> **With fever and rash, think—**
>
> **Tiny GERMS**
>
> **T**yphoid fever
> **G**onococcemia
> **E**ndocarditis
> **R**ocky Mountain spotted fever
> **M**eningococcemia
> **S**epsis (bacterial)

- A tick-borne disease caused by the spirochete *Borrelia burgdorferi*. Usually seen during the **summer months,** and carried by *Ixodes* ticks on white-tailed deer and white-footed mice. Endemic to the **Northeast,** northern Midwest, and Pacific coast.
- **Hx/PE:** Presents with the onset of rash with fever, malaise, fatigue, headache, myalgias, and/or arthralgias. Infection usually occurs after a tick feeds for > 18 hours.
  - **1° (early localized disease): Erythema migrans** begins as a small erythematous macule or papule that is found at the tick-feeding site and expands slowly over days to weeks. The border may be macular or raised, often with central clearing ("bull's eye").

Lyme disease is the most common vector-borne disease in North America.

246

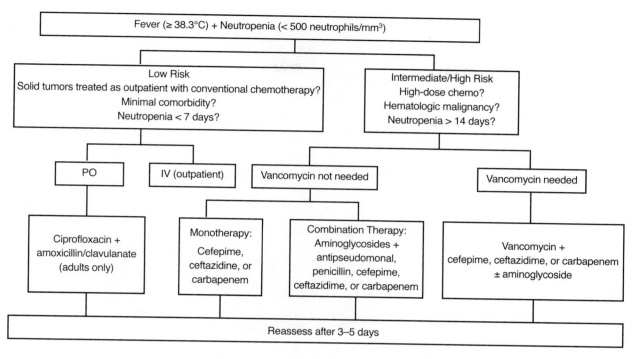

Fever (≥ 38.3°C) + Neutropenia (< 500 neutrophils/mm³)

Low Risk
Solid tumors treated as outpatient with conventional chemotherapy?
Minimal comorbidity?
Neutropenia < 7 days?

Intermediate/High Risk
High-dose chemo?
Hematologic malignancy?
Neutropenia > 14 days?

PO

IV (outpatient)

Vancomycin not needed

Vancomycin needed

Ciprofloxacin +
amoxicillin/clavulanate
(adults only)

Monotherapy:
Cefepime,
ceftazidine, or
carbapenem

Combination Therapy:
Aminoglycosides +
antipseudomonal,
penicillin, cefepime,
ceftazidime, or carbapenem

Vancomycin +
cefepime, ceftazidime, or carbapenem
± aminoglycoside

Reassess after 3–5 days

FIGURE 2.8-13. **Empiric treatment algorithm for a neutropenic fever patient.**

- **2° (early disseminated disease):** Presents with migratory polyarthropathies, neurologic phenomena (e.g., Bell's palsy), meningitis and/or myocarditis, and conduction abnormalities (third-degree heart block).
- **3° (late disease):** Arthritis and subacute encephalitis (memory loss and mood change).
- **Dx:** Clinical diagnosis of **erythema migrans** is as follows:
  - **ELISA** and **Western blot:** Use the Western blot to confirm a ⊕ or indeterminate ELISA. A ⊕ ELISA denotes **exposure** but is not specific for active disease. Western blots sent without ELISA have high rates of false positives.
  - **Tissue culture/PCR:** Extremely difficult to obtain; not routinely done.
- **Tx:** Treat early disease with **doxycycline** and more advanced disease (e.g., CNS or arthritic disease) with **ceftriaxone.** Consider empiric therapy for patients with the characteristic rash, arthralgias, or a tick bite acquired in an endemic area. Prevent with tick bite avoidance.

Lyme arthritis can be very subtle and minimally inflammatory and can wax and wane.

Rocky Mountain Spotted Fever

- A disease caused by **Rickettsia rickettsii** and carried by the American dog tick (**Dermacentor variabilis**). The organism invades the endothelial lining of capillaries and causes **small vessel vasculitis.**
- **Hx/PE:** Presents with **headache, fever,** malaise, and **rash.** The characteristic rash is initially macular (beginning on the wrists and ankles) but becomes petechial/purpuric as it spreads centrally (see Figure 2.8-14). Altered mental status or DIC may develop in severe cases.
- **Dx:** Clinical diagnosis should be confirmed with indirect immunofluorescence of rash biopsy.
- **Tx:** **Doxycycline** or chloramphenicol (for multidrug-resistant organisms).

Rocky Mountain spotted fever starts on the wrists and ankles and then spreads centrally.

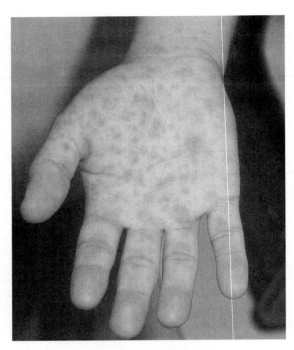

FIGURE 2.8-14. **Rocky Mountain spotted fever.**

These erythematous macular lesions will evolve into a petechial rash that will spread centrally. (Courtesy of Daniel Noltkamper, MD, as published in Knoop KJ et al. *Atlas of Emergency Medicine*, 2nd ed. New York: McGraw-Hill, 2002: 382.)

The condition can be rapidly fatal if left untreated. If clinical suspicion is high, begin treatment while awaiting testing. Prevent by avoiding tick bites.

Causes of red eye:

- *Conjunctivitis*
- *Uveitis*
- *Acute glaucoma*
- *Foreign body or corneal abrasion*
- *Keratitis*
- *Scleritis or episcleritis*
- *Trauma*
- *Subconjunctival hemorrhage*
- *Eyelid disorder*
- *Cluster headache*

► **INFECTIONS OF THE EYES AND EARS**

Infectious Conjunctivitis

A common complaint in the emergency room setting, inflammation of the conjunctiva is most often bacterial or viral but can also be fungal, parasitic, allergic, or chemical. It is essential to differentiate potentially vision-threatening infectious etiologies from allergic or other causes of conjunctivitis, as well as to identify other vision-threatening conditions that may mimic conjunctivitis. See Table 2.8-9 for the common etiologies of infectious conjunctivitis.

Orbital Cellulitis

- Commonly due to infection of the **paranasal sinuses**; can lead to endophthalmitis and blindness. Usually caused by **streptococci, staphylococci (including MRSA), and *H. influenzae*** (in children). In diabetic and immunocompromised patients, **mucormycosis and *Rhizopus*** are in the differential.
- **Hx/PE:** Presents with **acute-onset fever, proptosis, ↓ EOM, ocular pain, and ↓ visual acuity.** Look for a **history of ocular trauma or sinusitis.** Pala-

TABLE 2.8-9. **Common Causes of Infectious Conjunctivitis**

TYPE	PATHOGEN	CHARACTERISTIC	DIAGNOSIS	TREATMENT
Bacterial	Staphylococci, streptococci, *Haemophilus*, *Pseudomonas, Moraxella*	Foreign body sensation, purulent discharge.	Gram stain and culture if severe.	Antibiotic drops/ ointment.
	N. gonorrhoeae	**An emergency!** Corneal involvement can lead to perforation and blindness.	Gram stain shows gram-⊖ intracellular diplococci.	IM ceftriaxone, PO ciprofloxacin or ofloxacin. **Inpatient** treatment if complicated.
	C. trachomatis A–C	**Recurrent epithelial keratitis** in childhood, trichiasis, corneal scarring, and entropion. **The leading cause of preventable blindness worldwide.**	Giemsa stain, chlamydial cultures.	Azithromycin, tetracycline, or erythromycin × 3–4 weeks.
Viral	**Adenovirus** (most common)	Copious **watery discharge,** severe ocular irritation, preauricular lymphadenopathy. Occurs in epidemics.		**Contagious;** self-limited. Topical corticosteroids with supervision of an ophthalmologist.

tal or nasal mucosal ulceration with coexisting maxillary and/or ethmoid sinusitis suggests mucormycosis or *Rhizopus.*

- **Dx: Mostly clinical.** Blood and tissue fluid culture; CT scan (to rule out orbital abscess and intracranial involvement).
- **Tx: Admit. Immediate IV antibiotics;** request an **ophthalmologic/ENT** consult. Abscess formation may necessitate surgery. **Diabetic and immunocompromised patients** should be treated with **amphotericin B and surgical debridement** (often associated with **cavernous sinus thrombosis**) if *Mucor* or *Rhizopus* is diagnosed.

Neisseria conjunctivitis is an ocular emergency often requiring inpatient parenteral antibiotic therapy.

Otitis Externa

- An inflammation of the external auditory canal, also known as "swimmer's ear." *Pseudomonas* (from poorly chlorinated pools) and Enterobacteriaceae are the most common etiologic agents. Both grow in the presence of excess moisture.
- **Hx/PE:** Presents with pain, pruritus, and possible purulent discharge. Exam reveals **pain with movement of the tragus/pinna** (unlike otitis media) and an edematous and erythematous ear canal. See the Pediatrics chapter for a discussion of otitis media.
- **Dx:** A clinical diagnosis. Gram stain and culture are helpful if a fungal etiology is suspected. CT scan if the patient is toxic appearing.

Diabetics are at risk for malignant otitis externa.

■ **Tx: Antibiotic** and steroid eardrops. Use systemic antibiotics in patients with severe disease. Diabetics are at risk for malignant otitis externa and osteomyelitis of the skull base and thus require hospitalization and IV antibiotics.

Otitis media should not cause pain with movement of the tragus/pinna.

▶ **MISCELLANEOUS INFECTIONS**

Infective Endocarditis

Infection of the endocardium, usually 2° to bacterial or other infectious causes. Most commonly affects the heart valves, especially the mitral valve. Risk factors include rheumatic, congenital, or valvular heart disease; prosthetic heart valves; IV drug abuse; and immunosuppression. Etiologies are as follows:

■ *S. aureus* (both methicillin-sensitive and methicillin-resistant): The causative agent in > 80% of cases of acute bacterial endocarditis in patients with a history of IV drug abuse.
■ **Viridans streptococci:** The most common pathogens for left-sided subacute bacterial endocarditis.
■ **Coagulase-⊖ *Staphylococcus*:** The most common infecting organism in prosthetic valve endocarditis.
■ *Streptococcus bovis:* S. bovis endocarditis is associated with coexisting GI malignancy.
■ *Candida* and *Aspergillus* species: Account for most cases of fungal endocarditis. Predisposing factors include long-term indwelling IV catheters, malignancy, AIDS, organ transplantation, and IV drug use. Table 2.8-10 lists the causes of endocarditis.

HISTORY/PE

■ **Constitutional symptoms** are common (fever/FUO, weight loss, fatigue).
■ Exam reveals a **heart murmur.** The mitral valve is more commonly affected than the aortic valve in non–IV drug users; more right-sided involvement is found in IV drug users (tricuspid valve > mitral valve > aortic valve).
■ **Osler's nodes** (small, tender nodules on the finger and toe pads), **Janeway lesions** (small peripheral hemorrhages; see Figure 2.8-15), **splinter hemorrhages** (subungual petechiae; see Figure 2.8-16), **Roth's spots** (retinal hemorrhages), focal neurologic deficits from embolic stroke, and other embolic phenomena are also seen.

Presentation of endocarditis—

JR = NO FAME

Janeway lesions
Roth's spots
Nail-bed (splinter) hemorrhage
Osler's nodes
Fever
Anemia
Murmur
Emboli

TABLE 2.8-10. Causes of Endocarditis

ACUTE	SUBACUTE	MARANTIC	CULTURE-⊖ (INCLUDES HACEK)	SLE
S. aureus (IV drug abuse)	Viridans streptococci (native valve)	Cancer (poor prognosis).	Haemophilus parainfluenzae	Libman-Sacks endocarditis (autoantibody to valve)
S. pneumoniae	Enterococcus	Mets seed valves; emboli can cause cerebral infarcts.	Actinobacillus	
N. gonorrhoeae	S. epidermidis (prosthetic valve)		Cardiobacterium	
	S. bovis (GI insult)		Eikenella	
	Fungi		Kingella	
			Coxiella burnetii	
			Brucella	
			Bartonella	

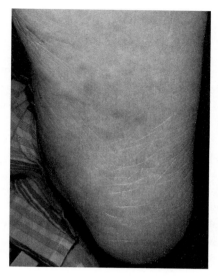

FIGURE 2.8-15. **Janeway lesions.**

Peripheral embolization to the sole leads to a cluster of erythematous macules known as Janeway lesions. (Courtesy of the Department of Dermatology, Wilford Hall USAF Medical Center and Brooke Army Medical Center, San Antonio, TX, as published in Knoop KJ et al. *Atlas of Emergency Medicine*, 2nd ed. New York: McGraw-Hill, 2002: 384.)

DIAGNOSIS

- Diagnosis is guided by risk factors, clinical symptoms, and the **Duke criteria** (see Table 2.8-11).
- **CBC** with leukocytosis and left shift; ↑ **ESR** and CRP.

TREATMENT

- **Early empiric IV antibiotic treatment** includes vancomycin or nafcillin + gentamicin. Ampicillin/sulbactam or ceftriaxone are alternative choices depending on the suspected organism. Tailor antibiotics once the causative agent is known. Acute valve replacement is sometimes necessary. The

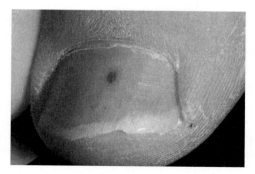

FIGURE 2.8-16. **Splinter hemorrhages.**

Note the splinter hemorrhages along the distal aspect of the nail plate, due to emboli from subacute bacterial endocarditis. (Courtesy of the Armed Forces Institute of Pathology, Bethesda, MD, as published in Knoop KJ et al. *Atlas of Emergency Medicine*, 2nd ed. New York: McGraw-Hill, 2002: 384.)

TABLE 2.8-11. Duke Criteria for the Diagnosis of Endocarditis

CRITERIA	COMPONENTS
Major	At least two separate ⊕ blood cultures for a typical organism, persistent bacteremia with any organism, or a single ⊕ culture of *Coxiella burnetii*. Evidence of endocardial involvement (via transesophageal echocardiography or new murmur).
Minor	Predisposing risk factors. Fever ≥ 38.3°C. **Vascular phenomena:** Septic emboli, septic infarcts, mycotic aneurysm, Janeway lesions. **Immunologic phenomena:** Glomerulonephritis, Osler's nodes. Roth's spots. Microbiological evidence that does not meet major criteria.

> **Endocarditis: indications for surgery—**
>
> **PUS RIVER**
>
> **P**rosthetic valve endocarditis (most cases)
> **U**ncontrolled infection
> **S**uppurative local complications with conduction abnormalities
> **R**esection of mycotic aneurysm
> **I**neffective antimicrobial therapy (e.g., vs. fungi)
> **V**alvular damage (significant)
> **E**mbolization (repeated systemic)
> **R**efractory CHF (or sudden onset)

The anthrax-associated pruritic papule forms an ulcer with an edematous halo and then a black eschar.

prognosis for prosthetic valve endocarditis is poor. See the mnemonic **PUS RIVER** for indications for surgery.

■ Give antibiotic prophylaxis before dental work in patients with high-risk valvular disease (e.g., those with previous endocarditis or a prosthetic valve).

Anthrax

Caused by the spore-forming gram-⊕ bacterium *Bacillus anthracis*. Its natural incidence is rare, but infection is an occupational hazard for veterinarians, farmers, and individuals who handle **animal wool, hair, hides, or bone meal products**. Also a biological weapon. *B. anthracis* can cause cutaneous (most common), inhalation (most deadly), or GI anthrax.

HISTORY/PE

■ **Cutaneous:** Presents 1–7 days after skin exposure and penetration of spores. The lesion begins as a **pruritic papule** that enlarges to form an ulcer surrounded by a satellite bulbus/lesion with an edematous halo and a round, regular, and raised edge. **Regional lymphadenopathy** is also characteristic. The lesion evolves into a **black eschar** within 7–10 days.
■ **Inhalational:** Presents with fever, dyspnea, hypoxia, hypotension, or symptoms of pneumonia (1–3 days after exposure), classically due to **hemorrhagic mediastinitis.**
■ **GI:** Occurs after the ingestion of poorly cooked, contaminated meat; can present with dysphagia, nausea/vomiting, bloody diarrhea, and abdominal pain.

DIAGNOSIS

CXR is the most sensitive test for inhalational disease (**widened mediastinum,** pleural effusions, infiltrates). Aerobic culture and Gram stain of ulcer exudate show nonmotile short chains of bacilli. Antibody tests are also useful in confirming the diagnosis.

TREATMENT

■ **Ciprofloxacin** or doxycycline plus one or two additional antibiotics for at least 14 days are first-line therapy for inhalational disease or cutaneous disease of the face, head, or neck. Many strains express β-lactamases that confer resistance to penicillin; therefore, penicillin and amoxicillin are no longer recommended as single agents for inhalational disease.

- For cutaneous disease, treat for 7–10 days. Postexposure prophylaxis (**ciprofloxacin**) to prevent inhalation anthrax should be continued for 60 days.

Osteomyelitis

Bone or bone marrow infection 2° to **direct spread** from a soft tissue infection (80% of cases) is most common in adults, whereas infection due to **hematogenous seeding** (20% of cases) is more common in children (metaphyses of the long bones) and IV drug users **(vertebral bodies)**. Common pathogens are outlined in Table 2.8-12.

History/PE

Presents with **localized bone pain and tenderness** along with warmth, swelling, erythema, and limited motion of the adjacent joint. Systemic symptoms (fevers, chills) and purulent drainage may be present.

Diagnosis

- **Labs:** ↑ WBC count, **ESR** (> 100), and **CRP** levels. Blood cultures may be ⊕.
- **Imaging:**
  - X-rays are often ⊖ initially but may show **periosteal elevation** within 10–14 days. Bone scans are also used and are sensitive for osteomyelitis but lack specificity.
  - **MRI** (test of choice) will show ↑ signal in the bone marrow and associated soft tissue infection.
- Definitive diagnosis is made by bone aspiration with Gram stain and culture. Clinical diagnosis made by probing through the soft tissue to bone is usually sufficient, as aspiration carries a risk of infection.

Penicillin and amoxicillin are no longer recommended as single agents for the treatment of disseminated anthrax. Treat with ciprofloxacin plus one or two other antibiotics.

Osteomyelitis is associated with peripheral vascular disease, diabetes, penetrating soft tissue injuries, chronic decubitus ulcers, and IV drug abuse.

TABLE 2.8-12. Common Pathogens in Osteomyelitis

If	Think
Most people	*S. aureus*
IV drug user	*S. aureus* or *Pseudomonas*
Sickle cell disease	*Salmonella*
Hip replacement	*S. epidermidis*
Foot puncture wound	*Pseudomonas*
Chronic	*S. aureus, Pseudomonas,* Enterobacteriaceae
Diabetic	Polymicrobial, *Pseudomonas, S. aureus,* streptococci, anaerobes

Diabetic osteomyelitis should be treated with antibiotics targeting gram-⊕ organisms and anaerobes.

TREATMENT

- **Surgical debridement** of necrotic, infected bone followed by **IV antibiotics** × 4–6 weeks. Empiric antibiotic selection is based on the suspected organism and Gram stain.
- Consider clindamycin + ciprofloxacin, ampicillin/sulbactam, or oxacillin/nafcillin (for methicillin-sensitive S. *aureus*); vancomycin (for MRSA); or ceftriaxone or ciprofloxacin (for gram-⊖ bacteria).

COMPLICATIONS

Chronic osteomyelitis, sepsis, septic arthritis. Long-standing chronic osteomyelitis with a draining sinus tract may eventually lead to **squamous cell carcinoma** (Marjolin's ulcer).

Musculoskeletal

Table 2.9-1 outlines the presentation and treatment of orthopedic injuries that commonly affect adults.

► **COMPARTMENT SYNDROME**

- ↑ **pressure** within a confined space that compromises nerve, muscle, and soft tissue perfusion. Occurs primarily in the anterior compartment of the lower leg and forearm 2° to trauma (fracture or muscle injury) to the affected compartment.
- **Hx/PE:** Presents with pain out of proportion to physical findings; **pain with passive motion** of the fingers and toes; and paresthesias, pallor, poikilothermia, pulselessness, and paralysis. Pulselessness occurs late.
- **Dx:** Measure compartment pressures (usually ≥ 30 mmHg); measure delta pressures (diastolic pressure – compartment pressure).
- **Tx: Immediate fasciotomy** to ↓ pressures and ↑ tissue perfusion.

► **CARPAL TUNNEL SYNDROME (CTS)**

Entrapment of the median nerve at the wrist caused by ↓ size or space of the carpal tunnel, leading to paresthesias, pain, and occasionally paralysis. Can be precipitated by overuse of wrist flexors, diabetes mellitus, or thyroid dysfunction. Commonly occurs in pregnant and middle-aged women.

HISTORY/PE

- Presents with aching over the **thenar area of the hand** and proximal forearm. Pain may extend to the shoulder.
- Paresthesia or numbness is seen in a median nerve distribution.
- Symptoms **worsen at night** or when the wrists are held in flexion or extension.
- Patients may report frequently dropping objects or inability to open jars.
- Exam shows thenar atrophy (if CTS is long-standing).
- **Phalen's maneuver** and **Tinel's sign** are ⊕.

DIAGNOSIS

A clinical diagnosis, although EMG testing can be used to confirm.

TREATMENT

- Splint the wrist in a neutral position at night and during the day if possible. Administer NSAIDs.
- Conservative treatment can include corticosteroid injection of the carpal canal.
- Work-related CTS may benefit from ergonomic aids.
- CTS of pregnancy usually resolves after delivery.
- Surgical release of the carpal tunnel is a widely accepted treatment, particularly for fixed sensory loss, thenar weakness, or intolerable symptoms.

COMPLICATIONS

Permanent loss of sensation, hand strength, and fine motor skills.

Volkmann's contracture of the wrist and fingers is caused by compartment syndrome due to supracondylar fractures.

The 6 P's of compartment syndrome:

Pain
Pallor
Paresthesias
Poikilothermia
Paralysis
Pulselessness

Phalen's maneuver: placing the wrists in flexion reproduces aching and numbness in < 60 seconds.

Tinel's sign: tapping over the median nerve at the wrist elicits tingling in the median nerve distribution.

TABLE 2.9-1. **Common Adult Orthopedic Injuries**

INJURY	MECHANICS	TREATMENT
Shoulder dislocation	**Anterior dislocation:** Most common; the axillary artery and nerve are at risk. Patients hold the arm in slight abduction and external rotation. **Posterior dislocation:** Rare; associated with seizure and electrocutions; can injure the radial artery. Patients hold the arm in adduction and internal rotation.	Reduction followed by a sling and swath. Recurrent dislocations may need surgical repair.
Hip dislocation	**Posterior dislocation:** Most common (> 90%); occurs via a posteriorly directed force on an internally rotated, flexed, adducted hip ("dashboard injury"). Associated with a risk of sciatic nerve injury and avascular necrosis (AVN). **Anterior dislocation:** Can injure the obturator nerve.	Closed reduction followed by abduction pillow/bracing. Evaluate with CT scan after reduction.
Colles' fracture	Involves the distal radius. Often results from a fall onto an outstretched hand, leading to a dorsally displaced, dorsally angulated fracture. Commonly seen in the elderly (osteoporosis) and children.	Closed reduction followed by application of a long-arm cast; open reduction if the fracture is intra-articular.
Scaphoid fracture	The **most commonly fractured carpal bone.** May take two weeks for radiographs to show the fracture. Assume a fracture if there is tenderness in the anatomical snuff box.	Thumb spica cast. If displacement or navicular nonunion is present, treat with open reduction. With proximal third scaphoid fractures, AVN may result from disruption of blood flow.
Boxer's fracture	Fracture of the fifth metacarpal neck. Due to forward trauma of a closed fist (e.g., punching a wall).	Closed reduction and ulnar gutter splint; percutaneous pinning if the fracture is excessively angulated. If skin is broken, assume infection by human oral pathogens and treat with surgical irrigation, debridement, and IV antibiotics (covering *Eikenella*).
Humerus fracture	Direct trauma. May have radial nerve palsy leading to wrist drop and loss of thumb abduction (see Figure 2.9-1).	Hanging-arm cast vs. coaptation splint and sling. Functional bracing.
"Nightstick fracture"	Ulnar shaft fracture resulting from self-defense with the arm against a blunt object.	Open reduction and internal fixation (ORIF) if significantly displaced.
Monteggia's fracture	Diaphyseal fracture of the proximal ulna with subluxation of the radial head.	ORIF of the shaft fracture (due to poor fracture diaphyseal blood supply) and closed reduction of the radial head.

HIGH-YIELD FACTS

MUSCULOSKELETAL

TABLE 2.9-1. **Common Adult Orthopedic Injuries** *(continued)*

INJURY	MECHANICS	TREATMENT
Galeazzi's fracture	Diaphyseal fracture of the radius with dislocation of the distal radioulnar joint. Results from a direct blow to the radius.	ORIF of the radius and casting of the fractured forearm in supination to reduce the distal radioulnar joint.
Hip fracture	↑ risk with osteoporosis. Presents with a shortened and externally rotated leg. **Displaced femoral neck fractures:** Associated with an ↑ risk of AVN, nonunion, and DVTs.	ORIF with parallel pinning of the femoral neck. Displaced fractures in elderly patients may require a hip hemiarthroplasty. Anticoagulate to ↓ the likelihood of DVTs.
Femoral fracture	Direct trauma. Beware of fat emboli, which present with fever, change in mental status, dyspnea, hypoxia, petechiae, and ↓ platelets.	Intramedullary nailing of the femur. Irrigate and debride open fractures.
Tibial fracture	Direct trauma. Watch for compartment syndrome.	Casting vs. intramedullary nailing.
Open fractures	An orthopedic emergency; patients must be taken to the OR in < 6 hours owing to ↑ infection risk.	OR emergently to repair fracture. Treat with antibiotics and tetanus prophylaxis.
Achilles tendon rupture	Presents with a sudden "pop" like a rifle shot. More likely with ↓ physical conditioning. Exam shows limited plantar flexion and a ⊕ Thompson's test (pressure on the gastrocnemius leading to absent foot plantar flexion).	Treat surgically followed by long leg cast for six weeks.
Knee injuries	Present with knee instability, edema, and hematoma. **ACL:** ▪ Results from a noncontact twisting mechanism, forced hyperextension, or impact to an extended knee. ▪ ⊕ anterior drawer and Lachman tests. ▪ Rule out a meniscal or MCL injury. **PCL:** ▪ Results from forced hyperextension. ▪ ⊕ posterior drawer test. **Meniscal tears:** ▪ Result from an acute twisting injury or a degenerative tear in elderly patients. ▪ Clicking or locking may be present. ▪ Exam shows joint line tenderness and a ⊕ McMurray's test.	Treatment of MCL/LCL and meniscal tears is usually conservative. Treatment of ACL injuries is generally surgical with graft from the patellar or hamstring tendons. Operative PCL repair is reserved for highly competitive athletes. Operative meniscal repair is for younger patients with significant tears or older patients whose symptoms do not respond to conservative treatment.

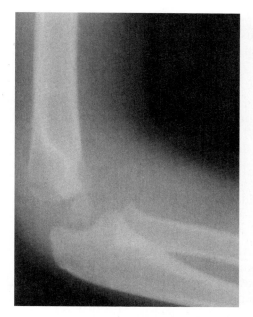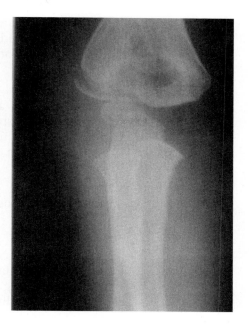

FIGURE 2.9-1. Lateral condyle fracture of the humerus.

(Reproduced, with permission, from Skinner HB. *Current Diagnosis & Treatment in Orthopedics*, 2nd ed. Stamford, CT: Appleton & Lange, 2000: 572.)

▶ BURSITIS

Inflammation of the bursa by **repetitive use, trauma, infection, or systemic inflammatory disease.** A bursa is a flattened sac filled with a small amount of synovial fluid that serves as a protective buffer between bones and overlapping muscles. Common sites of bursitis include subacromial, olecranon, trochanteric, prepatellar, and infrapatellar bursae. Septic bursitis is more common in superficial bursae (olecranon, prepatellar, and infrapatellar bursae).

HISTORY/PE

Presents with localized tenderness, ↓ range of motion (ROM), edema, and erythema; patients may have a history of trauma or inflammatory disease.

DIAGNOSIS

Needle aspiration is indicated if septic bursitis is suspected; no labs or imaging is needed.

TREATMENT

- Conservative treatment includes rest, heat and ice, elevation, and NSAIDs.
- Intrabursal corticosteroid injection can be considered (**contraindicated if septic bursitis** is suspected).
- Septic bursitis should be treated with 7–10 days of antibiotics.

▶ TENDINITIS

An **inflammatory condition** characterized by pain at tendinous insertions into bone associated with swelling or impaired function. It commonly occurs

Oral fluoroquinolones are associated with an ↑ risk of tendon rupture and tendinitis.

in the supraspinatus, **biceps,** wrist extensor, **patellar,** iliotibial band, posterior tibial, and **Achilles tendons.** Overuse is the most common cause and includes work-related activities or an ↑ in activity level.

HISTORY/PE

- Presents with pain at a tendinous insertion that worsens with **repetitive stress** and **resisted strength testing** of the affected muscle group.
- Wrist flexor tendinitis (lateral epicondylitis, or tennis elbow) worsens with resisted dorsiflexion of the wrist.

DIAGNOSIS

A clinical diagnosis. Consider a radiograph if there is a history of trauma.

TREATMENT

- Treat with rest and NSAIDs; apply ice for the first 24–48 hours.
- Consider splinting or immobilization.
- Begin strengthening exercises once pain has subsided.
- If conservative treatment fails, consider peritendinous injection of lidocaine and corticosteroids. **Never inject the Achilles tendon** in view of the ↑ risk of rupture. Avoid repetitive injection.

Most lower back pain is mechanical; bed rest is contraindicated.

▶ **LOW BACK PAIN (LBP)**

Table 2.9-2 outlines the motor, reflex, and sensory deficits with which low back pain is associated.

Herniated Disk

Causes include degenerative changes, trauma, or neck/back strain or sprain. Most common (95%) in the lumbar region, especially at L4–L5 and L5–S1.

HISTORY/PE

- Presents with sudden onset of severe, electricity-like LBP, usually preceded by several months of aching, "discogenic" pain.
- Common among middle-aged and older men.
- Exacerbated by ↑ intra-abdominal pressure or Valsalva (e.g., coughing).
- Associated with **sciatica,** paresthesias, muscle weakness, atrophy, contractions, or spasms.

Red flags for lower back pain include age > 50, > 6 weeks of pain, previous cancer history, severe pain, constitutional symptoms, and loss of anal sphincter tone.

TABLE 2.9-2. Motor and Sensory Deficits in Back Pain

NERVE ROOT	ASSOCIATED DEFICIT		
	MOTOR	REFLEX	SENSORY
L4	Foot dorsiflexion (tibialis anterior)	Patellar	Medial aspect of the lower leg.
L5	Big toe dorsiflexion (extensor hallucis longus), foot eversion (peroneus muscles)	None	Dorsum of the foot and lateral aspect of the lower leg.
S1	Plantar flexion (gastrocnemius/soleus), hip extension (gluteus maximus).	Achilles	Plantar and lateral aspects of the foot.

- A **passive straight leg raise** ↑ **pain** (highly sensitive but not specific).
- A crossed straight leg raise ↑ pain (highly specific but not sensitive). Large midline herniations can cause **cauda equina syndrome.**

DIAGNOSIS

- Obtain an ESR and a plain radiograph if other causes of back pain are suspected (e.g., infection, trauma, compression fracture).
- Order a stat MRI for cauda equina syndrome or for a severe or rapidly progressing neurologic deficit.
- Order an MRI if symptoms are refractory to conservative management. MRI may show disk herniation (see Figure 2.9-2).

TREATMENT

- NSAIDs in scheduled doses, physical therapy, and local heat lead to resolution within four weeks in 80% of cases.
- Epidural or nerve block may be of benefit.
- Severe or rapidly evolving neurologic deficits and cauda equina syndrome are indications for discectomy.

Spinal Stenosis

Narrowing of the lumbar or cervical spinal canal, leading to compression of the nerve roots. Most commonly due to degenerative joint disease; typically occurs in middle-aged or elderly patients.

HISTORY/PE

- Presents with neck pain, back pain that radiates to the buttocks and legs, and leg numbness/weakness.

Lung, breast, and prostate cancer can metastasize to the vertebrae and cause back pain.

Bowel or bladder dysfunction (urinary overflow incontinence), impotence, and saddle-area anesthesia are consistent with cauda equina syndrome, which is a surgical emergency.

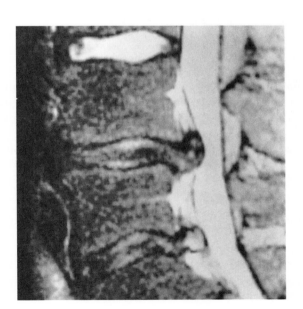

FIGURE 2.9-2. Disk herniation.

MRI reveals herniations of L4–L5 and L5–S1. (Reproduced, with permission, from Skinner HB. *Current Diagnosis & Treatment in Orthopedics*, 1st ed. Stamford, CT: Appleton & Lange, 1995: 186.)

HIGH-YIELD FACTS

MUSCULOSKELETAL

- Leg cramping is worse at rest, with standing, and with walking (pseudo- or neurogenic claudication).
- Symptoms **improve** with **flexion at the hips** and bending forward.

DIAGNOSIS

- Radiographs show degenerative changes that include disk space narrowing, facet hypertrophy, and spondylolisthesis, leading to a narrowed spinal canal.
- MRI or CT shows spinal stenosis.

TREATMENT

- **Mild to moderate:** NSAIDs and abdominal muscle strengthening.
- **Advanced:** Epidural corticosteroid injections can provide relief.
- **Refractory:** Surgical laminectomy may achieve significant short-term success, but many patients will have a recurrence of symptoms.

▶ OSTEOSARCOMA

The most common benign bone tumor is osteochondroma.

The second most common 1° malignant tumor of bone (after multiple myeloma). Tends to occur in the **metaphyseal** regions of the **distal femur, proximal tibia,** and proximal humerus; often metastasizes to the lungs. Some cases are preceded by Paget's disease. Risk factors include male gender and age 20–30.

HISTORY/PE

- Presents as progressive and eventually intractable **pain that is worse at night.**
- Constitutional symptoms such as fever, weight loss, and night sweats may be present.
- Erythema and enlargement over the site of the tumor may be seen.
- See the Endocrinology chapter for a discussion of osteosarcoma vs. Paget's disease.

DIAGNOSIS

- Radiographs show **Codman's triangle** (periosteal new bone formation at the diaphyseal end of the lesion) or a **"sunburst pattern"** of the osteosarcoma (see Figure 2.9-3)—in contrast to multilayered **"onion skinning,"** which is classic for Ewing's sarcoma.
- MRI and CT facilitate staging (soft tissue and bony invasion) and planning for surgery.

TREATMENT

- Limb-sparing surgical procedures and pre- and postoperative chemotherapy (e.g., methotrexate, doxorubicin, cisplatin, ifosfamide).
- Amputation may be necessary.

▶ OSTEOARTHRITIS (OA)

A common, chronic, noninflammatory arthritis of the synovial joints. Characterized by deterioration of the articular cartilage and osteophyte bone formation at the joint surfaces. Risk factors include a ⊕ family history, **obesity,** and a **history of joint trauma.**

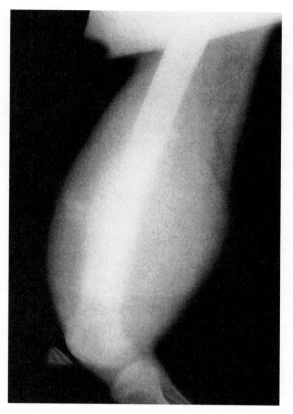

FIGURE 2.9-3.   Osteosarcoma.

"Sunburst" appearance of neoplastic bone formation in the femur of a 15-year-old girl. Amputation was required owing to the size of the tumor. (Reproduced, with permission, from Skinner HB. *Current Diagnosis & Treatment in Orthopedics*, 2nd ed. Stamford, CT: Appleton & Lange, 2000: 272.)

HISTORY/PE

Presents with **crepitus,** ↓ ROM, and initially **pain that worsens with activity and weight bearing but improves with rest.** Morning stiffness lasts for < 30 minutes. Stiffness is also experienced after periods of rest ("gelling").

DIAGNOSIS

- Radiographs show **joint space narrowing,** osteophytes, subchondral sclerosis, and subchondral bone cysts (see Figure 2.9-4). Radiograph severity does not correlate with symptomatology.
- Synovial fluid shows straw-colored fluid, normal viscosity, and a WBC count < 2000 cells/μL.

TREATMENT

Physical therapy, **weight reduction,** and **NSAIDs.** Intra-articular corticosteroid injections may provide temporary relief. **Consider joint replacement** (e.g., total hip/knee arthroplasty) in advanced cases.

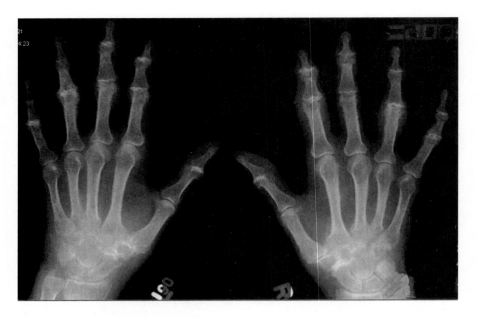

FIGURE 2.9-4. **Osteoarthritis.**

Plain radiographs show joint space narrowing, osteophytes, and subchondral degenerative cysts involving the DIP and PIP joints, with sparing of the MCP. (Reproduced, with permission, from USMLERx.com.)

▶ COMPLEX REGIONAL PAIN SYNDROME

A **pain syndrome** accompanied by **loss of function and autonomic dysfunction,** usually occurring after trauma. Formerly known as reflex sympathetic dystrophy. The disease has three phases: acute sympathetic denervation and underactivity → dystrophic phase → atrophic phase.

HISTORY/PE
- **Diffuse pain occurs** out of proportion to the initial injury, often in a **nonanatomic** distribution.
- Pain can occur at any time relative to the initial injury.
- **Loss of function** of the affected limb is seen.
- **Sympathetic dysfunction** occurs and may be documented by skin, soft tissue, or blood flow changes.
- Skin temperature, hair growth, and nail growth may ↑ or ↓. Edema may be present.

DIAGNOSIS
A clinical diagnosis, but objective evidence of changes in skin temperature, hair growth, or nail growth may be present.

TREATMENT
- Medications include NSAIDs, corticosteroids, low-dose TCAs, gabapentin, pregabalin, and calcitonin (no oral medications are consistently effective).
- Physical therapy modalities such as heat, ice, desensitization techniques, and gentle ROM exercises may be helpful.
- **Chemical sympathetic blockade** may relieve symptoms.
- Referral to a chronic pain specialist is appropriate for complicated cases.

- A centrally mediated chronic pain disorder characterized by soft tissue and axial skeletal pain in the absence of joint pain. Inflammation is notably absent.
- **Hx/PE:** Most common in **women 30–50 years of age**; associated with depression, anxiety, sleep disorders, IBS, and cognitive disorders ("fibro fog").
- **Dx:** Multiple (≥ 11 of 18), diffuse tender points over all four body quadrants and the axial skeleton must be present for diagnosis (see Figure 2.9-5). The presence of < 11 of 18 tender points or non-fibromyalgia-associated tender points is known as **myofascial pain syndrome.**
- **Tx: Antidepressants** (an SSRI/TCA combination has proven efficacy), gabapentin, pregabalin, muscle relaxants, and **physical therapy** (stretching, heat application, hydrotherapy). Avoid narcotics.

▶ **GOUT**

Recurrent attacks of **acute monoarticular arthritis** resulting from intra-articular deposition of **monosodium urate crystals** due to disorders of urate metabolism. Risk factors include male gender, obesity, and postmenopausal status in females.

HISTORY/PE

- Presents with excruciating joint pain of sudden onset that can awaken the patient from sleep.

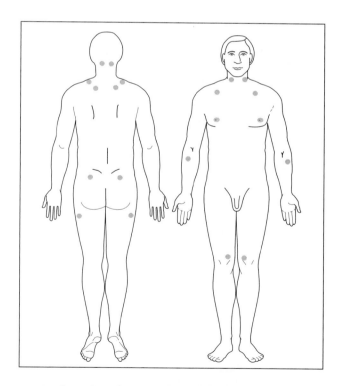

FIGURE 2.9-5. **Tender points characteristic of fibromyalgia.**

Causes of hyperuricemia:

↑ cell turnover (hemolysis, blast crisis, tumor lysis, myelodysplasia, psoriasis)
Cyclosporine
Dehydration
Diabetes insipidus
Diet (e.g., ↑ red meat, alcohol)
Diuretics
Lead poisoning
Lesch-Nyhan syndrome
Salicylates (low dose)
Starvation

Colchicine inhibits neutrophil chemotaxis and is most effective when used early during a gout flare (use is limited by a narrow therapeutic window).

- Most commonly affects the **first MTP joint** (podagra) and the midfoot, knees, ankles, and wrists; the hips and shoulders are generally spared.
- Joints are erythematous, swollen, and exquisitely tender.
- **Tophi** (urate crystal deposits in soft tissue) may be seen with chronic disease.

DIAGNOSIS

- Joint fluid aspirate shows **needle-shaped, negatively birefringent crystals** (see Table 2.9-3 and Clinical Images).
- An elevated WBC count in the joint aspirate or peripheral blood may be seen during flares.
- Serum uric acid is usually ↑ (≥ 7.5), but patients may have normal levels.
- Punched-out erosions with overhanging cortical bone (**"rat-bite" erosions**) are seen in advanced gout.

TREATMENT

- **Acute attacks:** High-dose **NSAIDs** (e.g., indomethacin), colchicine, and/or **steroids.**
- **Maintenance therapy: Allopurinol** for overproducers, those with contraindications to probenecid treatment (tophi, renal stones, chronic renal failure), and refractory cases; **probenecid** for undersecretors.
- Weight loss and avoidance of triggers of hyperuricemia will prevent recurrent attacks in many patients.

▶ ANKYLOSING SPONDYLITIS

A chronic inflammatory disease of the spine and pelvis that causes sacroiliitis leading to fusion of the affected joints. Strongly associated with **HLA-B27.** Risk factors include male gender and a ⊕ family history.

HISTORY/PE

- Typical onset is in the late teens and early 20s. Presents with fatigue, intermittent hip pain, and LBP that **worsens with inactivity and in the mornings.**
- ↓ spine flexion (⊕ Schober test), loss of lumbar lordosis, hip pain and stiffness, and ↓ chest expansion are seen as the disease progresses.
- Anterior **uveitis** and **heart block** may occur.
- Other forms of seronegative spondyloarthropathy must be ruled out, including the following:
    - **Reactive arthritis** (formerly known as **Reiter's syndrome**): A disease of young men. The characteristic arthritis, uveitis, conjunctivitis, and urethritis usually follow an infection with *Campylobacter, Shigella, Salmonella, Chlamydia,* or *Ureaplasma.*
    - **Psoriatic arthritis:** An oligoarthritis that can include the **DIP joints.**

TABLE 2.9-3. Gout vs. Pseudogout

DISORDER	CRYSTAL SHAPE	CRYSTAL BIREFRINGENCE
Gout	Needle shaped	⊖
Pseudogout	Rhomboid	⊕

Associated with psoriatic skin changes and **sausage-shaped digits** (dactylitis).
- **Enteropathic spondylitis:** An ankylosing spondylitis–like disease characterized by sacroiliitis that is usually asymmetric and is associated with IBD.

DIAGNOSIS

- $\oplus$ **HLA-B27** is found in 85–95% of cases.
- Radiographs may show **fused sacroiliac joints,** squaring of the lumbar vertebrae, development of vertical syndesmophytes, and bamboo spine.
- ESR or CRP is ↑ in 75% of cases.
- $\ominus$ **RF;** $\ominus$ ANA.

TREATMENT

- **NSAIDs** (e.g., indomethacin) for pain; exercise to improve posture and breathing.
- **Tumor necrosis factor (TNF) inhibitors** or sulfasalazine can be used in refractory cases.

▶ POLYMYOSITIS AND DERMATOMYOSITIS

Polymyositis is a progressive, systemic connective tissue disease characterized by immune-mediated striated muscle inflammation. **Dermatomyositis** presents with symptoms of polymyositis plus cutaneous involvement, although the pathogenesis is different. Most often affect patients 50–70 years of age; the male-to-female ratio is 1:2. African-Americans are affected more often than Caucasians.

HISTORY/PE

- Distinguished as follows:
    - **Polymyositis:** Presents with **symmetric,** progressive **proximal** muscle weakness, pain, and difficulty breathing or swallowing (advanced disease).
    - **Dermatomyositis:** Patients may have **heliotrope rash** (a violaceous periorbital rash), **"shawl sign"** (a rash involving the shoulders, upper chest, and back), and/or **Gottron's papules** (a papular rash with scales located on the dorsa of the hands, over bony prominences).
- Patients may also develop myocarditis and cardiac conduction deficits.
- Can be associated with an underlying malignancy, especially lung and breast carcinoma.

DIAGNOSIS

- ↑ **serum CK and anti-Jo-1 antibodies** are seen (see Table 2.9-4).
- **Muscle biopsy** reveals inflammation and muscle fibers in varying stages of necrosis and regeneration.

TREATMENT

- High-dose corticosteroids with taper after 4–6 weeks to ↓ the maintenance dose.
- Azathioprine and/or methotrexate can be used as steroid-sparing agents.

TABLE 2.9-4.   Common Antibodies and Their Disease Associations

ANTIBODY	DISEASE ASSOCIATION
ANA	SLE
Anti-CCP	RA
Anticentromere	CREST syndrome
Anti-dsDNA	SLE
Antihistone	Drug-induced SLE
Anti-Jo-1	Polymyositis/dermatomyositis
Antimitochondrial	Primary biliary cirrhosis
Anti-Scl-70	Scleroderma
Anti-Sm	SLE
Anti-TSHR	Graves' disease
c-ANCA	Vasculitis, especially Wegener's
p-ANCA	Vasculitis, microscopic polyangiitis
Rheumatoid factor	RA
U1RNP antibody	Mixed connective tissue disease

▶ RHEUMATOID ARTHRITIS (RA)

A systemic autoimmune disorder characterized by chronic, destructive, inflammatory arthritis with **symmetric** involvement of both large and small joints that results in synovial hypertrophy and pannus formation, ultimately leading to erosion of adjacent cartilage, bone, and tendons. Risk factors include female gender, age 35–50, and **HLA-DR4.**

HISTORY/PE

- Presents with insidious onset of **morning stiffness** for > 1 hour along with painful, warm swelling of multiple symmetric joints (**wrists, MCP joints,** ankles, knees, shoulders, hips, and elbows) for > 6 weeks.
- Fever, fatigue, malaise, anorexia, and weight loss may also be seen.
- Ulnar deviation of the fingers is seen with MCP joint hypertrophy (see Figure 2.9-6).
- Also presents with ligament and tendon deformations (e.g., swan-neck and boutonnière deformities), vasculitis, atlantoaxial subluxation (intubation risk), and keratoconjunctivitis sicca.

Sjögren's syndrome (keratoconjunctivitis sicca) is a common ocular manifestation of rheumatoid arthritis.

Felty's syndrome is characterized by rheumatoid arthritis, splenomegaly, and neutropenia.

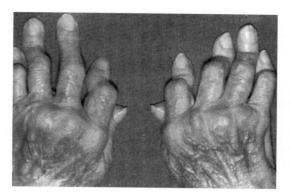

FIGURE 2.9-6. Rheumatoid arthritis.

Note the boutonnière deformities of the digits, ulnar deviation of the fingers, MCP joint hypertrophy, and severe involvement of the PIP joints. (Reproduced, with permission, from Chandrasoma P. *Concise Pathology*, 3rd ed. Stamford, CT: Appleton & Lange, 1998: 978.)

DIAGNOSIS

- **Labs:**
    - ↑ **RF** (IgM antibodies against Fc IgG) is seen in > 75% of cases.
    - The presence of anti-CCP (cyclic citrullinated peptide) is more specific than RF.
    - ↑ ESR may also be seen.
    - Anemia of chronic disease.
    - Synovial fluid aspirate shows turbid fluid, ↓ viscosity, and an ↑ WBC count (3000–50,000 cells/μL).
- **Radiographs:**
    - **Early:** Soft tissue swelling and juxta-articular demineralization.
    - **Late:** Joint space narrowing and erosions.

TREATMENT

- **NSAIDs** (can be reduced or discontinued following successful treatment with **disease-modifying antirheumatic drugs [DMARDs]**).
- DMARDs should be started early and include hydroxychloroquine, sulfasalazine, and methotrexate. Second-line agents include TNF inhibitors, rituximab (anti-CD20), and leflunomide.

▶ SCLERODERMA

Also called systemic sclerosis; characterized by inflammation that leads to progressive tissue fibrosis through excessive deposition of type I and type III collagen. Commonly manifests as **CREST syndrome** (limited form), but can also occur in a diffuse form involving the skin as well as the GI, GU, renal, pulmonary, and cardiovascular systems. Risk factors include female gender and age 35–50.

HISTORY/PE

- Exam may reveal symmetric thickening of the skin of face and/or distal extremities.
- **CREST syndrome** involves Calcinosis, Raynaud's phenomenon, Esophageal dysmotility, Sclerodactyly, and Telangiectasias.

CREST syndrome:

Calcinosis
Raynaud's phenomenon
Esophageal dysmotility
Sclerodactyly
Telangiectasias

- The diffuse form can lead to **pulmonary fibrosis,** cor pulmonale, acute renal failure, and malignant hypertension.

DIAGNOSIS

- RF and ANA may be ⊕.
- **Anticentromere antibodies** are specific for CREST syndrome (see Table 2.9-4).
- **Anti-Scl-70** (antitopoisomerase 1) **antibodies** are associated with diffuse disease and a poor prognosis (see Table 2.9-4).
- Eosinophilia may be seen.

TREATMENT

- Corticosteroids for acute flares; penicillamine can be used for skin changes.
- **Calcium channel blockers** for Raynaud's phenomenon.
- ACEIs for renal disease and prevention of a scleroderma renal crisis.

COMPLICATIONS

Mortality is due to pulmonary hypertension and complications of pulmonary hypertension.

▶ SYSTEMIC LUPUS ERYTHEMATOSUS (SLE)

A multisystem autoimmune disorder related to antibody-mediated cellular attack and deposition of antigen-antibody complexes. African-American women are at highest risk. Usually affects women of childbearing age.

HISTORY/PE

- Presents with nonspecific symptoms such as fever, anorexia, weight loss, and symmetric joint pain.
- The mnemonic **DOPAMINE RASH** summarizes the criteria for diagnosing SLE (see also Figure 2.9-7 and Clinical Images). Patients with four of the criteria are likely to have SLE (96% sensitive and specific).

DIAGNOSIS

- A ⊕ ANA is highly sensitive but not specific. **Anti-dsDNA** and **anti-Sm antibodies** are highly specific but not as sensitive (see Table 2.9-4).
    - **Drug-induced SLE:** ⊕ antihistone antibodies are seen **in 100% of cases** but are nonspecific.
    - **Neonatal SLE:** Associated with ⊕ anti-Ro antibodies transmitted from mother to neonate.
- The following may also be seen:
    - Antiphospholipid antibodies.
    - Anemia, leukopenia, and/or thrombocytopenia.
    - Proteinuria and/or casts.

TREATMENT

- **NSAIDs** for mild joint symptoms.
- **Corticosteroids** for **acute exacerbations.**
- Corticosteroids, hydroxychloroquine, cyclophosphamide, and azathioprine for progressive or refractory cases.

Criteria for SLE—

DOPAMINE RASH

Discoid rash
Oral ulcers
Photosensitivity
Arthritis
Malar rash
Immunologic criteria
Neurologic symptoms (lupus cerebritis, seizures)
Elevated ESR
Renal disease
ANA ⊕
Serositis (pleural or pericardial effusion)
Hematologic abnormalities

Drugs that can cause a lupus syndrome:

Chlorpromazine
Hydralazine
INH
Methyldopa
Penicillamine
Procainamide
Quinidine

Libman-Sacks endocarditis: noninfectious vegetations often seen on the mitral valve in association with SLE and antiphospholipid syndrome.

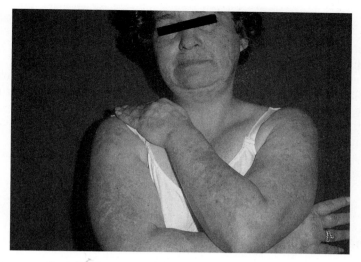

FIGURE 2.9-7. Systemic lupus erythematosus.

Erythematous patches and plaques of SLE, predominantly in sun-exposed areas. Note the malar rash across the bridge of the nose. (Reproduced, with permission, from Hurwitz RM. *Pathology of the Skin: Atlas of Clinical-Pathological Correlation*, 2nd ed. Stamford, CT: Appleton & Lange, 1998: 39.)

Also called giant cell arteritis; due to subacute granulomatous inflammation of the large vessels, including the aorta, external carotid (especially the **temporal branch**), and vertebral arteries. The most feared manifestation is **blindness** 2° to occlusion of the **central retinal artery** (a branch of the internal carotid artery). Risk factors include polymyalgia rheumatica (affects almost half of TA patients), age > 50, and female gender.

HISTORY/PE

- Presents with new headache (unilateral or bilateral); scalp pain and **temporal tenderness;** and **jaw claudication.**
- Fever, permanent **monocular blindness,** weight loss, and myalgias/arthralgias (especially of the shoulders and hips) are also seen.

DIAGNOSIS

- **ESR** > 50 (usually > 100).
- Ophthalmologic evaluation.
- **Temporal artery biopsy:** Look for thrombosis; necrosis of the media; and lymphocytes, plasma cells, and giant cells.

TREATMENT

High-dose prednisone begun immediately to prevent ocular involvement (or involvement of the remaining eye after onset of monocular blindness). Obtain a biopsy, but do not delay treatment. Conduct a follow-up eye exam.

- Risk factors include female gender and age > 50.
- **Hx/PE:**
    - Presents with pain and stiffness of **the shoulder and pelvic girdle** musculature with difficulty getting out of a chair or lifting the arms above the head.
    - Other symptoms include **fever,** malaise, and weight loss. Weakness is generally not appreciated on exam.
- **Dx:** Labs reveal a markedly ↑ **ESR, often associated with anemia.**
- **Tx: Low-dose prednisone** (10–20 mg/day).

Common Pediatric Orthopedic Injuries

Table 2.9-5 outlines the presentation and treatment of common pediatric orthopedic injuries.

Duchenne Muscular Dystrophy (DMD)

An **X-linked recessive disorder** resulting from a deficiency of **dystrophin,** a cytoskeletal protein. Onset is usually at 3–5 years of age.

HISTORY/PE

- Affects axial and proximal muscles more than distal muscles.
- May present with progressive **clumsiness, fatigability,** difficulty standing or walking, difficulty walking on toes (gastrocnemius shortening), **Gowers' maneuver** (using the hands to push off the thighs when rising from the floor), and waddling gait.
- **Pseudohypertrophy of the gastrocnemius muscles** is also seen.
- Mental retardation is common.
- Table 2.9-6 outlines the differential diagnosis of DMD and Becker muscular dystrophy.

DIAGNOSIS

- ⊖ **dystrophin immunostain;** ↑ CK.
- EMG shows polyphasic potentials and ↑ recruitment.
- **Muscle biopsy** shows necrotic muscle fibers from degeneration and variation in fiber size with fibrosis from regeneration.

TREATMENT

- Physical therapy is necessary to maintain ambulation and to prevent contractures.
- Liberal use of tendon release surgery may prolong ambulation.

COMPLICATIONS

Mortality is due to pulmonary congestion caused by high-output cardiac failure; cardiac fibrosis → arrhythmias and weak skeletal muscles → cardiopulmonary complications → pneumonia and respiratory failure.

TABLE 2.9-5. Orthopedic Injuries in Children

INJURY	MECHANICS	TREATMENT
Clavicular fracture	The most commonly fractured long bone in children. May be birth related (especially in large infants) and can be associated with brachial nerve palsies. Usually involves the middle third of the clavicle, with the proximal fracture end displaced superiorly owing to the pull of the sternocleidomastoid.	Figure-of-eight sling vs. arm sling.
Greenstick fracture	Incomplete fracture involving the cortex of only one side of the bone.	Reduction with casting. Order films at 10–14 days.
Nursemaid's elbow	Radial head subluxation that typically occurs as a result of being pulled or lifted by the hand. Presents with pain and refusal to bend the elbow.	Manual reduction by gentle supination of the elbow at 90 degrees of flexion. No immobilization.
Torus fracture	Buckling of the cortex of a long bone 2° to trauma. Usually occurs in the distal radius or ulna.	Cast immobilization for 3–5 weeks.
Supracondylar humerus fracture	Tends to occur at 5–8 years of age. Proximity to the brachial artery ↑ the risk of Volkmann's contracture (results from compartment syndrome of the forearm).	Cast immobilization; closed reduction with percutaneous pinning if significantly displaced.
Osgood-Schlatter disease	Overuse apophysitis of the tibial tubercle. Causes localized pain, especially with quadriceps contraction, in active young boys.	↓ activity for 2–3 months or until asymptomatic. A neoprene brace may provide symptomatic relief.
Salter-Harris fracture	Fractures of the growth plate in children. Classified by fracture location: ■ I: Physis (growth plate). ■ II: Metaphysis and physis. ■ III: Epiphysis and physis. ■ IV: Epiphysis, metaphysis, and physis. ■ V: Crush injury of the physis.	**Types I and II:** Conservative. **Types III–V:** Surgical repair to prevent complications such as leg length inequality.

Developmental Dysplasia of the Hip

Also called congenital hip dislocation; can result in subluxed, dislocatable, or dislocated femoral heads, leading to early degenerative joint disease of the hips. Dislocations result from poor development of the acetabulum and hip due to lax musculature and from **excessive uterine packing** in the flexed and adducted position (e.g., breech presentation), leading to excessive stretching of the posterior hip capsule and adductor muscle contracture.

TABLE 2.9-6. DMD vs. Becker Muscular Dystrophy

	DMD	BECKER MUSCULAR DYSTROPHY
Onset	3–5 years.	5–15 years and beyond.
Life expectancy	Teens.	30s–40s.
Mental retardation	Common.	Uncommon.
Western blot	Dystrophin is markedly ↓ or absent.	Dystrophin levels are normal, but protein is abnormal.

HISTORY/PE

- Most commonly found in **first-born females** born in the **breech position.**
- **Barlow's maneuver:** Pressure is placed on the inner aspect of the abducted thigh, and the hip is then adducted, leading to an audible "clunk" as the femoral head dislocates posteriorly.
- **Ortolani's maneuver:** The thighs are gently abducted from the midline with anterior pressure on the greater trochanter. A **soft click** signifies reduction of the femoral head into the acetabulum.
- **Allis' (Galeazzi's) sign:** The knees are at unequal heights when the hips and knees are flexed (the dislocated side is lower).
- **Asymmetric skin folds** and limited abduction of the affected hip are also seen.

DIAGNOSIS

- **Early detection is critical** to allow for proper hip development.
- Ultrasound may be helpful, especially after 10 weeks of age.
- Radiographs are unreliable until patients are > 4 months of age because of the radiolucency of the neonatal femoral head.

TREATMENT

- Begin treatment early.
- **< 6 months:** Splint with a **Pavlik harness** (maintains the hip flexed and abducted). To prevent AVN, do not flex the hips > 60 degrees.
- **6–15 months:** Spica cast.
- **15–24 months:** Open reduction followed by spica cast.

COMPLICATIONS

- Joint contractures and AVN of the femoral head.
- Without treatment, a significant defect is likely in patients < 2 years of age.

Legg-Calvé-Perthes Disease

Idiopathic AVN of the femoral head (see Figure 2.9-8). Most commonly found in boys 4–10 years of age. Usually a self-limited disease, with symptoms lasting < 18 months.

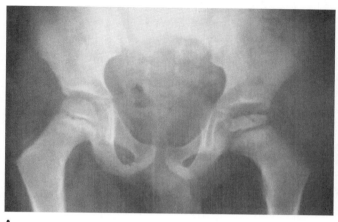

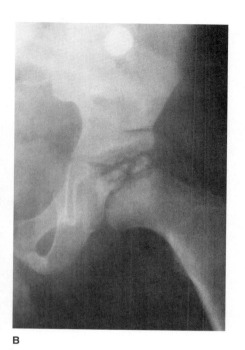

A

B

FIGURE 2.9-8   **Legg-Calvé-Perthes disease.**

AVN of the femoral head. (Reproduced, with permission, from Skinner HB. *Current Diagnosis & Treatment in Ortho-pedics*, 2nd ed. Stamford, CT: Appleton & Lange, 2000: 543.)

HISTORY/PE

- Generally asymptomatic at first, but patients can develop a painless limp.
- If pain is present, it can be in the groin or anterior thigh, or it may be referred to the knee.
- **Limited abduction and internal rotation;** atrophy of the affected leg.
- Usually unilateral (85–90%).

TREATMENT

- **Observation** is sufficient if there is limited femoral head involvement or if full ROM is present.
- If extensive or if there is ↓ ROM, consider bracing, hip abduction with a Petrie cast, or an osteotomy.
- The prognosis is good if the patient is < 5 years of age and has full ROM, ↓ femoral head involvement, and a stable joint.

Slipped Capital Femoral Epiphysis (SCFE)

Separation of the proximal femoral epiphysis through the growth plate, leading to medial and posterior displacement of the femoral head (relative to the femoral neck). May be due to an imbalance between growth hormone and sex hormones. Risk factors include obesity, age 11–13, male gender, and African-American ethnicity. Associated with hypothyroidism and other endocrinopathies.

HISTORY/PE

- Typically presents with acute or insidious **thigh** or **knee pain** and a **painful limp.**

> *Differential diagnosis of pediatric limp—*
>
> **STARTSS HOTT**
>
> **S**eptic joint
> **T**umor
> **A**vascular necrosis
>   (Legg-Calvé-Perthes)
> **R**heumatoid arthritis/JIA
> **T**uberculosis
> **S**ickle cell disease
> **S**CFE
> **H**enoch-Schönlein
>   purpura
> **O**steomyelitis
> **T**rauma
> **T**oxic synovitis

- Acute cases present with restricted ROM and, commonly, **inability to bear weight.**
- Bilateral in 40–50% of cases.
- Characterized by limited internal rotation and abduction of the hip. Flexion of the hip results in an obligatory external rotation 2° to physical displacement that is observed as further loss of internal rotation with hip flexion.

DIAGNOSIS

- Radiographs of **both** hips in **AP and frog-leg lateral views** reveal **posterior and medial displacement** of the femoral head (see Figure 2.9-9).
- Rule out hypothyroidism with TSH.

TREATMENT

- The disease is progressive, so treatment should begin promptly.
- **No weight bearing** should be allowed until the defect is surgically stabilized.
- **Gentle closed reduction** is appropriate only in acute slips.

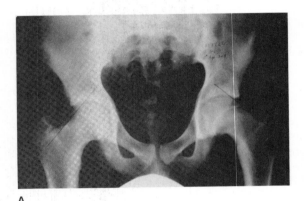

A

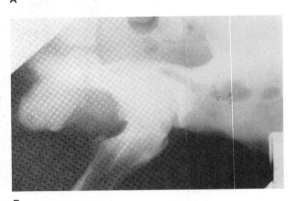

B

FIGURE 2.9-9.   **Slipped capital femoral epiphysis.**

(A) AP x-ray. The medial displacement of the left femoral epiphysis is best seen with a line drawn up the lateral femoral neck. The abnormal epiphysis does not protrude beyond this line. (B) Frog-leg lateral x-ray. Posterior displacement of the femoral epiphysis is characteristic. (Reproduced, with permission, from Skinner HB. *Current Diagnosis & Treatment in Orthopedics*, 2nd ed. Stamford, CT: Appleton & Lange, 2000: 546.)

Chondrolysis, AVN of the femoral head, and premature hip osteoarthritis leading to hip arthroplasty.

Scoliosis

A **lateral curvature of the spine** of > 10 degrees occurring in the thoracic and/or lumbar spine and associated with rotation of the vertebrae and sometimes excessive kyphosis or lordosis. **Most commonly idiopathic,** developing in early adolescence. Other etiologies are congenital or associated with neuromuscular, vertebral, or spinal cord disease. The male-to-female ratio is 1:7 for curves that progress and require treatment.

HISTORY/PE

- Idiopathic disease is usually identified during school physical screening.
- Vertebral and rib rotation deformities are accentuated by a forward bending test.

DIAGNOSIS

Radiographs of the spine (posterior, anterior, and full-length views).

TREATMENT

- Close observation for < 20 degrees of curvature.
- Spinal bracing for 20–49 degrees of curvature. **Curvature may progress even with bracing.**
- Surgical correction for > 50 degrees of curvature.

COMPLICATIONS

Severe scoliosis can create restrictive lung disease.

Juvenile Idiopathic Arthritis (JIA)

A nonmigratory, nonsuppurative mono- and polyarthritis with bony destruction that occurs in patients ≤ 16 years of age and lasts > 6 weeks. Formerly known as juvenile rheumatoid arthritis. Approximately 95% of cases resolve by puberty. More common in girls than in boys.

HISTORY/PE

- Can be accompanied by **fever, nodules, erythematous rashes, pericarditis,** and **fatigue.**
- Subtypes are as follows:
  - **Pauciarticular:** An asymmetric arthritis that involves weight-bearing joints. Associated with an ↑ risk of **iridocyclitis** that leads to blindness if left untreated.
  - **Polyarticular:** Resembles RA with symmetric involvement of multiple (≥ 5) small joints. Systemic features are less prominent; carries a ↓ risk of iridocyclitis.
  - **Acute febrile:** The least common subtype; manifests as arthritis with **daily high, spiking fevers** and a maculopapular, **evanescent, salmon-colored rash.** Hepatosplenomegaly and serositis may also be seen. No

iridocyclitis is present; remission may occur within one year. Occurs equally in girls and boys.

DIAGNOSIS

- There is **no diagnostic test for JIA.**
- **Labs:**
    - A ⊕ RF is found in 15% of cases.
    - ANA may be ⊕, especially in the pauciarticular subtype.
    - ↑ ESR, WBC count, and platelets.
- **Imaging:** Soft tissue swelling and osteoporosis may be seen.

TREATMENT

NSAIDs or corticosteroids; methotrexate is second-line therapy.

Neurology

Tables 2.10-1 through 2.10-5 and Figure 2.10-1 outline critical aspects of clinical neuroanatomy, including cranial nerve functions; the clinical presentation of common facial nerve lesions; spinal cord anatomy and functions; UMN and LMN signs; and pertinent clinical reflexes.

▶ VASCULAR DISORDERS

Stroke

Acute onset of focal neurologic deficits resulting from disruption of cerebral circulation. Many classifications exist, but the most common comparison involves

Stroke is the third most common cause of death and the leading cause of major disability in the United States.

TABLE 2.10-1. Cranial Nerve Functions

NERVE	CN	FUNCTION	TYPE	MNEMONIC
Olfactory	I	Smell	Sensory	Some
Optic	II	Sight	Sensory	Say
Oculomotor	III	Eye movement, pupillary constriction, lens accommodation, eyelid opening	Motor	Marry
Trochlear	IV	Eye movement	Motor	Money
Trigeminal	V	Mastication, facial sensation (including orbits, sinuses, tongue, teeth, and buccal mucosa), intracranial sensation (including meninges and blood vessels)	Both	But
Abducens	VI	Eye movement	Motor	My
Facial	VII	Facial movement, taste from the anterior two-thirds of the tongue, lacrimation, salivation (submandibular and sublingual glands), eyelid closing	Both	Brother
Vestibulocochlear	VIII	Hearing, balance	Sensory	Says
Glossopharyngeal	IX	Taste from the posterior third of the tongue, oropharyngeal sensation, swallowing (stylopharyngeus), salivation (parotid gland), monitoring carotid body and sinus chemo- and baroreceptors	Both	Big
Vagus	X	Taste from the epiglottic region, swallowing, palatal elevation, talking, thoracoabdominal viscera, monitoring aortic arch chemo- and baroreceptors.	Both	Brains
Accessory	XI	Head turning, shoulder shrugging	Motor	Matter
Hypoglossal	XII	Tongue movement	Motor	Most

Adapted, with permission, from Le T, Bhushan V et al. *First Aid for the USMLE Step 1 2009*. New York: McGraw-Hill, 2009: 394.

TABLE 2.10-2.   **Facial Nerve Lesions**

TYPE	DESCRIPTION	COMMENTS
UMN lesion	Lesion of the motor cortex or the connection between the cortex and the facial nucleus. Contralateral paralysis of the lower face only.	**AL**exander **Bell** with **STD**: **A**IDS, **L**yme, **S**arcoid, **T**umors, **D**iabetes.
LMN lesion	Ipsilateral paralysis of the upper and lower face.	
Bell's palsy	Complete destruction of the facial nucleus itself or its branchial efferent fibers (facial nerve proper).	
	Peripheral ipsilateral facial paralysis with inability to close the eye on the involved side. Can occur idiopathically; gradual recovery is seen in most cases.	
	Seen as a complication in **A**IDS, **L**yme disease, **S**arcoidosis, **T**umors, and **D**iabetes.	

Adapted, with permission, from Le T, Bhushan V et al. *First Aid for the USMLE Step 1 2009*. New York: McGraw-Hill, 2009: 397.

ischemic (80%) vs. hemorrhagic (20%). Table 2.10-6 contrasts modifiable and nonmodifiable risk factors associated with stroke. Etiologies are as follows:

- **Atherosclerosis** of the extracranial vessels (internal/common carotid, basilar, and vertebral arteries).
- **Lacunar infarcts** in regions supplied by perforating vessels (result from hypertension, hypercholesterolemia, or diabetes).
- **Cardiac or aortic emboli: Thromboemboli** (AF, ventricular hypokinesis, prosthetic valves, marantic endocarditis), **atheroemboli** (aortic arch atherosclerosis), **infectious emboli** (bacterial endocarditis), **paradoxical emboli** (via patent foramen ovale).
- **Hypercoagulable states:** Include those associated with antiphospholipid antibodies, activated protein C resistance, malignancy, and OCPs in the context of smoking.
- **Craniocervical dissection:** Trauma, fibromuscular dysplasia (young females), inflammatory/infectious diseases.

TABLE 2.10-3.   **Spinal Tract Functions**

TRACT	FUNCTION	DECUSSATION	ORIGIN
Lateral corticospinal	Movement of contralateral limbs	Pyramidal, at the cervicomedullary junction	1° motor cortex
Dorsal column medial lemniscus	Fine touch, vibration, conscious proprioception	Arcuate fibers at the medulla	Pacini's and Meissner's tactile disks, muscle spindles, and Golgi tendon organs
Spinothalamic	Pain, temperature	Ventral white commissure at spinal cord level	Free nerve endings, pain fibers

Adapted, with permission, from Le T, Bhushan V et al. *First Aid for the USMLE Step 1 2009*. New York: McGraw-Hill, 2009: 105.

TABLE 2.10-4. **UMN vs. LMN Signs**

Clinical Features	UMN	LMN
Pattern of weakness	Pyramidal (arm extensors, leg flexors)	Variable
Tone	Spastic ($\uparrow$); initially flaccid ($\downarrow$)	Flaccid ($\downarrow$)
DTRs	$\uparrow$ (initially $\downarrow$ or normal)	$\downarrow$
Miscellaneous signs	Babinski's, other CNS signs	Atrophy, fasciculations

- **Other causes:** Venous sinus thrombosis, sickle cell anemia, vasculitis (e.g., giant cell arteritis).

HISTORY/PE

Symptoms are dependent on the vascular territory affected:

- **Middle cerebral artery (MCA):** Aphasia (dominant hemisphere), neglect (nondominant hemisphere), contralateral paresis and sensory loss in the face and arm, gaze preference toward the side of the lesion, homonymous hemianopia.
- **Anterior cerebral artery (ACA):** Contralateral paresis and sensory loss in the leg; cognitive or personality changes.
- **Posterior cerebral artery (PCA):** Homonymous hemianopia, memory deficits, dyslexia/alexia.
- **Basilar artery:** Coma, "locked-in" syndrome, cranial nerve palsies (e.g., diplopia), apnea, visual symptoms, drop attacks, dysphagia, dysarthria, vertigo, "crossed" weakness and sensory loss affecting the ipsilateral face and contralateral body.
- **Lacunar:** Pure motor or sensory stroke, dysarthria–clumsy hand syndrome, ataxic hemiparesis.
- **TIA:** A transient neurologic deficit that lasts < **24 hours** (most last < 1 hour) and is determined to be of ischemic etiology. Many TIAs (~30–50%) are associated with small, asymptomatic strokes on diffusion-weighted MRI.

DIAGNOSIS

- **Emergent head CT without contrast** (see Figure 2.10-2) to differentiate ischemic from hemorrhagic stroke and to identify potential candidates for thrombolytic therapy.

> **The 4 "deadly D's" of posterior circulation strokes—**
>
> **D**iplopia
> **D**izziness
> **D**ysphagia
> **D**ysarthria

> **MCA stroke can cause CHANGes:**
>
> **C**ontralateral paresis and sensory loss in the face and arm
> **H**omonymous hemianopia
> **A**phasia (dominant)
> **N**eglect (nondominant)
> **G**aze preference toward the side of the lesion

TABLE 2.10-5. **Clinical Reflexes**

Distribution	Location	Comments
	Biceps = C5 nerve root.	Reflexes count up in order.
	Triceps = C7 nerve root.	S1, 2
	Patella = L4 nerve root.	L3, 4
	Achilles = S1 nerve root.	C5, 6
	Babinski––dorsiflexion of the big toe and fanning of other toes; sign of UMN lesion, but normal reflex in the first year of life.	C7, 8

Adapted, with permission, from Le T, Bhushan V et al. *First Aid for the USMLE Step 1 2009.* New York: McGraw-Hill, 2009: 392.

Poliomyelitis and Werdnig-Hoffmann disease: lower motor neuron lesions only, due to destruction of anterior horns; flaccid paralysis

Multiple sclerosis: mostly white matter of cervical region; random and asymmetric lesions, due to demyelination; scanning speech, intention tremor, nystagmus

ALS: combined upper and lower motor neuron deficits with no sensory deficit; both upper and lower motor neuron signs

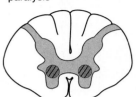 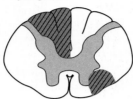 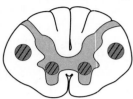

Complete occlusion of ventral artery; spares dorsal columns and tract of Lissauer

Tabes dorsalis (3° syphilis): degeneration of dorsal roots and dorsal columns; impaired proprioception, locomotor ataxia

Syringomyelia: crossing fibers of corticospinal tract damaged; bilateral loss of pain and temperature sensation

Vitamin B_{12} neuropathy and Friedreich's ataxia: demyelination of dorsal columns, lateral corticospinal tracts, and spinocerebellar tracts; ataxic gait, hyperreflexia, impaired position and vibration sense

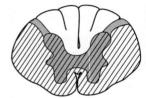 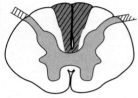 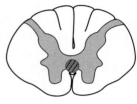 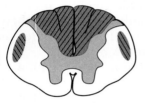

FIGURE 2.10-1. **Spinal cord lesions.**

(Reproduced, with permission, from Le T, Bhushan V et al. *First Aid for the USMLE Step 1 2009*. New York: McGraw-Hill, 2009: 389.)

- **MRI** to identify early ischemic changes (e.g., diffusion-weighted MRI is sensitive for acute stroke).
- **ECG** and an **echocardiogram** if embolic stroke is suspected.
- **Vascular studies** of intracranial and extracranial disease include carotid ultrasound, transcranial Doppler, MRA, and angiography (see Figure 2.10-3).

TABLE 2.10-6. **Modifiable and Nonmodifiable Risk Factors for Stroke**

MODIFIABLE RISK FACTORS	NONMODIFIABLE RISK FACTORS
"Live the way a **COACH SHoulDD**":	**FAME:**
CAD	**F**amily history of MI or stroke
Obesity	**A**ge > 60
Atrial fibrillation	**M**ale gender
Carotid stenosis	**E**thnicity (African-American,
Hypercholesterolemia	Hispanic, Asian)
Smoking	
Hypertension	
Diabetes	
Drug use (cocaine or IV drugs)	

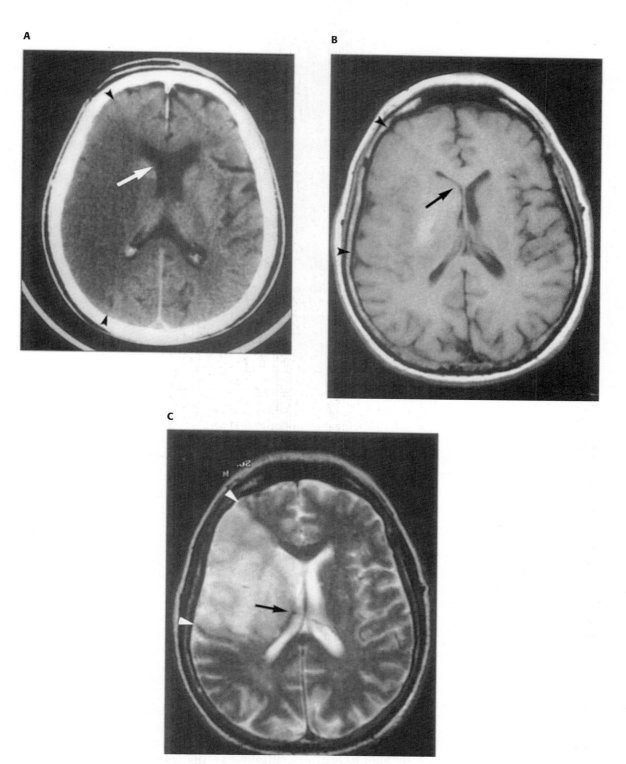

FIGURE 2.10-2. **CT/MRI findings in ischemic stroke in the right MCA territory.**

(A) CT shows low density and effacement of cortical sulci (between arrowheads) and compression of the anterior horn of the lateral ventricle (arrow). (B) T1-weighted MRI shows loss of sulcal markings (between arrowheads) and compression of the anterior horn of the lateral ventricle (arrow). (C) T2-weighted MRI scan shows increased signal intensity (between arrowheads) and ventricular compression (arrow). (Reproduced, with permission, from Aminoff MJ. *Clinical Neurology*, 3rd ed. Stamford, CT: Appleton & Lange, 1996: 275.)

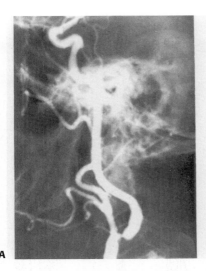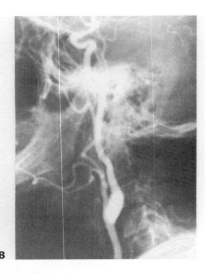

FIGURE 2.10-3. **Vascular studies pre- and postendarterectomy.**

(A) Carotid arteriogram showing stenosis of the proximal internal carotid artery. (B) Postoperative arteriogram with restoration of the normal luminal size following endarterectomy. (Reproduced, with permission, from Way LW. *Current Surgical Diagnosis & Treatment*, 10th ed. Stamford, CT: Appleton & Lange, 1994: 763.)

- **Screen for hypercoagulable states** with a history of thrombosis, in the setting of a first stroke, or in patients < 50 years of age.

TREATMENT

- Acute:
  - **Ischemic stroke: tPA** is indicated if administered within **three hours** of symptom onset, but first rule out contraindications. Be aware of potential bleeding or angioedema. **Intra-arterial thrombolysis** can be used for select patients within **six hours** of major stroke from MCA occlusion if such patients are not suitable candidates for IV tPA.
  - **Hemorrhagic stroke:** See the discussion of parenchymal hemorrhage.
  - ICU admission should be considered, especially for comatose patients or for those who are unable to protect their airways for possible intubation.
  - Monitor for signs and symptoms of brain swelling, ↑ ICP, and herniation. Serial CTs are helpful in the evaluation of deteriorating patients. As a temporizing measure, treat with **mannitol** and **hyperventilation.**
  - **ASA** is associated with ↓ morbidity and mortality in acute ischemic stroke presenting ≤ 48 hours from onset.
  - **Allow permissive hypertension and hypoxemia** to maintain perfusion of ischemic cerebral tissue. However, in the setting of severe hypertension (SBP > 220 or DBP >120) or hemorrhagic stroke, treat with IV **labetalol** or **nicardipine** infusion. Additionally, to administer tPA, SBP must be < 185 and DBP < 110.
  - **Treat fever and hyperglycemia,** as both are associated with worse prognoses in the setting of acute stroke.
  - Prevent and treat post-stroke complications such as aspiration pneumonia, UTI, and DVT.
  - **Immediate labs** to be obtained include CBC with platelets, cardiac enzymes and troponin, electrolytes, BUN, creatinine, serum glucose, PTT, PT, INR, lipid profile, and oxygen saturation.

Contraindications to tPA therapy—

SAMPLE STAGES

Stroke or head trauma within the last three months

Anticoagulation with INR > 1.7 or prolonged PTT

MI (recent)

Prior intracranial hemorrhage

Low platelet count (< 100,000/mm³)

Elevated BP: Systolic > 185 or diastolic BP > 110

Surgery in the past 14 days

TIA (mild symptoms or rapid improvement of symptoms)

Age < 18

GI or urinary bleeding in the past 21 days

Elevated (> 400) or ↓ (< 50 mg/dL) blood glucose

Seizures present at the onset of stroke

- **Prevention and long-term treatment:**
  - **ASA, clopidogrel:** If stroke is 2° to small vessel disease or thrombosis, or if anticoagulation is contraindicated.
  - **Carotid endarterectomy:** If stenosis is > 70% in symptomatic patients or > 60% in asymptomatic patients (contraindicated in 100% occlusion).
  - **Anticoagulation:** In new AF or hypercoagulable states, the target INR is 2–3. In cases involving a prosthetic valve, the target INR is 3–4 or add an antiplatelet agent.
  - **Management of hypertension, hypercholesterolemia,** and **diabetes** (hypertension is the single greatest risk factor for stroke).

Subarachnoid Hemorrhage (SAH)

Etiologies of SAH include **trauma, berry aneurysms,** AVM, and trauma to the circle of Willis.

HISTORY/PE

- Aneurysmal SAH presents with an **abrupt-onset, intensely painful "thunderclap" headache,** often followed by **neck stiffness** and other signs of meningeal irritation, including photophobia, nausea/vomiting, and meningeal stretch signs. Rapid development of obstructive hydrocephalus or seizures often leads to ↓ arousal or frank coma and death in the absence of neurosurgical intervention.
- More than one-third of patients will give a history of a **"sentinel bleed"** days to weeks earlier marked by an abrupt-onset headache, often with nausea/vomiting, or transient diplopia that completely resolved in a matter of minutes to hours.

DIAGNOSIS

- Immediate head **CT without contrast** (see Figure 2.10-4) to look for blood in the subarachnoid space. Sensitivity is > 95% in those with severe SAH but is much lower in patients with normal mental status.
- Immediate **LP if CT is** ⊖ to look for **RBCs, xanthochromia** (yellowish CSF due to breakdown of RBCs), ↑ protein (from the RBCs), and ↑ ICP. Note that LP results can be falsely ⊖ in the first 6–12 hours (because xanthochromia has not yet developed) and after the first 24–28 hours (because xanthochromia has resolved).
- **Four-vessel angiography** (or equivalent noninvasive angiography such as CT angiography with 3-D reconstructions) should be performed once SAH is confirmed. Noninvasive angiography is warranted in high-risk cases and in those with high clinical suspicion even if CT and LP are unrevealing.
- Call neurosurgery.

TREATMENT

- **Prevent rebleeding** (most likely to occur in the first 48 hours) by maintaining systolic BP < 150 until the aneurysm is clipped or coiled.
- **Prevent vasospasm and associated neurologic deterioration** (most likely to occur 5–7 days after SAH) by administering calcium channel blockers (CCBs), IV fluids, and pressors to maintain BP. Give phenytoin for **seizure prophylaxis.**
- ↓ **ICP** by raising the head of the bed and instituting hyperventilation.
- **Treat hydrocephalus** through a lumbar drain or serial LPs.

CN III palsy with pupillary involvement is associated with berry aneurysms.

Conditions associated with berry aneurysms that can MAKE an SAH more likely:

Marfan's syndrome
Aortic coarctation
Kidney disease (autosomal dominant, polycystic)
Ehlers-Danlos syndrome
Sickle cell anemia
Atherosclerosis
History (familial)

The characteristic "worst headache of my life" of SAH comes on quickly, in contrast to migraine (peak intensity > 30 minutes).

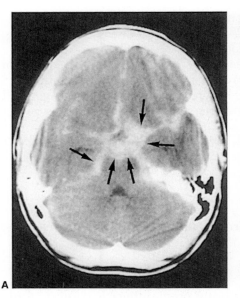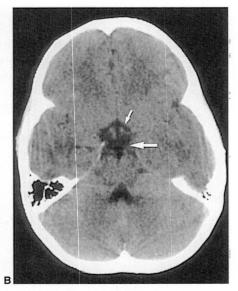

FIGURE 2.10-4. **Subarachnoid hemorrhage.**

(A) CT scan without contrast reveals blood in the subarachnoid space at the base of the brain (arrows). (B) A normal CT scan without contrast shows no density in this region (arrows). (Reproduced, with permission, from Aminoff MJ. *Clinical Neurology*, 3rd ed. Stamford, CT: Appleton & Lange, 1996: 78.)

- **Surgical clipping** is the **definitive treatment for aneurysms.** Endovascular coiling is an option for poor surgical candidates.

Intracerebral Hemorrhage

- Risk factors include hypertension, tumor, amyloid angiopathy (in the elderly), anticoagulation, and vascular malformations (AVMs, cavernous hemangiomas).
- **Hx/PE:** Presents with **focal motor and sensory deficits that often worsen as the hematoma expands.** Severe headache of sudden onset, nausea/vomiting, seizures, lethargy, or obtundation may also be seen.
- **Dx:** Immediate noncontrast head CT (see Figure 2.10-5). Look for mass effect or edema that may predict herniation.
- **Tx:** Similar to that of SAH. Elevate the head of the bed and institute antiseizure prophylaxis. Surgical evacuation may be necessary if mass effect is present. Several types of herniation may occur, including central, **uncal,** subfalcine, and tonsillar (see Figure 2.10-6 and Table 2.10-7).

Subdural Hematoma

- Typically occurs following head trauma (usually falls or assaults), leading to rupture of **bridging veins** and accumulation of blood between the dura and arachnoid membranes. Common in the **elderly** and **alcoholics.**
- **Hx/PE:** Presents with **headache, changes in mental status,** and **contralateral hemiparesis.** Changes may be subacute or chronic. May present as pseudodementia in the elderly.

Mental status changes associated with an expanding epidural hematoma occur within minutes to hours and classically have a lucid interval. With a subdural hematoma, mental status changes can occur within days to weeks.

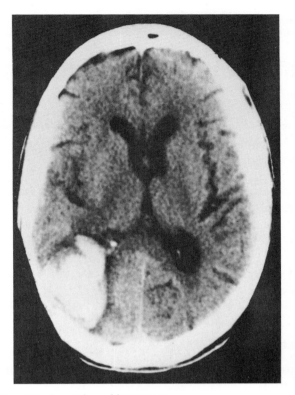

FIGURE 2.10-5. **Intraparenchymal hematoma.**

Head CT without contrast reveals the irregularly shaped hyperdensity with midline shift of the choroid plexus. (Reproduced, with permission, from Saunders CE. *Current Emergency Diagnosis & Treatment*, 4th ed. Stamford, CT: Appleton & Lange, 1992: 248.)

- **Dx:** CT demonstrates a **crescent-shaped, concave hyperdensity acutely** (isodense subacutely, hypodense chronically) that does **not cross the midline** (see Figure 2.10-7A).
- **Tx: Surgical evacuation if symptomatic.** Subdural blood may regress spontaneously if it is chronic.

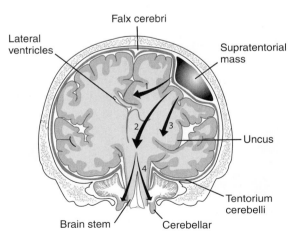

1. Cingulate herniation under falx cerebri
2. Downward transtentorial (central) herniation
3. Uncal herniation
4. Cerebellar tonsillar herniation into the foramen magnum

Coma and death result when these herniations compress the brain stem

FIGURE 2.10-6. **Sites of herniation syndromes.**

(Adapted, with permission, from Simon RP et al. *Clinical Neurology*, 4th ed. Stamford, CT: Appleton & Lange, 1999: 314.)

TABLE 2.10-7. Clinical Presentation of Herniation Syndromes

TYPE OF HERNIATION	PRESENTATION
Cingulate herniation	Occurs 2° to mass lesions of the frontal lobes. No specific signs or symptoms; frequently seen on head CT.
Downward transtentorial (central) herniation	Occurs when large supratentorial mass lesions push the midbrain inferiorly. Presents with a rapid change in mental status; bilaterally small and reactive pupils; Cheyne-Stokes respirations; and flexor or extensor posturing.
Uncal herniation	Occurs 2° to mass lesions of the middle fossa. CN III becomes entrapped, leading to a fixed and dilated ipsilateral pupil followed by an eye that is deviated "down and out." Ipsilesional hemiparesis ("false localizing") results from compression of the cerebral peduncle (opposite the mass lesion) against the tentorial edge.
Cerebellar tonsillar herniation into the foramen magnum	Occurs 2° to posterior fossa mass lesions. Tonsillar herniation → medullary compression → respiratory arrest. Usually rapidly fatal.

Epidural Hematoma

- Usually a result of a **lateral skull fracture** leading to a tear of the **middle meningeal artery.**
- Hx/PE: Obvious, severe **trauma** induces an **immediate loss of consciousness** followed by a **lucid interval (minutes to hours).** Uncal herniation

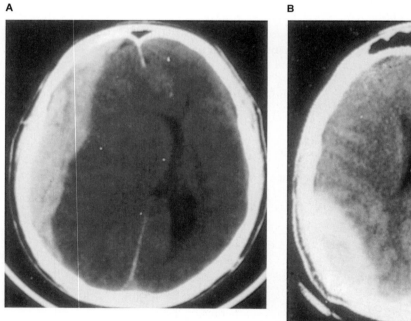
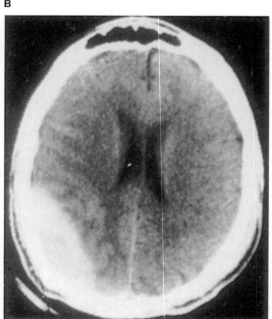

FIGURE 2.10-7. Subdural vs. epidural hematoma.

(A) Subdural hematoma. Note the crescent shape and the mass effect with midline shift. (B) Epidural hematoma with classic biconvex lens shape. (Reproduced, with permission, from Aminoff MJ. *Clinical Neurology*, 3rd ed. Stamford, CT: Appleton & Lange, 1996: 296.)

leads to **coma** with a **"blown pupil"** (fixed and dilated ipsilateral pupil) and ultimately ipsilateral hemiparesis.

- **Dx: CT shows a lens-shaped, convex hyperdensity limited by the sutures** (see Figure 2.10-7B).
- **Tx:** Emergent neurosurgical evacuation. May quickly evolve to brain herniation and death 2° to the arterial source of bleeding.

A "blown pupil" suggests impending brain stem compression.

▶ HEADACHES

Causes of headache include the following:

- **Acute** (new; onset seconds to minutes): New migraine/cluster headache, aneurysmal SAH, acutely ↑ ICP (e.g., colloid cyst, obstructive hydrocephalus), acute ocular disease (e.g., angle-closure glaucoma), cerebral venous thrombosis, cavernous sinus thrombosis, craniocervical dissection, pituitary apoplexy, acute severe hypertension (e.g., pheochromocytoma), angina (rare), ischemic stroke/intraparenchymal hemorrhage (headache is usually not the presenting manifestation).
- **Subacute** (new; onset hours to days): New migraine/tension-type headache or viral syndrome vs. meningitis, other cranial infections (acute sinusitis, dental infections, orbital infections, cavernous sinus infections, otitis media/mastoiditis), temporal arteritis, subacutely ↑ ICP (e.g., large tumor, progressive hydrocephalus, altitude sickness, pseudotumor cerebri), subacute ocular disease (e.g., keratitis, iritis, scleritis, orbital infection), subacute severe hypertension (e.g., hypertensive encephalopathy, eclampsia), intracranial hypotension (e.g., spontaneous, post-LP), subdural hematoma, carbon monoxide, lead poisoning in children (rare), encephalitis.
- **Chronic/episodic:** Migraine, cluster headache, tension-type headache, medication overuse headaches (e.g., caffeine withdrawal, "rebound" headaches from NSAID or analgesic overuse), trigeminal or other neuralgias (e.g., glossopharyngeal, postherpetic), TMJ disease, cervical arthritis, chronic sinusitis.

HISTORY/PE

- Conduct full general and neurologic exams, including a **funduscopic** exam.
- Evaluate the following:
  - **Chronicity:** Recent or recently changed headaches warrant immediate workup if they are not clearly migraines or other 1° headache disorders.
  - **Characteristics:**
    - **Intensity:** Severe headaches are more likely to be dangerous, but not all dangerous headaches are severely intense (e.g., temporal arteritis).
    - **Location:** Posterior headaches are less likely to be benign, especially in children.
    - **Duration:** Headaches lasting > 72 hours are not migraines.
    - **Diurnal variation:** Cluster headaches and those from elevated ICP usually occur or worsen at night.
    - **Triggers:** Examples include chocolate and red wine.
    - **Provocative factors:** Lying down may make high-ICP headaches worse; standing up may make low-ICP headaches worse.
    - **Palliative factors:** Sleep clears migraines.

Recent-onset headaches warrant immediate workup! If headache is associated with focal neurologic deficits, rule out more serious etiologies with CT or MRI. Rule out SAH with a CT and LP if symptoms are abrupt in onset; then consider other causes typically missed by CT (e.g., dural thrombosis, dissection, or apoplexy).

- **Associated symptoms/signs:** Significant findings include **fever or rash** (consider meningitis or other infectious causes), **jaw claudication** (specific for temporal arteritis), or constitutional symptoms such as **weight loss** (associated with neoplastic, inflammatory, or infectious conditions). **Photophobia, nausea, and vomiting** are associated with migraine, aneurysmal SAH, and meningitis, but neck stiffness is more likely to accompany the latter two.
  - **Neurologic sequelae:** Look for **diplopia**, mental status changes or associated symptoms (numbness, weakness, dizziness, ataxia, visual disturbances), **papilledema**, or pupillary abnormalities (partial CN III palsy or Horner's syndrome).
  - **Patient risk factors:** High-risk patients are > 50 years of age, immunocompromised, or with preexisting malignancy.

DIAGNOSIS

- **If SAH is suspected,** obtain a **head CT without contrast.**
- **If CT is** ⊖**, LP is mandatory.**
- Obtain a CBC.
- If temporal arteritis is suspected, obtain ESR.
- A CT/MRI is needed for suspected SAH, ↑ ICP, or focal neurologic findings. Use **CT without contrast** to evaluate acute hemorrhage.

Migraine Headache

- Affects **females** more often than males; may be familial. Associated with **vascular** and brain neurotransmitter (**serotonin**) changes. Pain is ultimately linked to trigeminal nucleus activation in the brain stem.
- Auras appear to result from a different pathomechanism (electrical spreading depression in the brain, possibly linked to ion channel dysfunction) and may occur with or without the pain of migraine headache. Onset usually occurs by the **early 20s.**
- **Triggers** include certain foods (e.g., red wine), fasting, stress, menses, OCPs, bright light, and disruptions in normal sleep patterns.
- **Hx/PE:**
  - Presents with a throbbing headache (> 2 hours but usually < 24 hours, and almost always < 72 hours in duration) that is associated with **nausea, vomiting, photophobia,** and noise sensitivity. Headache is usually relieved by **sleep and darkness.**
  - **Classic migraines:** Often **unilateral** and preceded by a visual **aura** in the form of either scintillating scotomas (bright or flashing lights) or visual field cuts.
  - **Common migraines:** May be **bilateral** and periorbital **without preceding auras.**
- **Dx:** Based on history.
- **Tx:**
  - **Avoid known triggers.**
  - **Abortive therapy** includes **triptans** (first line after OTC NSAIDs have failed), **metoclopramide,** and various analgesics. Consider symptomatic treatment for nausea.
  - **Prophylaxis** for frequent or severe migraines includes **anticonvulsants** (e.g., gabapentin, topiramate), **TCAs** (e.g., amitriptyline), **β-blockers** (propranolol), and **CCBs.**

If a 20-year-old female develops headaches after drinking red wine, think migraine.

Cluster Headache

- **Males** are affected more often than females; average age of onset is 25.
- Hx/PE:
  - Presents as a brief, **excruciating, unilateral periorbital headache** that lasts 30 minutes to three hours, during which the patient tends to be extremely restless.
  - Attacks tend to occur in **clusters,** affecting the same part of the head at the same time of day (commonly during sleep) and in a certain season of the year.
  - Associated symptoms include **ipsilateral lacrimation** of the eye, conjunctival injection, Horner's syndrome, and nasal stuffiness.
- **Dx:** Classic presentations with a history of repeated attacks over an extended period of time require no evaluation. First episodes require a workup to exclude disorders associated with Horner's syndrome (e.g., carotid artery dissection or cavernous sinus infection).
- **Tx:**
  - **Acute therapy:** High-flow O_2 (100% non-rebreather), dihydroergotamine, octreotide, sumatriptan or zolmitriptan.
  - **Prophylactic therapy:** Transitional (prednisone, ergotamine), maintenance (verapamil, methysergide, lithium, valproic acid, topiramate).

If a 25-year-old male wakes up repeatedly during the night with unilateral periorbital pain associated with ipsilateral lacrimation, think cluster headache.

Tension-Type Headache

- Considered by some to be a milder form of migraine headache. More common in females than in males.
- **Hx/PE:** Presents with **tight, bandlike pain** that is not associated with sensory phobia, nausea/vomiting, or auras and is brought on by fatigue or stress. Nonspecific symptoms (e.g., anxiety, poor concentration, difficulty sleeping) may also be seen. May be generalized or most intense in the **frontal, occipital, and neck regions.** Usually occurs at the end of the day.
- **Dx:** A diagnosis of exclusion. Be particularly aware of giant cell arteritis in patients > 50 years of age with new headaches; always obtain an ESR even if headaches are mild and unassociated with constitutional or vascular symptoms. There are no focal neurologic signs.
- **Tx:** Relaxation, massage, hot baths, and **avoidance of exacerbating factors. NSAIDs** and **acetaminophen** are first-line abortive therapy, but triptans may also be considered.

If a 30-year-old female complains of headaches at the end of the day that worsen with stress and improve with relaxation or massage, think tension-type headache.

Tension-type headaches are the most common type of headache diagnosed in adults.

Cavernous Sinus Thrombosis

The usual etiology involves a **suppurative process** of the orbit, nasal sinuses, or central face that leads to **septic thrombosis** of the cavernous sinus. Nonseptic thrombosis is rare; *S. aureus* is the most common causative agent. The syndrome can also be seen with nonbacterial agents, particularly fungi (*Mucor* or *Aspergillus* species). Current antibiotics have greatly ↓ both incidence and mortality.

HISTORY/PE

- **Headache is the most common presenting symptom.**
- Patients may present with orbital pain, edema, diplopia (2° to oculomotor, abducens, or trochlear nerve involvement), or visual disturbances and may describe a recent history of sinusitis or facial infection. On exam, they typically appear ill and have a **fever.**

- Additional signs may include red eye, proptosis, ptosis, or ophthalmoplegia of the affected eye (partial or complete). Diminished pupillary constriction (CN III) and/or dilation (Horner's) may also be present.
- Changes in mental status such as confusion, drowsiness, or coma suggest spread to the CNS or sepsis. Late findings include meningismus or systemic signs of sepsis.

DIAGNOSIS

- Lab studies show an ↑ WBC count.
- Blood cultures reveal the causative agent in up to 50% of cases.
- CSF exam may reveal ↑ protein consistent with a parameningeal reaction unless there is frank meningitis.
- **MRI** (with gadolinium, pituitary protocol) is the principal means of confirming the anatomic diagnosis; MR or CT venography may be important adjuncts.
- Biopsy of paranasal sinuses or other affected tissue is often necessary in fungal cases for organism identification by histology and culture.

TREATMENT

- Treat aggressively and empirically with a **penicillinase-resistant penicillin** (nafcillin or oxacillin) plus a **third- or fourth-generation cephalosporin** (e.g., ceftriaxone or cefepime) to provide broad-spectrum coverage pending blood culture results. Potential anaerobic infection from sinus or dental sources should be covered with **metronidazole. Vancomycin** can be added to address potential MRSA involvement. Antifungal therapy is required for fungal cases.
- IV antibiotics are recommended for at least 3–4 weeks.

▶ SEIZURE DISORDERS

Paroxysmal events associated with aberrant electrical activity in the brain detectable by EEG, leading to changes in neurologic perception or behavior. An aura is experienced by 50–60% of patients with epilepsy. See Table 2.10-8 for common etiologies by age. To further narrow down the etiology of a seizure, assess the following:

- Determine whether the patient has a history of epilepsy (i.e., a history of unprovoked and recurrent seizures). Other seizures may be self-limited and may resolve once an underlying medical condition has been treated. Elevated serum prolactin levels are consistent with an epileptic seizure in the immediate postictal period.

TABLE 2.10-8. Causes of Seizure by Age Group

INFANTS	CHILDREN (2–10)	ADOLESCENTS	ADULTS (18–35)	ADULTS (35+)
Perinatal injury	Idiopathic	Idiopathic	Trauma	Trauma
Infection	Infection	Trauma	Alcoholism	Stroke
Metabolic	Trauma	Drug withdrawal	Brain tumor	Metabolic disorders
Congenital	Febrile	AVM		Alcoholism
				Brain tumor

- Non-neurologic etiologies include **hypoglycemia, hyponatremia, hypocalcemia, hyperosmolar states, hepatic encephalopathy,** uremia, porphyria, **drug overdose** (cocaine, antidepressants, neuroleptics, methylxanthines, lidocaine), **drug withdrawal** (alcohol and other sedatives), eclampsia, hyperthermia, hypertensive encephalopathy, head trauma, and cerebral hypoperfusion.
- Seizures with a focal onset (or focal postictal deficit) suggest focal CNS pathology. They may be the presenting sign of a tumor, stroke, AVM, infection, hemorrhage, or developmental abnormality.
- First seizures that resolve after a single episode are frequently left untreated when the underlying cause is unknown.

Partial Seizures

Arise from a **discrete region,** or an "epileptogenic focus," in one cerebral hemisphere and **do not lead to loss of consciousness** unless they secondarily generalize.

History/PE

- **Simple partial seizures:** May include motor features (e.g., jacksonian march, or the progressive jerking of successive body regions) as well as sensory, autonomic, or psychic features (e.g., fear, déjà vu, hallucinations) **without alteration of consciousness.** A postictal focal neurologic deficit (e.g., hemiplegia/hemiparesis, or Todd's paralysis) is possible and usually resolves within 24 hours. Often confused with acute stroke (ruled out by MRI).
- **Complex partial seizures:** Typically involve the temporal lobe (70–80%) with bilateral spread of the aberrant electrical discharge. Characterized by an **impaired level of consciousness,** auditory or visual hallucinations, déjà vu, automatisms (e.g., lip smacking, chewing, or even walking), and postictal confusion/disorientation and amnesia.

Diagnosis

- Obtain an **EEG.**
- Rule out systemic causes with a CBC, electrolytes, calcium, fasting glucose, LFTs, a renal panel, RPR, ESR, and a toxicology screen.
- A focal seizure implies a focal brain lesion. Rule out a mass by MRI or CT with contrast.

Treatment

- **Treat the underlying cause.**
- **Recurrent partial seizures:** Phenytoin, oxcarbazepine, carbamazepine (Tegretol), phenobarbital, and valproic acid can be administered as monotherapy. In **children, phenobarbital** is the first-line anticonvulsant.
- **Intractable temporal lobe seizures:** Consider **anterior temporal lobectomy.**

Tonic-Clonic (Grand Mal) Seizures

Primarily idiopathic. Partial seizures can evolve into secondarily generalized tonic-clonic seizures.

If a patient presents wth progressive jerking of successive body regions and hallucinations but without loss of consciousness, think simple partial seizures.

If a patient presents with an episode of lip smacking associated with an impaired level of consciousness and followed by confusion, think complex partial seizures.

Both simple partial and complex partial seizures may evolve into 2° generalized tonic-clonic (grand mal) seizures.

HISTORY/PE

- Presents with sudden onset of loss of consciousness with tonic extension of the back and extremities, continuing with 1–2 minutes of repetitive, symmetric clonic movements.
- Marked by **incontinence** and **tongue biting**. Patients may appear **cyanotic** during the ictal period. Consciousness is slowly regained in the postictal period, but patients are confused and may prefer to sleep; muscle aches and headaches may be present.

DIAGNOSIS

EEG typically shows 10-Hz activity during the tonic phase and slow waves during the clonic phase.

TREATMENT

- **Protect the airway.**
- Treat the underlying cause if known.
- **1° generalized tonic-clonic seizures: Phenytoin,** fosphenytoin, or valproate constitutes first-line therapy. Lamotrigine or topiramate may be used as adjunctive therapy.
- **Secondarily generalized tonic-clonic seizures:** Treatment is the same as that for partial seizures.

Absence (Petit Mal) Seizures

- Begin in **childhood;** subside before adulthood. Often **familial.**
- **Hx/PE:** Present with brief (**5- to 10-second**), often unnoticeable episodes of **impaired consciousness** occurring up to hundreds of times per day. Patients are **amnestic** during and immediately after seizures and may appear to be **daydreaming** or **staring.** Eye fluttering or lip smacking is common.
- **Dx: EEG** shows classic three-per-second spike-and-wave discharges.
- **Tx:** Ethosuximide is the first-line agent.

Status Epilepticus

A **medical emergency** consisting of prolonged (> **10-minute**) or repetitive seizures that occur without a return to baseline consciousness. May be either convulsive (the more medically urgent form) or nonconvulsive.

- Common causes include anticonvulsant withdrawal/noncompliance, anoxic brain injury, EtOH/sedative withdrawal or other drug intoxication, metabolic disturbances (e.g., hyponatremia), head trauma, and infection.
- Death usually results from the underlying medical condition and may occur in 10% of cases of status epilepticus.

DIAGNOSIS

- Determine the underlying cause with pulse oximetry, CBC, electrolytes, calcium, glucose, ABGs, LFTs, BUN/creatinine, ESR, antiepileptic drug levels, and a toxicology screen.
- **Obtain an EEG and brain imaging, but defer testing until the patient is stabilized.**
- **Obtain a stat head CT** to evaluate for intracranial hemorrhage.
- Obtain an LP in the setting of fever or meningeal signs, but only after having done a CT scan to assess the safety of the LP.

TREATMENT

- Maintain **ABCs**; consider rapid intubation for airway protection.
- Administer **thiamine, glucose, and naloxone** to presumptively treat potential etiologies.
- Give **IV benzodiazepine** (lorazepam or diazepam) plus a loading dose of **fosphenytoin.**
- If seizures continue, intubate and load with **phenobarbital.** Consider an IV sedative (midazolam or pentobarbital) and initiate continuous EEG monitoring.
- Initiate a meticulous search for the underlying cause.

*Treatment of status epilepticus: First **ABCs**, Then Begin Giving Naloxone: Fosphenytoin, **ABCs**, Thiamine, **B**enzodiazepine, **G**lucose, **N**aloxone.*

Infantile Spasms (West Syndrome)

- A form of **generalized epilepsy** that typically begins within six months of birth. May be idiopathic or 2° to a variety of conditions, including PKU, perinatal infections, hypoxic-ischemic injury, and tuberous sclerosis.
- Affects males more often than females; associated with a ⊕ family history.
- **Hx/PE:** Presents with tonic, bilateral, symmetric **jerks of the head, trunk, and extremities** that tend to occur in clusters of 5–10; **arrest of psychomotor development** occurs at the age of seizure onset. The majority of patients have mental retardation.
- **Dx:** Look for an **abnormal interictal EEG** characterized by **hypsarrhythmia.**
- **Tx:** Hormonal therapy with **ACTH**, prednisone, and clonazepam or valproic acid. Medications may treat the spasms but have little impact on patients' long-term prognosis.

If a male infant is brought to the hospital with muscular jerks and an uncle who had the same problem, think infantile spasms (West syndrome).

> ▶ **VERTIGO AND DIZZINESS**

Benign Paroxysmal Positional Vertigo (BPPV)

- A common cause of recurrent **peripheral vertigo** resulting from a **dislodged otolith** that leads to disturbances in the semicircular canals (95% posterior, 5% horizontal).
- **Hx/PE:** Patients with posterior canal BPPV present with **transient, episodic vertigo (lasting < 1 minute)** and mixed upbeat-**torsional nystagmus triggered by changes in head position** (classically while turning in bed, getting in/out of bed, or reaching overhead). Some patients complain of nonvertiginous feelings of dizziness or lightheadedness. Nausea and vomiting are uncommon owing to the short-lived stimulus.
- **Dx:**
  - Have the patient turn his or her head 45 degrees right or left and go from a sitting to a supine position while quickly turning the head to the side (**Dix-Hallpike maneuver**). If vertigo and the typical nystagmus (upbeat and toward the affected shoulder) are reproduced, BPPV is the likely diagnosis.
  - Nystagmus that persists for > 1 minute, gait disturbance, or nausea/vomiting that is out of proportion to nystagmus should raise concern for a central lesion.
- **Tx:**
  - Some 80% of cases can be resolved at the bedside using the modified Epley maneuver (a 270-degree head rotation from the Dix-Hallpike testing position).

With BPPV, it's all in the name:

- *Benign = otolith (not a tumor).*
- *Paroxysmal = sudden, temporary episodes lasting < 1 minute.*
- *Positional = starts while turning in bed or reaching overhead.*
- *Vertigo = vertigo or dizziness is the main symptom.*

- The condition usually subsides spontaneously in weeks to months but often recurs months or years later. Antivertigo medications (e.g., meclizine) are generally contraindicated, as they tend to inhibit central compensation, which may lead to chronic unsteadiness and falls in the elderly.

Acute Peripheral Vestibulopathy (Labyrinthitis and Vestibular Neuritis)

- Typically a **diagnosis of exclusion** once the more serious causes of vertigo (e.g., cerebellar stroke) have been ruled out.
- **Hx/PE:** Presents with **acute onset of severe vertigo, head-motion intolerance, and gait unsteadiness** accompanied by **nausea, vomiting, and nystagmus.** Auditory or aural symptoms ("labyrinthitis") may include unilateral tinnitus, ear fullness, or hearing loss. Without auditory or aural symptoms (more common), the condition is known as "vestibular neuritis."
- **Dx:**
  - Acute peripheral vestibulopathy demonstrates the following:
    - An abnormal vestibulo-ocular reflex (VOR) as determined by a bedside head impulse test (i.e., rapid head rotation from lateral to center while staring at the examiner's nose).
    - A predominantly horizontal nystagmus that always beats in one direction, opposite the lesion.
    - No vertical eye misalignment by alternate cover testing.
  - If patients are "high risk" (i.e., if they have atypical eye findings or any neurologic symptoms or signs, cannot stand independently, have head or neck pain, are > 50 years of age, or have one or more stroke risk factors), they should be imaged by MRI with diffusion-weighted imaging.
  - For low-risk patients, consider caloric testing as ancillary support for the diagnosis.
  - Labyrinthitis (with auditory symptoms) is mimicked by lateral pontine/cerebellar stroke (AICA arterial territory). Vestibular neuritis (without auditory symptoms) is mimicked by lateral medullary/cerebellar stroke (PICA arterial territory).
- **Tx:** Acute treatment consists of corticosteroids given < 72 hours after symptom onset and vestibular sedatives (e.g., meclizine). The condition usually subsides spontaneously within weeks to months. Once the hyperacute stage has passed, cautious engagement in normal physical activities and exercise should be encouraged.

Ménière's Disease

- A cause of recurrent **vertigo with auditory symptoms** that affects at least 1 in 500 in the United States. More common among females.
- **Hx/PE:** Presents with **recurrent episodes of severe vertigo, hearing loss, tinnitus, or ear fullness,** often lasting hours to days. Nausea and vomiting are typical. Patients progressively lose low-frequency hearing over years and may become deaf on the affected side.
- **Dx: Diagnosis is made clinically** and is based on a thorough history and physical exam. **Two episodes** (lasting 20 minutes or more) with remission of symptoms between episodes, hearing loss documented at least once with audiometry, and tinnitus or aural fullness are needed to make the diagnosis once other causes (e.g., TIA, otosyphilis) have been ruled out. A brain

If you see a 27-year-old male who presents with vertigo and vomiting for one week after having been diagnosed with a viral infection, think acute vestibular neuritis.

MRI with vascular imaging (e.g., MRA) may help assess potential intracranial pathology, particularly cerebrovascular disease.

- **Tx:** Classically, a low-sodium diet and diuretic therapy were first-line treatments. As theories of pathogenesis have shifted, many clinicians have begun to treat patients with "migraine" diets, other lifestyle changes, prophylactic antimigraine medications, and occasionally benzodiazepines or antiemetics. For severe unilateral cases, ablative therapies (e.g., intratympanic gentamicin to damage the labyrinth, vestibular nerve section) have been used with some success.

Ménière's disease consists of recurrent episodes, but unlike BPPV, these usually last hours to days.

Vestibular Migraine

- A cause of recurrent **vertigo (usually without auditory symptoms)** that affects roughly 10% of migraine sufferers. More common among females. Its pathogenesis may be related to intermittent electrical (ion channel) dysfunction in the cerebellum.
- **Hx/PE:** Presents with **recurrent episodes of mild dizziness to severe vertigo** lasting minutes to days. Nausea, vomiting, and photophobia are common; headaches are variably present and may be mild or severe. Patients are left with no substantial deficits in between spells, although balance may deteriorate over decades.
- **Dx:**
  - **The diagnosis is usually made clinically** on the basis of a thorough history and physical exam to exclude other causes.
  - Patients who would otherwise qualify for a diagnosis of Ménière's save the absence of auditory symptoms and documented hearing loss are likely to have vestibular migraine. A history of photo- or phonophobia during the episode, particularly if dizziness is associated with headache, is highly suggestive in such patients.
  - The diagnosis is one of exclusion, and care should be taken to ensure that patients do not have intermittent dizziness due to TIA. In patients < 50 years of age, a history of recent trauma or of severe, abrupt-onset, or persistent pain (> 72 hours) should raise concern for vertebral artery dissection with TIAs.
  - A brain MRI with vascular imaging (e.g., MRA) is sometimes indicated to assess potential intracranial pathology, particularly cerebrovascular disease.
  - Episodic ataxia type 2 can be corroborated by genetic testing.
- **Tx:** Can usually be prevented through migraine medication, diet, or lifestyle changes. Benzodiazepines or antiemetics may be tried. Surgical therapies are not indicated.

Unlike Ménière's, vestibular migraine usually has no associated auditory or aural symptoms.

Rule out vertebral artery dissection in those with persistent head or neck pain and intermittent isolated dizziness or vertigo.

Syncope

- One of the **most common causes** of loss of consciousness 2° **to an abrupt drop in cerebral perfusion.** Etiologies include cardiac arrhythmias and cardiac outflow obstruction, vasovagal syncope, orthostatic hypotension, micturition-related syncope, basilar TIAs, and idiopathic causes. Presyncope is described as a feeling of imminent loss of consciousness without actual fainting. Commonly **confused with seizures.**
- **Hx/PE:**
  - Patients may report a **trigger** (e.g., standing for long period of time, fear/sight of blood, Valsalva maneuver).

- Typically follows a prodrome of **lightheadedness or dizziness, muffled sounds, constricting vision, diffuse weakness, diaphoresis,** or **pallor.** Leads to **loss of consciousness and muscle tone for < 30 seconds** and **recovery within seconds.**
- **Dx:**
  - Structural CNS causes (e.g., basilar TIA, intermittent obstructive hydrocephalus) are rare among patients who return to normal mental status and have a normal neurologic examination after a brief loss of consciousness.
  - Seizures are more likely if limb jerking is unilateral or lasts > 30 seconds; if there is prolonged confusion after the episode; or if the patient bites the lateral aspect of their tongue.
  - Unless there is a clear vasovagal faint in a young patient without cardiac disease or risk factors, place all patients on **telemetry** or **Holter monitoring** to evaluate for arrhythmia, and rule out myocardial ischemia with an **ECG** and **cardiac enzymes.** Obtain an **EEG** to rule out seizures. Consider an **echocardiogram,** a **tilt-table test,** or **neuroimaging,** especially vascular.
- **Tx:** Treat the underlying cause; avoid triggers.

▶ DISORDERS OF THE NEUROMUSCULAR JUNCTION

Myasthenia Gravis

An **autoimmune disorder** caused by antibodies that bind to **postsynaptic acetylcholine (ACh) receptors** located at the neuromuscular junction. Most often affects young adult females, and can be associated with **thyrotoxicosis, thymoma,** and other autoimmune disorders.

HISTORY/PE

- Presents with fluctuating **fatigable ptosis or double vision,** bulbar symptoms (e.g., dysarthria, dysphagia), and **proximal muscle weakness. Symptoms typically worsen as the day progresses but fluctuate dramatically.**
- Patients may report difficulty climbing stairs, rising from a chair, brushing their hair, and swallowing.
- **Myasthenic crisis** is rare but includes the potentially lethal complications of respiratory compromise and aspiration.

DIAGNOSIS

- **Edrophonium (Tensilon test): Anticholinesterase** leads to **rapid** amelioration of symptoms. Rarely used today owing to the risk of bradycardia.
- **Ice test:** Place a pack of ice on one eye for five minutes; ptosis resolves transiently.
- An abnormal **single-fiber EMG** and/or a **decremental response to repetitive nerve stimulation** can yield additional confirmation.
- ACh antibodies are ⊕ in 80% of patients; anti–muscle-specific kinase (anti-MuSK) antibodies are ⊕ in 5%.
- Chest CT is used to evaluate for thymoma. Eighty-five percent of patients with thymoma have ⊕ antibodies against striated muscle.
- Follow serial FVCs to determine the need to intubate.

TREATMENT

- Anticholinesterases (**pyridostigmine**) are used for symptomatic treatment.
- **Prednisone** and other immunosuppressants (e.g., azathioprine, cyclosporine, mycophenolate) are the mainstays of treatment.
- In severe cases, plasmapheresis or IVIG may provide temporary relief (days to weeks).
- **Resection of thymoma** can be curative.
- **Avoid giving certain antibiotics** (e.g., aminoglycosides) **and drugs** (e.g., β-blockers) to patients with myasthenia gravis.

Lambert-Eaton Myasthenic Syndrome

- An autoimmune disorder caused by antibodies directed toward presynaptic calcium channels in the neuromuscular junction. **Small cell lung carcinoma** is a significant risk factor (60% of cases).
- Hx/PE: Presents with weakness and fatigability of proximal muscles along with depressed or absent DTRs. Extraocular, respiratory, and bulbar muscles are typically spared.
- **Dx: Repetitive nerve stimulation** reveals a characteristic incremental response. Also diagnosed by autoantibodies to presynaptic calcium channels and a chest CT indicative of a lung neoplasm.
- **Tx:** Treat small cell lung carcinoma; tumor resection may reverse symptoms. 3,4-diaminopyridine or guanidine can be given; acetylcholinesterase inhibitors (pyridostigmine) can be added to either regimen. Corticosteroids and azathioprine can be combined or used alone for immunosuppression.

Repetitive nerve stimulation reveals a characteristic incremental response in Lambert-Eaton myasthenic syndrome, and a decremental response in myasthenia gravis.

Multiple Sclerosis (MS)

Although the pathogenesis of MS is unclear, there is evidence of an autoimmune etiology in genetically susceptible individuals who are exposed to environmental triggers such as viral infections. Such potential etiologies are thought to be **T-cell mediated.** The female-to-male ratio is 3:2, and onset is typically between 20 and 40 years of age. MS becomes more common as one moves farther away from the equator. Subtypes are **relapsing-remitting,** primary progressive, secondary progressive, and progressive relapsing (see Table 2.10-9).

HISTORY/PE

- Presents with **multiple neurologic complaints that are separated in time and space and are not explained by a single lesion.** As the disease progresses, permanent deficits may accumulate.
- Limb weakness, **optic neuritis,** paresthesias, diplopia, vertigo, nystagmus, gait unsteadiness, urinary retention, sexual and bowel dysfunction, depression, and cognitive impairment are also seen. Symptoms classically worsen transiently with hot showers.
- Attacks are unpredictable but on average occur every 1.5 years, lasting for 6–8 weeks.
- Neurologic symptoms can come and go or be progressive. The **prognosis is best with a relapsing and remitting history.**
- Lhermitte's sign, demonstrated by sharp pain traveling up or down the neck and back with flexion, generally suggests the presence of cervical myelitis.

The classic triad in MS is scanning speech, intranuclear ophthalmoplegia, and nystagmus.

Pregnancy may be associated with a ↓ in symptoms of MS.

TABLE 2.10-9. Subtypes of Multiple Sclerosis

	RELAPSING-REMITTING	PRIMARY PROGRESSIVE	SECONDARY PROGRESSIVE	PROGRESSIVE RELAPSING
Relapses	Yes.	No acute episodes.	Yes.	Yes.
Progression	None.	From onset.	Not at onset; begins to progress later.	From onset.
Course of symptoms	Full recovery, or deficits may remain after each episode.	Minor remissions and plateaus may take place during progression.	Relapses, minor remissions, and plateaus may take place during progression.	Full recovery, or progressive deficits may remain after each episode.
Percentage of cases at onset	66%	19%	Develops after relapsing-remitting type.	15%
Prognosis	Best.	Worse.	Worse.	Worse.

DIAGNOSIS

- MRI shows **multiple, asymmetric,** often **periventricular** white matter lesions (Dawson's fingers), especially in the **corpus callosum.** Active lesions enhance with gadolinium.
- CSF reveals mononuclear pleocytosis (> 5 cells/μL), an ↑ IgG index, or oligoclonal bands (nonspecific).
- Abnormal somatosensory or visual evoked potentials may also be present.

TREATMENT

- **Corticosteroids** should be given during acute exacerbations.
- Immunomodulators alter relapse rates in relapsing-remitting MS and include interferon-β_{1a} (**A**vonex/Rebif), interferon-β_{1b} (**B**etaseron), and co-polymer-1 (**C**opaxone).
- Mitoxantrone can be given for worsening relapsing/remitting or progressive MS.
- Alternative treatments include cyclophosphamide, IVIG, and plasmapheresis.
- **Symptomatic therapy** is crucial and includes baclofen for spasticity; cholinergics for urinary retention; anticholinergics for urinary incontinence; carbamazepine or amitriptyline for painful paresthesias; and antidepressants for clinical depression.

> **MS treatment—as easy as ABC**
>
> **A**vonex/Rebif
> **B**etaseron
> **C**opaxone

For optic neuritis, give IV, not oral, corticosteroids.

Guillain-Barré Syndrome (GBS)

An **acute, rapidly progressive,** acquired demyelinating autoimmune disorder of the peripheral nerves that results in weakness. Also known as acute inflammatory demyelinating polyneuropathy. Associated with recent *Campylobacter jejuni* infection, viral infection, or influenza vaccination. Approximately 85% of patients make a complete or near-complete recovery (may take up to one year). The mortality rate is < 5%.

HISTORY/PE

- Classically presents with progressive (over days), symmetric, **ascending paralysis** (distal to proximal) involving the trunk, diaphragm, and cranial nerves. Atypical presentations are common, including variants that begin with cranial involvement or progress unpredictably to involve the respiratory muscles.
- Autonomic dysregulation, areflexia, and dysesthesias may be present.

DIAGNOSIS

- Evidence of diffuse demyelination is seen on **EMG** and **nerve conduction studies,** which show ↓ nerve conduction velocity.
- Supported by a **CSF protein level > 55 mg/dL** with little or no pleocytosis (albuminocytologic dissociation).

TREATMENT

- Admit to the ICU for impending **respiratory failure.**
- **Plasmapheresis** and **IVIG** are first-line treatments. Corticosteroids are **not indicated.**
- Aggressive physical rehabilitation is imperative.

Amyotrophic Lateral Sclerosis (ALS)

A **chronic, progressive degenerative disease** of unknown etiology characterized by loss of **upper and lower motor neurons.** Also known as **Lou Gehrig's disease.** ALS has an unrelenting course and almost always progresses to respiratory failure and death, usually within five years of diagnosis. Males are more commonly affected than females, and onset is generally between ages 40 and 80.

HISTORY/PE

- Presents with **asymmetric,** slowly progressive weakness (over months to years) affecting the arms, legs, diaphragm, and lower cranial nerves. Some patients initially present with **fasciculations.** Weight loss is common.
- Associated with **UMN** and/or **LMN signs** (see Table 2.10-4). Eye movements and sphincter tone are generally spared. Tongue atrophy and fasciculation may be apparent.
- Emotional lability is a common feature.

DIAGNOSIS

- The clinical presentation is usually diagnostic.
- Involvement of the tongue (CN XII) or oropharyngeal muscles (CN IX, X), known as "bulbar" involvement, suggests pathology above the foramen magnum and generally excludes the most common differential, cervical spondylosis with compressive myelopathy, as a cause.
- **EMG/nerve conduction studies** reveal widespread denervation and fibrillation potentials. Such studies are principally performed to exclude other demyelinating motor neuropathies.
- CT/MRI of the cervical spine is done to exclude structural lesions, particularly in those without bulbar involvement.

The 5 A's of GBS:

Acute inflammatory demyelinating polyradiculopathy
Ascending paralysis
Autonomic neuropathy
Arrhythmias
Albuminocytologic dissociation

A 55-year-old male presents with slowly progressive weakness in his left upper extremity and later his right, associated with fasciculations but without bladder disturbance and with a normal cervical MRI. Think ALS.

TREATMENT

Supportive measures and patient education.

A chronic, progressive, global decline in multiple cognitive areas (see the mnemonic **the 5 A's of dementia**). Alzheimer's disease accounts for 60–80% of cases. The differential diagnosis is described in the mnemonic **DEMEN-TIAS**. Take care not to confuse delirium and dementia (see the Psychiatry chapter).

Alzheimer's Disease (AD)

Risk factors for AD include **age**, female gender, a **family history, Down syndrome,** and low educational status. Pathology involves **neurofibrillary tangles, neuritic plaques** with **amyloid** deposition, amyloid angiopathy, and neuronal loss.

HISTORY/PE

- **Amnesia** for newly acquired information is usually the first presenting sign, followed by language deficits, acalculia, depression, agitation, psychosis, and apraxia (inability to perform skilled movements).
- Mild cognitive impairment may precede AD by 10 years. **Survival is 5–10 years** from the onset of symptoms, with death usually occurring 2° to **aspiration pneumonia** or other infections. Except for the mental state, the physical exam is generally normal.

DIAGNOSIS

- **A diagnosis of exclusion** that can be **definitively diagnosed only on autopsy;** suggested by clinical features and by an insidiously progressive cognitive course without substantial motor impairment.
- MRI or CT may show atrophy and can rule out other causes, particularly vascular dementia, normal pressure hydrocephalus, and chronic subdural hematoma. PET imaging shows nonspecific bilateral temporoparietal hypometabolism. CSF is normal.
- Neuropsychological testing can help distinguish dementia from depression. Hypothyroidism, vitamin B_{12} deficiency, and neurosyphilis should be ruled out in atypical cases.

TREATMENT

- **Prevention of associated symptoms:**
  - Provide supportive therapy for the patient and family.
  - Treat depression, agitation, sleep disorders, hallucinations, and delusions.
- **Prevention of disease progression: Cholinesterase inhibitors** (donepezil, rivastigmine, galantamine, and tacrine) are first-line therapy. Tacrine is associated with hepatotoxicity and is less often used. Memantine, an NMDA receptor antagonist, may slow decline in moderate to severe disease.

The 5 A's of dementia:

Aphasia
Amnesia
Agnosia
Apraxia
Disturbances in **A**bstract thought

Differential diagnosis—

DEMENTIAS

Neuro**D**egenerative diseases
Endocrine
Metabolic
Exogenous
Neoplasm
Trauma
Infection
Affective disorders
Stroke/**S**tructural

Vascular Dementia

Dementia associated with a history of stroke and cerebrovascular disease is the second most common type of dementia. **Risk factors** include **age, hypertension, diabetes,** embolic sources, and a history of **stroke.**

DIAGNOSIS

Criteria for the diagnosis of vascular dementia include the presence of dementia and two or more of the following:

- Focal neurologic signs on exam.
- Symptom onset that was abrupt, **stepwise,** or related to stroke.
- Brain imaging showing evidence of old infarctions or extensive deep white matter changes 2° to chronic ischemia.

TREATMENT

Protocols for the prevention and treatment of vascular dementia are the same as those for stroke.

If a patient shows abrupt changes in symptoms over time rather than a steady decline, think vascular dementia.

Frontotemporal Dementia (Pick's Disease)

A **rare,** progressive form of dementia characterized by **atrophy of the frontal and temporal lobes.** Round intraneuronal inclusions known as **Pick bodies** are the classic pathologic finding.

HISTORY/PE

Patients present with **significant changes in behavior and personality early in the disease.** Other symptoms include speech disturbance, inattentiveness, and occasionally extrapyramidal signs. Unlike Parkinson's disease, frontotemporal dementia rarely begins after age 75.

DIAGNOSIS

The diagnosis is suggested by clinical features and by evidence of circumscribed frontotemporal atrophy revealed by MRI or CT.

TREATMENT

Treatment is symptomatic only; no curative therapy has yet been made available.

Normal Pressure Hydrocephalus (NPH)

A **potentially treatable** form of dementia that is thought to arise from impaired CSF outflow from the brain.

HISTORY/PE

Symptoms include the **classic triad of dementia, gait apraxia, and urinary incontinence.** Headaches and other signs of ↑ ICP (e.g., papilledema) typically do not appear, although continuous ICP monitoring may reveal spikes of elevated pressure.

DIAGNOSIS

- The diagnosis is suggested by clinical features. The gait is classically described as "magnetic" or with "feet glued to the floor," as the forefoot is not completely dorsally extended.
- LP or continuous lumbar CSF drainage for several days reveals normal pressure but may cause clinically significant improvement of the patient's symptoms.
- CT or MRI shows ventricular enlargement out of proportion to sulcal atrophy.

TREATMENT

Surgical CSF shunting is the treatment of choice.

Creutzfeldt-Jakob Disease (CJD)

Although it is the most common **prion disease**, CJD remains an extremely rare form of dementia. CJD is a member of the transmissible spongiform encephalopathies, all of which are characterized by spongy degeneration, neuronal loss, and astrocytic proliferation. In CJD, an abnormal protease-resistant prion protein accumulates in the brain.

HISTORY/PE

CJD causes a **subacute dementia** with ataxia or myoclonic jerks with rapid clinical decline that is noted weeks to months after symptom onset.

DIAGNOSIS

- Suggested by clinical features.
- The differential diagnosis often includes viral encephalitis, Hashimoto's (steroid-responsive) encephalopathy, and toxic encephalopathy (e.g., lithium or bismuth).
- EEG shows **pyramidal signs** and **periodic sharp waves**.
- MRI with diffusion-weighted imaging may show ↑ T2 and FLAIR intensity in the putamen and the head of the caudate and is also used to exclude structural brain lesions.
- CSF is usually normal.
- Definitive diagnosis can be made only by brain biopsy or autopsy. Specimens must be handled with special precautions to avoid transmission.

TREATMENT

Currently, there is no effective treatment. Most patients die within one year of symptom onset.

If a patient presents with rapid cognitive decline over the course of weeks to months, think CJD.

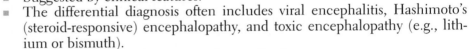

▶ **MOVEMENT DISORDERS**

Huntington's Disease (HD)

A rare, **hyperkinetic, autosomal-dominant** disease involving multiple **abnormal CAG triplet repeats** (< 29 is normal) within the *HD* gene on chromosome 4. The number of repeats typically expands in subsequent generations, leading to earlier expression and more severe disease (**anticipation**). Life expectancy is 20 years from the time of diagnosis.

HISTORY/PE

Presents at 30–50 years of age with gradual onset of **chorea** (sudden onset of purposeless, involuntary dancelike movements), **altered behavior,** and **dementia** (begins as irritability, clumsiness, fidgetiness, moodiness, and antisocial behavior). Weight loss and depression may also be seen.

DIAGNOSIS

- A **clinical diagnosis** confirmed by **genetic testing.**
- CT/MRI show cerebral atrophy (especially of the **caudate** and putamen). Molecular genetic testing is conducted to determine the number of CAG repeats.

TREATMENT

- There is no cure, and disease progression cannot be halted. Treat symptomatically.
- Reserpine or tetrabenazine can be given to minimize unwanted movements. Psychosis should preferably be treated with atypical antipsychotics to reduce the risk of extrapyramidal side effects or tardive dyskinesia. SSRIs are first-line therapy for depression.
- Genetic counseling should be offered to offspring.

Parkinson's Disease

An **idiopathic hypokinetic** disorder that usually begins after age 50–60 and is attributable to **dopamine depletion** in the **substantia nigra.** It is characterized pathologically by **Lewy bodies,** which are intraneuronal eosinophilic inclusions.

HISTORY/PE

- The "**Parkinson's tetrad**" consists of the following:
  - **Resting tremor** (e.g., "pill rolling").
  - **Rigidity:** "Cogwheeling" due to the combined effects of rigidity and tremor.
  - **Bradykinesia:** Slowed movements and difficulty initiating movements. Festinating gait (a wide leg stance with short accelerating steps) without arm swing is also seen.
  - **Postural instability:** Stooped posture, impaired righting reflexes, freezing, falls.
- Other manifestations include masked facies, memory loss, and micrographia.
- Parkinsonism is the broader clinical phenotype of bradykinesia and rigidity (with or without substantial tremor). It is often caused by disorders other than idiopathic Parkinson's disease, most commonly **multiple subcortical infarcts ("vascular parkinsonism").**
  - Nonidiopathic causes of parkinsonism include viral encephalitis (postencephalitic parkinsonism), trauma (dementia pugilistica), and numerous toxins (e.g., manganese, MPTP [designer drugs], and, iatrogenically, neuroleptics [tardive dyskinesia]). Some of these disorders are diagnosed on the basis of failure of levodopa/carbidopa to produce a clinical response.
  - Other idiopathic dementias may mimic Parkinson's disease and include progressive supranuclear palsy and multiple system atrophy.

If a 43-year-old male patient presents with sudden onset of chorea, irritability, and antisocial behavior and his father experienced these symptoms at a slightly older age, think Huntington's disease.

A significant difference between gait abnormalities in Parkinson's and that of NPH is preservation of arm swing in NPH.

There are four PaRTS to Parkinson's: Postural instability, Rigidity (cogwheeling), Tremor ("pill rolling"), and Slowed movements (bradykinesia).

TREATMENT

- **Levodopa** and **carbidopa,** both of which are dopamine precursors, are the mainstays of therapy.
- Dopamine agonists (ropinirole, pramipexole, bromocriptine) can be used for treatment in early disease. Apomorphine is another dopamine agonist that can be used for rescue therapy if a sudden additional dose is needed.
- Selegiline (an MAO-B inhibitor) may be neuroprotective and may ↓ the need for levodopa.
- Catechol-O-methyltransferase (COMT) inhibitors (entacapone or tolcapone) are not given alone but ↑ the availability of levodopa to the brain and may ↓ motor fluctuations.
- Amantadine has mild antiparkinsonian activity and may improve akinesia, rigidity, and tremor. It can be used for temporary, short-term monotherapy early in the course of the disease.
- If medical therapy fails, **surgical pallidotomy** or chronic **deep brain stimulation** may produce clinical benefit.

▶ NEOPLASMS

Intracranial neoplasms may be 1° (30%) or **metastatic (70%).**

- Of all 1° brain tumors, 40% are benign, and these rarely spread beyond the CNS.
- Metastatic tumors are most often from 1° **lung, breast, kidney, and GI tract neoplasms** and **melanoma.** They occur at the **gray-white junction; may be multiple discrete nodules;** and are characterized by rapid growth, invasiveness, necrosis, and neovascularization.
- More common in males than in females, except for meningiomas.

HISTORY/PE

- Symptoms depend on tumor type and location (see Table 2.10-10), local growth and **resulting mass effect,** cerebral edema, or elevated ICP 2° to ventricular obstruction. Although headaches are often thought of as the main presenting symptom, only 31% of patients present with headache at diagnosis and only 8% have headache as the sole presenting feature.
- Seizures or slowly progressive focal motor deficits are the most common presenting features. When ↑ ICP is the presenting feature, symptoms include headache, nausea/vomiting, and diplopia (false localizing CN VI palsies). However, in the era of neuroimaging, it is relatively rare for patients to present with ↑ ICP.
- Hemispheric tumors often produce visual field abnormalities and neuropsychiatric symptoms, including personality changes, lethargy, syncope, cognitive decline, aphasia, apraxia, and depression. Parasellar lesions usually present with visual loss and/or diplopia. Posterior fossa lesions tend to present with gait ataxia or cranial nerve deficits and/or ↑ ICP from obstructive hydrocephalus.
- Metastases that tend to present with intracranial hemorrhage include renal cell carcinoma, thyroid cancer, choriocarcinoma, and melanoma.

DIAGNOSIS

- Contrast CT and MRI with and without gadolinium to localize and determine the extent of the lesion. Gadolinium-enhanced MRI is generally better for visualizing soft tissue tumors and vascularity, but CT is better for

TABLE 2.10-10. Common 1° Neoplasms

Tumor	Pathology	Presentation	Treatment
Astrocytoma	Arises in brain parenchyma. Low-grade astrocytomas are relatively uncommon.	Presents with seizures, focal deficits, or headache. Has a **protracted course.** Has a better prognosis than glioblastoma multiforme (see below).	Resection if possible; radiation.
Glioblastoma multiforme (grade IV astrocytoma)	High mitotic activity and either endothelial proliferation or necrosis in tumor, leading to ring-enhancing lesions on MRI. There is a major difference between grade III and grade IV.	The most common 1° brain tumor. Presents with headache and ↑ seizures, focal deficits, or headache. Progresses rapidly and has a poor prognosis (< 1 year from the time of prognosis).	Surgical removal/resection. Radiation and chemotherapy have variable results.
Meningioma	Originates from the **dura mater or arachnoid.**	Presentation depends on location; often related to cranial neuropathy or is an incidental finding. Good prognosis. Incidence ↑ with age. Imaging may reveal **dural tail.**	Surgical resection; radiation for unresectable tumors.
Acoustic neuroma (schwannoma)	Derived from **Schwann cells.**	Presents with ipsilateral tinnitus, hearing loss, vertigo, and late signs of CN V–VII or brain stem compression.	Surgical removal.
Medulloblastoma	A primitive neuroectodermal tumor. Arises from the fourth ventricle and causes ↑ ICP.	**Common in children. Highly malignant;** may seed the subarachnoid space. May cause obstructive hydrocephalus.	Surgical resection coupled with radiation and chemotherapy.
Ependymoma	May arise from the ependyma of a ventricle (commonly the fourth) or the spinal cord.	Common in children; low grade. May cause obstructive hydrocephalus.	Surgical resection; radiation.

evaluating skull base lesions and for emergencies (e.g., obstructive hydrocephalus) when an MRI cannot be rapidly acquired.
- Histologic diagnosis via CT-guided biopsy or surgical tumor debulking/removal.

TREATMENT

- **Resection** (if possible), **radiation,** and **chemotherapy.**
- Therapy is highly dependent on tumor type, histology, progression, and site (see Table 2.10-10).
- **Corticosteroids** can be used to ↓ vasogenic edema and ↓ ICP. Management is often palliative.
- Seizure prophylaxis can be used in patients who have had a seizure.

Symptoms of ↑ ICP:

- *Nausea*
- *Vomiting*
- *Diplopia*
- *Headache that is worse in the morning or with recumbency*

Neurofibromatosis (NF)

The most common neurocutaneous disorder. There are **two major types:** neurofibromatosis 1 (NF1, or von Recklinghausen's syndrome) and neurofibromatosis 2 (NF2). Both obey **autosomal-dominant inheritance.** The *NF* genes are located on **chromosome 17 and 22,** respectively, for NF1 and NF2.

History/PE

- Diagnostic criteria for **NF1** include two or more of the following:
    - Six **café au lait spots** (each ≥ 5 mm in children or ≥ 15 mm in adults).
    - Two neurofibromas of any type.
    - **Freckling in the axillary or inguinal area.**
    - **Optic glioma.**
    - Two **Lisch** nodules (pigmented iris hamartomas).
    - Bone abnormality (e.g., kyphoscoliosis).
    - A **first-degree relative** with NF1.
- Diagnostic criteria for NF2 are as follows:
    - **Bilateral acoustic neuromas or** a first-degree relative with NF2 and **either** unilateral acoustic neuromas or two of any of the following: neurofibromas, meningiomas, gliomas, or schwannoma.
    - Other features include seizures, skin nodules, and café au lait spots.

Diagnosis

- **MRI** of the brain, brain stem, and spine with gadolinium.
- Obtain a complete dermatologic exam, ophthalmologic exam, and family history. Auditory testing is recommended.

Treatment

- There is no cure; treatment is symptomatic (e.g., surgery for kyphoscoliosis or debulking of tumors).
- Acoustic neuromas and optic gliomas can be treated with surgery or radiosurgery. Meningiomas may be resected.

Tuberous Sclerosis

Affects **many organ systems,** including the CNS, skin, heart, retina, and kidneys. Obeys **autosomal-dominant** inheritance.

History/PE

- Presents with **convulsive seizures** (infantile spasms in infants), "ash-leaf" **hypopigmented lesions** on the trunk and extremities, and **mental retardation** (↑ likelihood with early age of onset).
- Other skin manifestations include **sebaceous adenomas** (small red nodules on the nose and cheeks in the shape of a butterfly) and a **shagreen patch** (a rough papule in the lumbosacral region with an orange-peel consistency).
- Two retinal lesions are recognized: (1) mulberry tumors, which arise from the nerve head; and (2) phakomas, which are round, flat, gray lesions located peripherally in the retina.
- Symptoms are 2° to small benign tumors that grow on the face, eyes, brain, kidney, and other organs.

In NF1, you—

CANNOT FAIL 2 B 1st

CA (6 **CA**fé au lait spots)
NN (2 **N**eurofibromas)
OT (**O**p**T**ic glioma)
FAI (**F**reckling, **A**xillary or **I**nguinal)
L 2 (2 **L**isch nodules)
B (**B**one abnormality)
1st (**1st**-degree relative with NF1)

NF1 and NF2 are clinically evident by ages 15 and 20, respectively.

If you see infantile spasms in the setting of a hypopigmented lesion on the child's trunk, consider tuberous sclerosis.

- Mental retardation and CHF from cardiac rhabdomyoma may also be seen.
- Renal involvement may include hamartomas, angiomyolipomas, or, rarely, renal cell carcinoma.

DIAGNOSIS

- Diagnosis is usually clinical.
- Skin lesions are enhanced by a Wood's UV lamp.
- **Imaging:**
  - **Head CT:** Reveals calcified tubers within the cerebrum in the periventricular area. Lesions may on rare occasion transform into malignant astrocytomas.
  - **ECG:** Evaluate for rhabdomyoma of the heart, especially in the apex of the left ventricle (affects > 50% of patients).
  - **Renal ultrasound:** May reveal renal hamartomas, masses, or polycystic disease.
  - **Renal CT:** May show angiomyolipomas (causing cystic or fibrous pulmonary changes).
  - **CXR:** May reveal pulmonary lesions or cardiomegaly 2° to rhabdomyoma.

TREATMENT

- Treatment should be based on symptoms (e.g., cosmetic surgery for adenoma sebaceum).
- Simple partial or complex partial seizures can be controlled with oxcarbazepine or carbamazepine; lamotrigine can be given for generalized seizures. Treat infantile spasms with ACTH or vigabatrin.
- Surgical intervention may be indicated in the setting of ↑ ICP or for seizures associated with an epileptogenic focus or severe developmental delay.

▶ APHASIA

A general term for speech and language disorders. Usually results from insults (e.g., strokes, tumors, abscesses) to the "dominant hemisphere" (the left hemisphere in > 95% of right-handed people and 60–80% of left-handed people).

Broca's Aphasia

- A **disorder of language production, including writing,** with **intact comprehension.** Due to an insult to Broca's area in the **posterior inferior frontal gyrus.** Often 2° to a left superior **MCA stroke.** Also known as **motor aphasia.**
- **Hx/PE:** Presents with **impaired repetition, frustration** with awareness of deficits, arm and facial **hemiparesis,** hemisensory loss, and apraxia of the oral muscles. Speech is described as "telegraphic" and agrammatical with frequent pauses.
- **Tx: Speech therapy** (varying outcomes with intermediate prognosis).

Wernicke's Aphasia

- A **disorder of language comprehension** with **intact yet nonsensical production.** Also known as **sensory aphasia.**

Broca's aphasia is also known as expressive or nonfluent aphasia.

Wernicke's aphasia is also known as fluent or receptive aphasia.

- Due to an insult to Wernicke's area in the left posterior superior temporal (perisylvian) gyrus. Often 2° to left **inferior/posterior MCA** embolic stroke.
- **Hx/PE:** Presents with **preserved fluency** of language with impaired repetition and comprehension, leading to "**word salad.**" Patients are unable to follow commands; make frequent use of **neologisms** (made-up words) and paraphasic errors (word substitutions); show **lack of awareness** of deficits; and exhibit right upper homonymous quadrantanopia 2° to involvement of Meyer's loop.
- **Tx:** Treat the underlying etiology and institute speech therapy.

▶ COMA

A state of unconsciousness marked by a profound suppression of responses to external and internal stimuli (i.e., a state of unarousable unresponsiveness). Lesser states of impaired arousal are known as "obtundation" or "stupor." Coma is due to either catastrophic structural CNS injury or diffuse metabolic dysfunction. Coma indicates bilateral dysfunction of both cerebral hemispheres or the brain stem (pons or higher); when structural, coma usually results from bilateral pathology. Causes include the following:

- Diffuse **hypoxic/ischemic encephalopathy** (e.g., postcardiac arrest).
- **Diffuse axonal injury** from high-acceleration trauma (e.g., MVA).
- **Brain herniation** (e.g., cerebral mass lesion, SAH with obstructive hydrocephalus).
- **Widespread infection** (e.g., viral encephalitis or advanced bacterial meningitis).
- **Massive brain stem hemorrhage or infarction** (e.g., pontine myelinolysis).
- **Electrolyte disturbances** (e.g., hypoglycemia).
- **Exogenous toxins** (e.g., opiates, benzodiazepines, EtOH, other drugs).
- Generalized **seizure** activity or postictal states.
- **Endocrine** (e.g., severe hypothyroidism) or **metabolic dysfunction** (e.g., thiamine deficiency).

HISTORY/PE

- Obtain a complete medical history from witnesses, including current medications (e.g., **sedatives**).
- Conduct thorough medical and neurologic exams, including assessments of mental status, spontaneous motor activity, muscular tone, breathing pattern, funduscopy, pupillary response, eye movements (including the doll's-eye maneuver if the neck has been cleared from fracture), corneal reflex, cold-water caloric testing, gag reflex, and motor or autonomic responses to noxious stimuli applied to limbs, trunk and face (e.g., retromandibular pressure, nasal tickle).

DIAGNOSIS

- Typically made by a combination of the history/physical and laboratory tests or neuroimaging.
- Check glucose, electrolytes, calcium, a renal panel, LFTs, ABG, a toxicology screen, and blood and CSF cultures. Other metabolic tests (e.g., TSH) may be performed based on the clinical index of suspicion.
- Obtain a **head CT without contrast** before other imaging to evaluate for

hemorrhage or structural changes. Imaging should **precede LP** in light of the risk of herniation.

- Obtain an MRI to exclude structural changes and ischemia (e.g., brain stem). **EEG** may be both diagnostic and prognostic.
- Rule out catatonia, hysterical or conversion unresponsiveness, **"locked-in" syndrome,** or **persistent vegetative state** (PVS), all of which can be confused with true coma (see Table 2.10-11).
  - **"Locked-in" syndrome:** Patients are awake and alert but can move only their eyes and eyelids. Associated with central pontine myelinolysis, brain stem stroke, and advanced ALS.
  - **PVS:** Characterized by normal wake-sleep cycles but lack of awareness of self or the environment. The most common causes are trauma with diffuse cortical injury or hypoxic ischemic injury.

TREATMENT

Initial treatment should consist of the following measures:

- **Stabilize the patient:** Attend to **ABCs.**
- **Reverse the reversible:** Administer **DONT**—Dextrose, Oxygen, Naloxone, and Thiamine.
- **Identify and treat the underlying cause** and associated complications.
- **Prevent further damage.**

▶ NUTRITIONAL DEFICIENCIES

Table 2.10-12 describes the neurologic symptoms commonly associated with nutritional deficiencies.

▶ OPHTHALMOLOGY

Visual Field Defects

Figure 2.10-8 illustrates common visual field defects and the anatomic areas with which they are associated.

TABLE 2.10-11. **Differential Diagnosis of Coma**

	"LOCKED-IN" SYNDROME	**PVS**	**COMA**	**BRAIN DEATH**
Alertness	Wakeful and alert with retained cognitive abilities.	Wakefulness without awareness.	Unconscious; no sleep-wake cycles.	Unconscious; no sleep-wake cycles.
Most common causes	Central pontine myelinolysis, brain stem stroke, advanced ALS.	Diffuse cortical injury or hypoxic ischemic injury.	See above.	Same as coma.
Voluntary motor ability	Eyes and eyelids.	None.	None.	None.
Respiratory drive	Yes.	Yes.	Yes.	None.

TABLE 2.10-12. Neurologic Syndromes Associated with Nutritional Deficiencies

VITAMIN	SYNDROME	SIGNS/SYMPTOMS	CLASSIC PATIENTS	TREATMENT
Thiamine (vitamin B$_1$)	Wernicke's encephalopathy	The classic triad consists of **encephalopathy** (disorientation, inattentiveness, confusion, coma), **ophthalmoplegia** (nystagmus, lateral rectus palsy, conjugate gaze palsy, vertical gaze palsy), and **ataxia** (polyneuropathy; cerebellar and vestibular dysfunction leading to problems standing or walking).	**Alcoholics, hyperemesis, starvation, renal dialysis,** AIDS. **Can be brought on or exacerbated by high-dose glucose administration.**	Reversible almost immediately with thiamine administration. Always give thiamine before glucose.
	Korsakoff's dementia	Above, plus anterograde and retrograde amnesia, horizontal nystagmus, and confabulations.	Same as above. Usually occurs in the "resolution" phase of Wernicke's syndrome that was treated late or inadequately.	Irreversible.
Cyanocobalamin (vitamin B$_{12}$)[a]	Combined system disease (CSD) or subacute combined degeneration of the posterior and lateral columns of the spinal cord (see the discussion of clinical neuroanatomy); peripheral neuropathy.	Gradual, progressive onset. Symmetric paresthesias, stocking-glove sensory neuropathy, leg stiffness, spasticity, paraplegia, bowel and bladder dysfunction, sore tongue. Dementia.	Patients with pernicious anemia; strict vegetarians; status post gastric or ileal resection; ileal disease (e.g., Crohn's); alcoholics or others with malnutrition.	B$_{12}$ injections or large oral doses.
Folate[a]	Folate deficiency	Irritability; personality changes without the neurologic symptoms of CSD.	Alcoholics; patients with pernicious anemia.	Reversible if corrected early.

[a] Associated with ↑ homocysteine and ↑ risk of vascular events.

Glaucoma

In the eye, aqueous humor is produced by the ciliary body on the iris, travels through the pupil into the anterior chamber, and is then drained via the trabecular meshwork in the angle of the anterior chamber.

- Any process that disrupts this natural flow can ↑ intraocular pressure (IOP), damaging the optic nerve and causing visual field deficits. Glaucoma is the result of such damage to the nerve.

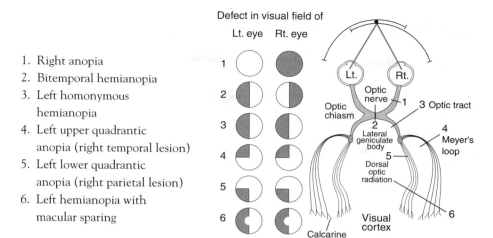

1. Right anopia
2. Bitemporal hemianopia
3. Left homonymous hemianopia
4. Left upper quadrantic anopia (right temporal lesion)
5. Left lower quadrantic anopia (right parietal lesion)
6. Left hemianopia with macular sparing

FIGURE 2.10-8. **Visual field defects.**

- Open-angle glaucoma is much more common in the United States than closed-angle glaucoma.

CLOSED-ANGLE GLAUCOMA

- Occurs when the iris dilates and pushes against the lens of the eye, disrupting flow of aqueous humor into the anterior chamber. Pressure in the posterior chamber then pushes the peripheral iris forward and blocks the angle.
- Risk factors include family history, older age, Asian ethnicity, hyperopia, prolonged **pupillary dilation** (prolonged time in a dark area, stress, medications), anterior uveitis, and lens dislocation.
- **Hx/PE:** Classically presents with extreme eye pain, blurred vision, headache, nausea, and vomiting. A hard, red eye is seen (from acute closure of a narrow anterior chamber angle); the pupil is dilated and nonreactive to light. IOP is ↑. If it resolves spontaneously prior to presentation (e.g., with pupillary constriction in sunlight), ophthalmologic examination may reveal narrow angles in one or both eyes.
- **Dx:** Diagnosis is based on clinical history and examination. Those that resolve may mimic a migraine headache with blurred vision; the distinction is that the headaches and blurred vision are more likely to be triggered by darkness (due to pupillary dilation) rather than by bright lights (migraine).
- **Tx:** This is a **medical emergency** that can cause blindness. Treatment to ↓ IOP may include eyedrops (timolol, pilocarpine, apraclonidine) or systemic medications (oral or IV acetazolamide, IV mannitol). **Laser peripheral iridotomy**, which creates a hole in the peripheral iris, is curative and may be performed prophylactically.

OPEN-ANGLE GLAUCOMA

- Flow of aqueous humor through the trabecular meshwork is limited, increasing IOP. A diseased trabecular meshwork obstructs proper drainage of the eye, leading to a gradual ↑ in pressure and progressive vision loss.

Open-angle glaucoma generally occurs bilaterally, but angle-closure glaucoma occurs unilaterally.

- Risk factors include age > 40 years, **African-American ethnicity**, diabetes, and myopia.
- **Hx/PE:** Usually asymptomatic until late in the clinical course, when patients may begin to notice visual deficits. Should be suspected in patients > 35 years of age who need **frequent lens changes** and have mild headaches, visual disturbances, and impaired adaptation to darkness. The earliest visual defect is seen in the peripheral nasal fields. **Cupping** of the optic nerve head is seen on funduscopic exam.
- **Dx:** Tonometry, ophthalmoscopic visualization of the optic nerve, and visual field testing are most important. A diseased trabecular meshwork obstructs proper drainage of the eye, gradually increasing pressure and leading to progressive vision loss.
- **Tx:** Treat with topical β-blockers (timolol, betaxolol) to ↓ aqueous humor production or with pilocarpine to ↑ aqueous outflow. Carbonic anhydrase inhibitors may also be used. If medication fails, laser trabeculoplasty or a trabeculectomy can improve aqueous drainage.

In the United States, macular degeneration is the leading cause of permanent bilateral visual loss in the elderly.

Age-Related Macular Degeneration (AMD)

More common among Caucasians, females, smokers, and those with a ⊕ family history.

HISTORY/PE

- Presents with **painless loss of central vision.**
- **Atrophic ("dry") macular degeneration:** Responsible for 80% of cases. Causes gradual vision loss.
- **Exudative or neovascular ("wet") macular degeneration:** Much less common, but associated with more rapid and severe vision damage.

DIAGNOSIS

Funduscopy by an ophthalmologist reveals drusen and/or pigmentary changes in patients with atrophic AMD. Hemorrhage and subretinal fluid are suggestive of exudative AMD.

TREATMENT

- **Atrophic AMD:**
  - No treatment is currently available, although a combination of vitamins (vitamin C, vitamin E, beta-carotene, and zinc) has been found to slow disease progression.
  - An ↑ mortality rate from high doses of vitamin E and an elevated lung cancer incidence among individuals on beta-carotene supplementation may require modification of this regimen for smokers.
- **Exudative AMD:**
  - VEGF inhibitors have been shown to improve vision (ranibizumab, bevacizumab) or slow visual loss (pegaptanib) in patients with exudative AMD.
  - Photodynamic therapy with verteporfin, which involves use of a laser to selectively target retinal vessels, may be useful in conjunction with VEGF inhibitors.

Retinal Vascular Occlusion

- Occurs in **elderly patients** and is often idiopathic.
- Hx/PE:
    - **Central retinal artery occlusion:** Presents with sudden, painless, **unilateral blindness.** The pupil reacts to a near stimulus but is sluggishly reactive to direct light. Patients present with a **cherry-red spot** on the fovea, retinal swelling (whitish appearance to the nerve fiber layer), and retinal arteries that may appear bloodless.
    - **Central retinal vein occlusion:** Characterized by rapid, painless vision loss of variable severity. A choked, swollen optic disk with hemorrhages, venous stasis retinal hemorrhages, cotton-wool spots, and edema of the macula may be seen on funduscopic exam.
- Tx:
    - **Central retinal artery occlusion: Intra-arterial thrombolysis** of the ophthalmic artery within **eight** hours of onset of symptoms may produce benefit in some patients, although evidence remains controversial. Other treatments applied but of unclear benefit include increasing IOP through drainage of the anterior chamber or IV acetazolamide. If implemented, treatments should be applied immediately before irreversible retinal infarction and permanent blindness ensue.
    - **Central retinal vein occlusion:** Laser photocoagulation has variable results.

Obstetrics

The Basics of Pregnancy

The following terms and concepts are central to an understanding of the physiologic processes of pregnancy (see also Figure 2.11-1).

Nägele's rule: due date = last menstrual period + nine months + seven days.

- **Gravidity:** The number of times a woman has been pregnant.
- **Parity:** The number of pregnancies that led to a birth beyond 20 weeks' gestational age or an infant weighing > 500 g.
- **Developmental age (DA):** The number of weeks and days since fertilization. Typically used only in research, as the exact date of fertilization is not commonly known.
- **Gestational age (GA):** The number of weeks and days measured from the first day of the last menstrual period (LMP). GA can also be determined by:
  - **Fundal height:** At 20 weeks, the uterus is at the umbilicus and grows approximately 1 cm/week.
  - **Quickening, or appreciation of fetal movement:** Typically occurs at 17–18 weeks.
  - **Fetal heart tones:** Can be heard at 10–12 weeks by Doppler.
  - **Ultrasound:** Measures fetal crown-rump length (CRL) at 5–12 weeks and measures biparietal diameter (BPD), femur length (FL), and abdominal circumference (AC) from 13 weeks. Ultrasound measurement of GA is most reliable during the first trimester.

Normal Physiology of Pregnancy

The normal physiologic changes that occur during pregnancy are graphically illustrated according to system in Figures 2.11-2 and 2.11-3.

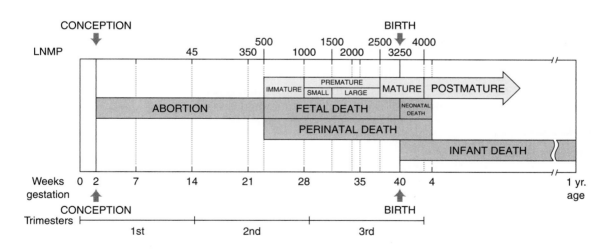

FIGURE 2.11-1. Perinatal nomenclature by date.

(Reproduced, with permission, from DeCherney AH, Nathan L. *Current Diagnosis & Treatment: Obstetrics & Gynecology,* 10th ed. New York: McGraw-Hill, 2007: Fig. 9-1.)

SYSTEM	PARAMETER	PATTERN
Renal	Renal flow	Increases 25–50%.
	Glomular filtration rate	Increases early, then plateaus.
Weight	Uterine weight	Increases from about 60–70 g to about 900–1200 g.
	Body weight	Average 11-kg (25-lb) increase.

FIGURE 2.11-2. Renal and uterine/body weight changes in normal pregnancy.

(Reproduced, with permission, from Gardner DG, Shoback D. *Greenspan's Basic & Clinical Endocrinology*, 8th ed. New York: McGraw-Hill, 2007: Fig. 17-2A.)

▶ **PRENATAL CARE**

The goal of prenatal care is to prevent, diagnose, and treat conditions that can lead to adverse outcomes in pregnancy. Expected weight gain, nutrition, and exercise recommendations are outlined in Table 2.11-1.

▶ **PRENATAL DIAGNOSTIC TESTING**

Table 2.11-2 outlines a typical prenatal diagnostic testing schedule by week. The sections that follow describe each recommended screening modality in further detail.

β-hCG

Get a quantitative β-hCG:
- *To diagnose and follow ectopic pregnancy.*
- *To monitor trophoblastic disease.*
- *To screen for fetal aneuploidy.*

- The **standard for diagnosing pregnancy.**
- Produced by the placenta; peaks at 100,000 mIU/mL by 10 weeks of gestation.
- ↓ throughout the second trimester; levels off in the third trimester.
- **hCG levels double approximately every 48 hours during early pregnancy.** This is often used to diagnose ectopic pregnancy when doubling is abnormal.

Quad Screening

*Still **UNDER**age at **18**: trisomy*

***18** = ↓ AFP, ↓ estriol, ↓ β-hCG, ↓ inhibin A.*

- Maternal serum α-fetoprotein (MSAFP), which is produced by the fetus, crosses the placenta in small amounts and enters the maternal circulation. Measurement results are reported as multiples of the median (MoMs) and depend on accurate gestational dating.
    - **Elevated MSAFP (> 2.5 MoMs):** Associated with open neural tube defects (anencephaly, spina bifida), abdominal wall defects (gastroschisis, omphalocele), multiple gestation, incorrect gestational dating, fetal death, and placental abnormalities (e.g., placental abruption).
    - **Decreased MSAFP (< 0.5 MoM):** Associated with trisomy 21 and 18, fetal demise, and inaccurate gestational dating.
- MSAFP is now **rarely performed alone** because its sensitivity for detecting chromosomal abnormalities is ↑ by adding inhibin A to estriol, β-hCG, and MSAFP (**quad screening**). Results of quad screening are as follows:

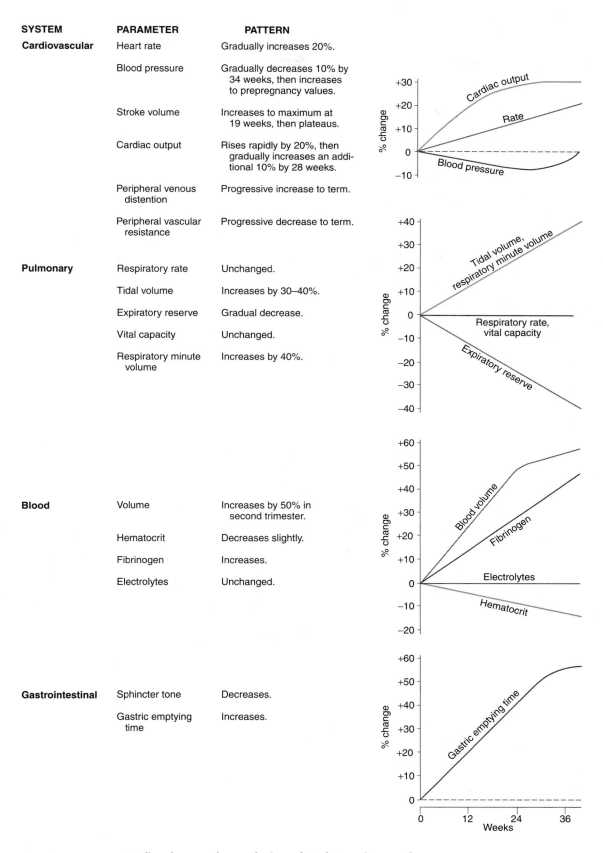

SYSTEM	PARAMETER	PATTERN
Cardiovascular	Heart rate	Gradually increases 20%.
	Blood pressure	Gradually decreases 10% by 34 weeks, then increases to prepregnancy values.
	Stroke volume	Increases to maximum at 19 weeks, then plateaus.
	Cardiac output	Rises rapidly by 20%, then gradually increases an additional 10% by 28 weeks.
	Peripheral venous distention	Progressive increase to term.
	Peripheral vascular resistance	Progressive decrease to term.
Pulmonary	Respiratory rate	Unchanged.
	Tidal volume	Increases by 30–40%.
	Expiratory reserve	Gradual decrease.
	Vital capacity	Unchanged.
	Respiratory minute volume	Increases by 40%.
Blood	Volume	Increases by 50% in second trimester.
	Hematocrit	Decreases slightly.
	Fibrinogen	Increases.
	Electrolytes	Unchanged.
Gastrointestinal	Sphincter tone	Decreases.
	Gastric emptying time	Increases.

FIGURE 2.11-3. **Cardiopulmonary, hematologic, and GI changes in normal pregnancy.**

(Reproduced, with permission, from Gardner DG, Shoback D. *Greenspan's Basic & Clinical Endocrinology*, 8th ed. New York: McGraw-Hill, 2007: Fig. 17-2B.)

TABLE 2.11-1. Standard Prenatal Care

CATEGORY	RECOMMENDATIONS
Weight gain	Guidelines for weight gain in pregnancy: ■ **Recommended gain:** An additional 100–300 kcal/day; 500 kcal/day during breastfeeding. ■ **Excessive gain:** > 1.5 kg/mo. ■ **Inadequate gain:** < 1 kg/mo. Guidelines according to prepregnancy body mass index (BMI): ■ **Underweight** (BMI < 19.8): 12–18 kg gain. ■ **Acceptable** (BMI 19.8–26.0): 11–16 kg gain. ■ **Overweight** (BMI 26.1–29.0): 7–11 kg gain. ■ **Severely overweight** (BMI > 29.0): 7 kg gain.
Nutrition	Guidelines for nutritional supplementation: ■ **Folic acid** supplements (↓ neural tube defects for **all** reproductive-age women): 0.4 mg/day, or 4 mg/day for women with a history of neural tube defects in prior pregnancies. ■ **Iron:** Starting at the first visit, 30 mg/day of elemental iron (or 150 mg of iron sulfate). ■ **Calcium:** 1300 mg/day for women < 19 years of age; 1000 mg/day for those > 19 years of age. Additional guidelines for complete vegetarians: ■ **Vitamin D:** 10 μg or 400 IU/day. ■ **Vitamin B$_{12}$:** 2 μg/day.
Exercise	Thirty minutes of moderate exercise daily is recommended.

■ **Trisomy 18:** All four are ↓.
■ **Trisomy 21:** ↓ AFP and estriol; ↑ β-hCG and inhibin A.

2 up, 2 down: trisomy 21 =
↓ AFP, ↓ estriol, ↑ β-hCG,
↑ inhibin A.

PAPP-A

■ Recommended at weeks 9–14.
■ Pregnancy-associated plasma protein A (PAPP-A) + ultrasound-determined nuchal transparency (a measure of fluid in the fetal neck) + free β-hCG can detect ~85% of cases of Down syndrome and ~97% of cases of trisomy 18.
■ **Advantages:** Screen of **low-risk** pregnant women (< 35 years of age); available earlier and less invasive than chorionic villus sampling (see below).

Chorionic Villus Sampling (CVS)

■ Recommended at weeks 10–12.
■ Involves transcervical or transabdominal aspiration of placental (chorionic villi) tissue.
  ■ **Advantages:** Has a diagnostic accuracy comparable to that of amniocentesis; available at 10–12 weeks' gestation.
  ■ **Disadvantages:** Carries a risk of fetal loss (1–2%); cannot detect open neural tube defects.
■ Limb defects have been associated with CVS performed at ≤ 9 weeks.

OBSTETRICS

HIGH-YIELD FACTS

TABLE 2.11-2. **Prenatal Diagnostic Testing Schedule**

WEEKS	PRENATAL DIAGNOSTIC TESTING
Prenatal visits	**Weeks 0–28:** Every four weeks. **Weeks 29–35:** Every two weeks. **Weeks 36–birth:** Every week.
Initial visit	**Heme:** CBC, Rh factor, type and screen. **Infectious disease:** UA and culture, rubella antibody titer, HBsAg, RPR/VDRL, cervical gonorrhea and chlamydia, PPD, HIV, Pap smear (to check for dysplasia). **If indicated:** HbA$_{1c}$, sickle cell screening. **Discuss genetic screening:** Tay-Sachs, CF.
9–14 weeks	Offer PAPP-A + nuchal transparency + free β-hCG +/− CVS.
15–20 weeks	Offer MSAFP or quad screen (AFP, estriol, β-hCG, and inhibin A) +/− amniocentesis.
18–20 weeks	Ultrasound for full anatomic screen.
24–28 weeks	One-hour glucose challenge test for gestational diabetes screen.
28–30 weeks	RhoGAM for Rh-⊖ women (after antibody screen).
32–36 weeks	Group B strep culture (GBS); repeat CBC.
34–40 weeks	Cervical chlamydia and gonorrhea cultures, HIV, RPR in high-risk patients.

Amniocentesis

- Recommended at 15–20 weeks.
- Consists of transabdominal aspiration of amniotic fluid using an ultrasound-guided needle and evaluation of fetal cells for genetic studies.
    - **Advantages:** Detects ~80% of open neural tube defects, ~85% of cases of Down syndrome, and ~60% of cases of trisomy 18.
    - **Disadvantages:** Risks include premature rupture of membranes (PROM), chorioamnionitis, and fetal-maternal hemorrhage, which can result in fetal loss (0.5%).
- Indicated for the following:
    - In women who will be > **35 years of age at the time of delivery.**
    - In conjunction with an abnormal quad screen.
    - In Rh-sensitized pregnancy to obtain fetal blood type or to detect fetal hemolysis.
    - To evaluate fetal lung maturity via a lecithin-to-sphingomyelin ratio ≥ 2.5 or to detect the presence of phosphatidylglycerol (done during the third trimester).

▶ TERATOLOGY

Major defects are apparent in about 3% of births and in roughly 4.5% of children by five years of age. Table 2.11-3 lists FDA risk classifications of pharmaceutical products for use during pregnancy. Table 2.11-4 outlines common teratogenic agents.

TABLE 2.11-3. FDA Risk Classification of Drugs for Use During Pregnancy

CATEGORY	DESCRIPTION	EXAMPLES
Category A	Adequate and well-controlled studies in women fail to demonstrate a risk to the fetus in the first trimester (and there is no risk in later trimesters). The possibility of fetal harm seems remote.	Vitamin B$_6$, vitamin E, folic acid (within the recommended daily allowances).
Category B	Either animal reproduction studies have not demonstrated risk to the fetus but no adequate and well-controlled studies in pregnant women have been reported, or animal reproduction studies have shown an adverse effect that was not confirmed in controlled studies in women in the first trimester (and there is no evidence of risk in later trimesters).	Ampicillin, acetaminophen, bupropion.
Category C	Either studies in animals have revealed adverse effects on the fetus but no controlled studies in women have been reported, or studies in women and animals are not available. Drugs should be given only if the potential benefit justifies the potential risk to the fetus.	Diphenhydramine, rifampin, zidovudine (AZT).
Category D	Positive evidence of human fetal risk exists, but the benefits from use in pregnant women may be acceptable despite the risk.	Alcohol, phenytoin, tetracycline.
Category X	Studies in animals or humans have demonstrated fetal abnormalities, or evidence exists of fetal risk based on human experience, or both, and the risk in pregnant women clearly outweighs any possible benefit.	Isotretinoin, thalidomide, warfarin.

▶ **MATERNAL-FETAL INFECTIONS**

Pregnant women should not change the cat's litterbox.

First-trimester toxoplasmosis infection is less common but more severe. Third-trimester infection is more common but less severe.

May occur at any time during pregnancy, labor, and delivery. Common sequelae include **premature delivery, CNS abnormalities**, anemia, **jaundice**, hepatosplenomegaly, and growth retardation. The most common pathogens can be remembered through use of the mnemonic **TORCHeS** (see also Table 2.11-5):

- **T**oxoplasmosis: Transplacental transmission, with 1° infection occurring via consumption of **raw meat** or contact with **cat feces**. Specific findings include hydrocephalus, **intracranial calcifications**, chorioretinitis, and **ring-enhancing lesions** on head CT.
- **O**ther: Parvovirus, varicella, *Listeria*, TB, malaria, fungi.
- **R**ubella: Transplacental transmission in the first trimester. Specific findings include a purpuric **"blueberry muffin" rash**, cataracts, mental retardation, hearing loss, and **patent ductus arteriosus (PDA)**.
- **C**MV: The **most common congenital infection**; primarily transmitted transplacentally. Specific findings include a petechial rash (similar to "blueberry muffin" rash) and **periventricular calcifications**.
- **H**erpes: Intrapartum transmission if the mother has **active lesions**. Can cause skin, eye, and mouth infections or life-threatening CNS/systemic infection.
- **H**IV: Transmission can occur in utero, at the time of delivery, or via breast milk. Occurs in 13–39% of births to infected mothers. The combination of AZT treatment (prenatally, intrapartum, and neonatally for the first six weeks of life) and cesarean delivery can lower transmission to 2%. Newborns with congenitally acquired HIV are often **asymptomatic**. Failure to

TABLE 2.11-4. **Common Teratogenic Agents and Their Associated Defects**

DRUGS AND CHEMICALS	DEFECTS
ACEIs	Fetal renal tubular dysplasia and neonatal renal failure, oligohydramnios, intrauterine growth restriction (IUGR), lack of cranial ossification.
Alcohol	Fetal alcohol syndrome (growth restriction before and after birth, mental retardation, midfacial hypoplasia, renal and cardiac defects). Consumption of > 6 drinks per day is associated with a 40% risk of fetal alcohol syndrome.
Androgens	Virilization of females; advanced genital development in males.
Carbamazepine	Neural tube defects, fingernail hypoplasia, microcephaly, developmental delay, IUGR.
Cocaine	Bowel atresias; congenital malformations of the heart, limbs, face, and GU tract; microcephaly; IUGR; cerebral infarctions.
Diethylstilbestrol (DES)	Clear cell adenocarcinoma of the vagina or cervix, vaginal adenosis, abnormalities of the cervix and uterus or testes, possible infertility.
Lead	↑ spontaneous abortion (SAB) rate; stillbirths.
Lithium	Congenital heart disease (Ebstein's anomaly).
Methotrexate	↑ SAB rate.
Organic mercury	Cerebral atrophy, microcephaly, mental retardation, spasticity, seizures, blindness.
Phenytoin	IUGR, mental retardation, microcephaly, dysmorphic craniofacial features, cardiac defects, fingernail hypoplasia.
Radiation	Microcephaly, mental retardation. Medical diagnostic radiation delivering < 0.05 Gy to the fetus has no teratogenic risk.
Streptomycin and kanamycin	Hearing loss; CN VIII damage.
Tetracycline	Permanent yellow-brown discoloration of deciduous teeth; hypoplasia of tooth enamel.
Thalidomide	Bilateral limb deficiencies, anotia and microtia, cardiac and GI anomalies.
Trimethadione and paramethadione	Cleft lip or cleft palate, cardiac defects, microcephaly, mental retardation.
Valproic acid	Neural tube defects (spina bifida); minor craniofacial defects.
Vitamin A and derivatives	↑ SAB rate, microtia, thymic agenesis, cardiovascular defects, craniofacial dysmorphism, microphthalmia, cleft lip or cleft palate, mental retardation.
Warfarin (wages **war** on the fetus)	Nasal hypoplasia and stippled bone epiphyses, developmental delay, IUGR, ophthalmologic abnormalities.

TABLE 2.11-5. Diagnosis and Treatment of Common Congenital Infections

DISEASE	DIAGNOSIS	TREATMENT	PREVENTION
Toxoplasmosis	Serologic testing	Pyrimethamine + sulfadiazine	Avoid exposure to cat feces during pregnancy. Spiramycin prophylaxis for the third trimester.
Rubella	Serologic testing		Immunize before pregnancy; vaccinate the mother after delivery if serologic titers remain $\ominus$.
CMV	Urine culture, PCR of amniotic fluid	Postpartum ganciclovir	
HSV	Serologic testing	Acyclovir	Perform a C-section if lesions are present at delivery.
HIV	ELISA, Western blot		AZT or nevirapine in pregnant women with HIV; perform elective C-section if viral load is > 1000; treat infants with prophylactic AZT; avoid breastfeeding.
Syphilis	Dark-field microscopy, VDRL/RPR, FTA-ABS	Penicillin	Penicillin in pregnant women who test $\oplus$.

thrive, bacterial infections with common organisms, and an ↑ incidence of upper and lower respiratory diseases may appear early or may be delayed for months to years. HIV-$\oplus$ mothers should be counseled not to breast-feed their infants.

- Syphilis: Primarily intrapartum transmission. Specific findings include a **maculopapular skin rash**, lymphadenopathy, hepatomegaly, **"snuffles"** (mucopurulent rhinitis), and osteitis. In childhood, late congenital syphilis is characterized by saber shins, saddle nose, CNS involvement, and Hutchinson's triad: **peg-shaped upper central incisors, deafness**, and **interstitial keratitis** (photophobia, lacrimation).

▶ SPONTANEOUS ABORTION (SAB)

Defined as loss of products of conception (POC) prior to the 20th week of pregnancy. Approximately 60% of chemically evident pregnancies and 15–20% of clinically diagnosed pregnancies terminate in a SAB. More than 80% will occur in the first trimester. Risk factors are as follows:

- **Chromosomal abnormalities:** A factor in approximately 50% of SABs in the first trimester, 20–30% in second-trimester losses, and 5–10% in third-trimester losses.
- **Maternal factors:**
  - Maternal trauma, ↑ maternal age, infection, dietary deficiencies.
  - **Inherited thrombophilias:** Factor V Leiden, prothrombin, antithrombin, proteins C and S, methylene tetrahydrofolate reductase (hyperhomocysteinemia).
  - **Immunologic issues:** Antiphospholipid antibodies, alloimmune factors.
  - **Anatomic issues:** Uterine abnormalities, incompetent cervix, cervical conization or loop electrosurgical excision procedure (LEEP), cervical injury, DES exposure, anatomical abnormalities of the cervix.

- **Endocrinologic issues:** Diabetes mellitus (DM), hypothyroidism, progesterone deficiency.
- **Environmental factors:** Tobacco (with > 14 cigarettes/day, the risk is two-fold), alcohol, caffeine (> 500 mg caffeine/day), toxins, drugs, radiation.
- **Fetal factors:** Anatomic malformation.

HISTORY/PE

See Table 2.11-6 for types of SAB.

DIAGNOSIS

- ↓ levels of hCG.
- **Ultrasound:**
  - Can identify the gestational sac 5–6 weeks from the LMP, a fetal pole at six weeks, and fetal cardiac activity at 6–7 weeks.
  - With accurate dating, a small, irregular intrauterine sac without a fetal pole on transvaginal ultrasound is diagnostic of an abnormal pregnancy.
- **Maternal Rh type should be determined and RhoGAM given if the type is Rh ⊖.**

▶ ELECTIVE TERMINATION OF PREGNANCY

It has been estimated that 50% of all pregnancies in the United States are unintended. Some 25% of **all** pregnancies end in elective abortion. Options for elective abortion depend on GA and patient preferences (see Table 2.11-7).

▶ NORMAL LABOR AND DELIVERY

Obstetric Examination

- Leopold's maneuvers are used to determine fetal lie (longitudinal or transverse) and, if possible, fetal presentation (breech or cephalic).
- **Cervical examination:**
  - Evaluate dilation, effacement, station, cervical position, and cervical consistency. Use the Bishop score (see Table 2.11-8) to evaluate the favorability of delivery and the probability of succeeding with an induction. Scoring is interpreted as follows:
    - **0–4:** Indicates a 45–50% chance of failure. Give prostaglandins for induction.
    - **5–9:** Points to a 10% chance of failure. Give pitocin for induction.
    - **10–13:** Associated with a very high probability of success. There is no need for intervention for induction.
  - Confirm or determine fetal presentation.
  - Determine fetal position through palpation of the fetal sutures and fontanelles.
  - Conduct a **sterile speculum exam if rupture of membranes (ROM) is suspected.**
- Table 2.11-9 and Figure 2.11-4 depict the normal stages of labor.

Fetal Heart Rate (FHR) Monitoring

FHR monitoring is the most common obstetric procedure and is used in 85% of live births in the United States. It may be performed with an electrode at-

TABLE 2.11-6. Types of Spontaneous Abortion

TYPE	SYMPTOMS/SIGNS	DIAGNOSIS	TREATMENT
Complete	POC is expelled. Pain ceases, but spotting may persist.	**Closed os.** Ultrasound shows an empty uterus. POC should be sent to pathology to confirm fetal tissue.	None.
Incomplete	Some POC is expelled. Bleeding/mild cramping. Visible tissue on exam.	**Open os.** Ultrasound shows retained fetal tissue.	Manual uterine aspiration (MUA) or D&C.
Threatened	No POC is expelled. Uterine bleeding +/− abdominal pain.	**Closed os** + intact membranes + fetal cardiac motion on ultrasound.	Pelvic rest for 24–48 hours and follow-up ultrasound to assess the viability of conceptus.
Inevitable	No POC is expelled. Uterine bleeding and cramps.	**Open os** +/− ROM.	MUA, D&C, misoprostol, or expectant management.
Missed	No POC is expelled. No fetal cardiac motion. No uterine bleeding. Brownish vaginal discharge.	**Closed os.** No fetal cardiac activity; retained fetal tissue on ultrasound.	MUA, D&C, or misoprostol.
Septic	Endometritis leading to septicemia. **Maternal mortality is 10–15%.**	Hypotension, hypothermia, ↑ WBC count.	MUA, D&C, and IV antibiotics.
Intrauterine fetal demise	Absence of fetal cardiac activity.	Uterus small for GA; no fetal heart tones or movement on ultrasound.	Induce labor; evacuate the uterus (D&E) to prevent DIC at GA > 16 weeks.
Recurrent[a]	If early in pregnancy, often due to chromosomal abnormalities. If later in pregnancy, often due to hypercoagulable states (e.g., SLE, factor V Leiden, protein S deficiency). Incompetent cervix should be suspected with a history of painless dilation of the cervix and delivery of a normal fetus between 18 and 32 weeks.	Karyotyping of both parents. Hypercoagulability workup of mother. **Evaluate for uterine abnormalities.**	Surgical cerclage procedures to suture the cervix closed until labor or ROM occurs with subsequent removal prior to delivery. Restriction of activities.

[a] Defined as two or more consecutive SABs or a total of three SABs in one year.

tached to the fetal scalp (a method that yields more precise results), or external monitoring can be conducted using Doppler ultrasound (a less invasive option). However, continuous electronic FHR monitoring has not been shown to be more effective than appropriate intermittent monitoring.

TABLE 2.11-7. Elective Termination of Pregnancy

	PROCEDURE	TIMING
First trimester (90% therapeutic abortions [TABs])	**Medical management:** ▪ Oral mifepristone (low dose) + oral/vaginal misoprostol ▪ IM/oral methotrexate + oral/vaginal misoprostol ▪ Vaginal or sublingual or buccal misoprostol (high dose), repeated up to three times **Surgical management:** ▪ Manual aspiration ▪ D&C with vacuum aspiration	**Up to:** 49 days' GA 49 days' GA 56 days' GA Up to 13 weeks' GA
Second trimester (10% TABs)	**Obstetric management:** Induction of labor (typically with prostaglandins, amniotomy, and oxytocin) **Surgical management:** D&E	13–24 weeks' GA (depending on state laws) Same as above

RECOMMENDATIONS FOR FHR MONITORING

- **Patients without complications:** Review FHR tracings every 30 minutes in the first stage of labor and every 15 minutes in the second stage of labor.
- **Patients with complications:** Review FHR tracings every 15 minutes in the first stage of labor and every 5 minutes in the second stage of labor.

COMPONENTS OF FHR EVALUATION

- **Rate** (normal = 110–160 bpm):
  - **FHR < 110 bpm:** Bradycardia. Can be caused by congenital heart malformations or severe hypoxia (2° to uterine hyperstimulation, cord prolapse, or rapid fetal descent).
  - **FHR > 160 bpm:** Tachycardia. Can be caused by hypoxia, maternal fever, or fetal anemia.
- **Variability** (normal beat-to-beat variability = 6–25 bpm): See Figures 2.11-5 and 2.11-6.
  - **Undetectable variability:** Indicates severe fetal distress.

TABLE 2.11-8. Bishop Score

	SCORE			
FACTOR	0	1	2	3
Cervical dilation	Closed	1–2	3–4	5+
Cervical effacement	0–30	40–50	60–70	80+
Fetal station	−3	−2	−1	+1 to +2
Cervical consistency	Firm	Medium	Soft	—
Cervical position	Posterior	Mid	Anterior	—

TABLE 2.11-9. Stages of Labor

		DURATION		
STAGE	**STARTS/ENDS**	**PRIMIPAROUS**	**MULTIPAROUS**	**COMMENTS**
First				
Latent	Onset of labor to 3–4 cm dilation	6–11 hrs	4–8 hrs	Prolongation seen with excessive sedation and hypertonic uterine contractions.
Active	4 cm to complete cervical dilation (10 cm)	4–6 hrs (1.2 cm/hr)	2–3 hrs (1.5 cm/hr)	Prolongation seen with **cephalopelvic disproportion.**
Second	Complete cervical dilation to delivery of infant	0.5–3.0 hrs	5–30 min	Baby goes through all cardinal movements of delivery.
Third	Delivery of infant to delivery of placenta	0–0.5 hr	0–0.5 hr	Uterus contracts and placenta separates to establish hemostasis.

- **Minimal variability:** < 6 bpm. Indicates **fetal distress or the effects of opioids or magnesium.**
- **Normal variability:** 6–25 bpm.
- **Marked variability:** > 25 bpm. **May indicate fetal distress; may occur before a ↓ in variability.**
- **Sinusoidal variability:** Points to serious fetal anemia; may also occur during maternal meperidine use.

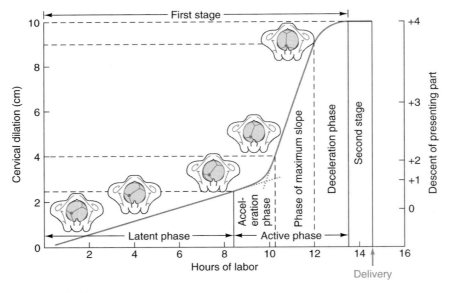

FIGURE 2.11-4. Stages of labor.

Cervical dilation, level of descent, and orientation of occipitoanterior presentation during various stages of labor. (Reproduced, with permission, from DeCherney AH. *Current Obstetric & Gynecologic Diagnosis & Treatment*, 8th ed. Stamford, CT: Appleton & Lange, 1994: 211.)

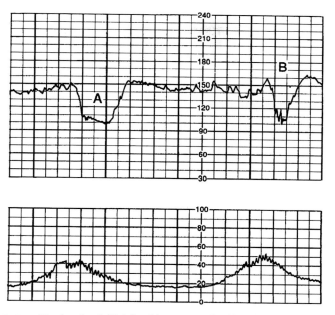

FIGURE 2.11-5. **Varying (variable) fetal heart rate decelerations.**

Deceleration B exhibits "shoulders" of acceleration compared with deceleration A. (Reproduced, with permission, from Cunningham FG et al. *Williams Obstetrics*, 22nd ed. New York: McGraw-Hill, 2005: Fig. 18-21.)

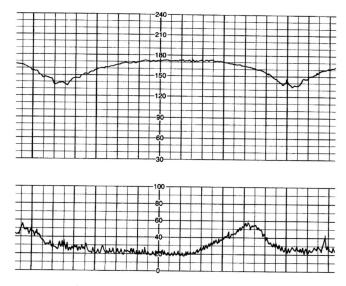

FIGURE 2.11-6. **Late fetal heart rate decelerations.**

Late decelerations due to uteroplacental insufficiency resulting from placental abruption. Immediate cesarean delivery was performed. Umbilical artery pH was 7.05 and PO_2 was 11 mmHg. (Reproduced, with permission, from Cunningham FG et al. *Williams Obstetrics*, 22nd ed. New York: McGraw-Hill, 2005: Fig. 18-17.)

- **Accelerations:** Onset of an ↑ in FHR to a peak in < 30 seconds. **Reassuring because they indicate fetal ability to appropriately respond to the environment.**
- **Decelerations:** See Table 2.11-10.

Antepartum Fetal Surveillance

In general, antepartum fetal surveillance is used in pregnancies in which the risk of antepartum fetal demise is ↑. Testing is initiated in most at-risk patients

TABLE 2.11-10. **Types of Fetal Deceleration**

TYPE	DESCRIPTION	ETIOLOGY	SCHEMATIC
Early	A visually apparent, gradual (onset to nadir in > 30 sec) ↓ in FHR with a return to baseline that mirrors the uterine contraction.	Head compression from the uterine contraction (normal).	
Late	A visually apparent, gradual (onset to nadir in > 30 sec) ↓ in FHR with return to baseline whose onset, nadir, and recovery occur after the beginning, peak, and end of uterine contraction, respectively.	Uteroplacental insufficiency and fetal hypoxemia.	
Variable	An abrupt (onset to nadir in < 30 sec), visually apparent ↓ in FHR below baseline lasting ≥ 15 sec but < 2 min.	Umbilical cord compression.	

Illustrations reproduced, with permission, from Cunningham FG et al. *Williams Obstetrics,* 22nd ed. New York: McGraw-Hill, 2005: Figs.18-14, 18-16, and 18-18.

at 32–34 weeks (or 26–28 weeks if there are multiple worrisome risk factors present). The following assessments are made:

- **Fetal movement assessment:** Assessed by the mother as the number of fetal movements over one hour. The average time to obtain 10 movements is 20 minutes. Maternal reports of ↓ fetal movements should be evaluated by means of the tests described below.
- **Nonstress test (NST):** Performed with the mother resting in the lateral tilt position (to prevent supine hypotension). FHR is monitored externally by Doppler along with a tocodynamometer to detect uterine contractions. Acoustic stimulation may be used.
  - **"Reactive" (normal response):** Two accelerations of ≥ **15 bpm above baseline lasting for at least 15 seconds** over a 20-minute period (see Figure 2.11-7).
  - **"Nonreactive":** Fewer than two accelerations over a 20-minute period. Perform further tests (e.g., a biophysical profile). Lack of FHR accelerations may occur with any of the following: GA < 32 weeks, fetal sleeping, fetal CNS anomalies, and maternal sedative or narcotic administration.
- **Contraction stress test (CST):** Performed in the lateral recumbent position. FHR is monitored during spontaneous or induced (via nipple stimulation or oxytocin) contractions. Reactivity is determined from fetal heart monitoring, as with the NST. The procedure is contraindicated in women with preterm membrane rupture or known placenta previa; women with a history of uterine surgery; and women who are at high risk for preterm labor.

HIGH-YIELD FACTS

OBSTETRICS

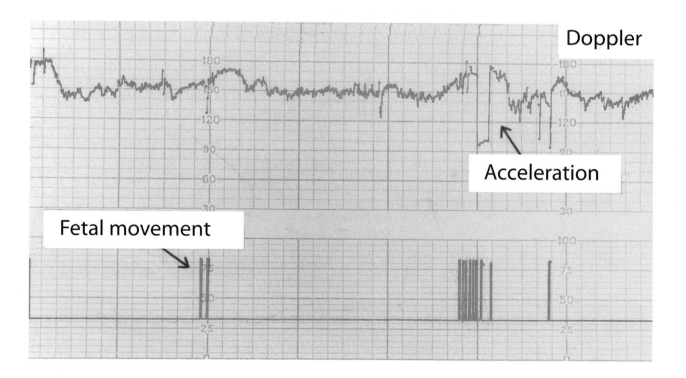

FIGURE 2.11-7. **Reactive nonstress test.**

(Reproduced, with permission, from Cunningham FG et al. *Williams Obstetrics*, 22nd ed. New York: McGraw-Hill, 2005: Fig. 15-7.)

- ■ **"Positive" CST:** Defined by late decelerations following 50% or more of contractions in a 10-minute window; raises concerns about fetal compromise. Delivery is usually warranted.
- ■ **"Negative" CST:** Defined as no late or significant variable decelerations within 10 minutes and at least three contractions. Highly predictive of fetal well-being in conjunction with a normal NST.
- ■ **"Equivocal" CST:** Defined by intermittent late decelerations or significant variable decelerations.
- ■ **Biophysical profile (BPP):** Uses real-time ultrasound to assign a score of 2 (normal) or 0 (abnormal) to five parameters: fetal tone, breathing, movement, amniotic fluid volume, and NST. Scoring is as follows:
  - ■ **8–10:** Reassuring for fetal well-being.
  - ■ **6:** Considered equivocal. Term pregnancies are usually delivered with this profile.
  - ■ **0–4:** Extremely worrisome for fetal asphyxia; strong consideration should be given to immediate delivery if no other explanation is found.
- ■ **Modified biophysical profile (mBPP):** Combines the NST with the amniotic fluid index (AFI, or the sum of the measurements of the deepest cord-free amniotic fluid measured in each of the abdominal quadrants). The test is considered normal with a reactive NST and an AFI > 5 cm.
- ■ **Umbilical artery Doppler velocimetry:** With IUGR, there is reduction and even reversal of umbilical artery diastolic flow. The test is of benefit only when IUGR is suspected.
- ■ **Oligohydramnios (AFI < 5 cm) always warrants further workup.**

> **When performing a BPP, remember to–**
>
> **Test the Baby, MAN!**
>
> Fetal **T**one
> Fetal **B**reathing
> Fetal **M**ovement
> **A**mniotic fluid volume
> **N**onstress test

Obstetric Analgesia and Anesthesia

Uterine contractions and cervical dilation result in visceral pain (T10–L1). Descent of the fetal head and pressure on the vagina and perineum result in somatic pain (pudendal nerve, S2–S4). In the absence of a medical contraindication, maternal request is a sufficient medical indication for pain relief during labor. Absolute contraindications to regional anesthesia (epidural, spinal, or combination) include the following (see also Table 2.11-11):

- ■ Refractory maternal hypotension
- ■ Maternal coagulopathy
- ■ Maternal use of a once-daily dose of low-molecular-weight heparin (LMWH) within 12 hours
- ■ Untreated maternal bacteremia
- ■ Skin infection over the site of needle placement
- ■ ↑ ICP caused by a mass lesion

▶ MEDICAL COMPLICATIONS OF PREGNANCY

Hyperemesis Gravidarum

Persistent vomiting not related to other causes, **acute starvation** (usually large ketonuria), and weight loss (usually at least a 5% ↓ from prepregnancy weight). Occurs in 0.5–2.0% of pregnancies. More common in first pregnancies, multiple gestations, and molar pregnancies. ↑ β-hCG and ↑ estradiol have been implicated in its pathophysiology.

TABLE 2.11-11. Available Methods of Anesthesia and Analgesia

METHOD	ADVANTAGES	DISADVANTAGES
Nonpharmacologic (social support, massages, breathing, aromatherapy, ambulation and repositioning)	No known ⊖ side effects. Works by increasing coping with pain rather than eliminating pain.	Limited pain relief.
Opioids	Provide an adequate level of pain relief for some women without the risks associated with regional anesthesia.	The sedative effect of opioids ↓ FHR variability and ↑ the possible need for neonatal naloxone administration and five-minute Apgar scores < 7.
Local block (lidocaine)	Excellent anesthesia before episiotomy and during repair of lacerations; can be used to perform a pudendal block.	Rarely, may cause seizures, hypotension, and cardiac arrhythmias.
Epidural	The most effective form of pain relief; can also be used for cesarean delivery or postpartum tubal ligation.	Can result in pruritus, fever, hypotension, and transient FHR deceleration.
Spinal	Rapid-onset analgesia that provides excellent pain relief for procedures of limited duration (30–250 minutes).	**Limited duration;** puts patients at risk for hypotension, postdural puncture headache, and transient neurologic symptoms.
Combined spinal epidural	Offers rapid onset of spinal analgesia combined with the ability to prolong the duration of analgesia with continuous epidural infusion.	Carries the risks of both procedures; may ↑ the risk of bradycardia and emergent cesarean delivery over epidural analgesia alone.
General	Used in emergent cesarean delivery and indicated in some cases of FHR abnormality; can be useful in cases where regional anesthesia is absolutely contraindicated or fails.	Requires airway control; carries a significant risk of **maternal aspiration** and **neonatal depression** (inhaled anesthetic agents readily cross the placenta); associated with higher maternal morbidity rates than epidural anesthesia.

HISTORY/PE

Distinguish from "morning sickness," acid reflux, gastroenteritis, hyperthyroidism, and neurologic conditions.

DIAGNOSIS

- **Rule out molar pregnancy:** Check β-hCG level and ultrasound.
- **Determine severity:** Evaluate for ketonemia, ketonuria, hyponatremia, and hypokalemic, hypochloremic metabolic alkalosis. Measure liver enzymes, serum bilirubin, and serum amylase/lipase.

*The first step in the diagnosis of hyperemesis gravidarum is to **rule out molar pregnancy** with ultrasound +/– β-hCG.*

TREATMENT

- **First step:** Administer vitamin B_6.
- **Second step:** Doxylamine (an antihistamine) PO.
- **Third step:** Promethazine or dimenhydrinate PO/PR.
- **If severe:** Metoclopramide, ondansetron, prochlorperazine, or promethazine IM/PO.
- **If dehydrated:** IV fluids, IV nutritional supplementation, and dimenhydrinate IV.

The first step in the management of hyperemesis gravidarum is vitamin B_6 and doxylamine if not severe or antiemetics and IV fluids if severe.

Diabetes in Pregnancy

Diabetes in pregnancy is divided into two categories: gestational diabetes, in which onset occurs during pregnancy, and pregestational diabetes. The White classification (see Table 2.11-12) is commonly used to classify women according to the nature of their diabetes and the associated risk.

GESTATIONAL DIABETES MELLITUS

Carbohydrate intolerance of variable severity that is first diagnosed during pregnancy. Occurs in **3–5% of all pregnancies, usually in late pregnancy.**

HISTORY/PE

Typically asymptomatic. Edema, polyhydramnios, or a **large-for-GA infant (> 90th percentile) may be warning signs.**

DIAGNOSIS

- **First step: One-hour 50-g glucose challenge test;** venous plasma glucose is measured one hour later (at 24–28 weeks). Values ≥ 140 mg/dL are considered abnormal.
- **Next step:** Confirm with an oral three-hour (100-g) glucose tolerance test showing any two of the following: fasting > 95 mg/dL; one hour > 180 mg/dL; two hours > 155 mg/dL; three hours > 140 mg/dL.

Gestational diabetes is typically asymptomatic, so the first step in diagnosis is a one-hour glucose challenge at 24–28 weeks. If ≥ 140 mg/dL, perform a three-hour glucose challenge test.

TREATMENT

- **Mother:**
    - **First step:** Start with the **ADA diet,** regular exercise, and strict glucose monitoring (four times a day). Tight maternal glucose control (fasting glucose < 100; one- to two-hour postprandial glucose < 150) improves outcomes.
    - **Next step: Add insulin** if dietary control is insufficient.
    - Give intrapartum insulin and dextrose to maintain tight control during delivery.
- **Fetus:**
    - Obtain periodic ultrasound and NSTs to assess fetal growth and well-being.
    - It may be necessary to induce labor at 39–40 weeks.

Keys to the management of gestational diabetes: (1) the ADA diet; (2) insulin if needed; (3) ultrasound for fetal growth; and (4) NST beginning at 30–32 weeks.

COMPLICATIONS

More than 50% of patients go on to **develop glucose intolerance and/or type 2 DM** later in life.

TABLE 2.11-12. White Classification of Diabetes in Pregnancy

CLASS	CRITERION
A1	Gestational diabetes; insulin not required.
A2	Gestational diabetes; insulin required.
B	Age of onset 20 years or older or duration < 10 years.
C	Age of onset 10–19 years or duration 10–19 years.
D	Age of onset < 10 years or duration > 20 years.
F	Nephropathy.
H	Cardiomyopathy.
R	Proliferating retinopathy.
RF	Retinopathy and nephropathy.
T	Renal transplant.

PREGESTATIONAL DIABETES AND PREGNANCY

Observed in 1% of all pregnancies. Insulin requirements may ↑ as much as threefold. Poorly controlled DM is associated with an ↑ **risk of congenital malformations,** fetal loss, and maternal/fetal morbidity during labor and delivery.

TREATMENT

- **Mother:**
  - Renal, ophthalmologic, and cardiac evaluation to assess for end-organ damage.
  - Strict glucose control (with diet, exercise, insulin therapy, and frequent self-monitoring for type 1 and type 2 DM) to minimize fetal defects.
    - **Fasting morning:** ≤ 90 mg/dL.
    - **Two-hour postprandial:** < 120 mg/dL.
- **Fetus:**
  - **18–20 weeks:** Ultrasound to determine fetal age and growth; evaluate for cardiac anomalies and polyhydramnios; quad screen to screen for developmental anomalies.
  - **32–34 weeks:** Close fetal surveillance (e.g., NST, CST, BPP). Admit if maternal DM has been poorly controlled or fetal parameters are a concern. Serial ultrasounds for fetal growth.
- **Delivery and postpartum:**
  - Maintain normoglycemia (80–100 mg/dL) during labor with an IV insulin drip and hourly glucose measurements.
  - Consider early delivery in the setting of poor maternal glucose control, preeclampsia, macrosomia, or evidence of fetal lung maturity.
  - Cesarean delivery should be considered for an estimated fetal weight (EFW) > 4500 g.

Greater than eight, investigate! If HbA₁c is > 8%, look for congenital abnormalities.

If UA before 20 weeks reveals glycosuria, think pregestational diabetes.

Hyperglycemia in the first trimester suggests preexisting diabetes and should be managed as pregestational diabetes.

- Encourage breastfeeding with an appropriate ↑ in caloric intake.
- Continue glucose monitoring postpartum. Insulin needs rapidly ↓ after delivery.

COMPLICATIONS

See Table 2.11-13.

Gestational and Chronic Hypertension

- Distinguished as follows:
  - **Gestational hypertension** (formerly known as pregnancy-induced hypertension): Idiopathic hypertension **without** significant proteinuria (< 300 mg/L) that develops at > 20 weeks' gestation. As many as 25% of patients may go on to develop preeclampsia.
  - **Chronic hypertension:** Present before conception and at < 20 weeks' gestation, or may persist for > 12 weeks postpartum. Up to one-third of patients may develop superimposed preeclampsia.
- **Tx:** Monitor BP closely and treat with appropriate antihypertensives (e.g., methyldopa, labetalol, nifedipine). **Do not give ACEIs or diuretics,** as ACEIs are known to lead to uterine ischemia, and diuretics can aggravate low plasma volume to the point of uterine ischemia.
- **Cx:** Complications are similar to those of preeclampsia (see below).

Preeclampsia and Eclampsia

Distinguished as follows:

- **Preeclampsia: New-onset hypertension** (SBP ≥ 140 mmHg or DBP ≥ 90 mmHg) **and proteinuria** (> 300 mg of protein in a 24-hour period) occurring at **> 20 weeks' gestation.**
- **Eclampsia:** New-onset **grand mal seizures** in women with preeclampsia.
- **HELLP syndrome (hemolytic anemia, elevated liver enzymes, and low platelets):** A variant of preeclampsia with a poor prognosis.
  - The etiology is unknown, but clinical manifestations are explained by vasospasm leading to hemorrhage and organ necrosis.

> **HELLP** *syndrome:*
>
> **H**emolysis
> **E**levated **L**FTs
> **L**ow **P**latelets

TABLE 2.11-13. **Complications of Pregestational Diabetes Mellitus**

MATERNAL COMPLICATIONS	FETAL COMPLICATIONS
DKA (type 1) or HHNK (type 2)	Macrosomia or IUGR
Preeclampsia/eclampsia	Cardiac and renal defects
Cephalopelvic disproportion (from macrosomia) and need for C-section	Neural tube defects (e.g., sacral agenesis)
Preterm labor	Hypocalcemia
Infection	Polycythemia
Polyhydramnios	Hyperbilirubinemia
Postpartum hemorrhage	IUGR
Maternal mortality	Hypoglycemia from hyperinsulinemia
	Respiratory distress syndrome (RDS)
	Birth injury (e.g., shoulder dystocia)
	Perinatal mortality

- Risk factors include nulliparity, African-American ethnicity, extremes of age (< 20 or > 35), multiple gestation, molar pregnancy, renal disease (due to SLE or type 1 DM), a family history of preeclampsia, and chronic hypertension.

HISTORY/PE

See Table 2.11-14 for the signs and symptoms of preeclampsia and eclampsia.

TREATMENT

The only cure for preeclampsia/eclampsia is delivery of the fetus.

- Preeclampsia:
    - If the patient is close to term or preeclampsia worsens, **induce delivery with IV oxytocin, prostaglandin, or amniotomy.**
    - If far from term, treat with modified bed rest and expectant management.
- Severe preeclampsia:
    - **First step: Control BP** with labetalol and/or hydralazine (goal < 160/110 with a DBP of 90–100 to maintain fetal blood flow).
    - **Second step: Prevent seizures with continuous magnesium sulfate drip.** Watch for signs of magnesium toxicity (loss of DTRs, respiratory paralysis, coma). **Continue seizure prophylaxis for 24 hours postpartum.** Treat magnesium toxicity with IV calcium gluconate.
    - **Third step:** Deliver by induction or C-section when mother is stable.
- Eclampsia:
    - **First step:** ABCs with supplemental O_2.
    - **Second step:** Seizure control/prophylaxis with **magnesium.** If seizures recur, give IV diazepam. Monitor magnesium blood levels and magnesium toxicity; monitor fetal status. Control BP (labetalol and/or hydralazine). Limit fluids; Foley for strict I/Os.

The classic triad of preeclampsia—

It's not just HyPE

Hypertension
Proteinuria
Edema

Signs of severe preeclampsia are persistent headache or other cerebral or visual disturbances, persistent epigastric pain, and hyperreactive reflexes.

TABLE 2.11-14. Presentation of Preeclampsia and Eclampsia

	SIGNS AND SYMPTOMS
Mild preeclampsia	Usually asymptomatic. BP ≥ **140/90** on two occasions > 6 hours apart. Proteinuria (> 300 mg/24 hrs or 1–2 ⊕ urine dipsticks). Edema.
Severe preeclampsia	BP > **160/110** on two occasions > 6 hours apart. **Renal:** Proteinuria (> 5 g/24 hrs or 3–4 ⊕ urine dipsticks) or oliguria (< 500 mL/24 hrs). **Cerebral changes:** Headache, somnolence. **Visual changes:** Blurred vision, scotomata. **Hyperactive reflexes/clonus.** **RUQ pain.** **Hemolysis, elevated liver enzymes, thrombocytopenia (HELLP syndrome).**
Eclampsia	The most common signs preceding an eclamptic attack are **headache, visual changes, and RUQ/epigastric pain.** **Seizures** are severe if not controlled with anticonvulsant therapy.

- **Third step:** Initiate delivery if the patient is stable and convulsions are controlled. Postpartum management is the same as that for preeclampsia. Seizures may occur antepartum (25%), intrapartum (50%), or postpartum (25%); most occur within 48 hours after delivery.

COMPLICATIONS

- **Preeclampsia:** Prematurity, fetal distress, stillbirth, placental abruption, seizure, DIC, cerebral hemorrhage, serous retinal detachment, fetal/maternal death.
- **Eclampsia:** Cerebral hemorrhage, aspiration pneumonia, hypoxic encephalopathy, thromboembolic events, fetal/maternal death.

Antepartum Hemorrhage

- Defined as any bleeding that occurs after 20 weeks' gestation.
- Complicates 3–5% of pregnancies (prior to 20 weeks, bleeding is referred to as threatened abortion).
- The most common causes are **placental abruption** and **placenta previa** (see Table 2.11-15 and Figure 2.11-8). Other causes include other forms of abnormal placentation (e.g., placenta accreta), ruptured uterus, genital tract lesions, and trauma.

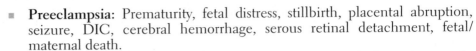

> ▶ **OBSTETRIC COMPLICATIONS OF PREGNANCY**

Ectopic Pregnancy

Most often tubal, but can be abdominal, ovarian, or cervical.

HISTORY/PE

- Presents with abdominal pain and vaginal spotting/bleeding, although some patients are asymptomatic.
- Associated with etiologies that cause scarring to the fallopian tubes, including a history of PID, pelvic surgery, DES use, or endometriosis.
- The differential includes surgical abdomen, abortion, ovarian torsion, PID, and ruptured ovarian cyst.

DIAGNOSIS

Approach a woman of reproductive age presenting with abdominal pain as a ruptured ectopic pregnancy until proven otherwise. Proceed as follows:

- **First step:** ⊕ pregnancy test and a transvaginal ultrasound showing an empty uterus.
- **Second step:** Confirm with a serial hCG without appropriate hCG doubling.

TREATMENT

- Medical treatment (methotrexate) is sufficient for small, unruptured tubal pregnancies.
- Surgical options for salpingectomy or salpingostomy with evacuation (laparoscopy vs. laparotomy).

COMPLICATIONS

Tubal rupture and hemoperitoneum (an obstetric emergency).

With third-trimester bleeding, think anatomically:

- *Vagina: bloody show, trauma*
- *Cervix: cervical cancer, cervical/vaginal lesion*
- *Placenta: placental abruption, placenta previa*
- *Fetus: fetal bleeding*

The classic triad of ectopic pregnancy PAVEs the way for diagnosis:

Pain (abdominal)
Amenorrhea
Vaginal bleeding
Ectopic pregnancy

TABLE 2.11-15. Placental Abruption vs. Placenta Previa

	PLACENTAL ABRUPTION	PLACENTA PREVIA
Pathophysiology	**Premature** (before delivery) **separation** of normally implanted placenta.	**Abnormal placental implantation:** ■ **Total:** Placenta covers the cervical os. ■ **Marginal:** Placenta extends to the margin of the os. ■ **Low-lying**: Placenta is in close proximity to the os.
Incidence	1 in 100.	1 in 200.
Risk factors	Hypertension, abdominal/pelvic trauma, tobacco or cocaine use, previous abruption, rapid decompression of an overdistended uterus, excessive stimulation.	Prior C-sections, grand multiparity, advanced maternal age, multiple gestation, prior placenta previa.
Symptoms	**Painful, dark** vaginal bleeding that does not spontaneously cease. Abdominal pain, uterine hypertonicity. Fetal distress.	**Painless, bright red** bleeding that often ceases in 1–2 hours with or without uterine contractions. Usually no fetal distress.
Diagnosis	**Primarily clinical.** Transabdominal/transvaginal ultrasound sensitivity is only 50%; look for retroplacental clot; most useful for ruling out previa.	**Transabdominal/transvaginal ultrasound sensitivity is > 95%;** look for an abnormally positioned placenta.
Management	Stabilize patients with mild abruption and a premature fetus; **manage expectantly** (hospitalize; start IV and fetal monitoring; type and cross blood; bed rest). **Moderate to severe abruption:** Immediate delivery (vaginal delivery with amniotomy if mother and fetus are stable and delivery is expected soon; C-section for maternal or fetal distress).	**No vaginal exam!** **Stabilize patients with a premature fetus;** manage expectantly. Give tocolytics. Serial ultrasound to assess fetal growth; resolution of partial previa. Give betamethasone to help with fetal lung maturity. **Deliver by C-section. Indications for delivery include labor, life-threatening bleeding, fetal distress, documented fetal lung maturity, and 36 weeks' GA.**
Complications	Hemorrhagic shock. Coagulopathy: **DIC** in 10%. Recurrence risk is 5–16% and rises to 25% after two previous abruptions. Fetal hypoxia.	↑ risk of placenta accreta. Vasa previa (fetal vessels crossing the internal os). Preterm delivery, PROM, IUGR, congenital anomalies. Recurrence risk is 4–8%.

HIGH-YIELD FACTS

OBSTETRICS

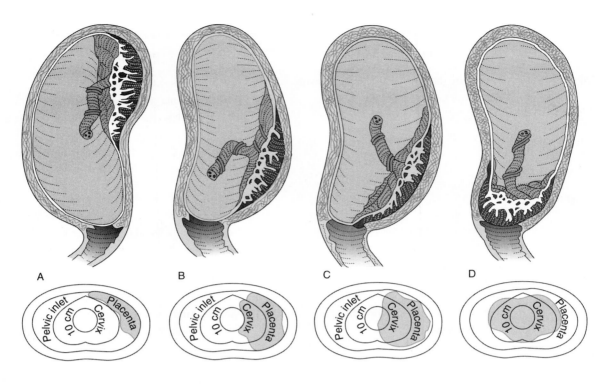

FIGURE 2.11-8. **Placental implantation.**

(A) Normal placenta. (B) Low implantation. (C) Partial placenta previa. (D) Complete placenta previa. (Adapted, with permission, from DeCherney AH. *Current Obstetric & Gynecologic Diagnosis & Treatment*, 8th ed. Stamford, CT: Appleton & Lange, 1994: 404.)

Intrauterine Growth Restriction (IUGR)

Defined as an EFW less than the 10th percentile for GA.

HISTORY/PE

- Affected infants are commonly born to women with systemic diseases that lead to uteroplacental insufficiency (intrauterine infection, hypertension, anemia).
- Other risk factors include maternal substance abuse, placenta previa, and multiple gestations.

DIAGNOSIS

- **First step:** Diagnose by confirming serial fundal height measurements with ultrasound.
- **Second step:** Ultrasound the fetus for EFW (although as pregnancy advances, ultrasound fetal weight estimates become increasingly unreliable).

TREATMENT

- **First step:** Explore the underlying etiology and correct if possible.
- **If near due date:** Administer steroids (e.g., betamethasone) to accelerate fetal lung maturity.
- **Then:** Perform fetal monitoring with NST, CST, BPP, and umbilical artery Doppler velocimetry. A nonreassuring status near term may prompt delivery.

↑ perinatal morbidity and mortality.

Fetal Macrosomia

- Defined as a birth weight > 90th percentile. A common sequela of gestational diabetes.
- **Dx:** Diagnose by weighing the newborn at birth (prenatal diagnosis is imprecise).
- **Tx:** Planned cesarean delivery may be considered for an EFW > 5000 g in women without diabetes and for an EFW > 4500 g in women with diabetes.
- **Cx:** ↑ risk of shoulder dystocia (leading to brachial plexus injury and Erb-Duchenne palsy) as birth weight ↑.

Polyhydramnios

- Defined as an AFI > 20 on ultrasound. May be present in normal pregnancies, but fetal chromosomal developmental abnormalities must be considered.
- Etiologies include maternal DM, multiple gestation, isoimmunization, pulmonary abnormalities (e.g., cystic lung malformations), fetal anomalies (e.g., duodenal atresia, tracheoesophageal fistula, anencephaly), and twin-twin transfusion syndrome.
- **Hx/PE:** Usually asymptomatic.
- **Dx:** Fundal height greater than expected. Evaluation includes ultrasound for fetal anomalies, glucose testing for DM, and Rh screen.
- **Tx:** Etiology specific.
- **Cx:** Preterm labor, fetal malpresentation, cord prolapse.

Oligohydramnios

- An AFI < 5 cm on ultrasound. Usually asymptomatic, but IUGR or fetal distress may be present. Etiologies include fetal urinary tract abnormalities (e.g., renal agenesis, GU obstruction), chronic uteroplacental insufficiency, and ROM.
- **Dx:** The sum of the deepest amniotic fluid pocket in all four abdominal quadrants on ultrasound.
- **Tx:** Rule out inaccurate gestational dates. Treat the underlying cause if possible.
- **Cx:** Associated with a 40-fold ↑ in perinatal mortality. Other complications include musculoskeletal abnormalities (e.g., clubfoot, facial distortion), pulmonary hypoplasia, umbilical cord compression, and IUGR.

Rh Isoimmunization

In this condition, fetal RBCs leak into the maternal circulation, and maternal anti-Rh IgG antibodies form that can cross the placenta, leading to hemolysis of fetal Rh RBCs (**erythroblastosis fetalis**). There is an ↑ risk among an Rh-⊖ women who have had a previous SAB or TAB as well as among those who have undergone a previous delivery with no RhoGAM given.

HIGH-YIELD FACTS

OBSTETRICS

DIAGNOSIS

Sensitized Rh-$\ominus$ mothers with titers $> 1:16$ should be closely monitored with serial ultrasound and amniocentesis for evidence of fetal hemolysis.

TREATMENT

In severe cases, initiate preterm delivery when fetal lungs are mature. Prior to delivery, intrauterine blood transfusions may be given to correct a low fetal hematocrit.

PREVENTION

- If the mother is Rh $\ominus$ at 28 weeks and the father is Rh $\oplus$ or unknown, give **RhoGAM** (Rh immune globulin).
- If the baby is Rh $\oplus$, give RhoGAM postpartum.
- Give RhoGAM to Rh-$\ominus$ mothers who undergo abortion or who have had an ectopic pregnancy, amniocentesis, vaginal bleeding, or placenta previa/placental abruption. Type and screen is critical; follow β-hCG closely and prevent pregnancy for one year.

COMPLICATIONS

- Hydrops fetalis occurs when fetal hemoglobin drops to < 7 g/dL.
- Other complications include fetal hypoxia and acidosis, kernicterus, prematurity, and death.

Gestational Trophoblastic Disease (GTD)

A range of proliferative trophoblastic abnormalities that can be benign or malignant.

- **Complete moles:** Usually result from sperm fertilization of an empty ovum; **46,XX** (paternally derived).
- **Incomplete (partial) moles:** Occur when a normal ovum is fertilized by two sperm (or a haploid sperm that duplicates its chromosomes); usually **69,XXY** and contain fetal tissue.

HISTORY/PE

- Presents with first-trimester **uterine bleeding** (most common), hyperemesis gravidarum, preeclampsia/eclampsia at < 24 weeks, and uterine size greater than dates.
- Risk factors include extremes of age (< 20 or > 40 years) and a diet deficient in folate or beta-carotene.

DIAGNOSIS

- No fetal heartbeat is detected. Pelvic exam may reveal enlarged ovaries (bilateral theca-lutein cysts) or expulsion of **grapelike molar clusters** into the vagina.
- Labs show markedly $\uparrow$ serum β-hCG (usually $> 100,000$ mIU/mL), and pelvic ultrasound reveals a "snowstorm" appearance with no gestational sac or fetus present (see Figure 2.11-9).
- CXR may show lung metastases; D&C reveals **"cluster-of-grapes"** tissue (see Figure 2.11-10).

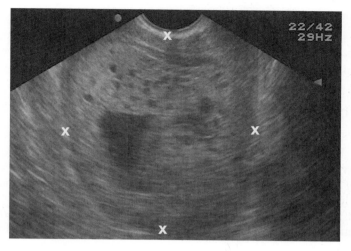

FIGURE 2.11-9.   Molar pregnancy.

Transvaginal ultrasound shows a large, complex intrauterine mass with cystic regions that have the characteristic appearance of grapes.(Reproduced, with permission, from Tintinalli JE et al. *Tintinalli's Emergency Medicine: A Comprehensive Study Guide*, 6th ed. New York: McGraw-Hill, 2004: Fig. 113-27.)

TREATMENT

Evacuate the uterus and follow with weekly β-hCG. Treat malignant disease with chemotherapy (methotrexate or dactinomycin) and residual uterine disease with hysterectomy; chemotherapy and irradiation are highly effective for metastases.

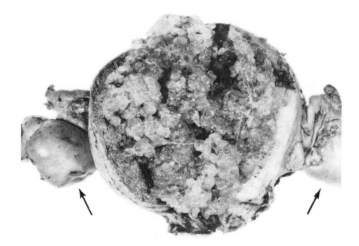

FIGURE 2.11-10.   Gross specimen of hydatidiform mole.

A complete or classical hydatidiform mole is characterized grossly by an abundance of edematous enlarged chorionic villi but no fetus or fetal membranes. There are theca-lutein cysts in both ovaries (arrows). (Reproduced, with permission, from Cunningham FG et al. *Williams Obstetrics*, 22nd ed. New York: McGraw-Hill, 2005: Fig.11-1.)

Molar pregnancy may progress to malignant GTD, including invasive moles (10–15%) and choriocarcinoma (2–5%) with pulmonary or CNS metastases. Trophoblastic pulmonary emboli may also be seen.

Multiple Gestations

- Affect 3% of all live births.
- Since 1980, there has been a 65% ↑ in the frequency of dizygotic (fraternal) twins and a 500% ↑ in triplet and high-order births (most due to the advent of assisted reproductive technology). The incidence of monozygotic (identical) twins has remained steady.
- **Hx/PE:** Characterized by rapid uterine growth, excessive maternal weight gain, and palpation of three or more large fetal parts on Leopold's maneuvers.
- **Dx:** Ultrasound; hCG, HPL, and MSAFP are elevated for GA.
- **Tx:** Multifetal reduction and selective fetal termination is an option for higher-order multiple pregnancies; antepartum fetal surveillance for IUGR. Management by a high-risk specialist is recommended.
- **Cx:**
  - **Maternal:** Patients are six times more likely to be hospitalized with complications—e.g., preeclampsia, preterm labor, preterm PROM (PPROM), placental abruption, pyelonephritis, and postpartum hemorrhage.
  - **Fetal:** Complications include twin-to-twin transfusion syndrome, IUGR, and preterm labor.

▶ ABNORMAL LABOR AND DELIVERY

Shoulder Dystocia

Affects 0.6–1.4% of all deliveries in the United States. Risk factors include obesity, diabetes, a history of a macrosomic infant, and a history of prior shoulder dystocia.

DIAGNOSIS

Diagnosed by a prolonged second stage of labor, recoil of the perineum ("turtle sign"), and lack of spontaneous restitution.

TREATMENT

In the event of dystocia, be the mother's **HELPER:**

- **H**elp reposition.
- **E**pisiotomy.
- **L**eg elevated (McRoberts' maneuver).
- **P**ressure (suprapubic).
- **E**nter the vagina and attempt rotation (Wood's screw).
- **R**each for the fetal arm.

Failure to Progress

Associated with chorioamnionitis, occiput posterior position, nulliparity, and elevated birth weight.

DIAGNOSIS

- **First-stage protraction or arrest:** Labor that fails to produce adequate rates of progressive cervical change.
- **Prolonged second-stage arrest:**
  - **Nulliparous:** Inadequate cervical dilation after > 3 hours with regional anesthesia; > 2 hours without.
  - **Multiparous:** Inadequate cervical dilation after > 2 hours with regional anesthesia; > 1 hour without.

TREATMENT

See Table 2.11-16.

COMPLICATIONS

- Chorioamnionitis leads to fetal infection, pneumonia, and bacteremia.
- Some 10% of those affected have permanent injury, 11% have a risk of postpartum hemorrhage, and 3.8% are at risk of fourth-degree laceration.

Rupture of Membranes (ROM)

Distinguished as follows:

- **Spontaneous ROM:** Occurs > 1 hour before onset of labor. May be precipitated by vaginal or cervical infections, abnormal membrane physiology, or cervical incompetence.
- **PPROM:** Rupture of membranes occurring at < 37 weeks' gestation.
- **Prolonged ROM:** Defined as rupture > 18 hours prior to delivery. Risk factors include low socioeconomic status (SES), young maternal age, smoking, and STDs.

HISTORY/PE

Patients often report a **"gush" of clear or blood-tinged amniotic fluid.** Uterine contractions may be present.

TABLE 2.11-16. Failure to Progress

STAGE	DEFINITION	TREATMENT[a]
First	Failure to have progressive cervical change:	
Latent	■ **Prima:** > 20 hours	Therapeutic rest via parenteral analgesia; oxytocin;
	■ **Multi:** > 14 hours	amniotomy; cervical ripening.
Active	■ **Prima:** > 2 hrs	Amniotomy; oxytocin; C-section if the previous interventions
	■ **Multi:** > 2 hrs after reaching 3–4 cm	are ineffective.
Second	Arrest of fetal descent:	Close observation with ↓ in epidural rate and continued
	■ **Prima:** > 2 hrs; > 3 hours with epidural	oxytocin.
	■ **Multi:** > 1 hr; > 2 hrs with epidural	Assisted vaginal delivery (forceps or vacuum).
		C-section.

[a] Augmentation with oxytocin should be considered when contraction frequency is < 3 in a 10-minute period or intensity of contraction is < 25 mmHg above baseline.

HIGH-YIELD FACTS

OBSTETRICS

DIAGNOSIS

- First step:
  - A **sterile speculum exam** reveals **pooling** of amniotic fluid in the vaginal vault.
  - **Nitrazine paper test** is ⊕ (paper turns blue, indicating alkaline pH of amniotic fluid).
  - **Fern test** is ⊕ (a ferning pattern is seen under a microscope after amniotic fluid dries on a glass slide).
- **Second step:** Ultrasound to assess amniotic fluid volume.
- **If unsure:** Ultrasound-guided transabdominal instillation of indigo carmine dye to check for leakage (unequivocal test).
- Minimize infection risk; **do not perform digital vaginal exams on women who are not in labor or for whom labor is not planned immediately.**
- Check fetal heart tracing, maternal temperature, WBC count, and uterine tenderness for evidence of chorioamnionitis.

TREATMENT

- **Depends on GA and fetal lung maturity.**
  - **Term:** First check GBS status and fetal presentation; **then** labor may be induced or the patient can be observed for 24–72 hours.
  - **> 34–36 weeks' gestation:** Labor induction may be considered.
  - **< 32 weeks' gestation:** Expectant management with bed rest and pelvic rest.
- **Antibiotics:** Given to prevent infection and to prolong the latency period in the absence of infection.
- **Antenatal corticosteroids** (e.g., betamethasone or dexamethasone × 48 hours): Can be given to promote fetal lung maturity in the absence of intra-amniotic infection prior to 32 weeks' GA.
- If signs of infection or fetal distress develop, give antibiotics (ampicillin and gentamicin) and induce labor.

COMPLICATIONS

Preterm labor and delivery, chorioamnionitis, placental abruption, cord prolapse.

Preterm Labor

- Defined as onset of labor between **20 and 37 weeks' gestation.**
- Occurs in > 10% of all U.S. pregnancies and is the 1° cause of neonatal morbidity and mortality.
- Risk factors include multiple gestation, infection, PROM, uterine anomalies, previous preterm labor or delivery, polyhydramnios, placental abruption, poor maternal nutrition, and low SES. **Most patients have no identifiable risk factors.**

HISTORY/PE

Patients may have menstrual-like cramps, onset of low back pain, pelvic pressure, and new vaginal discharge or bleeding.

DIAGNOSIS

- Requires **regular uterine contractions** (≥ 3 contractions of 30 seconds each over a 30-minute period) and **concurrent cervical change** at < 37 weeks' gestation.

- **Assess for contraindications to tocolysis** (e.g., infection, nonreassuring fetal testing, placental abruption).
- Perform a **sterile speculum exam** to rule out PROM.
- Obtain an **ultrasound** to rule out fetal or uterine anomalies, verify GA, and assess fetal presentation and amniotic fluid volume.
- Obtain cultures for chlamydia, gonorrhea, and GBS. Obtain a UA and urine culture.

TREATMENT

- Hydration and bed rest.
- Unless contraindicated, begin **tocolytic therapy** (β-mimetics, $MgSO_4$, CCBs, PGIs) and give **steroids** to accelerate fetal lung maturation. Give **penicillin or ampicillin for GBS prophylaxis** if preterm delivery is likely.

COMPLICATIONS

RDS, intraventricular hemorrhage, **PDA**, necrotizing enterocolitis, retinopathy of prematurity, bronchopulmonary dysplasia, death.

Fetal Malpresentation

Defined as any presentation other than vertex (i.e., head closest to birth canal, chin to chest, occiput anterior). Risk factors include **prematurity,** prior breech delivery, uterine anomalies, poly- or oligohydramnios, multiple gestations, PPROM, hydrocephalus, anencephaly, and placenta previa.

HISTORY/PE

Breech presentations are the most common form (affect 3% of all deliveries) and involve presentation of the fetal lower extremities or buttocks into the maternal pelvis (see Figure 2.11-11). Subtypes include the following:

- **Frank breech (50–75%):** The thighs are flexed and the knees are extended.
- **Footling breech (20%):** One or both legs are extended below the buttocks.
- **Complete breech (5–10%):** The thighs and knees are flexed.

Breech presentation is the most common fetal malpresentation.

TREATMENT

- **Follow:** Up to 75% spontaneously change to vertex by week 38.
- **External version:** If the fetus has not reverted spontaneously, a version may be attempted by applying directed pressure to the maternal abdomen to turn the infant to vertex. The success rate is roughly 50%. Risks of version are placental abruption and cord compression, so be prepared for an emergency C-section if needed.
- **Trial of breech vaginal delivery:** Attempt **only if delivery is imminent;** otherwise contraindicated. Complications include cord prolapse and/or head entrapment.
- **Elective C-section:** Recommended given the lower risk of fetal morbidity.

Indications for Cesarean Section

See Table 2.11-17 for indications. For both elective and indicated cesarean delivery, **sodium citrate** should be used to ↓ gastric acidity and prevent acid aspiration syndrome.

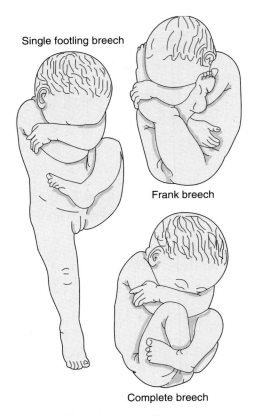

Single footling breech

Frank breech

Complete breech

FIGURE 2.11-11. Types of breech presentations.

(Reproduced, with permission, from DeCherney AH. *Current Obstetric & Gynecologic Diagnosis & Treatment*, 8th ed. Stamford, CT: Appleton & Lange, 1994: 411.)

TABLE 2.11-17. Indications for Cesarean Section

MATERNAL FACTORS	FETAL AND MATERNAL FACTORS	FETAL FACTORS
Prior classical C-section (vertical incision predisposes to uterine rupture with vaginal delivery)	Cephalopelvic disproportion (most common cause of 1° C-section)	Fetal malposition (e.g., posterior chin, transverse lie, shoulder presentation)
Active genital herpes infection	Placenta previa/placental abruption	Fetal distress
Cervical carcinoma	Failed operative vaginal delivery	Cord compression/prolapse
Maternal trauma/demise	Post-term pregnancy (relative indication)	Erythroblastosis fetalis (Rh incompatibility)
HIV infection		
Prior transverse C-section (relative indication)		

HIGH-YIELD FACTS

OBSTETRICS

Episiotomy

- Surgical extension of the vaginal opening into the perineum.
- There are two types: **median** (midline) and **mediolateral.**
- Complications include extension to the anal sphincter (third degree) or rectum (fourth degree), which is more common with midline episiotomy, as well as bleeding, infection, dyspareunia, and, in rare cases, rectovaginal fistula formation or maternal death.
- Routine use of episiotomy is **not recommended.**

▶ PUERPERIUM

Postpartum Hemorrhage

- Defined as a loss of **> 500 mL of blood for vaginal delivery** or **> 1000 mL for C-section** occurring before, during, or after delivery of the placenta. Table 2.11-18 summarizes common causes.
- Complications include acute blood loss (potentially fatal), anemia due to chronic blood loss (predisposes to puerperal infection), and **Sheehan's syndrome** (pituitary ischemia and necrosis; the 1° cause of anterior pituitary insufficiency in adult females, most commonly presenting as **failure to lactate**).

TABLE 2.11-18. **Common Causes of Postpartum Hemorrhage**

	UTERINE ATONY	**GENITAL TRACT TRAUMA**	**RETAINED PLACENTAL TISSUE**
Risk factors	Uterine overdistention (multiple gestation, macrosomia, polyhydramnios). Exhausted myometrium (rapid or prolonged labor, oxytocin stimulation). Uterine infection. Conditions interfering with contractions (anesthesia, myomas, MgSO$_4$).	Precipitous labor. Operative vaginal delivery (forceps, vacuum extraction). Large infant. Inadequate episiotomy repair.	Placenta accreta/increta/percreta. Placenta previa. Uterine leiomyomas. Preterm delivery. Previous C-section/ curettage.
Diagnosis	Palpation of a soft, enlarged, "boggy" uterus. The most common cause of **postpartum hemorrhage** (90%).	Manual and visual inspection of the lower genital tract for any laceration > 2 cm long.	Manual and visual inspection of the placenta and uterine cavity for missing cotyledons. Ultrasound may also be used to inspect the uterus.
Treatment[a]	Bimanual **uterine massage** (usually successful). **Oxytocin** infusion. **Methergine** (methylergonovine) if not hypertensive. **Prostaglandin** (PGF$_{2a}$).	Surgical repair of the physical defect.	Manual removal of remaining placental tissue. Curettage with suctioning (take care not to perforate the uterine fundus).

[a] For all uterine causes, when bleeding persists after conventional therapy, uterine/internal iliac artery ligation or hysterectomy can be lifesaving.

The 7 W's of postpartum fever (10 days postdelivery):

Womb (endomyometritis)
Wind (atelectasis, pneumonia)
Water (UTI)
Walk (DVT, pulmonary embolism)
Wound (incision, episiotomy)
Weaning (breast engorgement, abscess, mastitis)
Wonder drugs (drug fever)

Postpartum Infections

■ Characterized by a temperature ≥ 38°C **for at least two of the first ten postpartum days (not including the first 24 hours).**

■ Risk factors for postpartum endometritis include emergent C-section, PROM, prolonged labor, multiple intrapartum vaginal exams, intrauterine manipulations, delivery, low SES, young age, prolonged ruptured membranes, bacterial colonization, and corticosteroid use.

■ For endometritis, hospitalize and give **broad-spectrum empiric IV antibiotics** (e.g., clindamycin and gentamicin) **until patients have been afebrile for 48 hours** (24 hours for chorioamnionitis). Add ampicillin for complicated cases.

■ For persistent postpartum fever that is not responsive to broad-spectrum antibiotics, think **septic pelvic thrombophlebitis,** in which pelvic infection leads to infection of the vein wall and intimal damage, leading in turn to thrombogenesis. The clot is then invaded by microorganisms. Suppuration follows, with liquefaction, **fragmentation, and, finally, septic embolization.**
  ■ Presents with abdominal and back pain and a picket-fence fever curve ("hectic" fevers) with wide swings from normal to as high as 41°C (105.8°F).
  ■ Diagnose with blood cultures and CT looking for a pelvic abscess.
  ■ Treat with broad-spectrum antibiotics and **anticoagulation** with heparin × 7–10 days.

Sheehan's Syndrome (Postpartum Pituitary Necrosis)

■ Defined as pituitary ischemia and necrosis that leads to anterior pituitary insufficiency 2° to massive obstetric hemorrhage and shock.

■ **Hx/PE:**
  ■ The 1° cause of anterior pituitary insufficiency in adult females. The **most common presenting syndrome is failure to lactate** (due to ↓ prolactin levels).
  ■ Other symptoms include weakness, lethargy, cold insensitivity, genital atrophy, and menstrual disorders.

■ **Dx:** The diagnosis is established with provocative hormonal testing and MRI of the pituitary and hypothalamus to rule out tumor or other pathology.

■ **Tx:** Treatment consists of the replacement of all deficient hormones. However, some patients may recover TSH and even gonadotropin function after cortisol replacement alone.

Lactation and Breastfeeding

■ During pregnancy, ↑ estrogen and progesterone result in breast hypertrophy and inhibition of prolactin release. After delivery of the placenta, hormone levels ↓ markedly and prolactin is released, stimulating milk production. Periodic infant suckling leads to further release of **prolactin** and **oxytocin,** which stimulate myoepithelial cell contraction and milk ejection ("let-down reflex").

■ Colostrum ("early breast milk") contains protein, fat, **secretory IgA,** and minerals. Within one week postpartum, mature milk with protein, fat, lactose, and water is produced.

■ High IgA levels in colostrum provide passive immunity for the infant and protect against enteric bacteria.

- Other benefits include ↓ incidence of infant allergies, early upper respiratory tract infections, and GI infections; facilitation of mother-child bonding; and maternal weight loss.
- Contraindications to breastfeeding include HIV infection, active HBV and HCV infection, and use of certain medications (e.g., tetracycline, chloramphenicol, warfarin).

Mastitis

Cellulitis of the periglandular tissue caused by nipple trauma from breastfeeding coupled with the introduction of bacteria, usually *S. aureus*, from the infant's pharynx into the nipple ducts. Affects 2–3% of nursing women.

HISTORY/PE

- Symptoms often begin 2–4 weeks postpartum.
- Breast symptoms are **usually unilateral** and include breast tenderness, a palpable mass, erythema, edema, warmth, and possible purulent nipple drainage. Significant fever, chills, and malaise may also be seen.

DIAGNOSIS

- Differentiate from simple breast swelling.
- Infection is suggested by focal symptoms, a ⊕ breast milk culture, an ↑ WBC count, and fever.

TREATMENT

The treatment of mastitis includes antibiotics and continued breastfeeding.

- **First step: Continued breastfeeding** to prevent the accumulation of infected material (or use of a breast pump in patients who are no longer breastfeeding) **and** PO antibiotics (dicloxacillin, cephalexin, amoxicillin/clavulanate, azithromycin, clindamycin).
- **Next step:** If abscess is present, treat with incision and drainage.

Gynecology

- Breast development **(thelarche)** **precedes** menarche and usually begins between the ages of 8 and 11.
- **Menarche** usually occurs between the ages of 10 and 16.
- Figure 2.12-1 graphically illustrates the stages of normal female development.

▶ **NORMAL MENSTRUAL CYCLE**

The progression of a normal menstrual cycle is as follows (see also Figure 2.12-2):

- **Follicular phase (days 1–13):** Typically lasts about 13 days but may vary. ↑ FSH → growth of follicles → ↑ estrogen production. Results in the development of straight glands and thin secretions of the uterine lining **(proliferative phase)**.
- **Ovulation (day 14):**
  - LH and FSH spike results in rupture of the ovarian follicle and release of a mature ovum.
  - Ruptured follicular cells involute and create the corpus luteum.
- **Luteal phase (days 15–28):** This phase is the length of time (14 days) that the corpus luteum can survive without further LH stimulation.

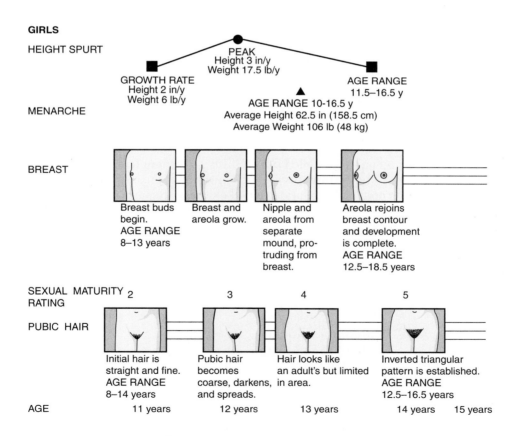

FIGURE 2.12-1. **Normal female development.**

(Reproduced, with permission, from Hay WW Jr et al. *Current Diagnosis & Treatment: Pediatrics*, 19th ed. New York: McGraw-Hill, 2008: Fig. 3-4.)

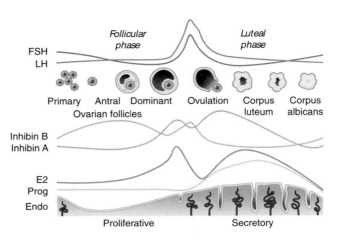

FIGURE 2.12-2. Normal menstrual cycle.

(Reproduced, with permission, from Fauci AS et al. *Harrison's Principles of Internal Medicine*, 17th ed. New York: McGraw-Hill, 2008: Fig. 341-8.)

- The corpus luteum produces estrogen and progesterone, allowing the endometrial lining to develop thick endometrial glands with thick secretions (secretory phase).
- In the absence of implantation, the corpus luteum cannot be sustained, and the endometrial lining sloughs off.

 MENOPAUSE

Cessation of menses for a minimum of 12 months as a result of cessation of follicular development. Average age of onset is 51. "Premature menopause" is defined as ovarian failure and menstrual cessation before age 40.

HISTORY/PE

- The mnemonic **HAVOC** lists prominent features of menopause.
- Other symptoms include insomnia, anxiety/irritability, vaginal bleeding, poor concentration, mood changes, dyspareunia, and loss of libido.

DIAGNOSIS

- Labs first show ↑ **FSH** and then show ↑ **LH.**
- DEXA scan to follow bone density for osteoporosis.
- Lipid profile (↑ total cholesterol, ↓ HDL).

TREATMENT

- **Vasomotor symptoms:**
  - **HRT (combination estrogen and progestin):**
    - HRT has been shown to ↑ cardiovascular morbidity and mortality and may ↑ the incidence of breast and endometrial cancers. For this reason, clinicians should thoroughly review the risks and benefits of HRT before initiating treatment.
    - Posthysterectomy patients do not need progestin. Unopposed estrogen in patients with a uterus predisposes to endometrial cancer.
    - Contraindications to HRT include vaginal bleeding, suspected or known breast cancer, endometrial cancer, and a history of thromboembolism, chronic liver disease, or hypertriglyceridemia.

Menopause wreaks—

HAVOC

Hot flashes (vasomotor instability)
Atrophy of the
Vagina
Osteoporosis
Coronary artery disease

*Currently, HRT is **not** recommended as first-line treatment for menopausal symptoms.*

- **Non-HRT:** Venlafaxine and, less commonly, clonidine can be given to ↓ the frequency of hot flashes.
- **Vaginal atrophy:**
  - **Long term: Estradiol vaginal ring.**
  - **Short term:** Estrogen vaginal cream will relieve symptoms.
- **Osteoporosis:** Treat with daily calcium supplementation and exercise; possibly bisphosphonates.

Once a woman is postmenopausal, she should be routinely screened for osteoporosis.

► CONTRACEPTION

- Of women who are sexually active and do not use a contraceptive method, **85% will become pregnant within one year.**
- Absolute contraindications to various methods are as follows:
  - **Estrogen-containing hormonal methods** (OCPs, NuvaRing, "the patch"):
    - Pregnancy
    - A history of CAD or DVT
    - Breast cancer
    - Undiagnosed abnormal vaginal bleeding
    - Estrogen-dependent cancer
    - A benign or malignant liver neoplasm
    - Current tobacco use **and** age > 35
  - **Mirena and Copper T IUDs:**
    - Known or suspected pregnancy
    - Unexplained vaginal bleeding until diagnosed
    - Current purulent cervicitis
    - PID that is active (within three months) or recurrent
    - Confirmed symptomatic actinomycosis on culture (but not asymptomatic colonization)
    - A bicornuate or septate uterus
    - Cervical or uterine cancer
    - A Pap smear with squamous intraepithelial lesions or two atypical Pap smears
    - A history of heart valve replacement or artificial joints
  - **Copper T alone:** Copper intolerance (allergy to copper, Wilson's disease); severe dysmenorrhea and/or menorrhagia.
  - **Mirena alone:** Levonorgestrel allergy, breast cancer, acute liver disease or liver tumor, or a history of ⊕ *BRCA*.
- Table 2.12-1 describes the effectiveness of contraceptive methods along with their relative advantages and disadvantages.
- Emergency contraception (EC) methods prevent pregnancy after unprotected sex or contraceptive failure. Table 2.12-2 describes the various methods of EC.

*More than one sexual partner and nulliparity are **not** absolute contraindications to IUD use.*

The most effective methods of contraception are longer-term methods that ↓ user error.

Combined hormonal methods of contraception protect against endometrial, ovarian, and breast cancer.

► SEXUAL ASSAULT

Sexual assault is the most frequently unreported crime in the United States. Physicians are often required to evaluate rape victims and collect evidence. Most rape victims are women; however, men may also be victims of rape.

HISTORY/PE

- Take a full history, including contraceptive use, last time of coitus, condom use prior to the assault, drug or alcohol use, history of STDs, history of mental illness or deficiency, description of the assailant, location and

TABLE 2.12-1. Contraceptive Methods

METHOD	ADVANTAGES	DISADVANTAGES
Most effective: > 99% (1 in 100 women will become pregnant using these methods)		
Implanon ("the implant"): Progestin-only implant	Lasts up to three years. Immediate fertility with removal. Safe with breastfeeding.	Associated with weight gain, depression, irregular bleeding (no period; spotting; heavier, more frequent periods).
Intrauterine device with progestin (Mirena): Inflammation from foreign body; cervical thickening and endometrial decidualization with progesterone	Effective for up to five years. Lighter periods; less cramping. Immediate fertility with removal. Safe with breastfeeding.	Spotting (up to six months). Associated with acne. Risk of uterine puncture (1/1000).
Intrauterine device— ParaGard (Copper T): Inflammation from foreign body; copper exerts a spermicidal effect	Effective for up to 10 years. Immediate fertility with removal. Safe with breastfeeding.	↑ cramping and bleeding (5–10%). Risk of uterine puncture (1/1000).
Surgical sterilization (vasectomy, tubal ligation)	Permanently effective. Safe with breastfeeding.	**Tubal ligation:** Irreversible; ↑ ectopic pregnancy. **Vasectomy:** Most failures are due to not waiting for two ⊖ semen samples.
Very effective: 90–99% (1–10 in 100 women will become pregnant using these methods)		
Depo-Provera (medroxy-progesterone): IM injection every three months	Lighter or no periods. Each shot works for three months. Safe with breastfeeding.	Associated with irregular bleeding and weight gain. Decreases in bone mineral density (reversible). Delayed fertility after discontinuation (one shot can last 10 months).
Ortho Evra ("the patch"): Combined weekly estrogen and progestin dermal patch	Can make periods more regular. Not administered daily.	Risk of thromboembolism (especially for smokers and those > 35 years of age).
NuvaRing ("the ring"): Combined low-dose progestin and an estrogen vaginal ring	Can make periods more regular. Can improve acne. Used continuously for three weeks; then one week without the ring. Safe to use continuously to skip periods.	May ↑ vaginal discharge. Spotting occurs in the first 1–2 months.

HIGH-YIELD FACTS

GYNECOLOGY

TABLE 2.12-1. Contraceptive Methods *(continued)*

METHOD	ADVANTAGES	DISADVANTAGES
Oral contraceptive pills (combination estrogen and progestin): Inhibit FSH/LH, suppressing ovulation; thicken cervical mucus; decidualize endometrium	↓ risk of ovarian and endometrial cancers.[a] Predictable, lighter, less painful menses. Often improve acne. Immediate fertility upon cessation.	Require daily compliance. Breakthrough bleeding (10–30%). Risk of thromboembolism (especially for smokers and those > 35 years of age).
Progestin-only "minipills": Thicken cervical mucus	Safe with breastfeeding.	Requires strict compliance (taking pill at the same time each day).
Moderately effective: 75–90% (up to 10–25 women in 100 will become pregnant using these methods)		
Male condoms: A latex sheath covers the penis	**The only method that effectively protects against pregnancy and STDs, including HIV.**	Possible allergy to latex or spermicides.
Diaphragm with spermicide	Some protection against STDs.	Must be fitted by provider.
Female condom	Some protection against STDs.	Can be clumsy and difficult.
Fertility awareness methods	No side effects. Often used by women who have a cultural, religious, or personal preference for "natural" contraception.	Requires partner's participation. No STD/HIV protection.
Less effective: 68–74% (26–32 women in 100 will become pregnant using these methods)		
Withdrawal	No side effects.	No STD/HIV protection.
Spermicide	Frequent use may protect against HIV. May be used as a 2° method.	Not recommended as a 1° method.

[a] Other combined hormonal methods (e.g., patch, ring) may also protect against endometrial, breast, and ovarian cancer; however, data are still lacking given their relatively recent introduction.

time of the assault, circumstances of the assault (e.g., penile penetration, use of condoms, extragenital acts, use or display of weapons), and the patient's actions since the assault (e.g., douching, bathing, brushing teeth, urination/defecation, changing clothes).

■ Conduct a complete physical exam, making note of any signs of trauma, along with a detailed pelvic exam, including a survey of the external genitals, vagina, cervix, and anus.

DIAGNOSIS

■ Saline prep for sperm.
■ Gonorrhea and chlamydia smear/culture (including rectal if appropriate).

TABLE 2.12-2. Emergency Contraceptive Methods

METHOD	ADVANTAGES	DISADVANTAGES
"Morning-After Pill"—used within 120 hours of unprotected sex		
Combined estrogen/progestin (75% effective)	Available over the counter. Does not disrupt embryo postimplantation. Can be used as bridge contraception. Safe for all women.	Nausea, vomiting, fatigue, headache, dizziness, breast tenderness. No protection against STDs.
Progestin only (80% effective)	Same as above. Fewer nausea/vomiting side effects than combined EC.	Same as above.
Copper T IUD—used within 7 days of unprotected sex (99% effective)	Can be used as EC and continued for up to 10 years of contraception.	High initial cost of insertion. Must be inserted by provider. No protection against STDs.

- Serologic testing for HIV, syphilis, HSV, HBV, and CMV.
- Serum pregnancy test.
- Blood alcohol level; urine toxicology screen.

TREATMENT

- STD treatment (ceftriaxone plus doxycycline).
- HIV risk assessment and possible postexposure prophylaxis.
- EC for pregnancy prevention.
- Refer for psychological counseling.
- Arrange for follow-up with the same physician or with another provider if more appropriate.
- Follow-up should include repeat screening for STDs, repeat screening for pregnancy, and a discussion of coping methods with appropriate referrals for psychiatric care if needed.

► **ABNORMALITIES OF THE MENSTRUAL CYCLE**

Pediatric Vaginal Discharge

Pediatric vaginal discharge is caused by a variety of factors and may be normal, but STDs resulting from sexual abuse must be ruled out.

Etiologies of vaginal discharge in pediatric patients include the following:

- **Infectious vulvovaginitis:**
  - May present with a malodorous, yellow-green, purulent discharge; most often caused by group A streptococcus.
  - May also be caused by any STD resulting from sexual abuse (STDs **must be ruled out and, if found, reported to child protective services**).
- **Foreign objects.**
- **Candidal infection:** May be associated with diabetes; measure glucose and/or check for glycosuria.
- **Sarcoma botryoides (rhabdomyosarcoma):** A malignancy with lesions that have the appearance of "bunches of grapes" within the vagina.

Precocious Puberty

Onset of 2° sexual characteristics before the age of eight. Subtypes are as follows (see also Table 2.12-3):

- **Central precocious puberty:** Results from early activation of hypothalamic GnRH production. Most commonly idiopathic (also known as constitutional or true); may be related to obesity. May also be caused by CNS tumors.
- **Peripheral precocious puberty:** Also called pseudo-precocious puberty. Results from nonhypothalamic GnRH production.

HISTORY/PE

- Signs of **estrogen excess** (breast development and possibly vaginal bleeding) point to ovarian cysts or tumors.
- Signs of **androgen excess** (pubic and/or axillary hair, enlarged clitoris, acne, and/or ↑ body odor) suggest adrenal tumors or congenital adrenal hyperplasia (CAH).

DIAGNOSIS

- **First step:** Obtain a radiograph of the wrist and hand to determine bone age.
  - If bone age is within one year of chronological age, puberty has not started or has just recently begun.
  - If bone age exceeds chronological age by > 2 years, puberty has been present for at least one year or is progressing rapidly.
- **Next step:** Conduct a GnRH agonist (leuprolide) stimulation test.
  - **Central precocious puberty:** If LH response is ⊕, obtain a **cranial MRI** to look for CNS tumors.
    - In girls 6–8 years of age with signs of precocious puberty, the incidence of CNS tumor is 2% in the absence of other CNS signs.
    - If CNS tumors are ruled out, constitutional precocious puberty is the likely etiology.
  - **Peripheral precocious puberty:** If LH response is ⊖, order the following:
    - **Ultrasound of the ovaries and/or adrenals:** To look for ovarian or adrenal cysts/tumors.
    - **Estradiol:** Levels will be ↑ in ovarian cysts or tumors.

If onset of 2° sexual characteristics is seen by age eight, work up for precocious puberty by determining bone age and conducting a GnRH stimulation test to distinguish central from peripheral precocious puberty.

TABLE 2.12-3.   Causes of Precocious Pubertal Development

CENTRAL (GnRH-DEPENDENT)	PERIPHERAL (GnRH-INDEPENDENT)
Constitutional (idiopathic)	Congenital adrenal hyperplasia
Hypothalamic lesions (hamartomas, tumors, congenital malformations)	Adrenal tumors
	McCune-Albright syndrome (polyostotic fibrous dysplasia)
Dysgerminomas	
Hydrocephalus	Gonadal tumors
CNS infections	Exogenous estrogen, oral (OCPs) or topical
CNS trauma/irradiation	Ovarian cysts (females)
Pineal tumors (rare)	
Neurofibromatosis with CNS involvement	
Tuberous sclerosis	

- **Androgen (DHEA, DHEAS):** Especially critical in the setting of advanced bone age or signs of adrenarche.
- **17-OH progesterone:** To screen for advanced bone age or adrenarche.

TREATMENT

- **Central precocious puberty: Leuprolide** is first-line therapy. With treatment, physical changes regress or cease to progress.
- **Peripheral precocious puberty:** Treat the cause.
  - **Ovarian cysts:** No intervention is necessary, as cysts will usually regress spontaneously.
  - **CAH:** Treat with glucocorticoids. Surgery is **not** required for the treatment of ambiguous genitalia.
  - **Adrenal or ovarian tumors:** Require surgical resection.
  - **McCune-Albright syndrome:** Antiestrogens (tamoxifen) or estrogen synthesis blockers (ketoconazole or testolactone) may be effective.

1° Amenorrhea/Delayed Puberty

1° amenorrhea is defined as **the absence of menses by age 16 with 2° sexual development present, or the absence of 2° sexual characteristics by age 14.**

HISTORY/PE

- **Absence of 2° sexual characteristics** (no estrogen production): Etiologies are as follows:
  - **Constitutional growth delay:** The **most common cause.**
  - **1° ovarian insufficiency:** Most commonly Turner's syndrome. Look for a history of radiation and chemotherapy.
  - **Central hypogonadism:** May be caused by a variety of factors, including the following:
    - Undernourishment, stress, prolactinemia, or exercise.
    - CNS tumor or cranial irradiation.
    - Kallmann's syndrome (isolated gonadotropin deficiency) associated with anosmia.
- **Presence of 2° sexual characteristics** (evidence of estrogen production but other anatomic or genetic problems): Etiologies include the following:
  - **Müllerian agenesis:** Absence of two-thirds of the vagina; uterine abnormalities.
  - **Imperforate hymen:** Presents with hematocolpos (blood in the vagina) that cannot escape, along with a bulging hymen. Requires surgical opening.
  - **Complete androgen insensitivity:** Patients present with breast development (aromatization of testosterone to estrogen) but are amenorrheic and lack pubic hair.

DIAGNOSIS

- **First step:** Get a pregnancy test.
- **Next step:** Obtain a radiograph to determine if bone age is consistent with pubertal onset (> 12 years in girls).
  - If the patient is of short stature (bone age < 12 years) with normal growth velocity, **constitutional growth delay** (the most common cause of 1° amenorrhea) is the probable cause.

- If bone age is > 12 years but there are no signs of puberty, obtain **LH/FSH** and consider where the problem is on the HPA axis (see Figure 2.12-3).
  - **↓ GnRH, ↓ LH/FSH, ↓ estrogen/progesterone at prepuberty levels:** Points to constitutional growth delay (puberty has not yet started).
  - **↓ GnRH, ↓ LH/FSH, ↓ estrogen/progesterone:** Hypogonadotropic hypogonadism. Suggests a hypothalamic or pituitary problem.
  - **↑ GnRH, ↑ LH/FSH, ↓ estrogen/progesterone:** Hypergonadotropic hypogonadism. Points to a condition in which the ovaries fail to produce estrogen.
  - **↑ GnRH, ↑ LH/FSH, high estrogen or testosterone:** Suggests PCOS or a problem with estrogen receptors.
  - **Normal pubertal hormone levels:** Indicates an anatomic problem (menstrual blood can't get out).

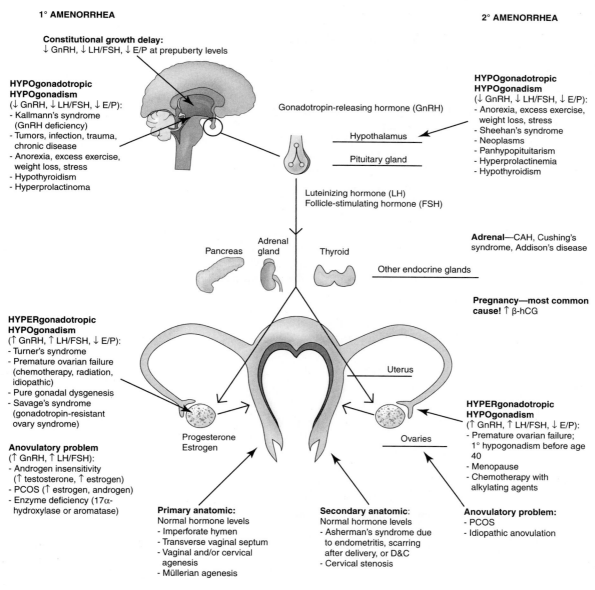

1° AMENORRHEA

Constitutional growth delay:
↓ GnRH, ↓ LH/FSH, ↓ E/P at prepuberty levels

HYPOgonadotropic HYPOgonadism
(↓ GnRH, ↓ LH/FSH, ↓ E/P):
- Kallmann's syndrome (GnRH deficiency)
- Tumors, infection, trauma, chronic disease
- Anorexia, excess exercise, weight loss, stress
- Hypothyroidism
- Hyperprolactinoma

HYPERgonadotropic HYPOgonadism
(↑ GnRH, ↑ LH/FSH, ↓ E/P):
- Turner's syndrome
- Premature ovarian failure (chemotherapy, radiation, idiopathic)
- Pure gonadal dysgenesis
- Savage's syndrome (gonadotropin-resistant ovary syndrome)

Anovulatory problem
(↑ GnRH, ↑ LH/FSH):
- Androgen insensitivity (↑ testosterone, ↑ estrogen)
- PCOS (↑ estrogen, androgen)
- Enzyme deficiency (17α-hydroxylase or aromatase)

2° AMENORRHEA

HYPOgonadotropic HYPOgonadism
(↓ GnRH, ↓ LH/FSH, ↓ E/P):
- Anorexia, excess exercise, weight loss, stress
- Sheehan's syndrome
- Neoplasms
- Panhypopituitarism
- Hyperprolactinemia
- Hypothyroidism

Gonadotropin-releasing hormone (GnRH)

Hypothalamus

Pituitary gland

Luteinizing hormone (LH)
Follicle-stimulating hormone (FSH)

Pancreas

Adrenal gland

Thyroid

Adrenal—CAH, Cushing's syndrome, Addison's disease

Other endocrine glands

Pregnancy—most common cause! ↑ β-hCG

Uterus

Progesterone
Estrogen

Ovaries

HYPERgonadotropic HYPOgonadism
(↑ GnRH, ↑ LH/FSH, ↓ E/P):
- Premature ovarian failure; 1° hypogonadism before age 40
- Menopause
- Chemotherapy with alkylating agents

Anovulatory problem:
- PCOS
- Idiopathic anovulation

Primary anatomic:
Normal hormone levels
- Imperforate hymen
- Transverse vaginal septum
- Vaginal and/or cervical agenesis
- Müllerian agenesis

Secondary anatomic:
Normal hormone levels
- Asherman's syndrome due to endometritis, scarring after delivery, or D&C
- Cervical stenosis

FIGURE 2.12-3. Causes of primary and secondary amenorrhea.

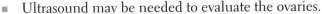

- Ultrasound may be needed to evaluate the ovaries.
- **Normal breast development and no uterus:** Obtain a **karyotype** to evaluate for androgen insensitivity syndrome.
- **Stigmata of Turner's syndrome:** Obtain a **karyotype.**
- **Normal breast development and uterus:** Measure prolactin and obtain a cranial MRI.

TREATMENT

- **Constitutional growth delay:** No treatment is needed.
- **Hypogonadism:** Begin HRT with estrogen alone at the lowest dose. Twelve to eighteen months later, begin cyclic estrogen/progesterone therapy (if the uterus is present).
- **Anatomic:** Generally requires surgical intervention.

The first step in the workup of 1° or 2° amenorrhea is a pregnancy test!

2° Amenorrhea

HISTORY/PE

Defined as the absence of menses for six consecutive months in women who have passed menarche.

DIAGNOSIS

- **First step:** Get a pregnancy test.
- **Second step:**
  - ⊖ β-hCG: Measure TSH and prolactin.
    - ↑ **TSH:** Indicates hypothyroidism.
    - ↑ **prolactin** (inhibits the release of LH and FSH): Points to a thyroid pathology. Order an MRI of the pituitary to rule out tumor.
    - ↑↑ **prolactin:** Suggests a prolactin-secreting pituitary adenoma.
  - **Normal β-hCG:** Initiate a progestin challenge (10 days of progestin).
    - ⊕ **progestin challenge (withdrawal bleed):** Indicates anovulation that is likely due to noncyclic gonadotropin secretion, pointing to PCOS or idiopathic anovulation. Check LH levels, and if LH is moderately high, the etiology is likely **PCOS.** Marked elevation of LH can indicate premature menopause.
    - ⊖ **progestin challenge (no bleed):** Indicates uterine abnormality or estrogen deficiency. Check FSH levels.
      - ↑ **FSH:** Indicates hypergonadotropic hypogonadism/ovarian failure.
      - ↓ **FSH:** Obtain a cyclic estrogen/progesterone test. A ⊕ withdrawal bleed points to hypogonadotropic hypogonadism; a ⊖ withdrawal bleed suggests an endometrial or anatomic problem.
- **Signs of hyperglycemia (polydipsia, polyuria) or hypotension:** Conduct a 1-mg overnight dexamethasone suppression test to distinguish CAH, Cushing's syndrome, and Addison's syndrome.
- **If clinical virilization is present:** Measure testosterone, DHEAS, and 17–hydroxyprogesterone.
  - **Mild pattern:** PCOS, CAH, or Cushing's syndrome.
  - **Moderate to severe pattern:** Look for an ovarian or adrenal tumor.

TREATMENT

- **Hypothalamic:** Reverse the underlying cause and induce ovulation with gonadotropins.

- **Tumors:** Excision; medical therapy for prolactinomas (e.g., bromocriptine, cabergoline).
- **Premature ovarian failure (age < 40 years):** If the uterus is present, treat with estrogen plus progestin replacement therapy.

1° Dysmenorrhea

Menstrual pain associated with ovulatory cycles in the **absence of pathologic findings.** Caused by uterine vasoconstriction, anoxia, and sustained contractions mediated by an excess of prostaglandin ($PGF_{2\alpha}$).

HISTORY/PE

- Presents with low, midline, spasmodic pelvic pain that often radiates to the back or inner thighs.
- Cramps occur in the first 1–3 days of menstruation and may be associated with nausea, diarrhea, headache, and flushing.
- There are **no pathologic findings on pelvic exam.**

DIAGNOSIS

A diagnosis of exclusion. Rule out 2° dysmenorrhea (see workup below).

TREATMENT

NSAIDs; topical heat therapy; combined OCPs, Mirena IUD.

2° Dysmenorrhea

Menstrual pain for which an organic cause exists. Common causes include endometriosis and adenomyosis, tumors, fibroids, adhesions, polyps, and PID.

HISTORY/PE

- **Look for pathology.** Patients may have a palpable uterine mass, cervical motion tenderness, adnexal tenderness, a vaginal or cervical discharge, or visible vaginal pathology (mucosal tears, masses, prolapse). However, normal abdominal and pelvic exams do not rule out pathology.
- See Table 2.12-4 for distinguishing features of endometriosis vs. adenomyosis.

DIAGNOSIS

- **First step:** Obtain a β-hCG to exclude ectopic pregnancy.
- **Second step:** Order the following:
  - A CBC with differential to rule out infection or neoplasm.
  - UA to rule out UTI.
  - Gonococcal/chlamydial swabs to rule out STDs/PID.
  - Stool guaiac to rule out GI pathology.
- **Third step:** Look for pelvic pathology causing pain (see Table 2.12-4).

TREATMENT

Treatment is etiology specific.

TABLE 2.12-4. Endometriosis vs. Adenomyosis

	ENDOMETRIOSIS	ADENOMYOSIS
Definition	Functional endometrial glands and stroma **outside** the uterus.	Endometrial tissue **in** the myometrium of the uterus.
History/PE	Presents with **cyclical** pelvic and/or rectal pain and dyspareunia (painful intercourse).	Presents with the classic triad of **noncyclical** pain, menorrhagia, and an enlarged uterus.
Diagnosis	Requires direct visualization by laparoscopy or laparotomy. Classic lesions have a blue-black ("raspberry") or dark brown ("powder-burned") appearance. Ovaries may have endometriomas (the characteristic "chocolate cysts").	Ultrasound is useful but cannot distinguish between leiomyoma and adenomyosis. MRI can aid in diagnosis but is costly.
Treatment	**Pharmacologic:** Inhibit ovulation. Combination OCPs are first line; other options include GnRH analogs (leuprolide) and danazol. **Conservative surgical treatment:** Excision, cauterization, or ablation of the lesions and lysis of adhesions. Twenty percent of patients can become pregnant subsequent to treatment. **Definitive surgical treatment:** TAH/BSO +/− lysis of adhesions.	**Pharmacologic:** Largely symptomatic relief. **NSAIDs** (first line) plus OCPs or progestins. **Conservative surgical treatment:** Endometrial ablation or resection using hysteroscopy. Complete eradication of deep adenomyosis is difficult and results in high treatment failure. **Definitive surgical treatment:** Hysterectomy is the only definitive treatment.
Complications	Infertility (the most common cause among menstruating women > 30 years of age).	Rarely, can progress to endometrial carcinoma.

Abnormal Uterine Bleeding

Normal menstrual bleeding ranges from two to seven days. Vaginal bleeding that occurs **six or more months** following the cessation of menstrual function is **cancer related** until proven otherwise.

HISTORY/PE

- Assess the extent of bleeding:
    - **Menorrhagia:** ↑ amount of flow (> 80 mL of blood loss per cycle) or prolonged bleeding (flow lasting > 8 days); may lead to anemia.
    - **Oligomenorrhea:** An ↑ length of time between menses (35–90 days between cycles).
    - **Polymenorrhea:** Frequent menstruation (< 21-day cycle); anovular.
    - **Metrorrhagia:** Bleeding between periods.
    - **Menometrorrhagia:** Excessive and irregular bleeding.
- **Pelvic exam:** Look for an enlarged uterus, a cervical mass, or polyps to assess for myomas, pregnancy, or cervical cancer.

DIAGNOSIS

- **First step:** Obtain a β-hCG to rule out ectopic pregnancy.
- **Second step:** Order a CBC to rule out anemia.

Pregnancy is the most common cause of abnormal uterine bleeding and amenorrhea. Always check a pregnancy test!

- **Third step:**
  - Pap smear to rule out cervical cancer (which can present with bleeding).
  - TFTs to rule out hyper-/hypothyroidism and hyperprolactinemia.
  - Obtain platelet count, bleeding time, and PT/PTT to rule out von Willebrand's disease and factor XI deficiency.
  - Order an ultrasound to evaluate the ovaries, uterus, and endometrium. Look for uterine masses, polycystic ovaries, and thickness of the endometrium.
  - If the endometrium is ≥ 4 mm in a **postmenopausal woman,** obtain an endometrial biopsy. An endometrial biopsy should also be obtained if the patient is > 35 years of age, obese (BMI > 35), and diabetic.

TREATMENT

- **Heavy bleeding:** Since heavy or prolonged uterine bleeding has likely denuded the endometrial cavity, estrogen is needed to rapidly promote endometrial growth.
  - **First step:** For hemorrhage, high-dose estrogen IV stabilizes the endometrial lining and stops bleeding within one hour.
  - **Next step:** If bleeding is not controlled within 12–24 hours, a D&C is indicated.
- **Ovulatory bleeding:** The goal is to ↓ blood loss.
  - **First step:** NSAIDs to ↓ blood loss.
  - **Next step:** If the patient is hemodynamically stable, treat with OCPs or a Mirena IUD to thicken the endometrium and control the bleeding. If this is not effective within 24 hours, look for an alternative diagnosis.
- **Anovulatory bleeding: The goal is to convert proliferative endometrium to secretory endometrium.**
  - Give progestins × 10 days to stimulate withdrawal bleeding.
  - For young patients with anovulatory bleeding who may also have a bleeding disorder, give desmopressin followed by a rapid ↑ in von Willebrand's factor and factor VIII (lasts roughly six hours).
- **If medical management fails,** options include the following:
  - **D&C:** An appropriate diagnostic/therapeutic option.
  - **Hysteroscopy:** Can help identify endometrial polyps as well as aid in the performance of directed uterine biopsies.
  - **Hysterectomy or endometrial ablation:** Appropriate in women who fail or do not want hormonal treatment, have symptomatic anemia, and/or experience a disruption in their quality of life from persistent, unscheduled bleeding.

▶ REPRODUCTIVE ENDOCRINOLOGY

Congenital Adrenal Hyperplasia (CAH)

A 21-hydroxylase deficiency that can present in its most severe, classic form as a newborn female infant with ambiguous genitalia and life-threatening salt wasting (see the Endocrinology chapter for a discussion of early-onset CAH). Milder forms present later in life. 11β-hydroxylase deficiency is a less common cause of adrenal hyperplasia.

HISTORY/PE

Presents with excessive hirsutism, acne, amenorrhea and/or abnormal uterine bleeding, infertility, and, rarely, a palpable pelvic mass.

First-line treatment of abnormal uterine bleeding consists of NSAIDs to ↓ blood loss!

OCPs and the Mirena IUD are highly effective treatment options for menorrhagia.

Complications of abnormal uterine bleeding are anemia and endometrial hyperplasia +/– carcinoma.

- *Hirsutism = male hair pattern.*
- *Virilization = frontal balding, muscularity, clitoromegaly, and deepening of the voice.*
- *Defeminization = ↓ breast size; loss of feminine adipose tissue.*

DIAGNOSIS

- ↑ **androgens (testosterone > 2 ng; DHEAS > 7 μg/mL):** Rule out adrenal or ovarian neoplasm.
- ↑ **serum testosterone:** Suspect an ovarian tumor.
- ↑ **DHEAS:** Suspect an adrenal source (adrenal tumor, Cushing's syndrome, CAH).
- ↑ **17-OH progesterone levels** (either basally or in response to ACTH stimulation).
- Table 2.12-5 outlines the differential diagnosis of hyperandrogenism.

TREATMENT

Glucocorticoids (e.g., prednisone). Medical therapy for adrenal and ovarian disorders prevents new terminal hair growth but does not resolve hirsutism. Laser ablation, electrolysis, or conventional hair removal techniques must be used to remove unwanted hair.

*The most severe form of PCOS is **HAIR-AN syndrome**: **H**yper**A**ndrogenism, **I**nsulin **R**esistance, and **A**canthosis **N**igricans.*

Polycystic Ovarian Syndrome (PCOS)

One of the most common endocrine disorders in reproductive women, with a prevalence of 6–10% among U.S. women of reproductive age. Also known as Stein-Leventhal syndrome. Diagnosis requires two of the following three criteria:

1. Polycystic ovaries
2. Oligo-/anovulation
3. Clinical or biochemical evidence of hyperandrogenism

TABLE 2.12-5. Differential Diagnosis of Hyperandrogenism

DISORDER	HISTORY/PE	DIAGNOSIS
PCOS	Irregular menses, slow-onset hirsutism, obesity, infertility, hypertension, a ⊕ family history of PCOS or DM.	Fasting glucose, insulin/lipid profile, BP, ultrasound for ovarian cysts.
21-hydroxylase deficiency—nonclassic (late-onset) CAH	Severe hirsutism or virilization, a strong family history of CAH, short stature, signs of defeminization. More common among Ashkenazi Jews.	17-hydroxyprogesterone (17-HP) levels before and after ACTH stimulation test > 10 ng/dL; *CYP21* genotype.
21-hydroxylase deficiency—classic (congenital) CAH	Same as above but with congenital virilization.	17-HP levels > 30 ng/dL.
Hypothyroidism	Fatigue, weight gain, amenorrhea.	TSH.
Hyperprolactinemia	Amenorrhea, galactorrhea, infertility.	Prolactin.
Androgen-secreting neoplasm	Pelvic mass, rapid-onset hirsutism or virilization, > 30 with onset of symptoms.	Pelvic ultrasound or abdominal/pelvic CT.
Cushing's syndrome	Hypertension, buffalo hump, purple striae, truncal obesity.	Elevated BP plus dexamethasone suppression test.

HISTORY/PE

- High BP.
- BMI > 30 (obesity).
- Stigmata of hyperandrogenism or insulin resistance (menstrual cycle disturbances, hirsutism, obesity, acne, androgenic alopecia, acanthosis nigricans).
- Women with PCOS are also at ↑ risk for the following:
  - Type 2 DM
  - Insulin resistance
  - Infertility
  - Metabolic syndrome—insulin resistance, obesity, atherogenic dyslipidemia, and hypertension

DIAGNOSIS

- **Biochemical hyperandrogenemia:** ↑ testosterone (total +/– free); DHEAS, DHEA.
- **Exclude other causes of hyperandrogenism:**
  - TSH, prolactin.
  - 17-OH progesterone to rule out nonclassical CAH.
  - Consider screening in the setting of clinical signs of Cushing's syndrome (e.g., moon facies, buffalo hump, abdominal striae) or acromegaly (e.g., ↑ head size).
- **Evaluate for metabolic abnormalities:**
  - Two-hour oral glucose tolerance test.
  - Fasting lipid and lipoprotein levels (total cholesterol, HDL, LDL, triglycerides).
- **Optional tests:**
  - **Ultrasound:** Look for > 8 small, subcapsular follicles forming a "**pearl necklace" sign** (see Figure 2.12-4). Seen in roughly two-thirds of women with PCOS.
  - **Gonadotropins:** ↑ **LH/FSH ratio** (> 2:1).
  - **Fasting insulin levels.**
  - **24-hour urine for free cortisol:** Adult-onset CAH or Cushing's syndrome.

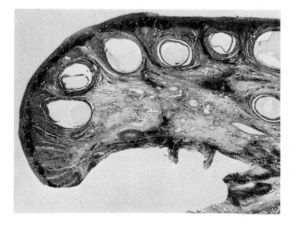

FIGURE 2.12-4. **Polycystic ovary with prominent multiple cysts.**

(Reproduced, with permission, from DeCherney AH. *Current Obstetric & Gynecologic Diagnosis & Treatment*, 8th ed. Stamford, CT: Appleton & Lange, 1994: 747.)

TREATMENT

- **Women who are not attempting to conceive:** Treat with a **combination of OCPs, progestin,** and **metformin** (or other insulin-sensitizing agents).
- **Women who are attempting to conceive:** Clomiphene +/– **metformin** is first-line treatment for ovulatory stimulation.
- **Symptom-specific treatment:**
  - **Hirsutism:** Combination OCPs are first line; antiandrogens (spironolactone, finasteride) and **metformin** may also be used.
  - **Cardiovascular risk factors and lipid levels:** Diet, weight loss, and exercise plus potentially lipid-controlling medication (e.g., statins).

COMPLICATIONS

↑ risk of early-onset type 2 DM; ↑ risk of miscarriages; ↑ long-term risk of breast and endometrial cancer due to unopposed estrogen secretion.

> *Combined hormonal contraception or progestin ↓ the risk of endometrial hyperplasia/carcinoma among women with PCOS.*

Infertility

Defined as inability to conceive after 12 months of normal, regular, unprotected sexual activity. 1° infertility is characterized by no prior pregnancies; 2° infertility occurs in the setting of at least one prior pregnancy. Etiologies are shown in Figure 2.12-5 and Table 2.11-6.

▶ GYNECOLOGIC INFECTIONS

Cyst and Abscess of Bartholin's Duct

Obstruction of the gland leads to pain, swelling, and abscess formation.

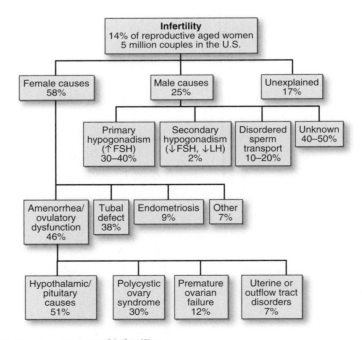

FIGURE 2.12-5. **Causes of infertility.**

(Reproduced, with permission, from Fauci AS et al. *Harrison's Principles of Internal Medicine,* 17th ed. New York: McGraw-Hill, 2008: Fig. 341-9.)

TABLE 2.12-6.   Infertility Workup

	HISTORY/PE	DIAGNOSIS	TREATMENT
Male causes	Testicular injury or infection Medications (corticosteroids, cimetidine, spironolactone) Thyroid or liver disease Signs of hypogonadism Varicocele	TSH Prolactin Karyotype (to rule out Klinefelter's syndrome) Semen analysis	Treatment of hormonal deficiency Intrauterine insemination (IUI) Donor insemination In vitro fertilization (IVF) Intracytoplasmic sperm injection
Ovulatory factors	Age (incidence ↑ with age) Symptoms of hyper-/ hypothyroidism Galactorrhea Menstrual cycle abnormalities	Basal body temperature Ovulation predictor Midluteal progesterone Early follicular FSH +/− estradiol level (ovarian reserve) TSH, prolactin, androgens Ovarian sonography (antral follicle count) Endometrial biopsy (luteal phase defect)	Treatment depends on the etiology (e.g., levothyroxine, dopamine) Induction of ovulation with **clomiphene**, gonadotropins, and pulsatile GnRH IUI IVF
Tubal/ pelvic factors	History of PID, appendicitis, endometriosis, pelvic adhesions, tubal surgery	Hysterosalpingogram, endometrial biopsy	Laparoscopic resection or ablation of endometriomas or fibroids IVF
Cervical factors	Abnormal Pap smears, postcoital bleeding, cryotherapy, conization, or DES exposure in utero	Pap smear Physical exam Antisperm antibodies	IUI with washed sperm IVF

HISTORY/PE

- Presents with periodic painful swelling on either side of the introitus and dyspareunia.
- A fluctuant swelling 1–4 cm in diameter is seen in the inferior portion of either labium minus.
- Tenderness is evidence of active infection.

TREATMENT

- Asymptomatic cysts do not require therapy. Frequent warm soaks may be helpful.
- If an abscess develops, treat with aspiration or incision and drainage. Culture for *Chlamydia* and other pathogens.
- Antibiotics are unnecessary unless cellulitis is present.

Vaginitis

A spectrum of conditions that cause vulvovaginal symptoms such as itching, burning, irritation, and abnormal discharge. The most common causes are bacterial vaginosis, vulvovaginal candidiasis, and trichomoniasis (see Table 2.12-7).

HISTORY/PE

- Presents with a change in discharge, malodor, pruritus, irritation, burning, swelling, dyspareunia, and dysuria.
- Normal secretions are as follows:
  - **Midcycle estrogen surge:** Clear, elastic, mucoid secretions.
  - **Luteal phase/pregnancy:** Thick and white secretions; adhere to the vaginal wall.

TABLE 2.12-7. Causes of Vaginitis

	BACTERIAL VAGINOSIS	**TRICHOMONAS**	**YEAST**
Incidence	15–50% (most common).	5–50%.	15–30%.
Etiology	Reflects a shift in vaginal flora.	Protozoal flagellates (**an STD**).	Usually *Candida albicans.*
Risk factors	Pregnancy, > 1 sexual partner, female sexual partner, frequent douching.	An STD. Unprotected sex with multiple partners.	**DM, broad-spectrum antibiotic use, pregnancy, corticosteroids,** HIV, OCP use, IUD use, young age at first intercourse, ↑ frequency of intercourse.
History	Odor, ↑ discharge.	↑ discharge, odor, pruritus, dysuria.	Pruritus, dysuria, burning, ↑ discharge.
Exam	Mild vulvar irritation.	"Strawberry petechiae" in the upper vagina/cervix (rare).	Erythematous, excoriated vulva/ vagina.
Discharge	Homogenous, **grayish-white, fishy**/stale odor.	Profuse, malodorous, **yellow-green, frothy.**	Thick, white, curdy texture without odor.
Wet mount[a]	**"Clue cells"** (epithelial cells coated with bacteria; see Figure 2.12-6); shift in vaginal flora (↑ cocci, ↓ lactobacilli).	**Motile trichomonads** (flagellated organisms that are slightly larger than WBCs).	–
KOH prep	⊕ whiff test (fishy smell).	–	Hyphae (see Figure 2.12–6).
Treatment	PO or vaginal metronidazole or clindamycin.	Single-dose PO metronidazole or tinidazole. Treat partners; test for other STDs.	Topical azole or PO fluconazole.
Complications	Chorioamnionitis/endometritis, infection, preterm delivery, miscarriage, PID.	Same as for bacterial vaginosis.	Oral azoles should be avoided in pregnancy.

[a] If there are many WBCs and no organism on saline smear, suspect *Chlamydia.*

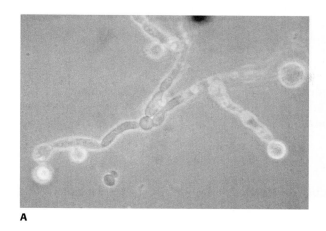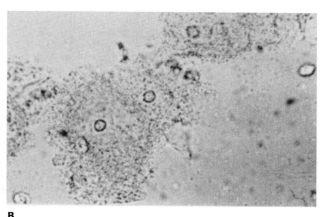

A   **B**

FIGURE 2.12-6.   Causes of vaginitis.

(A) Candidal vaginitis. *Candida albicans* organisms are evident on KOH wet mount. (B) *Gardnerella vaginalis*. Note the granular epithelial cells ("clue cells") and indistinct cell margins. (Image A reproduced, with permission, from Wolff K et al. *Fitzpatrick's Color Atlas & Synopsis of Clinical Dermatology*, 5th ed. New York: McGraw-Hill, 2005: 717. Image B reproduced, with permission, from Kasper DL et al. *Harrison's Principles of Internal Medicine*, 16th ed. New York: McGraw-Hill, 2005: 767.)

- Conduct a thorough examination of the vulva, vaginal walls, and cervix.
- If there are many WBCs and no organism on saline smear, suspect *Chlamydia*.

DIAGNOSIS/TREATMENT

- Samples from the speculum exam should be obtained for vaginal pH, amine ("whiff") test, wet mount (with saline), and 10% hydroxide (KOH) microscopy.
- To rule out cervicitis, DNA tests or cultures for *Neisseria gonorrhoeae* or *Chlamydia trachomatis* should be obtained in patients with a purulent discharge, numerous leukocytes on wet prep, cervical friability, and any symptoms of PID.
- Treatment is etiology specific (see Table 2.12-7).

Cervicitis

- **Inflammation of the uterine cervix.** Because the female genital tract is contiguous from the vulva to the fallopian tubes, there is some overlap between vulvovaginitis and cervicitis. Etiologies are as follows:
    - **Infectious (most common):** *Chlamydia*, gonococcus, *Trichomonas*, HSV, HPV.
    - **Noninfectious:** Trauma, radiation exposure, malignancy.
- **Hx/PE:** Yellow-green mucopurulent discharge; ⊕ **cervical motion tenderness; absence of other signs of PID.**
- **Dx/Tx:** See the discussion of STDs in the Infectious Disease chapter.

Pelvic Inflammatory Disease (PID)

A polymicrobial infection of the **upper genital tract** that is associated with *Neisseria gonorrhoeae* (one-third of cases), *Chlamydia trachomatis* (one-third of cases), and endogenous aerobes/anaerobes. The lifetime risk is 1–3%. Risk

Criteria for the clinical diagnosis of bacterial vaginosis (three of four are required):

- *Abnormal whitish-gray discharge*
- *Vaginal pH > 4.5*
- *Positive amine ("whiff") test*
- *Clue cells comprise > 20% of epithelial cells on wet mount*

IUDs do not ↑ PID risk.

Acute causes of pelvic pain—

A ROPE

Appendicitis
Ruptured ovarian cyst
Ovarian torsion/abscess
PID
Ectopic pregnancy

The chandelier sign is defined as severe cervical motion tenderness that makes the patient "jump for the chandelier" on exam.

factors include non-Caucasian ethnicity, douching, smoking, multiple sex partners, and prior STDs and/or PID.

HISTORY/PE

- Presents with lower abdominal pain, **fever** and chills, menstrual disturbances, and a purulent cervical discharge.
- **Cervical motion tenderness (chandelier sign) and adnexal tenderness** are also seen.

DIAGNOSIS

- Diagnosed by the presence of acute lower abdominal or pelvic pain plus one of the following:
  - Uterine tenderness
  - Adnexal tenderness
  - Cervical motion tenderness
- A WBC count > 10,000 has **poor positive and negative predictive value** for PID.
- Order a β-hCG and ultrasound to rule out pregnancy and to evaluate for the possibility of tubo-ovarian abscess.
- Ultrasound is a noninvasive means of diagnosing PID. Look for:
  - Thickening or dilation of the fallopian tubes
  - Fluid in the cul-de-sac
  - Multicystic ovary
  - Tubo-ovarian abscess

TREATMENT

- **Antibiotic treatment should not be delayed** while awaiting culture results. All sexual partners should be examined and treated appropriately.
- **Outpatient regimens:**
  - **Regimen A:** Ofloxacin **or** levofloxacin × 14 days +/– metronidazole × 14 days.
  - **Regimen B:** Ceftriaxone IM × 1 dose **or** cefoxitin **plus** probenecid **plus** doxycycline × 14 days +/– metronidazole × 14 days.
  - **Inpatient antibiotic regimens:**
    - Cefoxitin or cefotetan plus doxycycline × 14 days.
    - Clindamycin plus gentamicin × 14 days.
- **Surgery:**
  - Drainage of a tubo-ovarian/pelvic abscess is appropriate if the mass persists after antibiotic treatment; the abscess is > 4–6 cm; or the mass is in the cul-de-sac in the midline and drainable through the vagina.
  - If the abscess is dissecting the rectovaginal septum and is fixed to the vaginal membrane, colpotomy drainage is appropriate.
  - If the patient's condition deteriorates, perform exploratory laparotomy.
  - Surgery may range from TAH/BSO with lysis of adhesions in severe cases to conservative surgery for women who desire to maintain fertility.

Mild and subclinical PID is a major cause of tubal factor infertility, ectopic pregnancy, and chronic pelvic pain due to pelvic scarring.

COMPLICATIONS

- Some 25% of women with acute disease develop repeated episodes of infection, chronic pelvic pain, dyspareunia, **ectopic pregnancy,** or **infertility.**
- RUQ pain (Fitz-Hugh–Curtis syndrome) may indicate an associated perihepatitis (abnormal liver function, shoulder pain).
- The risk of infertility ↑ with repeated episodes of salpingitis and is esti-

mated to approach 10% after the first episode, 25% after the second episode, and 50% after a third episode.

Toxic Shock Syndrome (TSS)

Caused by preformed *S. aureus* toxin (TSST-1); often occurs within five days of the onset of a menstrual period in women who have used **tampons**. The incidence in menstruating women is now 6–7:100,000 annually. Nonmenstrual cases are nearly as common as menstrual cases.

HISTORY/PE

- Presents with **abrupt onset of fever, vomiting,** and watery diarrhea, with fever 38.9°C (102°F) or higher.
- A **diffuse macular erythematous rash** is also seen.
- Nonpurulent conjunctivitis is common.
- **Desquamation, especially of the palms and soles,** generally occurs during recovery within 1–2 weeks of illness.

DIAGNOSIS

Blood cultures are ⊖ because symptoms result from preformed toxin and are not due to the invasive properties of the organism.

TSS is a rare but potentially fatal reaction to S. aureus toxin. Diagnosis is clinical because reaction is to the toxin produced by the bacteria, not to the bacterium itself. The first steps in treatment are rapid rehydration and antibiotic treatment.

TREATMENT

- **Rapid rehydration.**
- **Antistaphylococcal drugs** (nafcillin, oxacillin); vancomycin for women with penicillin allergy.
- Corticosteroids can reduce the severity of illness and ↓ fever.
- Manage renal or cardiac failure.

COMPLICATIONS

- The mortality rate associated with TSS is 3–6%.
- Three major causes of death are ARDS, intractable hypotension, and hemorrhage 2° to DIC.

▶ GYNECOLOGIC NEOPLASMS

Gynecologic cancers include uterine, endometrial, ovarian, cervical, and vulvar neoplasms. Ovarian cancer carries the highest mortality.

Uterine Leiomyoma (Fibroids)

The most common **benign** neoplasm of the female genital tract. The tumor is discrete, round, firm, and often multiple and is composed of smooth muscle and connective tissue. Tumors are estrogen and progesterone sensitive, so they often ↑ in size during pregnancy and ↓ after menopause. Malignant transformation to **leiomyosarcoma is rare (0.1–0.5%).** Prevalence is 25% among Caucasian women and 50% among African-American women.

HISTORY/PE

- The majority of cases are asymptomatic.
- Symptomatic patients may present with the following:

Uterine myomas are benign but can cause infertility or menorrhagia.

- **Bleeding:** Longer, heavier periods; anemia.
- **Pressure:** Pelvic pressure and bloating; constipation and rectal pressure; urinary frequency or retention.
- **Pain:** 2° dysmenorrhea, dyspareunia.
- **Pelvic symptoms:** A firm, nontender, irregular enlarged ("lumpy-bumpy"), or cobblestone uterus may be seen.

DIAGNOSIS

If a uterine mass continues to grow after menopause, malignancy must be ruled out with a biopsy.

- **CBC:** To look for anemia.
- **Ultrasound:** To look for **uterine myomas;** can also exclude ovarian masses.
- **MRI:** Can delineate intramural and submucous myomas.

TREATMENT

- **Pharmacologic:**
  - NSAIDs.
  - Combined hormonal contraception.
  - Medroxyprogesterone acetate or danazol to slow or stop bleeding.
  - GnRH analogs (leuprolide or nafarelin) to ↓ **the size of myomas, suppress further growth,** and ↓ **surrounding vascularity.** Also used prior to surgery.
- **Surgery:** Emergent surgery is indicated for torsion of a pedunculated myoma.
  - **Women of childbearing years:** Myomectomy or hysteroscopy with leiomyoma resection.
  - **Women who have completed childbearing:** Total or subtotal abdominal or vaginal hysterectomy.
  - **Uterine artery embolization** (~ 25% will need further invasive treatment).

COMPLICATIONS

Infertility may be due to a myoma that distorts the uterine cavity and plays a role similar to that of an IUD.

Endometrial Cancer

Type I endometrioid adenocarcinomas derive from **atypical endometrial hyperplasia** and are the most common female reproductive cancer in the United States (~35,000 cases/year). Type II cancers derive from serous or clear cell histology (see Table 2.12-8).

HISTORY/PE

Eighty percent of women with endometrial carcinoma have vaginal bleeding, but only 5–10% of women with abnormal vaginal bleeding have endometrial cancer.

- **Type I:** Vaginal bleeding (early finding); pain (late finding); metabolic syndrome.
- **Type II:** No vaginal bleeding.

DIAGNOSIS

- Endometrial/endocervical biopsy.
- Vaginal ultrasound shows a thickened endometrium leading to hypertrophy and neoplastic change.

TABLE 2.12-8.   Types of Endometrial Cancer

	TYPE I: ENDOMETRIOID	TYPE II: SEROUS
Epidemiology	75% of endometrial cancers.	25% of endometrial cancers.
Etiology	Unopposed estrogen stimulation (e.g., tamoxifen use, exogenous estrogen-only therapy).	Unrelated to estrogen; the p53 mutation is present in 90% of cases.
Precursor lesion	Hyperplasia and atypical hyperplasia.	None.
Mean age at diagnosis	55 years.	67 years.
Prognosis	Favorable.	Poor.

TREATMENT

- **Type I:** High-dose progestins for women of childbearing age; TAH/BSO +/– radiation for postmenopausal women.
- **Type II:** TAH/BSO with adjuvant chemotherapy for advanced-stage cancer.

Cervical Cancer

The upper third of the cervix is made up of columnar cells (similar to the lower uterine segment). The lower two-thirds of the cervix is made up of squamous cells (similar to the vagina). The exposure of columnar cells to an acidic vaginal pH results in metaplasia to squamous cells. The **normal squamocolumnar junction (transformation zone)** is located in the ectocervix and can be exposed to carcinogens, resulting in cervical intraepithelial neoplasia (CIN), an abnormal proliferation or overgrowth of the basal cell layer.

- HPV DNA is found in 99.7% of all cervical carcinomas. HPV 16 is the most prevalent type in squamous cell carcinoma; HPV 18 is most prevalent in adenocarcinoma.
- Additional risk factors for cervical cancer include immunosuppression, infection with HIV or a history of STDs, tobacco use, high parity, and OCPs.
- The Gardasil vaccine may protect against HPV types 6, 11, 16, and 18 and may also prevent the development of cervical cancer.

HISTORY/PE

- Metrorrhagia, postcoital spotting, and cervical ulceration are the most common signs.
- A bloody or purulent, malodorous, nonpruritic discharge may appear after invasion.

SCREENING

- Starting at age 21 or no more than three years after becoming sexually active, women should have a **Pap smear with conventional cervical cytology on a yearly basis or liquid-based cervical cytology once every two years.** Table 2.12-9 outlines the classification of Pap smear results.

Hormonal contraceptives are protective against endometrial cancer.

*Screening of asymptomatic women for endometrial cancer is **not** recommended.*

Fifty percent of women with cervical cancer had not had a Pap smear in the three years preceding their diagnosis, and another 10% had not been screened in five years.

HIGH-YIELD FACTS

GYNECOLOGY

TABLE 2.12-9. **Classification Systems for Pap Smears**

NUMERICAL	DYSPLASIA	CIN	BETHESDA SYSTEM
1	Benign	Benign	Normal
2	Benign with inflammation	Benign with inflammation	Normal, atypical squamous cells (ASC)
3	Mild dysplasia	CIN I	LSIL
3	Moderate dysplasia	CIN II	HSIL
3	Severe dysplasia	CIN II	HSIL
4	Carcinoma in situ	CIN II	HSIL
5	Invasive cancer	Invasive cancer	Invasive cancer

- Women ≥ 30 years of age who have had three consecutive normal tests may ↑ their screening interval to once every three years.
- For women ≥ 30 years of age, **HPV DNA testing** for high-risk strands may be used for screening as well.
- Screening should be discontinued for women ≥ 70 years of age who have had three or more normal Pap smears. Women with DES exposure and/or immunocompromised status (including HIV positivity) should continue as long as they do not have a life-limiting condition.
- Women who have had the HPV vaccine should continue cervical cancer screening according to established guidelines.

DIAGNOSIS

- Recent guidelines for the diagnosis and follow-up of cervical cancer distinguish women ≤ 21 from those > 21 years of age for all subtypes of cervical lesions except atypical glandular cells.
- The diagnosis and follow-up of specific subtypes of cervical lesions should thus proceed as follows:
  - **Atypical glandular cells (AGC):**
    - **< 35 years of age with no endometrial cancer risk factors:** Proceed to colposcopy, endocervical curettage (ECC), and HPV DNA testing.
    - **≥ 35 years of age, ⊕ endometrial cancer factors, or abnormal bleeding:** Add an endometrial biopsy.
  - **Atypical squamous cells of undetermined significance (ASC-US):**
    - **≤ 21 years of age:** Repeat Pap smear at 12 months. If Pap smear is ⊖ or reveals ASC-US or LSIL, repeat at 12 months.
    - **> 21 years of age:** Immediate colposcopy, HPV DNA testing, and repeat Pap smear at 6 months.
  - **Low-grade squamous intraepithelial lesions (LSIL):**
    - **≤ 21 years of age:** Same as ASC-US.
    - **> 21 years of age:** Immediate colposcopy.
  - **High-grade squamous intraepithelial lesions (HSIL) or atypical squamous cells suspicious of high-grade dysplasia (ASC-H):** Immediate colposcopy is indicated for **all age groups.**

- **Treatment is based on findings of colposcopy:**
    - If colposcopy is satisfactory, proceed to treatment based on findings.
    - If colposcopy is unsatisfactory, perform ECC and cervical biopsy and proceed to treatment based on findings.

TREATMENT

- **Noninvasive disease:** Treatment based on biopsy results for noninvasive lesions (stage 0 disease) is as follows (see Figure 2.12-7):
    - **CIN I:**
        - Untreated CIN I will regress in 60% of patients, progress in 10%, and persist in 30%. Thus, the mainstay of treatment for CIN I is **close observation.**
        - For women **> 21 years of age**, Pap smear screening at 6 and 12 months and/or HPV DNA testing at 12 months is indicated. For women **≤ 21 years of age, HPV testing is not recommended.**
        - After two ⊖ Pap smears or a ⊖ DNA test, patients can be managed with routine annual follow-up.
        - Persistent CIN I can be treated with **ablative** (cryotherapy or laser ablation) or **excisional therapy** (loop electrosurgical excision procedure [LEEP]; laser and cold-knife conization).

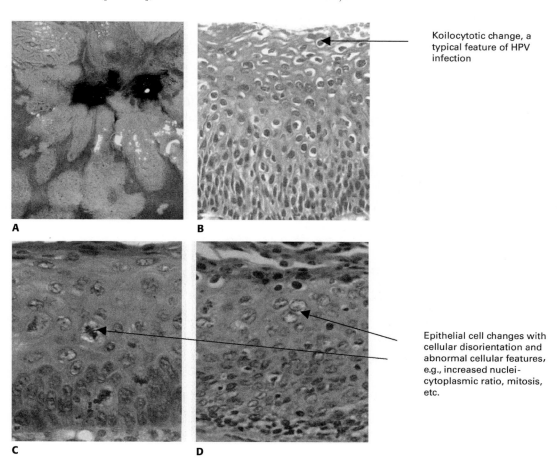

Koilocytotic change, a typical feature of HPV infection

Epithelial cell changes with cellular disorientation and abnormal cellular features, e.g., increased nuclei-cytoplasmic ratio, mitosis, etc.

A   B   C   D

FIGURE 2.12-7. Cervical intraepithelial neoplasia.

(A) Colpophotograph illustrating a low-grade cervical intraepithelial neoplasia (CIN) in the transformation zone. (B)–(D).Histopathology of CIN I, II, and III. (Reproduced, with permission, from Kantarjian HM et al. *MD Anderson Manual of Medical Oncology,* 1st ed. New York: McGraw-Hill: Fig. 24-4.)

- **CIN II and III:**
    - Untreated CIN II will regress in 43% of patients, progress in 22%, and persist in 35%. Untreated CIN III will regress in 32% of patients, progress in 14%, and persist in 56%.
    - CIN II and III should be treated with **ablative** (cryotherapy or laser ablation) or **excisional therapy** (LEEP; laser and cold-knife conization).
    - Hysterectomy is a treatment option for recurrent CIN II or III.
    - Postablative or excisional therapy follow-up is as follows:
        - **CIN I, II, or III with ⊖ margins:** Pap smear at 12 months and/or HPV testing.
        - **CIN II or III with ⊕ margins:** Pap smear at 6 months; consider repeat ECC.
        - If margins are unknown, obtain a Pap smear at 6 months and HPV DNA testing at 12 months.
- **Invasive disease:** Treatment based on biopsy results for **invasive carcinoma** is as follows (for staging, see Figure 2.12-8):
    - **Microinvasive carcinoma (stage IA1):** Treat with cone biopsy and close follow-up or simple hysterectomy.
    - **Stages IA2, IB1, and IIA:** May be treated either with radical hysterectomy with concomitant radiation and chemotherapy or with radiation plus chemotherapy alone.
    - **Stages IB2, IIB, III, and IV:** Treat with radiation therapy plus concurrent cisplatin-based chemotherapy.

PROGNOSIS

- The overall five-year relative survival rate for carcinoma of the cervix is 68% in Caucasian women and 55% in African-American women.

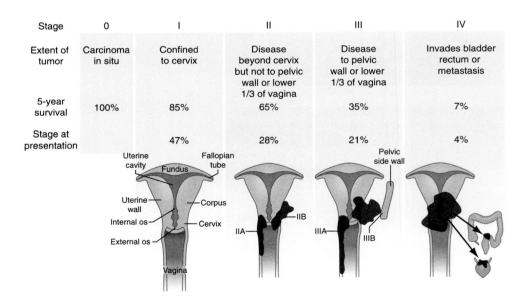

FIGURE 2.12-8. **Staging of cervical cancer.**

Anatomic display of the stages of cervix cancer, defined by location, extent of tumor, frequency of presentation, and five-year survival. (Reproduced, with permission, from Fauci AS et al. *Harrison's Principles of Internal Medicine*, 17th ed. New York: McGraw-Hill, 2008: Fig. 93-1.)

- Survival rates are inversely proportionate to the stage of cancer:
  - **Stage 0:** 99–100%.
  - **Stage IA:** > 95%.
  - **Stage IB-IIA:** 80–90%.
  - **Stage IIB:** 65%.
  - **Stage III:** 40%.
  - **Stage IV:** < 20%.
- Almost two-thirds of patients with untreated carcinoma of the cervix die of uremia when ureteral obstruction is bilateral.

Vulvar Cancer

Responsible for 1–4% of gynecologic malignancies. Some 90–95% are squamous lesions occurring in women > 50 years of age, followed by melanoma, basal cell carcinoma, adenocarcinoma, sarcoma, Bartholin's gland tumors, and metastatic disease. Risk factors include **HPV (types 16, 18, and 31)**, lichen sclerosus, infrequent medical exams, diabetes, obesity, hypertension, cardiovascular disease, and immunosuppression.

HISTORY/PE

- Presents with pruritus, pain, or ulceration of the mass.
- **Early:** Lesions may appear white, pigmented, raised, thickened, nodular, or ulcerative.
- **Late:** Presents with a large, cauliflower-like or hard ulcerated area in the vulva.

DIAGNOSIS

- The first step is vulvar punch biopsy for any suspicious lesions.
- Vulvar intraepithelial neoplasia (VIN) is considered precancerous and more commonly occurs in premenopausal women.
  - **VIN I and II:** Associated with mild and moderate dysplasia.
  - **VIN III:** Carcinoma in situ.

TREATMENT

- **Precancerous lesions:** Reduce irritative or other predisposing causes. Topical corticosteroids (e.g., betamethasone, clobetasol) and crotamiton are particularly effective for pruritus.
- **High-grade VIN:** Topical chemotherapy, laser ablation, wide local excision, skinning vulvectomy, and simple vulvectomy.
- **Invasive:** Treated with (1) radical vulvectomy and regional lymphadenectomy or (2) wide local excision of the 1° tumor with inguinal lymph node dissection +/− preoperative radiation, chemotherapy, or both.

Vaginal Cancer

Accounts for 1–2% of all gynecologic malignancies. Squamous cell carcinoma usually occurs in postmenopausal woman, whereas other histologic types (rhabdosarcoma, endodermal sinus tumor, adenocarcinoma, and clear cell adenocarcinoma from DES) usually affect younger women. Risk factors include immunosuppression, chronic irritation (e.g., long-term pessary use or prolapse of female organs), low socioeconomic status, radiation for cervical cancer, hysterectomy for dysplasia, multiple sexual partners, and DES exposure.

HISTORY/PE

- Characterized by abnormal vaginal bleeding, an abnormal discharge, or postcoital bleeding.
- Presents in the upper third of the vagina in 75% of patients.

DIAGNOSIS

Cytology, colposcopy, and biopsy.

TREATMENT

- Local excision of involved areas when they are few and small.
- Extensive involvement of the vaginal mucosa may require partial or complete vaginectomy.
- Invasive disease requires radiation therapy or radical surgery.

Ovarian Cancer

Most ovarian tumors are benign, but malignant tumors are the leading cause of death from reproductive tract cancer. Risk factors include the following:

- Age, low parity, ↓ fertility, or delayed childbearing.
- A ⊕ family history. Patients with one affected first-degree relative have a 5% lifetime risk. With two or more affected first-degree relatives, the risk is 7%.
- The *BRCA1* mutation carries a 45% lifetime risk of ovarian cancer. The *BRCA2* mutation is associated with a 25% lifetime risk.
- **Lynch II syndrome,** or hereditary nonpolyposis colorectal cancer (HNPCC), is associated with an ↑ risk of colon, ovarian, endometrial, and breast cancer.
- **OCPs** taken for five years or more ↓ risk by 29%.

HISTORY/PE

- Both benign and malignant ovarian neoplasms are generally asymptomatic.
- Mild, nonspecific GI symptoms or pelvic pressure/pain may be seen.
- Early disease is typically not detected on routine pelvic exam.
- Some 75% of woman present with **advanced malignant disease,** as evidenced by abdominal pain and bloating, a palpable abdominal mass, and ascites.
- Table 2.12-10 differentiates the benign and malignant characteristics of pelvic masses.

DIAGNOSIS

- **Tumor markers** (see Table 2.12-11): ↑ **CA-125** is associated with epithelial cell cancer (90% of ovarian cancers) but is used only as a marker for progression and recurrence.
  - **Premenopausal women:** ↑ CA-125 may point to benign disease such as endometriosis.
  - **Postmenopausal women:** ↑ CA-125 (> 35 units) indicates an ↑ likelihood that the ovarian tumor is malignant.
- **Transvaginal ultrasound:** Used to screen **high-risk women.**

Frequency of female genital tract cancers: endometrial > ovarian > cervical. Number of deaths: ovarian > endometrial > cervical.

Any palpable ovarian or adnexal mass in a premenarchal or postmenopausal patient is suggestive of an ovarian neoplasm.

TABLE 2.12-10.   **Benign vs. Malignant Pelvic Masses**

FINDING	BENIGN	MALIGNANT
Exam: pelvic mass		
Mobility	Mobile	Fixed
Consistency	Cystic	Solid or firm
Location	Unilateral	Bilateral
Cul-de-sac	Smooth	Nodular
Transvaginal ultrasound: **adnexal mass**		
Size	< 8 cm	> 8 cm
Consistency	Cystic	Solid or cystic and solid
Septations	Unilocular	Multilocular
Location	Unilateral	Bilateral
Other	Calcifications	Ascites

TREATMENT

Treatment of **ovarian masses** is as follows:

- **Premenarchal women:** Masses > 2 cm require exploratory laparotomy.
- **Premenopausal women:**
  - Observation for 4–6 weeks is sufficient for asymptomatic, mobile, unilateral, simple cystic masses < 8–10 cm. Most resolve spontaneously.
  - Surgical evaluation is warranted for masses > 8–10 cm as well as for those that are unchanged on repeat pelvic exam and ultrasound.
- **Postmenopausal women:**
  - Asymptomatic, unilateral simple cysts < 5 cm in diameter with a **normal CA-125** should be **closely followed with ultrasound.**
  - Palpable masses warrant surgical evaluation by exploratory laparotomy.

Treatment of **ovarian cancer** is as follows:

- **Surgery:**
  - Surgical staging followed by TAH/BSO with omentectomy and pelvic and para-aortic lymphadenectomy.

TABLE 2.12-11.   **Ovarian Tumor Markers**

TUMOR	MARKER
Epithelial	CA-125
Endodermal sinus	AFP
Embryonal carcinoma	AFP, hCG
Choriocarcinoma	hCG
Dysgerminoma	LDH
Granulosa cell	Inhibin

HIGH-YIELD FACTS

GYNECOLOGY

- Benign neoplasms warrant tumor removal or unilateral oophorectomy.
- **Postoperative chemotherapy** is routine except for women with early-stage or low-grade ovarian cancer.
- Radiation therapy is effective for dysgerminomas.

PREVENTION

- Women with the *BRCA1* gene mutation should be screened annually with ultrasound and CA-125 testing. Prophylactic oophorectomy is recommended by age 35 or whenever childbearing is completed.
- OCP use ↓ risk.

▶ PELVIC ORGAN PROLAPSE

Risk factors for pelvic organ prolapse include vaginal birth (particularly with use of forceps), genetic predisposition, advancing age, prior pelvic surgery, connective tissue disorders, and ↑ intra-abdominal pressure associated with obesity or straining with chronic constipation.

HISTORY/PE

- Presents with the sensation of a bulge or protrusion in the vagina.
- Urinary or fecal incontinence, a sense of incomplete bladder emptying, and dyspareunia are also seen.

DIAGNOSIS

The degree of prolapse can be evaluated by having the woman perform the Valsalva maneuver while in the lithotomy position.

TREATMENT

- Supportive measures include a high-fiber diet and weight reduction in obese patients and limitation of straining and lifting.
- Pessaries may temporarily reduce prolapse and are helpful in women who do not wish to undergo surgery or who are chronically ill.
- The most common surgical procedure is vaginal or abdominal hysterectomy with vaginal vault suspension.

▶ URINARY INCONTINENCE

Defined as the involuntary loss of urine due to either bladder or sphincteric dysfunction.

HISTORY/PE

- Table 2.12-12 outlines the types of incontinence along with their distinguishing features and treatment (see also the mnemonic **DIAPPERS**).
- Exclude fistula in cases of total incontinence. Look for neurologic abnormalities in cases of urge incontinence (spasticity, flaccidity, rectal sphincter tone) or distended bladder in overflow incontinence.

DIAGNOSIS/TREATMENT

- **First step:** Obtain a UA and urine culture to exclude UTI.
- **Next step:**
  - Voiding diary; possible urodynamic testing.

Causes of urinary incontinence without specific urogenital pathology—

DIAPPERS

Delirium/confusional state
Infection
Atrophic urethritis/ vaginitis
Pharmaceutical
Psychiatric causes (especially depression)
Excessive urinary output (hyperglycemia, hypercalcemia, CHF)
Restricted mobility
Stool impaction

TABLE 2.12-12. **Types of Incontinence**

TYPE	HISTORY OF URINE LOSS	MECHANISM	TREATMENT
Total	Uncontrolled loss at all times and in all positions.	Loss of sphincteric efficiency (previous surgery, nerve damage, cancer infiltration). Abnormal connection between the urinary tract and the skin (fistula).	Surgery.
Stress	After ↑ intra-abdominal pressure (coughing, sneezing, lifting).	Urethral sphincteric insufficiency due to laxity of pelvic floor musculature; common in multiparous women or after pelvic surgery.	Kegel exercises and pessary. Vaginal vault suspension surgery.
Urge[a]	Strong, unexpected urge to void that is unrelated to position or activity.	Detrusor hyperreflexia or sphincter dysfunction due to inflammatory conditions or neurogenic disorders of the bladder.	Anticholinergic medications or TCAs; behavioral training (biofeedback).
Overflow[b]	Chronic urinary retention.	Chronically distended bladder with ↑ intravesical pressure that just exceeds the outlet resistance, allowing a small amount of urine to dribble out.	Placement of urethral catheter in acute settings. Treat underlying diseases. Timed voiding.

[a] Etiologies include inhibited contractions, local irritation (cystitis, stone, tumor), and CNS causes.

[b] Etiologies include physical agents (tumor, stricture), neurologic factors (lesions), and medications.

- Serum creatinine to exclude renal dysfunction.
- Cystogram to demonstrate fistula sites and descensus of the bladder neck.
- Table 2.12-12 outlines treatment options according to subtype.

▶ BREAST DISORDERS

Fibrocystic Change

The most common of all benign breast conditions. Involves exaggerated stromal tissue response to hormones and growth factors. Findings include cysts (gross and microscopic), papillomatosis, adenosis, fibrosis, and ductal epithelial hyperplasia. Primarily affects women 30–50 years of age; rarely found in postmenopausal woman. Associated with trauma and caffeine use.

HISTORY/PE

- Presents with cyclic bilateral mastalgia and swelling, with symptoms most prominent just before menstruation.
- Rapid **fluctuation** in the size of the masses is common.
- Other symptoms include an irregular, bumpy consistency to the breast tissue ("oatmeal with raisins").

The differential diagnosis of a breast mass includes fibrocystic disease, fibroadenoma, mastitis/abscess, fat necrosis, and breast cancer.

DIAGNOSIS

- See Figure 2.12-9 for an algorithm of a breast mass workup.
- Mammography is of limited use. Ultrasound can help differentiate a cystic from a solid mass.
- Fine-needle aspiration (FNA) of a discrete mass that is suggestive of a cyst is indicated to alleviate pain as well as to confirm the cystic nature of the mass.
- Perform an excisional biopsy if no fluid is obtained or if the fluid is bloody on aspiration.
- There is an ↑ risk of **breast cancer** if ductal epithelial hyperplasia or cellular atypia is present.

TREATMENT

- Dietary modifications (e.g., caffeine restriction).
- Danazol may be given for severe pain but is rarely used in view of its side effects (acne, hirsutism, edema).
- Consider use of OCPs, which ↓ hormonal fluctuations.

Fibroadenoma

A benign, slow-growing breast tumor with epithelial and stromal components. **The most common breast lesion in women < 30 years of age.** Cystosarcoma phyllodes is a large fibroadenoma.

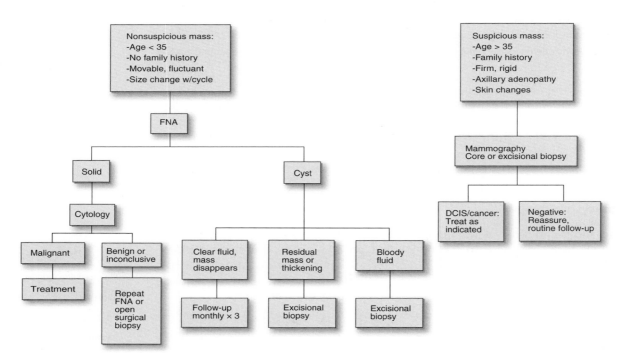

FIGURE 2.12-9.   Workup of a breast mass.

- Presents as a round or ovoid, rubbery, discrete, relatively mobile, non-tender mass 1–3 cm in diameter.
- Usually solitary, although up to 20% of patients develop multiple fibroadenomas.
- Tumors do not change during the menstrual cycle.
- Does not occur after menopause unless the patient is on HRT.

DIAGNOSIS

- **Breast ultrasound** can differentiate cystic from solid masses.
- **Needle biopsy or FNA.**
- Excision with pathologic exam if the diagnosis remains uncertain.

TREATMENT

Excision is curative, but recurrence is common.

Breast Cancer

The most common cancer (affects one in eight women) and the second most common cause of cancer death in women (after lung cancer). **Sixty percent occur in the upper outer quadrant.** Risk factors include the following (**most women have no risk factors**):

- Female gender, older age.
- A personal history of breast cancer.
- Breast cancer in a first-degree relative.
- *BRCA1* and *BRCA2* mutations (associated with early onset).
- A high-fat and low-fiber diet.
- A history of fibrocystic change with cellular atypia.
- ↑ exposure to estrogen (nulliparity, early menarche, late menopause, first full-term pregnancy after age 35).

↑ *exposure to estrogen (early menarche, late menopause, nulliparity) ↑ the risk of breast cancer.*

HISTORY/PE

Ninety percent of breast cancers are found by the patient. Clinical manifestations include the following:

- **Early findings:** May present as a single, nontender, firm-to-hard mass with ill-defined margins or as mammographic abnormalities with no palpable mass.
- **Later findings:** Skin or nipple retraction, axillary lymphadenopathy, breast enlargement, redness, edema, pain, fixation of the mass to the skin or chest wall.
- **Late findings:**
  - Ulceration; supraclavicular lymphadenopathy; edema of the arm; metastases to the bone, lung, and liver.
  - Prolonged unilateral scaling erosion of the nipple with or without discharge (Paget's disease of the nipple).
- **Metastatic disease:**
  - Back or bone pain, jaundice, weight loss.
  - A firm or hard axillary node > 1 cm.
  - Axillary nodes that are matted or fixed to the skin (stage III); ipsilateral supraclavicular or infraclavicular nodes (stage IV).

DIAGNOSIS

- Diagnostic measures differ for postmenopausal and premenopausal women.
  - **Postmenopausal women:** The first step is **mammography.** Look for ↑ density with microcalcifications and irregular borders. Mammography can detect lesions roughly two years before they become clinically palpable (see Figure 2.12-10A).
  - **Premenopausal women:** The first step for women < 30 years of age is **ultrasound,** which can distinguish a solid mass from a benign cyst (see Figure 2.12-10B).
- Additional measures include the following:
  - **Tumor markers for recurrent breast cancer:** Include **CEA and CA 15-3 or CA 27-29.**
  - **Receptor status of tumor:** Determine estrogen receptor (ER), progesterone receptor (PR), and *HER2/neu* status.
  - **Metastatic disease:**
    - **Labs:** ↑ ESR, ↑ alkaline phosphatase (liver and bone metastases), ↑ calcium.
    - **Imaging:** CXR; CT of the chest, abdomen, pelvis, and brain; bone scan.

TREATMENT

- **Pharmacologic:**
  - **All hormone receptor–⊕ patients should receive tamoxifen.**
  - **ER-⊖ patients should receive chemotherapy.**
  - **Trastuzumab,** a monoclonal antibody that binds to *HER2/neu* receptors on the cancer cell, is highly effective in *HER2/neu*-expressive cancers.
- **Surgical options** include the following:
  - Partial mastectomy (lumpectomy) plus axillary dissection followed by radiation therapy.
  - Modified radical mastectomy (total mastectomy plus axillary dissection).
  - **Contraindications to breast-conserving therapy** include large tumor size, subareolar location, multifocal tumors, fixation to the chest wall, or involvement of the nipple or overlying skin.
  - **Stage IV disease** should be treated with radiotherapy and hormonal therapy; mastectomy may be required for local symptom control.

PROGNOSIS

- **TNM staging (I–IV) is the most reliable indicator of prognosis.**
- ER- and PR-⊕ status is associated with a favorable course.
- Cancer localized to the breast has a 75–90% cure rate. With spread to the axilla, the five-year survival is 40–50%.
- Aneuploidy is associated with a poor prognosis.

COMPLICATIONS

Pleural effusion occurs in 50% of patients with metastatic breast cancer; edema of the arm is common.

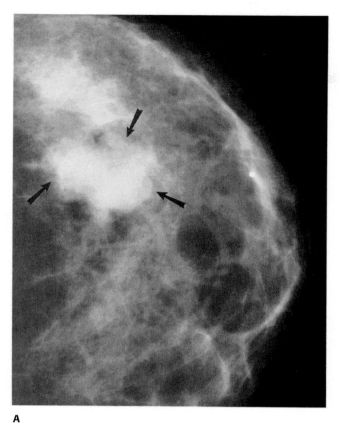

A

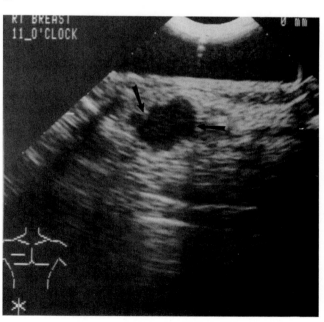

B

FIGURE 2.12-10. **Palpable breast mass on mammography and ultrasound.**

(A) Craniocaudal mammography of a palpable mass (arrows). (B) Ultrasound image demonstrating a solid mass with irregular borders (arrows) consistent with cancer. (Reproduced, with permission, from Brunicardi FC et al. *Schwartz's Principles of Surgery*, 8th ed. New York: McGraw-Hill, 2005: Fig. 16-26.)

HIGH-YIELD FACTS

GYNECOLOGY

Pediatrics

Also known as nonaccidental trauma; includes neglect as well as physical, sexual, and psychological maltreatment of children. Suspect abuse if the history is discordant with physical findings or if there is a delay in obtaining appropriate medical care. Certain injuries in children such as retinal hemorrhages and specific fracture types are pathognomonic for abuse.

HISTORY/PE

- Abuse or neglect in infants may present as apnea, seizures, feeding intolerance, excessive irritability or somnolence, or failure to thrive (FTT).
- Neglect in older children may present as poor hygiene or behavioral abnormalities.
- Exam findings may include the following:
    - Injuries in atypical places (e.g., the face or thighs) or patterns (stocking-glove burns, cigarette burns, belt marks).
    - Spiral fractures of the humerus and femur (strongly suggest abuse in children < 3 years of age) or epiphyseal/metaphyseal "bucket fractures," which suggest shaking or jerking of the child's limbs.
    - Posterior rib fractures.
    - Genital trauma, bleeding, or discharge.

Consider abuse if the caretaker's story and the child's injuries don't match.

DIAGNOSIS

- Rule out conditions that mimic abuse—e.g., bleeding disorders or Mongolian spots (bruises), osteogenesis imperfecta (fractures), bullous impetigo (cigarette burns), and "coining" (an alternative treatment in certain cultures).
- A skeletal survey and bone scan can show **fractures in various stages of healing.**
- Test for gonorrhea, syphilis, chlamydia, and HIV if sexual abuse is suspected.
- Rule out shaken baby syndrome (SBS) by performing an ophthalmologic exam for retinal hemorrhages and a noncontrast CT for subdural hematomas. Infants with SBS often do not exhibit external signs of abuse.
- Consider an MRI to visualize white matter changes (diffuse axonal injury associated with violent shaking) and the extent of intra- and extracranial bleeds. MRI often requires the young patient to be sedated and/or intubated, while CT usually does not.

TREATMENT

- Document injuries, including location, size, shape, color, and the nature of all lesions, bruises, or burns.
- Notify child protective services (CPS) for evaluation and possible removal of the child from the home.
- Hospitalize if necessary to stabilize injuries or to protect the child.

Reporting any suspicion of child abuse is mandatory; you cannot be sued for doing so.

▶ **CONGENITAL HEART DISEASE**

Intrauterine risk factors for congenital heart disease include maternal drug use (alcohol, lithium, thalidomide, phenytoin), maternal infections (rubella), and maternal illness (DM, PKU). Disease is classified by the presence or absence of cyanosis:

VSD is the most common congenital heart defect.

- **Acyanotic conditions ("pink babies"):** Have left-to-right shunts in which oxygenated blood from the lungs is shunted back into the pulmonary circulation.
- **Cyanotic conditions ("blue babies"):** Have right-to-left shunts in which deoxygenated blood is shunted into the systemic circulation.

Ventricular Septal Defect (VSD)

A condition in which an opening in the ventricular septum allows blood to flow between ventricles. VSD is the **most common congenital heart defect.** It is more common among patients with Apert's syndrome (cranial deformities, fusion of the fingers and toes), Down syndrome, fetal alcohol syndrome, TORCH syndrome (toxoplasmosis, other agents, rubella, CMV, HSV), cri du chat syndrome, and trisomies 13 and 18.

HISTORY/PE

- Small defects are usually asymptomatic at birth, but exam reveals a **harsh holosystolic murmur** heard best at the lower left sternal border.
- Large defects can present with **frequent respiratory infections, dyspnea, FTT, and CHF.** If present, the holosystolic murmur is softer and more blowing but can be accompanied by a systolic thrill, crackles, a narrow S_2 with an ↑ P_1, and a mid-diastolic apical rumble reflecting ↑ flow across the mitral valve.

DIAGNOSIS

Echocardiogram is diagnostic. ECG and CXR can demonstrate LVH with small defects and show both LVH and RVH with larger VSDs. CXR may show ↑ pulmonary vascular markings.

TREATMENT

- Most small VSDs close spontaneously; patients should be monitored via echocardiography.
- Surgical repair is indicated in symptomatic patients who fail medical management, children < 1 year of age with signs of pulmonary hypertension, and older children with large VSDs that have not ↓ in size over time.
- Treat existing CHF with diuretics, inotropes, and ACEIs; treat respiratory infections as needed.

Atrial Septal Defect (ASD)

A condition in which an opening in the atrial septum allows blood to flow between the atria, leading to left-to-right shunting. Associated with Holt-Oram syndrome (absent radii, ASD, first-degree heart block), fetal alcohol syndrome, and Down syndrome.

HISTORY/PE

- Ostium primum defects present in early childhood with findings of a murmur or fatigue with exertion. Ostium secundum defects (most common) tend to present in late childhood or early adulthood. Symptom onset and severity depend on the size of the defect.
- Symptoms of easy fatigability, frequent respiratory infections, and FTT can be observed, but patients are **frequently asymptomatic.**

ASD has a fixed, widely split S_2.

- Exam reveals a right ventricular heave; a **wide and fixed, split S$_2$**; and a systolic ejection murmur at the upper left sternal border (from ↑ flow across the pulmonary valve). There may also be a mid-diastolic rumble at the left lower sternal border.

DIAGNOSIS

- Echocardiogram with color flow Doppler reveals blood flow between the atria (diagnostic), paradoxical ventricular wall motion, and a dilated right ventricle.
- ECG most commonly shows right axis deviation and RVH, although other patterns are possible depending on the type of defect. PR prolongation is common.
- CXR reveals cardiomegaly and ↑ pulmonary vascular markings.

TREATMENT

- Most lesions are small defects that may close spontaneously and do not require treatment.
- Surgical closure is indicated in infants with CHF and in patients with more than a 2:1 ratio of pulmonary to systemic blood flow. Early correction prevents complications such as arrhythmias, right ventricular dysfunction, and Eisenmenger's syndrome.

Patent Ductus Arteriosus (PDA)

Failure of the ductus arteriosus to close in the first few days of life, leading to a left-to-right shunt from the aorta to the pulmonary artery. Risk factors include maternal first-trimester **rubella** infection, prematurity, and female gender.

HISTORY/PE

- Typically asymptomatic; patients with large defects may present with FTT, recurrent lower respiratory tract infections, lower extremity clubbing, and CHF.
- Exam reveals a wide pulse pressure; a **continuous "machinery murmur"** at the second left intercostal space at the sternal border; a loud S$_2$; and bounding peripheral pulses.

DIAGNOSIS

- A color flow Doppler demonstrating blood flow from the aorta into the pulmonary artery is diagnostic.
- With larger PDAs, echocardiography shows left atrial and left ventricular enlargement.
- ECG may show LVH, and CXR may show cardiomegaly if large lesions.

TREATMENT

- Give indomethacin unless the PDA is needed for survival (e.g., transposition of the great vessels, tetralogy of Fallot, hypoplastic left heart) or if indomethacin is contraindicated (e.g., intraventricular hemorrhage).
- If indomethacin fails or if the child is > 6–8 months of age, surgical closure is required.

In Eisenmenger's syndrome, left-to-right shunt leads to pulmonary hypertension and shunt reversal.

In infants presenting in a shocklike state within the first few weeks of life, look for:
1. Sepsis
2. Inborn error of metabolism
3. Ductal-dependent congenital heart disease, usually left-sided lesions (as the ductus is closing)
4. Congenital adrenal hyperplasia

Come **IN** and **CLOSE** the door: give **IN**domethacin to **CLOSE** a PDA.

What maternally ingested drug is associated with **Ebstein's anomaly** (tricuspid valve displacement into the right ventricle)? Lithium.

Coarctation of the Aorta

Constriction of a portion of the aorta, leading to ↑ flow proximal to and ↓ flow distal to the coarctation. Occurs just below the left subclavian artery in 98% of patients. The condition is associated with **Turner's** syndrome, berry aneurysms, and male gender. **More than two-thirds of patients have a bicuspid aortic valve.**

Coarctation is a cause of 2°
hypertension in children.

HISTORY/PE

- Often presents in childhood with **asymptomatic hypertension.**
- Lower extremity claudication, syncope, epistaxis, and headache may be present.
- The classic physical exam finding is a systolic BP that is higher in the upper extremities; the difference in BP between the left and right arm can indicate the point of coarctation.
- Additional findings include weak femoral pulses, radiofemoral delay, a short systolic murmur in the left axilla, and a forceful apical impulse.
- In infancy, critical coarctation requires a patent PDA for survival. Such infants may present in the first few weeks of life in a shocklike state when the PDA closes. Differential cyanosis may be seen with lower oxygen saturation in the left arm and lower extremities (postductal areas) as compared to the right arm (preductal area).

DIAGNOSIS

- Echocardiography and color flow Doppler are diagnostic.
- CXR in young children may demonstrate cardiomegaly and pulmonary congestion.
- In older children, the following compensatory changes may be seen: LVH on ECG; the **"3" sign on CXR** due to pre- and postdilatation of the coarctation segment with aortic wall indentation; and **"rib notching"** due to collateral circulation through the intercostal arteries.

TREATMENT

- If severe coarctation presents in infancy, the ductus arteriosus should be kept open with prostaglandin E_1 (PGE_1).
- Surgical correction or balloon angioplasty (controversial).
- Monitor for restenosis, aneurysm development, and aortic dissection.

Transposition of the Great Vessels

The most common cyanotic congenital heart lesion in the newborn. In this condition, the aorta is connected to the right ventricle and the pulmonary artery to the left ventricle, creating parallel pulmonary and systemic circulations. **Without a septal defect or a PDA, it is incompatible with life.** Risk factors include diabetic mothers and, rarely, DiGeorge syndrome (see the mnemonic **CATCH 22**).

DiGeorge
syndrome–

CATCH 22

Cardiac abnormalities
Abnormal facies
Thymic aplasia
Cleft palate
Hypocalcemia
22q11 deletion

HISTORY/PE

- Critical illness and cyanosis typically occur immediately after birth. Reverse differential cyanosis may be seen if left ventricular outflow tract obstruction (e.g., coarctation, aortic stenosis) is also present.

- Exam reveals tachypnea, progressive hypoxemia, and extreme cyanosis. Some patients have signs of CHF, and a single loud S_2 is often present. There may not be a murmur if no VSD is present.

DIAGNOSIS

- Echocardiography.
- CXR may show a narrow heart base, absence of the main pulmonary artery segment ("egg-shaped silhouette"), and ↑ pulmonary vascular markings.

TREATMENT

- Start IV PGE_1 to maintain or open the PDA.
- If surgery is not feasible within the first few days of life or if the PDA cannot be maintained with prostaglandin, perform balloon atrial septostomy to create or enlarge an ASD.
- Surgical correction (arterial or atrial switch).

Tetralogy of Fallot

Consists of pulmonary stenosis, overriding aorta, RVH, and VSD. **The most common cyanotic congenital heart disease in children.** Early cyanosis results from right-to-left shunting across the VSD. As right-sided pressures ↓ in the weeks after birth, the shunt direction reverses and cyanosis may ↓. If the degree of pulmonary stenosis is severe, the right-sided pressures may remain high and cyanosis may worsen over time. Risk factors include maternal PKU and DiGeorge syndrome.

HISTORY/PE

- Presents in infancy or early childhood with dyspnea and fatigability. Cyanosis is often not present at birth but develops over the first two years of life; the degree of cyanosis often reflects the extent of pulmonary stenosis.
- Infants are often asymptomatic until 4–6 months of age, when CHF may develop and may manifest as diaphoresis with feeding or tachypnea.
- Children often squat for relief (↑ systemic vascular resistance) during hypoxemic episodes ("tet spells").
- Hypoxemia may lead to FTT or mental status changes.
- Exam reveals a systolic ejection murmur at the left upper sternal border (right ventricular outflow obstruction), a right ventricular heave, and a single S_2.

DIAGNOSIS

- Echocardiography and catheterization.
- CXR shows a "boot-shaped" heart with ↓ pulmonary vascular markings. Remember that a VSD may result in ↑ pulmonary vascular markings.
- ECG shows right-axis deviation and RVH.

TREATMENT

- Lesions with severe pulmonary stenosis or atresia require immediate PGE_1 to keep the PDA open along with urgent surgical consultation.
- Treat hypercyanotic "tet spells" with O_2, propranolol, phenylephrine, knee-chest position, fluids, and morphine.
- Temporary palliation can be achieved through the creation of an artificial shunt (e.g., balloon atrial septostomy) before definitive surgical correction (Blalock-Taussig shunt).

*Coarctation in infancy may present with differential cyanosis, while transposition of the great arteries may present with **reverse** differential cyanosis.*

> **Tetralogy of Fallot—**
>
> **PROVe**
>
> **P**ulmonary stenosis
> **R**VH
> **O**verriding aorta
> **V**SD

*Transposition of the great vessels is the most common cyanotic heart disease of **newborns.** Tetralogy of Fallot is the most common cyanotic heart disease of **childhood.***

Both transposition of the great vessels and tetralogy of Fallot are initially treated with PGE_1 and are definitively treated with surgical correction.

Developmental Milestones

Table 2.13-1 highlights major developmental milestones. Commonly tested milestones appear in bold.

TABLE 2.13-1. **Developmental Milestones**

Ageª	Gross Motor	Fine Motor	Language	Social/Cognitive
2 months	**Lifts head/chest when prone.**	Tracks past midline.	Alerts to sound; coos.	Recognizes parent; **social smile.**
4–5 months	**Rolls front to back,** back to front (5 months).	Grasps rattle.	Orients to voice; begins to make consonant sounds; razzes.	Enjoys looking around; laughs.
6 months	Sits unassisted.	Transfers objects; raking grasp.	Babbles.	**Stranger anxiety.**
9–10 months	Crawls; pulls to stand.	Uses **three-finger (immature) pincer grasp.**	Says "mama/dada" (nonspecific).	Waves bye-bye; plays pat-a-cake.
12 months	Cruises (11 months); **walks alone.**	Uses **two-finger (mature) pincer grasp.**	Says "mama/dada" (specific).	Imitates actions; **separation anxiety.**
15 months	Walks backward.	Uses cup.	Uses 4–6 words.	Temper tantrums.
18 months	Runs; kicks a ball.	Builds tower of 2–4 cubes.	Names common objects.	May start toilet training.
2 years	Walks up/down steps with help; jumps.	Builds tower of six cubes.	Uses **two-word phrases.**	Follows two-step commands; removes clothes.
3 years	Rides tricycle; climbs stairs with alternating feet (3–4 years).	Copies a circle; uses utensils.	Uses **three-word sentences.**	Brushes teeth with help; washes/dries hands.
4 years	Hops.	Copies a square.	Knows colors and some numbers.	Cooperative play; plays board games.
5 years	Skips; walks backward for long distances.	Ties shoelaces; knows left and right; prints letters.	Uses five-word sentences.	Domestic role playing; plays dress-up.

ª For premature infants < 2 years of age, chronological age must be adjusted for gestational age. For example, an infant born at seven months' gestation (two months early) would be expected to perform at the four-month level at the chronological age of six months.

Growth

At each well-child check, height, weight, and head circumference are plotted on growth charts specific for gender and age:

- **Head circumference:** Measured routinely in the first two years. ↑ head circumference can indicate hydrocephalus or tumor; ↓ head circumference can point to microcephaly (e.g., TORCH infections).
- **Height and weight:** Measured routinely until adulthood. The pattern of growth is more important than the raw numbers. Infants may lose 5–10% of birth weight (BW) over the first few days but should return to their BW by 14 days. Infants can be expected to double their BW by 4–5 months, triple by one year, and quadruple by two years.
- **Failure to thrive:** Persistent weight less than the 5th percentile for age or "falling off the growth curve" (i.e., crossing two major percentile lines on a growth chart). Classified as follows:
    - **Organic:** Due to an underlying medical condition such as cystic fibrosis, congenital heart disease, celiac sprue, pyloric stenosis, chronic infection (e.g., HIV), and GERD.
    - **Nonorganic:** Primarily due to psychosocial factors such as maternal depression, neglect, or abuse.
- A careful dietary history and close observation of maternal-infant interactions (especially preparation of formula and feeding) are critical to diagnosis.
- Children should be hospitalized if there is evidence of neglect or severe malnourishment. Calorie counts and supplemental nutrition (if breastfeeding is inadequate) are mainstays of treatment.

Sexual Development

- **Tanner staging:** Performed to assess physical development in boys and girls. Stage 1 is preadolescent; stage 5 is adult. Increasing stages are assigned for testicular and penile growth in boys and breast growth in girls; pubic hair development is used for both stages.
    - **Girls:** The average age of puberty is 10.5 years. Generally the order of progression is **thelarche** (breast bud development) → **pubarche** (pubic hair development) → growth spurt → **menarche** (first menstrual bleeding). The average age of menarche in United States girls is 12.5 years.
    - **Boys:** The average age of puberty is 11.5 years. Generally the order of progression is **gonadarche** (testicular enlargement) → **pubarche** → **adrenarche** (axillary hair, facial hair, vocal changes) → growth spurt.
- Variants of normal sexual development are as follows:
    - **Delayed puberty:** No testicular enlargement in boys by age 14, or no breast development or pubic hair in girls by age 13.
    - **Constitutional growth delay:** A normal variant, and the most common cause of delayed puberty. The growth curve lags behind others of the same age but is consistent. There is often a ⊕ family history, and children ultimately achieve target height potential.
    - **Pathological puberty delay:** Rarely, due to systemic disease (e.g., IBD), malnutrition (e.g., anorexia nervosa), gonadal dysgenesis (e.g., Klinefelter's syndrome, Turner's syndrome), or endocrine abnormalities (e.g., hypopituitarism, hypothyroidism, Kallmann's syndrome, androgen insensitivity syndrome, Prader-Willi syndrome)
    - **Precocious puberty:** Any sign of 2° sexual maturation in girls < 8 years or boys < 9 years of age. Often idiopathic; may be central or peripheral (see the Gynecology chapter).

Signs of autism include no babbling and/or gesturing by 12 months, no single words by 16 months, no two-word phrases by 24 months, failure to make eye contact, or any loss of language or social skills.

*Infants with FTT will first fall off of the **weight** curve, then the **height** curve, and finally the **head circumference** curve.*

Tables 2.13-2 and 2.13-3 outline common genetic diseases and their associated abnormalities.

TABLE 2.13-2. Genetic Diseases

DISEASE	GENETIC ABNORMALITY	COMMON CHARACTERISTICS
Down syndrome	Trisomy 21 (most common) or robertsonian translocation (higher risk of recurrence)	The most common chromosomal disorder and cause of mental retardation. Associated with advanced maternal age. Presents with mental retardation, a flat facial profile, prominent epicanthal folds, and a simian crease. Associated with duodenal atresia, Hirschsprung's disease, and congenital heart disease (the most common malformation is atrioventricular canal, which includes an ASD and VSD with mitral and tricuspid valve abnormalities due to endocardial cushion defects). Associated with an ↑ risk of acute lymphocytic leukemia (ALL), hypothyroidism, and early-onset Alzheimer's.
Edwards' syndrome	Trisomy 18	Presents with severe mental retardation, **rocker-bottom feet,** low-set ears, **micrognathia,** clenched hands, and a prominent occiput. Associated with congenital heart disease. May have horseshoe kidneys. Death usually occurs within one year of birth.
Patau's syndrome	Trisomy 13	Presents with severe mental retardation, **microphthalmia, microcephaly,** cleft lip/palate, abnormal forebrain structures (holoprosencephaly), "punched-out" scalp lesions, and **polydactyly.** Associated with congenital heart disease. Death usually occurs within one year of birth.
Klinefelter's syndrome (male)	45,XXY	Presence of an inactivated X chromosome (Barr body). One of the most common causes of hypogonadism in males. Presents with testicular atrophy, a eunuchoid body shape, tall stature, long extremities, and gynecomastia. Treat with **testosterone** (prevents gynecomastia; improves 2° sexual characteristics).
Turner's syndrome (female)	45,XO	The most common cause of 1° amenorrhea; due to **gonadal dysgenesis.** No Barr body. Features include short stature, shield chest, widely spaced nipples, webbed neck, **coarctation of the aorta,** and/or bicuspid aortic valve. May present with lymphedema of the hands and feet in the neonatal period. May have horseshoe kidney.
Double Y males	47,XYY	Observed with ↑ frequency among inmates of penal institutions. Phenotypically normal; patients are very tall with severe acne and antisocial behavior (seen in 1–2% of XYY males).

TABLE 2.13-2.   **Genetic Diseases** *(continued)*

DISEASE	GENETIC ABNORMALITY	COMMON CHARACTERISTICS
Phenylketonuria (PKU)	↓ phenylalanine hydroxylase or ↓ tetrahydrobiopterin cofactor	Screened for at birth; screening is valid only after the baby has had a protein meal (i.e., a normal breast or formula feed). Tyrosine becomes essential and phenylalanine builds up excess phenyl ketones. Presents with mental retardation, fair skin, eczema, and a musty or mousy urine odor. Blond-haired, blue-eyed infants. Associated with an ↑ risk of heart disease. Treat with ↓ phenylalanine and ↑ tyrosine in diet. A mother with PKU who wants to become pregnant must restrict her diet as above before conception.
Fragile X syndrome	An X-linked defect affecting the methylation and expression of the *FMR1* gene	The second most common cause of genetic mental retardation. Presents with **macro-orchidism;** a **long face** with a large jaw; large, everted ears; and **autism.** A triplet repeat disorder that may show genetic anticipation.

Cystic Fibrosis (CF)

An autosomal-recessive disorder caused by mutations in the *CFTR* gene (chloride channel) on chromosome 7 and characterized by widespread exocrine gland dysfunction. CF is the most common severe genetic disease in the United States and is most frequently found in Caucasians.

HISTORY/PE

- Fifty percent of patients present with **FTT** or **chronic sinopulmonary disease.**
- Characterized by recurrent pulmonary infections (especially with *Pseudomonas* and *S. aureus*) with subsequent cyanosis, digital clubbing, cough, dyspnea, bronchiectasis, hemoptysis, chronic sinusitis, rhonchi, rales, hyperresonance to percussion, and nasal polyposis.
- Fifteen percent of infants present with **meconium ileus.** Patients usually have greasy stools and flatulence; other prominent GI symptoms include pancreatitis, rectal prolapse, hypoproteinemia, biliary cirrhosis, jaundice, and esophageal varices.
- GI symptoms are more prominent in infancy, while pulmonary manifestations predominate thereafter.
- Additional symptoms include type 2 DM, a "salty taste," male infertility (agenesis of the vas deferens), and unexplained hyponatremia.
- Patients are at risk for fat-soluble vitamin deficiency (vitamins A, D, E, and K) 2° to malabsorption and may present with manifestations of these deficiencies.

DIAGNOSIS

- Sweat chloride test > 60 mEq/L for those < 20 years of age and > 80 mEq/L in adults; DNA probe test.
- Most states now perform mandatory newborn screening, but occasional false positives do occur, so children must be brought in for a sweat test to distinguish disease from a carrier state.

The sweat chloride test has traditionally been considered the gold standard for the diagnosis of CF, but confirmatory genetic analysis is now routinely done.

TABLE 2.13-3. **Lysosomal Storage Diseases**

DISEASE	ETIOLOGY	MODE OF INHERITANCE/NOTES
Fabry's disease	Caused by a deficiency of α-galactosidase A that leads to accumulation of ceramide trihexoside in the heart, brain, and kidneys. Findings include renal failure and an ↑ risk of stroke and MI.	X-linked recessive.
Krabbe's disease	Absence of galactosylceramide and galactoside (due to galactosylceramidase deficiency), leading to the accumulation of galactocerebroside in the brain. Characterized by optic atrophy, spasticity, and early death.	Autosomal recessive.
Gaucher's disease	Caused by a deficiency of glucocerebrosidase that leads to the accumulation of glucocerebroside in the brain, liver, spleen, and bone marrow (Gaucher's cells with characteristic "crinkled paper," enlarged cytoplasm). May present with hepatosplenomegaly, anemia, and thrombocytopenia. Type 1, the more common form, is compatible with a normal life span and does not affect the brain.	Autosomal recessive.
Niemann-Pick disease	A deficiency of sphingomyelinase that leads to the buildup of sphingomyelin cholesterol in reticuloendothelial and parenchymal cells and tissues. Patients with type A die by the age of three.	Autosomal recessive. No man **PICKs (Niemann-PICK)** his nose with his **sphinger.**
Tay-Sachs disease	An absence of hexosaminidase that leads to GM$_2$ ganglioside accumulation. Infants may appear normal until 3–6 months of age, when weakness begins and development slows and regresses. Exaggerated startle response. Death occurs by the age of three. A **cherry-red spot** is visible on the macula. The carrier rate is 1 in 30 Jews of European descent (1 in 300 for others).	**Tay-SaX lacks heXosaminidase.**
Metachromatic leukodystrophy	A deficiency of arylsulfatase A that leads to the accumulation of sulfatide in the brain, kidney, liver, and peripheral nerves.	Autosomal recessive.
Hurler's syndrome	A deficiency of α-L-iduronidase that leads to corneal clouding and mental retardation.	Autosomal recessive.
Hunter's syndrome	A deficiency of iduronate sulfatase. A mild form of Hurler's with no corneal clouding and mild mental retardation.	X-linked recessive. **Hunters need to see (no corneal clouding) to aim for the X.**

TREATMENT

- Pulmonary manifestations are managed with chest physical therapy, bronchodilators, corticosteroids, antibiotics, and DNase.
- Administer pancreatic enzymes and fat-soluble vitamins A, D, E, and K for malabsorption.
- Nutritional counseling and support with a high-calorie and high-protein diet are essential for health maintenance.

- Patients who have severe disease (but who can tolerate surgery) may be candidates for lung or pancreas transplants. Life expectancy was once around 20 years, but with newer treatments it is increasing to past age 30.

Intussusception

A condition in which one portion of the bowel invaginates or "telescopes" into an adjacent segment, usually proximal to the ileocecal valve (see Figure 2.13-1). The most common cause of bowel obstruction in the first two years of life (males > females); usually seen between three months and three years of age. The cause is often unknown. Risk factors include conditions with potential lead points, including Meckel's diverticulum, intestinal lymphoma (> 6 years of age), Henoch-Schönlein purpura, parasites, polyps, adenovirus or rotavirus infection, celiac disease, and CF.

HISTORY/PE

- Presents with abrupt-onset, colicky abdominal pain in apparently healthy children, often accompanied by flexed knees and vomiting. The child may appear well in between episodes if intussusception is released.
- The classic triad is abdominal pain, vomiting, and blood per rectum (affects only one in three patients).
- Late signs include bloody mucus in stools (red **"currant jelly" stool**), lethargy, and fever. The condition may progress to shock as blood flow to the affected segment is compromised.
- On exam, look for abdominal tenderness, a ⊕ stool guaiac, and a palpable **"sausage-shaped"** RUQ abdominal mass.

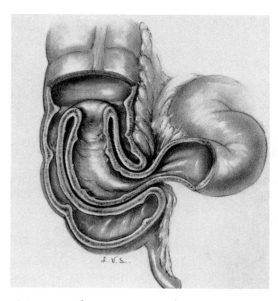

FIGURE 2.13-1.   Intussusception.

A segment of bowel telescopes into an adjacent segment, causing obstruction. (Reproduced, with permission, from Way LW. *Current Surgical Diagnosis & Treatment*, 10th ed. Stamford, CT: Appleton & Lange, 1994: 1222.)

HIGH-YIELD FACTS

PEDIATRICS

DIAGNOSIS/TREATMENT

- Correct any volume or electrolyte abnormalities and check CBC (for leukocytosis).
- Abdominal plain films are often normal early in the disease, but later they may show small bowel obstruction, perforation, or a soft tissue mass. Ultrasound may show a "target sign."
- In the setting of high clinical suspicion, an **air-contrast barium enema** should be performed without delay, as it is diagnostic in > 95% of cases and curative in > 80%. If the child is unstable or has peritoneal signs or if enema reduction is unsuccessful, perform surgical reduction and resection of gangrenous bowel.

Pyloric Stenosis

Hypertrophy of the pyloric sphincter, leading to gastric outlet obstruction. More common in firstborn males; associated with tracheoesophageal fistula and with a maternal history of pyloric stenosis.

HISTORY/PE

- **Nonbilious** emesis typically begins around three weeks of age and progresses to **projectile emesis** after most to all feedings.
- Babies initially feed well but eventually suffer from malnutrition and dehydration.
- Exam may reveal a palpable **olive-shaped,** mobile, nontender epigastric mass and visible gastric peristaltic waves.

DIAGNOSIS

- Abdominal ultrasound is the imaging modality of choice and reveals a hypertrophic pylorus.
- Barium studies reveal a narrow pyloric channel ("string sign") or a pyloric beak.

TREATMENT

- Correct existing dehydration and acid-base/electrolyte abnormalities.
- Surgical correction with **pyloromyotomy.**

Meckel's Diverticulum

Caused by failure of the omphalomesenteric (or vitelline) duct to obliterate. The most common congenital abnormality of the small intestine, affecting up to 2% of children. Most frequently occurs in children < 2 years of age.

HISTORY/PE

- Typically asymptomatic, and often discovered incidentally.
- Classically presents with sudden, **painless rectal bleeding.**
- Abdominal pain typically signifies complications such as diverticulitis, volvulus, and intussusception.

DIAGNOSIS

A Meckel scintigraphy scan (technetium-99m pertechnetate) is diagnostic; plain films have limited value but can be useful in diagnosing obstruction or perforation.

TREATMENT

- In the presence of active bleeding, treatment is excision of the diverticulum together with the adjacent ileal segment (ulcers frequently develop in adjacent ileum).
- If the condition is asymptomatic but discovered intraoperatively, treatment is controversial but often involves excision.

Hirschsprung's Disease

Congenital lack of ganglion cells in the distal colon, leading to uncoordinated peristalsis and ↓ motility. Associated with male gender, Down syndrome, Waardenburg's syndrome, and multiple endocrine neoplasia (MEN) type 2.

HISTORY/PE

- Neonates present with **failure to pass meconium** within 48 hours of birth, accompanied by bilious vomiting and FTT; children with less severe lesions may present later in life with chronic constipation.
- Physical exam may reveal abdominal distention and explosive discharge of stool following rectal exam.

DIAGNOSIS

- Barium enema is the imaging study of choice and reveals a narrowed distal colon with proximal dilation. Plain films reveal distended bowel loops with a paucity of air in the rectum.
- Anorectal manometry detects a failure of the internal sphincter to relax after distention of the rectal lumen. It is typically used in atypical presentations or older children.
- **Full-thickness rectal biopsy** confirms the diagnosis and reveals absence of the myenteric (Auerbach's) plexus and submucosal (Meissner's) plexus along with hypertrophied nerve trunks enhanced with acetylcholinesterase stain.

TREATMENT

Traditionally a two-stage surgical repair is used involving the creation of a diverting colostomy at the time of diagnosis, followed several weeks later by a definitive "pull-through" procedure connecting the remaining colon to the rectum.

Malrotation with Volvulus

Congenital malrotation of the midgut results in abnormal positioning of the small intestine (cecum in the right hypochondrium) and formation of fibrous bands (Ladd's bands). Bands predispose to obstruction and constriction of blood flow.

HISTORY/PE

- Often presents in the newborn period with **bilious emesis,** crampy abdominal pain, distention, and the passage of blood or mucus in stool.
- Postsurgical adhesions can lead to obstruction and volvulus at any point in life.

The definitive diagnosis of Hirschsprung's disease requires a full-thickness rectal biopsy.

DIAGNOSIS

- AXR may reveal the absence of intestinal gas but may also be normal.
- If the patient is stable, an **upper GI** is the study of choice and shows an abnormal location of the ligament of Treitz. Ultrasound may be used, but sensitivity is determined by the experience of the ultrasonographer.

TREATMENT

- NG tube insertion to decompress the intestine.
- IV fluid hydration.
- Surgical repair (emergent when volvulus is present).

Necrotizing Enterocolitis (NEC)

A condition in which a portion of the bowel undergoes necrosis. The most common GI emergency in neonates; most commonly occurs in **premature infants** but can occur in full-term infants as well.

HISTORY/PE

- Symptoms are nonspecific and include feeding intolerance, delayed gastric emptying, abdominal distention, and bloody stools.
- Symptoms may rapidly progress to intestinal perforation, peritonitis, abdominal erythema, and shock. Maintain a high index of suspicion.

DIAGNOSIS

- Lab findings are nonspecific and may show hyponatremia, metabolic acidosis, leukopenia or leukocytosis with left shift, thrombocytopenia, and coagulopathy (DIC with prolonged PT, aPTT, and a ⊕ D-dimer).
- Plain abdominal radiographs may show dilated bowel loops, **pneumatosis intestinalis** (intramural air bubbles representing gas produced by bacteria within the bowel wall), portal venous gas, or abdominal free air. Serial abdominal plain films should be taken every six hours.
- Ultrasound may also be helpful in discerning free air, areas of loculation or walled-off abscesses, and bowel necrosis.

Pneumatosis intestinalis on plain films is pathognomonic for necrotizing enterocolitis in neonates.

TREATMENT

- Initiate supportive measures, including NPO, an orogastric tube for gastric decompression, correction of dehydration and electrolyte abnormalities, TPN, and IV antibiotics.
- Indications for surgery are perforation or radiographic worsening on serial abdominal plain films. An ileostomy with mucous fistula is typically performed, with a reanastomosis later.
- Complications include formation of intestinal **strictures** and **short-bowel syndrome**.

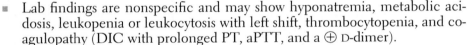

▶ **IMMUNOLOGY**

Immunodeficiency Disorders

Congenital immunodeficiencies are rare and often present with chronic or recurrent infections (e.g., chronic thrush), unusual or opportunistic organisms, incomplete treatment response, or FTT. Categorization is based on the one immune system component that is abnormal (see also Table 2.13-4).

TABLE 2.13-4. Pediatric Immunodeficiencies

DISORDER	DESCRIPTION	INFECTION RISK/TYPE	DIAGNOSIS/TREATMENT
B cell			
X-linked agamma-globulinemia (**B**ruton's)	A **B-cell** deficiency in **boys** only.	Life threatening; encapsulated *Pseudomonas, Streptococcus pneumoniae,* and *Haemophilus* infections after six months (passive immunity through maternal antibodies wanes).	Quantitative immunoglobulin levels. If low, confirm diagnosis with B- and T-cell subsets (absent B cells; T cells are often high); absent tonsils and other lymphoid tissue may be a clue. Treat with prophylactic antibiotics and IVIG.
Common variable immunodeficiency	Immunoglobulin level drops in the **20s and 30s; usually a combined B- and T-cell defect.**	↑ pyogenic upper and lower respiratory infections; ↑ risk of lymphoma and autoimmune disease.	Quantitative immunoglobulin levels; confirm with B- and T-cell subsets; treat with IVIG.
IgA deficiency	Mild; the most common immunodeficiency.	Usually asymptomatic; patients may develop recurrent respiratory or GI infections. Anaphylactic transfusion reaction due to anti-IgA antibodies is a common presentation.	Quantitative IgA levels; treat infections. Do **not** give immunoglobulins (can lead to the production of anti-IgA antibodies).
T cell			
Thymic aplasia (DiGeorge syndrome)	See mnemonic. Presents with **tetany** (2° to **hypocalcemia**) in the first days of life.	Variable risk of infection. ↑↑↑ infections with fungi and *Pneumocystis jiroveci* pneumonia (formerly *P. carinii*).	Absolute lymphocyte count; mitogen stimulation response; delayed hypersensitivity skin testing. Treat with bone marrow transplantation and IVIG for antibody deficiency; PCP prophylaxis. Thymus transplantation is an alternative.
Combined			
Ataxia-telangiectasia	**Oculocutaneous telangiectasias** and progressive **cerebellar ataxia.** Caused by a **DNA repair defect.**	↑ incidence of non-Hodgkin's lymphoma, leukemia, and gastric carcinoma.	No specific treatment; may require IVIG depending on the severity of the Ig deficiency.
Severe combined immunodeficiency (SCID)	Severe lack of B and T cells.	Severe, frequent bacterial infections; chronic candidiasis; and opportunistic organisms.	Treat with bone marrow transplant or stem cell transplant and IVIG for antibody deficiency. **Needs PCP prophylaxis.**

TABLE 2.13-4. Pediatric Immunodeficiencies *(continued)*

DISORDER	DESCRIPTION	INFECTION RISK/TYPE	DIAGNOSIS/TREATMENT
Combined (continued)			
Wiskott-Aldrich syndrome	An **X-linked** disorder with less severe B- and T-cell dysfunction. Patients have **eczema,** ↑ IgE/IgA, ↓ IgM, and **thrombocytopenia.** The classic presentation involves bleeding, eczema, and recurrent otitis media.	↑↑ risk of atopic disorders, lymphoma/leukemia, and infection from *S. pneumoniae, S. aureus,* and *H. influenzae* type b.	Treatment is supportive (IVIG and antibiotics). Patients rarely survive to adulthood. Patients with severe infections may be treated with a bone marrow transplant.
Phagocytic			
Chronic granulomatous disease (CGD)	An X-linked (2/3) or autosomal-recessive (1/3) disease with deficient superoxide production by PMNs and macrophages. Anemia, lymphadenopathy, and hypergamma-globulinemia may be present.	Chronic skin, pulmonary, GI, and urinary tract infections; osteomyelitis and hepatitis. Infecting organisms are catalase ⊕. ↑ risk of infection with *Aspergillus.* May have granulomas of the skin and GI/GU tracts.	Absolute neutrophil count with neutrophil assays. **The nitroblue tetrazolium test is diagnostic for CGD. Treat with daily TMP-SMX;** judicious use of antibiotics during infections. IFN-γ can ↓ the incidence of serious infection. Bone marrow transplantation and gene therapy are new therapies.
Leukocyte adhesion deficiency	A defect in the chemotaxis of leukocytes.	Recurrent skin, mucosal, and pulmonary infections. May present as omphalitis in the newborn period with delayed separation of the umbilical cord.	No pus with minimal inflammation in wounds (due to a chemotaxis defect). High WBCs in blood. Bone marrow transplantation is curative.
Chédiak-Higashi syndrome	An autosomal-recessive disorder that leads to a defect in neutrophil chemotaxis/microtubule polymerization. The syndrome includes oculocutaneous albinism, neuropathy, and neutropenia.	↑↑ incidence of overwhelming infections with *S. pyogenes, S. aureus,* and *Pseudomonas* species.	Look for giant granules in neutrophils. Bone marrow transplant is the treatment of choice.

TABLE 2.13-4. Pediatric Immunodeficiencies (continued)

DISORDER	DESCRIPTION	INFECTION RISK/TYPE	DIAGNOSIS/TREATMENT
Complement			
C1 esterase deficiency (hereditary angioedema)	An autosomal-dominant disorder with recurrent episodes of angioedema lasting 2–72 hours and provoked by stress or trauma.	Can lead to life-threatening airway edema.	Total hemolytic complement (CH50) to assess the quantity and function of complement. Purified C1 esterase and FFP can be used prior to surgery.
Terminal complement deficiency (C5–C9)	Inability to form membrane attack complex (MAC).	Recurrent meningococcal or gonococcal infections. Rarely, lupus or glomerulonephritis.	Meningococcal vaccine and appropriate antibiotics.

- **B-cell deficiencies:** Most common (50%). Typically present **after six months of age** with recurrent sinopulmonary, GI, and urinary tract infections with encapsulated organisms (*H. influenzae, S. pneumoniae, Neisseria meningitidis*). Treated with IVIF (except for IgA deficiencies).
- **T-cell deficiencies:** Tend to present earlier (1–3 months) with **opportunistic and low-grade fungal, viral, and intracellular bacterial infections** (e.g., mycobacteria). 2° B-cell dysfunction may also be seen.
- **Phagocyte deficiencies:** Characterized by mucous membrane infections, abscesses, and poor wound healing. **Infections with catalase-⊕ organisms** (e.g., *S. aureus*), **fungi, and gram-⊖ enteric organisms are common.**
- **Complement deficiencies:** Present in children with congenital asplenia or splenic dysfunction (sickle cell disease). Characterized by recurrent **bacterial** infections with **encapsulated organisms.**

Kawasaki Disease

A multisystemic acute vasculitis that primarily affects young children (80% are < 5 years of age), particularly those of Asian ancestry. Divided into acute, subacute, and chronic phases.

DIAGNOSIS

- **Acute phase:** Lasts 1–2 weeks and presents with the following symptoms (fever plus four or more of the criteria below are required for diagnosis):
  - Fever (usually > 40°C) for at least **five** days.
  - Bilateral, nonexudative, painless conjunctivitis sparing the limbic area.
  - Polymorphous rash (primarily truncal).
  - Cervical lymphadenopathy (often painful and unilateral, with at least one node > 1.5 cm).
  - Diffuse mucous membrane erythema (e.g., "strawberry tongue"); dry, red, chapped lips.
  - Erythema of the palms and soles; indurative edema of the hands and feet; late desquamation of the fingertips (in the subacute phase).
  - Other manifestations include sterile pyuria, gallbladder hydrops, hepatitis, and arthritis.

Untreated Kawasaki disease can lead to coronary aneurysms and even myocardial infarction!

Kawasaki disease symptoms—

CRASH and BURN

Conjunctivitis
Rash
Adenopathy
Strawberry tongue
Hands and feet (red, swollen, flaky skin)
BURN (fever > 40°C for ≥ 5 days)

- **Subacute phase:** Begins after the abatement of fever and typically lasts for an additional 2–3 weeks. Manifestations are thrombocytosis and elevated ESR. Untreated children may begin to develop coronary artery aneurysms (40%); all patients should be assessed by echocardiography at diagnosis.
- **Chronic phase:** Begins when all clinical symptoms have disappeared; lasts until ESR returns to baseline. **Untreated children are at risk of aneurysmal expansion and MI.**

TREATMENT

- High-dose **ASA** (for inflammation and fever) and **IVIG** (to prevent aneurysms).
- Low-dose ASA is then continued, usually for six weeks. Children who develop coronary aneurysms may require chronic anticoagulation with ASA or other antiplatelet medications.
- Corticosteroids may be used in IVIG-refractory cases, but **routine use is not recommended.**
- Referral to a pediatric cardiologist and routine follow-up echocardiograms to assess for progression of coronary artery aneurysms are important parts of ongoing management.

Juvenile Idiopathic Arthritis (JIA)

An autoimmune disorder manifesting as arthritis with "morning stiffness" and gradual loss of motion that is present for at least six weeks in a patient < 16 years of age. Formerly known as juvenile rheumatoid arthritis (JRA).

DIAGNOSIS

- **Pauciarticular (oligoarthritis):** Most common; four or fewer joints are involved (usually weight-bearing); usually ANA ⊕ and RF ⊖. Involves young females; **uveitis** is common and requires slit-lamp exam for evaluation. No systemic symptoms.
- **Polyarthritis:** Involves five or more joints; symmetric. RF positivity is rare and indicates severe disease; younger children may be ANA ⊕ with milder disease. Systemic symptoms are rare.
- **Systemic-onset (Still's disease):** May present with recurrent high fever (usually > 39°C), hepatosplenomegaly, and a salmon-colored macular rash; usually RF ⊖ and ANA ⊖.

TREATMENT

- NSAIDs and strengthening exercises.
- Corticosteroids and immunosuppressive medications (methotrexate; anti-TNF agents such as etanercept) are second-line agents.
- Corticosteroids are used in the presence of carditis.

▶ **INFECTIOUS DISEASE**

Acute Otitis Media

A suppurative infection of the middle ear cavity that is common in children. Up to 75% of children have at least three episodes by the age of two. Common pathogens include **S. pneumoniae, nontypable H. influenzae, Moraxella catarrhalis,** and viruses such as influenza A, RSV, and parainfluenza virus.

HISTORY/PE

Symptoms include ear pain, fever, crying, irritability, difficulty feeding or sleeping, vomiting, and diarrhea. Young children may tug on their ears.

DIAGNOSIS

Signs on otoscopic exam reveal an erythematous tympanic membrane (TM), bulging or retraction of the TM, loss of TM light reflex, and ↓ TM mobility (test with an insufflator bulb).

TREATMENT

- **High-dose amoxicillin** (80–90 mg/kg/day) × 10 days for empiric therapy. Resistant cases may require amoxicillin/clavulanic acid.
- Complications include TM perforation, mastoiditis, meningitis, cholesteatomas, and chronic otitis media. Recurrent otitis media can cause hearing loss with resultant speech and language delay. Chronic otitis media may require tympanostomy tubes.

Bronchiolitis

An acute inflammatory illness of the small airways that primarily affects infants and children < 2 years of age, often in the fall or winter months. **RSV is the most common cause;** others include parainfluenza, influenza, and metapneumovirus. Progression to respiratory failure is a potentially fatal complication. For severe RSV, risk factors include age < 6 months, male gender, prematurity, heart or lung disease, and immunodeficiency.

RSV is the most common cause of bronchiolitis.

HISTORY/PE

- Presents with low-grade fever, rhinorrhea, cough, and apnea (in young infants).
- Exam reveals **tachypnea, wheezing,** intercostal retractions, crackles, prolonged expiration, expiratory wheezing, and hyperresonance to percussion.

DIAGNOSIS

- Predominantly a clinical diagnosis; routine cases do not need blood work or a CXR.
- CXR may be obtained to rule out pneumonia and may show hyperinflation of the lungs with flattened diaphragms, interstitial infiltrates, and atelectasis.
- Nasopharyngeal aspirate to test for RSV is highly sensitive and specific but has little effect on management (infants should be treated for bronchiolitis regardless of whether RSV is ⊕ or not).

TREATMENT

- Treatment is primarily supportive; treat mild disease with outpatient management using fluids and nebulizers if needed.
- Hospitalize in the setting of marked respiratory distress, O₂ saturation of < 92%, toxic appearance, dehydration/poor oral feeding, a history of prematurity (< 34 weeks), age < 3 months, underlying cardiopulmonary disease, or unreliable parents.
- Treat inpatients with contact isolation, hydration, and O₂. A trial of aerosolized albuterol may be attempted; continue albuterol therapy only if effective.

- Ribavirin is an antiviral drug that has a controversial role in bronchiolitis treatment. It is sometimes used in high-risk infants with underlying heart, lung, or immune disease.
- RSV prophylaxis with injectable poly- or monoclonal antibodies (RespiGam or Synagis) is recommended in winter for high-risk patients ≤ 2 years of age (e.g., those with a history of prematurity, chronic lung disease, or congenital heart disease).

Croup (Laryngotracheobronchitis)

An acute viral inflammatory disease of the larynx, primarily within the subglottic space. Pathogens include **parainfluenza** virus type 1 (most common), 2, and 3; RSV; influenza; and adenovirus. Bacterial superinfection may progress to tracheitis.

HISTORY/PE

Prodromal URI symptoms are typically followed by low-grade fever, mild dyspnea, inspiratory stridor that worsens with agitation, a hoarse voice, and a characteristic **barking cough** (usually at night).

DIAGNOSIS

- Diagnosed by clinical impression; often based on the degree of stridor and respiratory distress.
- AP neck film may show the **classic "steeple sign" from subglottic narrowing** (see Figure 2.13-2), but the finding is **neither sensitive nor specific.**
- Table 2.13-5 differentiates croup from epiglottitis and tracheitis.

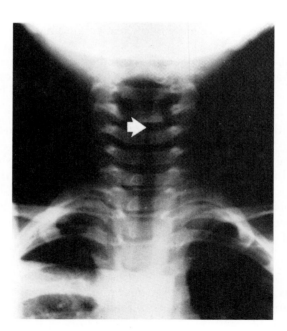

FIGURE 2.13-2. Croup.

The x-ray shows marked subglottic narrowing of the airway ("steeple sign"). (Reproduced, with permission, from Saunders CE. *Current Emergency Diagnosis & Treatment*, 4th ed. Stamford, CT: Appleton & Lange, 1992: 448.)

TABLE 2.13-5. **Characteristics of Croup, Epiglottitis, and Tracheitis**

	CROUP	EPIGLOTTITIS	TRACHEITIS
Age group affected	3 months to 3 years	3–7 years	3 months to 2 years
Incidence in children presenting with stridor	88%	8%	2%
Pathogen	Parainfluenza virus	*H. influenzae*	Often *S. aureus*
Onset	Prodrome (1–7 days)	Rapid (4–12 hours)	Prodrome (3 days) leading to acute decompensation (10 hours)
Fever severity	Low grade	High grade	Intermediate grade
Associated symptoms	Barking cough, hoarseness	Muffled voice, drooling	Variable respiratory distress
Position preference	None	Seated, neck extended	None
Response to racemic epinephrine	Stridor improves	None	None
CXR findings	"Steeple sign" on AP film	"Thumbprint sign'" on lateral film	Subglottic narrowing

TREATMENT

- **Mild cases:** Outpatient management with cool mist therapy and fluids.
- **Moderate cases:** May require supplemental O_2, oral and IM corticosteroids, and nebulized racemic epinephrine.
- **Severe cases** (e.g., respiratory distress at rest, inspiratory stridor): Hospitalize and give nebulized racemic epinephrine.

Epiglottitis

A serious and rapidly progressive infection of supraglottic structures (e.g., the epiglottis and aryepiglottic folds). Prior to immunization, *H. influenzae* type b was the 1° pathogen. Common causes now include *Streptococcus* species, nontypable *H. influenzae*, and viral agents.

HISTORY/PE

- Presents with acute-onset high fever (39–40°C), dysphagia, drooling, a muffled voice, inspiratory retractions, cyanosis, and soft stridor.
- Patients sit with the neck hyperextended and the chin protruding ("sniffing dog" position) and lean forward in a "tripod" position to maximize air entry.
- Untreated infection can lead to life-threatening airway obstruction and respiratory arrest.

Epiglottitis can lead to life-threatening airway obstruction.

DIAGNOSIS

- Diagnosed by clinical impression. The differential diagnosis must include diffuse and localized causes of airway obstruction (see Tables 2.13-5 and 2.13-6).
- **The airway must be secured before definitive diagnosis.** In light of potential laryngospasm and airway compromise, **do not examine the throat unless an anesthesiologist or otolaryngologist is present.**
- Definitive diagnosis is made via direct fiberoptic visualization of a cherry-red, swollen epiglottis and arytenoids.
- Lateral x-ray shows a swollen epiglottis obliterating the valleculae ("thumbprint sign"; see Figure 2.13-3).

TREATMENT

- This disease is a true emergency. Keep the patient (and parents) calm, call anesthesia, and transfer the patient to the OR.
- Treat with endotracheal intubation or tracheostomy and IV antibiotics (ceftriaxone or cefuroxime).

Meningitis

Bacterial meningitis most often occurs in children < 3 years of age; common organisms include S. *pneumoniae*, N. *meningitidis*, and E. *coli*. Enteroviruses are the most common agents of viral meningitis and occur in children of all ages. Risk factors include sinofacial infections, trauma, and sepsis.

Don't be fooled—neonates and young children rarely have meningeal signs on exam!

HISTORY/PE

- Bacterial meningitis classically presents with the triad of **headache, high fever, and nuchal rigidity.**

TABLE 2.13-6. **Comparison of Retropharyngeal Abscess and Peritonsillar Abscess**

	RETROPHARYNGEAL ABSCESS	PERITONSILLAR ABSCESS
Age group affected	Six months to six years.	Usually > 10 years of age.
History/PE	Muffled "hot potato" voice; trismus; drooling; cervical lymphadenopathy. Usually unilateral; may see mass in the posterior pharyngeal wall on visual inspection.	Muffled "hot potato" voice; trismus; drooling; displacement of the affected tonsil medially and laterally.
Pathogen	Group A streptococcus (most common); S. *aureus*; *Bacteroides*.	Group A streptococcus (most common); S. *aureus*; S. *pneumoniae*; anaerobes.
Preferred position	Supine with the neck extended (sitting up or flexing the neck worsens symptoms).	None.
Diagnosis	On lateral neck x-ray, the soft tissue plane should be ≤ 50% of the width of the corresponding vertebral body. Contrast CT of the neck helps differentiate abscess from cellulitis.	Usually clinical.
Treatment	Aspiration or incision and drainage of abscess; antibiotics.	Incision and drainage +/– tonsillectomy; antibiotics.

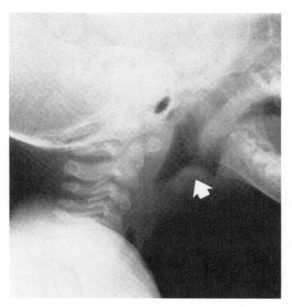

FIGURE 2.13-3. Epiglottitis.

The classic swollen epiglottis ("thumbprint sign"; arrow) and obstructed airway are seen on lateral neck x-ray. (Reproduced, with permission, from Saunders CE. *Current Emergency Diagnosis & Treatment*, 4th ed. Stamford, CT: Appleton & Lange, 1992: 447.)

- Viral meningitis is typically preceded by a prodromal illness that includes fever, sore throat, and fatigue.
- Kernig's sign (pain on knee extension when the hip is flexed) and Brudzinski's sign (pain with passive neck flexion) are nonspecific signs of meningeal irritation.
- Additional physical exam findings may include signs of ↑ ICP (papilledema, cranial nerve palsies) or petechial rash (*N. meningitidis*). Signs in neonates include lethargy, hyper- or hypothermia, poor tone, a bulging fontanelle, and vomiting.

DIAGNOSIS

- Head CT to rule out ↑ ICP (risk of brain stem herniation).
- Perform an LP; send cell count with differential, glucose and protein levels, Gram stain, and culture.

TREATMENT

- Empiric antibiotic therapy regimens (ceftriaxone, vancomycin, ampicillin) should be administered until bacterial meningitis can be excluded.
- Neonates should receive ampicillin and cefotaxime or gentamicin. Consider acyclovir if there is concern for herpes encephalitis (e.g., if the mother had HSV lesions at the time of the infant's birth).
- Older children should receive ceftriaxone and vancomycin.

Pertussis

A bacterial infection caused by *Bordetella pertussis* (whooping cough), a gram-⊖ bacillus. The DTaP vaccine (given in five doses in early childhood) is protective, but immunity wanes by adolescence. Adolescents and young adults serve as the primary reservoir for pertussis. Pertussis can be life threatening for young infants but is generally a milder infection in older children and adults.

HISTORY/PE

- Has three stages: (1) catarrhal (mild URI symptoms; lasts 1–2 weeks), (2) paroxysmal (paroxysms of cough with inspiratory whoop and post-tussive emesis; lasts 2–3 months), and (3) convalescent (symptoms wane).
- Patients most often present in the paroxysmal stage but are most contagious in the catarrhal stage.
- The classic presentation is an infant < 6 months of age with post-tussive emesis and apnea.

DIAGNOSIS

- Labs show an elevated WBC count with lymphocytosis (often ≥ 70%).
- Culture is the gold standard.

TREATMENT

- Hospitalize infants < 6 months of age.
- Give erythromycin × 14 days to patients and close contacts (including day care contacts).
- Patients should not return to school or day care until five days of antibiotics have been administered or until three weeks have elapsed if no therapy has been initiated.

Viral Exanthems

Table 2.13-7 outlines the clinical presentation of common viral exanthems.

TABLE 2.13-7. Viral Exanthems

DISEASE	CAUSE	CHARACTERISTICS	COMPLICATIONS
Erythema infectiosum (fifth disease)	Parvovirus B19	**Prodrome:** None; fever is often absent or low grade. **Rash:** "Slapped-cheek," erythematous rash. An erythematous, pruritic, maculopapular rash starts on the arms and spreads to the trunk and legs. **Worsens with fever and sun exposure.**	Arthritis, hemolytic anemia, encephalopathy. Congenital infection is associated with fetal hydrops and death. Aplastic crisis may be precipitated in children with ↑ RBC turnover (e.g., sickle cell anemia, hereditary spherocytosis) or in those with ↓ RBC production (e.g., severe iron deficiency anemia).
Measles	Paramyxovirus	**Prodrome:** Low-grade fever with **C**ough, **C**oryza, and **C**onjunctivitis (the "**3 C's**"); Koplik's spots (small irregular red spots with central gray specks) appear on the buccal mucosa after 1–2 days. **Rash:** An erythematous maculopapular rash spreads from the head toward the feet.	**Common:** Otitis media, pneumonia, laryngotracheitis. **Rare:** Subacute sclerosing panencephalitis.

TABLE 2.13-7. **Viral Exanthems** *(continued)*

DISEASE	CAUSE	CHARACTERISTICS	COMPLICATIONS
Rubella	Rubella virus	**Prodrome:** Asymptomatic or tender, generalized lymphadenopathy. **Rash:** Presents with an erythematous, tender maculopapular rash that also starts on the face and spreads distally. In contrast to measles, children with rubella often have only a low-grade fever and do not appear as ill. Polyarthritis may be seen in adolescents.	Encephalitis, thrombocytopenia (a rare complication of postnatal infection). Congenital infection is associated with congenital anomalies.
Roseola infantum	HHV-6	**Prodrome:** Acute onset of high fever (> 40°C); no other symptoms for 3–4 days. **Rash: A maculopapular rash appears as fever breaks** (begins on the trunk and quickly spreads to the face and extremities) and often lasts < 24 hours.	**Febrile seizures** may occur as a result of rapid fever onset.
Varicella	Varicella-zoster virus (VZV)	**Prodrome:** Mild fever, anorexia, and malaise precede the rash by 24 hours. **Rash:** Generalized, pruritic, "teardrop" vesicular periphery; lesions are often at different stages of healing. Infectious from 24 hours before eruption until lesions crust over.	Progressive varicella with meningoencephalitis and hepatitis occurs in immunocompromised children. Congenital infection is associated with congenital anomalies.
Varicella zoster	VZV	**Prodrome:** Reactivation of varicella infection; starts as pain along an affected sensory nerve. **Rash:** Pruritic "teardrop" vesicular rash in a dermatomal distribution. Uncommon unless the patient is immunocompromised.	Encephalopathy, aseptic meningitis, pneumonitis, TTP, Guillain-Barré syndrome, cellulitis, arthritis.
Hand-foot-and-mouth disease	Coxsackie A	**Prodrome:** Fever, anorexia, oral pain. **Rash:** Oral ulcers; maculopapular vesicular rash on the hands and feet and sometimes on the buttocks.	None (self-limited).

HIGH-YIELD FACTS

PEDIATRICS

Apgar scoring—

APGAR (0, 1, 2 in each category)

Appearance (blue/pale, pink trunk, all pink)
Pulse (0, < 100, > 100)
Grimace with stimulation (0, grimace, grimace and cough)
Activity (limp, some, active)
Respiratory effort (0, irregular, regular)

Direct hyperbilirubinemia is always pathologic.

Apgar Scoring

A rapid scoring system that helps evaluate the need for neonatal resuscitation. Each of five parameters (see the mnemonic **APGAR**) is assigned a score of 0–2 at one and five minutes after birth.

- **Scores of 8–10:** Typically reflect good cardiopulmonary adaptation.
- **Scores of 4–7:** Indicate the possible need for resuscitation. Infants should be observed, stimulated, and possibly given ventilatory support.
- **Scores of 0–3:** Indicate the need for immediate resuscitation.

Congenital Malformations

Table 2.13-8 describes selected congenital malformations.

Neonatal Jaundice

An elevated serum bilirubin concentration (> 5 mg/dL) due to ↑ hemolysis or ↓ excretion. Subtypes are as follows:

- **Conjugated (direct) hyperbilirubinemia:** Always pathologic.
- **Unconjugated (indirect) hyperbilirubinemia:** May be physiologic or pathologic. See Table 2.13-9 for differentiating characteristics.
- **Kernicterus:** A complication of unconjugated hyperbilirubinemia that results from irreversible bilirubin deposition in the basal ganglia, pons, and cerebellum. It typically occurs at levels of > 25–30 mg/dL and can be fatal. Risk factors include prematurity, asphyxia, and sepsis.

HISTORY/PE

- The differential includes the following:
    - **Conjugated:** Extrahepatic cholestasis (biliary atresia, choledochal cysts), intrahepatic cholestasis (neonatal hepatitis, inborn errors of metabolism, TPN cholestasis), Dubin-Johnson syndrome, Rotor's syndrome, TORCH infections (see the Infectious Disease chapter).
    - **Unconjugated:** Physiologic jaundice, hemolysis, breast milk jaundice, ↑ enterohepatic circulation (e.g., GI obstruction), disorders of bilirubin metabolism, hemolysis, sepsis, Crigler-Najjar syndrome, Gilbert's syndrome.
- The history should focus on diet (breast milk or formula), intrauterine drug exposure, and family history (hemoglobinopathies, enzyme deficiencies, RBC defects).
- Physical exam may reveal signs of hepatic or GI dysfunction (abdominal distention, delayed passage of meconium, light-colored stools, dark urine), infection, or hemoglobinopathies (cephalohematomas, bruising, pallor, petechiae, and hepatomegaly).
- **Kernicterus** presents with lethargy, poor feeding, a high-pitched cry, hypertonicity, and seizures; jaundice may follow a cephalopedal progression as bilirubin concentrations ↑.

DIAGNOSIS

- CBC with peripheral blood smear; blood typing of mother and infant (for ABO or Rh incompatibility); Coombs' test and bilirubin levels.
- Ultrasound and/or HIDA scan can confirm suspected cholestatic disease.

TABLE 2.13-8.   Selected Congenital Malformations

MALFORMATION	PRESENTATION/DIAGNOSIS/TREATMENT
Tracheoesophageal fistula	Tract between the trachea and esophagus. Associated with defects such as esophageal atresia and **VACTERL** (**V**ertebral, **A**nal, **C**ardiac, **T**racheal, **E**sophageal, **R**enal, **L**imb) anomalies. **Presentation:** Polyhydramnios in utero, ↑ oral secretions, inability to feed, gagging, aspiration pneumonia, respiratory distress. **Diagnosis:** CXR showing an NG tube coiled in the esophagus identifies esophageal atresia. The presence of air in the GI tract is suggestive; confirm with bronchoscopy. **Treatment:** Surgical repair.
Congenital diaphragmatic hernia	GI tract segments protrude through the diaphragm into the thorax; 90% are posterior left (Bochdalek). **Presentation:** Respiratory distress (from pulmonary hypoplasia and pulmonary hypertension); sunken abdomen; bowel sounds over the left hemithorax. **Diagnosis:** Ultrasound in utero; confirmed by postnatal CXR. **Treatment:** High-frequency ventilation or extracorporeal membrane oxygenation to manage pulmonary hypertension; surgical repair.
Gastroschisis	Herniation of the intestine only through the abdominal wall next to the umbilicus (usually on the right) with no sac. **Presentation:** Polyhydramnios in utero; often premature; associated with GI stenoses or atresia. **Treatment:** A surgical emergency! Single-stage closure is possible in only 10% of cases.
Omphalocele	Herniation of abdominal viscera through the abdominal wall at the umbilicus into a sac covered by peritoneum and amniotic membrane. **Presentation/diagnosis:** Polyhydramnios in utero; often premature; associated with other GI and cardiac defects. Seen in Beckwith-Wiedemann syndrome and trisomies. **Treatment:** C-section can prevent sac rupture; if the sac is intact, postpone surgical correction until the patient is fully resuscitated. Keep the sac covered/stable with petroleum and gauze. Intermittent NG suction to prevent abdominal distention.
Duodenal atresia	Complete or partial failure of the duodenal lumen to recanalize during gestational weeks 8–10. **Presentation:** Polyhydramnios in utero; bilious emesis within hours after first feeding; associated with Down syndrome and other cardiac/GI anomalies (e.g., annular pancreas, malrotation, imperforate anus). **Diagnosis:** Abdominal radiographs show the **"double-bubble"** sign (air bubbles in the stomach and duodenum) proximal to the site of the atresia. **Treatment:** Surgical repair.

- For direct hyperbilirubinemia, check LFTs, bile acids, blood cultures, sweat test, and tests for aminoacidopathies and α_1-antitrypsin deficiency.
- A jaundiced neonate who is febrile, hypotensive, and/or tachypneic needs a full sepsis workup and ICU monitoring.

TREATMENT

- Treat underlying causes (e.g., infection).
- Treat unconjugated hyperbilirubinemia with **phototherapy** (for mild elevations) or **exchange transfusion** (for severe elevations > 20 mg/dL). Start

TABLE 2.13-9. Physiologic vs. Pathologic Jaundice

PHYSIOLOGIC JAUNDICE	PATHOLOGIC JAUNDICE
Not present until 72 hours after birth.	Present in the first 24 hours of life.
Bilirubin $\uparrow$ < 5 mg/dL/day.	Bilirubin $\uparrow$ > 0.5 mg/dL/hour.
Bilirubin peaks at < 14–15 mg/dL.	Bilirubin $\uparrow$ to > 15 mg/dL.
Direct bilirubin is < 10% of total.	Direct bilirubin is > 10% of total.
Resolves by one week in term infants and two weeks in preterm infants.	Persists beyond one week in term infants and two weeks in preterm infants.

phototherapy earlier (10–15 mg/dL) for preterm infants. Phototherapy with conjugated hyperbilirubinemia can lead to skin bronzing.

Respiratory Distress Syndrome (RDS)

The most common cause of respiratory failure in **preterm** infants (affects > 70% of infants born at 28–30 weeks' gestation); formerly known as hyaline membrane disease. **Surfactant deficiency** leads to poor lung compliance, alveolar collapse, and atelectasis. Risk factors include maternal DM, male gender, and the second born of twins.

RDS is the most common cause of respiratory failure in preterm infants.

HISTORY/PE

Presents in the first 48–72 hours of life with a respiratory rate > 60/min, progressive hypoxemia, cyanosis, nasal flaring, intercostal retractions, and expiratory grunting.

DIAGNOSIS

- Check ABGs, CBC, and blood cultures to rule out infection.
- Diagnosis is based mainly on characteristic CXR findings:
    - **RDS:** "Ground-glass" appearance, diffuse atelectasis, and **air bronchograms** on CXR.
    - **Transient tachypnea of the newborn:** Retained amniotic fluid results in prominent perihilar streaking in interlobular fissures.
    - **Meconium aspiration:** Coarse, irregular infiltrates; hyperexpansion and pneumothoraces.
    - **Congenital pneumonia:** Nonspecific patchy infiltrates; neutropenia, tracheal aspirate, and Gram stain suggest the diagnosis.

TREATMENT

- Continuous positive airway pressure (CPAP) or intubation and mechanical ventilation.
- Artificial surfactant administration $\downarrow$ mortality.
- Pretreat mothers at risk for preterm delivery (< 30 weeks' gestation) with corticosteroids; if > 30 weeks, monitor fetal lung maturity via a lecithin-to-sphingomyelin (L/S) ratio and the presence of phosphatidylglycerol in amniotic fluid.

An L/S ratio < 2:1 indicates a need for maternal glucocorticoid administration.

Persistent PDA, **bronchopulmonary dysplasia,** retinopathy of prematurity, barotrauma from positive pressure ventilation, intraventricular hemorrhage, and NEC are complications of treatment.

▶ NEUROLOGY

Cerebral Palsy

A range of **nonhereditary, nonprogressive** disorders of movement and posture; the most common movement disorder in children. Often results from perinatal neurologic insult, but in most cases the cause is unknown. Risk factors include low birth weight, intrauterine exposure to maternal infection, prematurity, perinatal asphyxia, trauma, brain malformation, and neonatal cerebral hemorrhage. Categories include the following:

- **Pyramidal (spastic):** Spastic paresis of any or all limbs. Accounts for 75% of cases. Mental retardation is present in up to 90% of cases.
- **Extrapyramidal (dyskinetic):** A result of damage to extrapyramidal tracts. Subtypes are ataxic (difficulty coordinating purposeful movements), choreoathetoid, and dystonic (uncontrollable jerking, writhing, or posturing). Abnormal movements worsen with stress and disappear during sleep.

HISTORY/PE

- May be associated with seizure disorders, behavioral disorders, hearing or vision impairment, learning disabilities, and speech deficits.
- Affected limbs may show hyperreflexia, pathologic reflexes (e.g., Babinski), ↑ tone/contractures, weakness, and/or underdevelopment.
- Toe walking and scissor gait are common. Hip dislocations and scoliosis may be seen.

DIAGNOSIS

Diagnosed by clinical impression. Ultrasound or CT may be useful in infants to identify intracranial hemorrhage or structural malformations. MRI is diagnostic in older children. EEG may be useful in patients with seizures.

TREATMENT

- There is no cure for cerebral palsy. Special education, physical therapy, braces, and surgical release of contractures may help.
- Treat spasticity with diazepam, dantrolene, or baclofen. Baclofen pumps and posterior rhizotomy may alleviate severe contractures.

Febrile Seizures

Usually occur in children between six months and five years of age who have no evidence of intracranial infection or other causes. Risk factors include a rapid ↑ in temperature and a history of febrile seizures in a close relative. Febrile seizures recur in 30% of patients.

HISTORY/PE

- Seizures usually occur during the onset of fever and may be the first sign of an underlying illness (e.g., otitis media, roseola).

The most common presenting symptom of cerebral palsy is delayed motor development.

- Classified as simple or complex:
  - **Simple:** A **short-duration** (< 15-minute), **generalized** seizure with one seizure in a 24-hour period. High fever (> 39°C) and fever onset within hours of the seizure are typical.
  - **Complex:** A **long-duration** (> 15-minute) or **focal** seizure, or multiple seizures in a 24-hour period. Low-grade fever for several days before seizure onset may be present.

DIAGNOSIS

- Focus on finding a source of infection. LP is indicated if there are clinical signs of CNS infection (e.g., altered consciousness, meningismus, a tense/bulging anterior fontanelle) after ruling out ↑ ICP.
- No lab studies are needed if presentation is consistent with febrile seizures in children > 18 months of age. Infants < 12 months of age need a sepsis workup (CBC, UA, and blood, urine, and CSF culture).
- For atypical presentations, obtain electrolytes, serum glucose, blood cultures, UA, and CBC with differential.

TREATMENT

- Use antipyretic therapy (acetaminophen; avoid ASA in light of the risk of Reye's syndrome) and treat any underlying illness. Note that antipyretic therapy does not ↓ the recurrence of febrile seizures.
- For complex seizures, perform a thorough neurologic evaluation, including an EEG and MRI. Chronic anticonvulsant therapy (e.g., diazepam or phenobarbital) may be necessary.

COMPLICATIONS

- The risk of recurrence is < 30% and is highest within one year of the initial episode. For simple febrile seizures, there is no ↑ risk of developmental abnormalities or epilepsy.
- Risk factors for the development of epilepsy include complex febrile seizures (~10% risk), a ⊕ family history of epilepsy, and an abnormal neurologic exam or developmental delay.

Perform an LP if CNS infection is suspected in a patient with a febrile seizure.

*Simple febrile seizures do **not** cause brain damage, usually do **not** recur, and do **not** lead to an ↑ risk of epilepsy.*

ALL is the most common childhood malignancy, followed by CNS tumors and lymphomas.

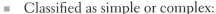

▶ **ONCOLOGY**

Leukemia

A hematopoietic malignancy of lymphocytic or myeloblastic origin. The most common childhood malignancy; 97% of cases are acute leukemias (ALL > AML). ALL is most common in male Caucasian children between two and five years of age; AML is seen most frequently in male African-American children throughout childhood. Associated with trisomy 21, Fanconi's anemia, prior radiation, severe combined immunodeficiency, and congenital bone marrow failure states.

HISTORY/PE

- Symptoms are abrupt in onset. They are initially nonspecific (anorexia, fatigue) and are followed by bone pain with refusal to bear weight, fever (from neutropenia), anemia, ecchymoses, petechiae, and/or hepatosplenomegaly.
- CNS metastases may be associated with headache, vomiting, and papilledema.

426

- AML can present with a chloroma, a greenish soft-tissue tumor on the skin or spinal cord.

DIAGNOSIS

- CBC, coagulation studies, and peripheral blood smear (high numbers of blast cells). Peripheral smears show lymphoblasts in 90% of cases. WBC counts can be low, normal, or high.
- Obtain a bone marrow aspirate for immunophenotyping (TdT assay and a panel of monoclonal antibodies to T- and B-cell antigens) and genetic analysis, which help confirm the diagnosis.
- CXR to rule out a mediastinal mass.

TREATMENT

- Chemotherapy based, including induction, consolidation, and maintenance phases.
- Tumor lysis syndrome (hyperkalemia, hyperphosphatemia, hyperuricemia) is common prior to and during the initiation of treatment. Treat with fluids, diuretics, allopurinol, urine alkalinization, and reduction of phosphate intake.

Watch for tumor lysis syndrome at the onset of any chemotherapy regimen.

Neuroblastoma

An embryonal tumor of neural crest origin. More than half of patients are < 2 years of age, and 70% of patients have distant metastases at presentation. Associated with neurofibromatosis, Hirschsprung's disease, and the N-*myc* oncogene.

HISTORY/PE

- Lesion sites are most commonly abdominal, thoracic, and cervical (in descending order).
- Symptoms may vary with location and may include a **nontender** abdominal mass (may cross the midline), Horner's syndrome, hypertension, or cord compression (from a paraspinal tumor).
- Patients may have anemia, FTT, and fever.
- More than 50% of patients will have metastases at diagnosis. Signs include bone marrow suppression, proptosis, hepatomegaly, subcutaneous nodules, and opsoclonus/myoclonus.

DIAGNOSIS

- CT scan; fine-needle aspirate of tumor. Histologically appears as small, round, blue tumor cells with a characteristic rosette pattern.
- Elevated 24-hour urinary catecholamines (VMA and HVA).
- Bone scan and bone marrow aspirate.
- CBC, LFTs, coagulation panel, BUN/creatinine.

TREATMENT

Local excision plus postsurgical chemotherapy and/or radiation.

Wilms' Tumor

A renal tumor of embryonal origin that is most commonly seen in children 2–5 years of age. Associated with Beckwith-Wiedemann syndrome (hemihy-

Wilms' tumor is associated with aniridia and hemihypertrophy.

pertrophy, macroglossia, visceromegaly), neurofibromatosis, and WAGR syndrome (**W**ilms', **A**niridia, **G**enitourinary abnormalities, mental **R**etardation).

HISTORY/PE

- Presents as an **asymptomatic, nontender,** smooth abdominal mass.
- Abdominal pain, fever, hypertension, and microscopic or gross hematuria are seen.

DIAGNOSIS

- CBC, BUN, creatinine, and UA.
- Abdominal ultrasound.
- CT scans of the chest and abdomen are used to detect metastases.

TREATMENT

Local resection and nephrectomy with postsurgical chemotherapy and radiation depending on stage and histology.

Childhood Bone Tumors

It is critical to distinguish between Ewing's sarcoma and osteosarcoma (see Table 2.13-10).

▶ PREVENTIVE CARE

Anticipatory Guidance

An important aspect of every well-child visit. Commonly tested advice includes the following:

TABLE 2.13-10. Ewing's Sarcoma vs. Osteosarcoma

	EWING'S SARCOMA	**OSTEOSARCOMA**
Origin	Sarcoma (neuroectoderm); associated with chromosome 11:22 translocation.	Osteoblasts (mesenchyme).
Epidemiology	Commonly seen in Caucasian male adolescents.	Commonly seen in male adolescents.
History/PE	Local pain and swelling. **Systemic symptoms** (fever, anorexia, fatigue) are common.	Local pain and swelling. Systemic symptoms are rare.
Location	**Midshaft** of long bones (femur, pelvis, fibula, humerus).	**Metaphyses** of long bones (distal femur, proximal tibia, proximal humerus). Metastases to lungs in 20%.
Diagnosis	Leukocytosis, ↑ ESR. Lytic bone lesion with **"onion skin"** periosteal reaction on plain x-ray.	↑ alkaline phosphatase. **"Sunburst" lytic bone lesions.** Chest CT to rule out pulmonary metastases.
Treatment	Local excision, chemotherapy, and radiation.	Local excision, chemotherapy.

- Keep the water heater at < 48.8°C (< 120°F).
- Babies should **sleep on their backs** without any stuffed animals or other toys in the crib (to ↓ the risk of SIDS).
- Car safety seats should be rear facing and should be placed in the back of the car (seats can face forward if the child is > 1 year of age and weighs > 20 lbs).
- No solid foods should be given prior to six months; they should then be introduced gradually and one at a time. Do not give cow's milk prior to 12 months.
- Syrup of ipecac (an emetic) is no longer routinely recommended for accidental poisoning. Poison control should be contacted immediately for assistance.

Hearing and Vision Screening

- Objective hearing screening (otoacoustic emissions and/or auditory brain stem response) for newborns prior to discharge is common.
- Objective hearing screening is indicated for children with a history of meningitis, TORCH infections, measles and mumps, and recurrent otitis media or chronic middle ear infections.
- The red reflex should be checked at birth. Leukocoria is the lack of a red reflex.
- **Strabismus** (ocular misalignment) is normal until three months of age; beyond three months, children should be evaluated by a pediatric ophthalmologist and may require corrective lenses, occlusion, and/or surgery to prevent **amblyopia** (suppression of retinal images in a misaligned eye, leading to permanent vision loss).

Leukocoria indicates retinoblastoma, congenital cataracts, or retinopathy of prematurity.

Childhood Vaccinations

The Epidemiology chapter summarizes CDC-recommended vaccinations for the pediatric population. Contraindications and precautions in this population are as follows:

- **Contraindications:**
    - Severe allergy to a vaccine component or a prior dose of vaccine. Patients who are allergic to eggs may not receive MMR or influenza vaccine.
    - Encephalopathy within seven days of prior pertussis vaccination.
    - Avoid live vaccines (oral polio vaccine, varicella, MMR) in immunocompromised and pregnant patients (exception: HIV patients may receive MMR and varicella).
- **Precautions:**
    - Current moderate to severe illness (with or without fever).
    - Prior reactions to pertussis vaccine (fever > 40.5°C, shocklike state, persistent crying for > 3 hours within 48 hours of vaccination, or seizure within three days of vaccination).
    - A history of receiving IVIG in the past year.
- The following are **not** contraindications to vaccination:
    - Mild illness and/or low-grade fever.
    - Current antibiotic therapy.
    - Prematurity.
- Pneumococcal polysaccharide vaccine (PPV) should be administered to high-risk groups (sickle cell disease or splenectomy, immunodeficient).

Lead Poisoning

Most exposure in children is due to lead-contaminated household dust from leaded paint. Screening should be routinely performed at 12 and 24 months for patients living in high-risk areas (pre-1950s homes or zip codes with high percentages of elevated blood lead levels).

HISTORY/PE

- Presents with irritability, hyperactivity or apathy, anorexia, intermittent abdominal pain, constipation, intermittent vomiting, and peripheral neuropathy (wrist or foot drop).
- Acute encephalopathy (usually with levels > 70 μg/dL) is characterized by ↑ ICP, vomiting, confusion, seizures, and coma.

DIAGNOSIS

- Blood lead level.
- CBC and peripheral blood smear show microcytic, hypochromic anemia and basophilic stippling.

TREATMENT

- **< 45 μg/dL and asymptomatic:** Retest at 1–3 months; remove sources of lead exposure.
- **45–69 μg/dL:** Chelation therapy (inpatient **EDTA** or outpatient oral succimer [**DMSA**]).
- **≥ 70 μg/dL:** Chelation therapy (inpatient EDTA + **BAL** [IM dimercaprol]).

New evidence has shown impaired intelligence and neurodevelopmental outcomes among children exposed to lead levels as low as 10 μg/dL.

Psychiatry

Generalized Anxiety Disorder

- **Uncontrollable, excessive anxiety or worry about activities or events in life** that leads to significant impairment or distress.
- The male-to-female ratio is 1:2; clinical onset is usually in the early 20s.
- Hx/PE: Presents with anxiety on most days (**six or more months**) and with **three or more somatic symptoms** (restlessness, fatigue, difficulty concentrating, irritability, muscle tension, disturbed sleep).
- **Tx:**
    - Lifestyle changes, psychotherapy, medication. SSRIs, venlafaxine, and buspirone are most often used (see Table 2.14-1). Benzodiazepines may be used for immediate symptom relief.
    - Taper benzodiazepines as soon as long-term treatment is initiated (e.g., with SSRIs) in light of the high risk of tolerance and dependence. Do not stop benzodiazepines "cold turkey," as patients may develop potentially lethal withdrawal symptoms similar to those of alcohol withdrawal.
    - Patient education is essential.

Buspirone is another drug, in addition to SSRIs, that should not be used with MAOIs.

Obsessive-Compulsive Disorder (OCD)

- Characterized by obsessions and/or compulsions that lead to significant distress and dysfunction in social or personal areas.
- Typically presents in late adolescence or early adulthood; prevalence is equal in males and females. Often a chronic condition that is difficult to treat.
- Hx/PE:
    - **Obsessions: Persistent, unwanted, and intrusive ideas, thoughts, impulses, or images** that lead to marked anxiety or distress (e.g., fear of contamination, fear of harm to oneself or to loved ones) and occur despite the patient's attempts to prevent them.

Many OCD patients initially present to a nonpsychiatrist—e.g., they may consult a dermatologist with a skin complaint 2° to overwashing hands.

TABLE 2.14-1. Anxiolytic Medications

DRUG CLASS	INDICATIONS	SIDE EFFECTS
SSRIs (fluoxetine, sertraline, paroxetine, citalopram, escitalopram)	First-line treatment for generalized anxiety disorder, OCD, and PTSD.	Nausea, GI upset, somnolence, sexual dysfunction, agitation.
Buspirone	Generalized anxiety disorder, OCD, PTSD.	Seizures with chronic use. No tolerance, dependence, or withdrawal.
β-blockers	Performance anxiety, PTSD.	Bradycardia, hypotension.
Benzodiazepines	Anxiety, insomnia, alcohol withdrawal, muscle spasm, night terrors, sleepwalking.	↓ sleep duration; risk of abuse, tolerance, and dependence; disinhibition in young or old patients; confusion.
Flumazenil (competitive antagonist at GABA receptor)	Antidote to benzodiazepine intoxication.	Resedation; nausea, dizziness, vomiting, and pain at the injection site.

- **Compulsions: Repeated mental acts or behaviors** that neutralize anxiety from obsessions (e.g., hand washing, elaborate rituals for ordinary tasks, counting, excessive checking).
    - Patients **recognize these behaviors as excessive and irrational products of their own minds** (vs. obsessive-compulsive personality disorder, or OCPD; see Table 2.14-2). Patients wish they could get rid of the obsessions and/or compulsions.
- **Tx:** Pharmacotherapy (SSRIs are first-line pharmacologic treatment; see Table 2.14-1); cognitive-behavioral therapy (CBT) using exposure and desensitization relaxation techniques. Patient education is imperative.

Panic Disorder

- Characterized by recurrent, unexpected panic attacks.
- Two to three times more common in females than in males. **Agoraphobia** is present in 30–50% of cases. The average age of onset is 25, but may occur at any age.
- **Hx/PE:**
    - **Panic attacks** are defined as discrete **periods of intense fear or discomfort** in which at least four of the following symptoms develop abruptly and peak within 10 minutes: tachypnea, chest pain, **palpitations, diaphoresis,** nausea, trembling, dizziness, **fear of dying** or "going crazy," depersonalization, or hot flashes.
    - Perioral and/or acral paresthesias, when present, are fairly specific to panic attacks, which produce hyperventilation and low oxygen saturation.
    - Patients present with **one or more months** of concern about having additional attacks or significant behavior change as a result of the attacks—e.g., avoiding situations that may precipitate attacks.
    - **Elucidate if a patient has panic disorder with or without agoraphobia** so that agoraphobia can also be addressed in the treatment plan.
    - The differential should include the following:
        - **Medical conditions:** Angina, MI, arrhythmias, hyperthyroidism, vitamin B_{12} deficiency, pheochromocytoma.
        - **Psychiatric conditions:** Substance-induced anxiety, generalized anxiety disorder, PTSD.
- **Tx:**
    - CBT, pharmacotherapy (e.g., SSRIs, TCAs).
    - Benzodiazepines (e.g., clonazepam) may be used for immediate relief, but long-term use should be avoided in light of the potential for addiction and tolerance (see Table 2.14-1).
    - Taper benzodiazepines as soon as long-term treatment is initiated (e.g., SSRIs).

Alprazolam (Xanax) is an SSRI that is sometimes used to treat panic disorder, but it has such a short half-life that patients can go into mild withdrawal within a day.

TABLE 2.14-2. OCD vs. OCPD

OCD	OCPD
Characterized by obsessions and/or compulsions.	Patients are excessively conscientious and inflexible.
Patients **recognize** the obsessions/compulsions and want to be rid of them (ego-dystonic).	Patients **do not recognize** their behavior as problematic (ego-syntonic).

Phobias (Social and Specific)

- Defined as follows:
  - **Social phobia:** Characterized by marked fear provoked by **social or performance situations** in which embarrassment may occur. It may be specific (e.g., public speaking, urinating in public) or general (e.g., social interaction) and often begins in adolescence.
  - **Specific phobia:** Anxiety is provoked by exposure to a **feared object or situation** (e.g., animals, heights, airplanes). Most cases begin in childhood.
- **Hx/PE:** Presents with excessive or unreasonable fear and/or avoidance of an object or situation that is persistent and leads to significant distress or impairment in function. A related history of traumatic events or panic attacks may be present. Patients recognize that their fear is excessive.
- **Tx:**
  - **Specific phobias:** CBT involving desensitization through incremental exposure to the feared object or situation and relaxation techniques. Other options include supportive, family, and insight-oriented psychotherapy.
  - **Social phobias:** CBT, SSRIs, low-dose benzodiazepines, or β-blockers (for performance anxiety) may be used (see Table 2.14-1).

Post-traumatic Stress Disorder (PTSD)

- Follows exposure to an extreme, life-threatening traumatic event (e.g., assault, combat, witnessing a violent crime) that evoked intense fear, helplessness, or horror.
- **Hx/PE:**
  - Characterized by **reexperiencing of the event** (e.g., nightmares), **avoidance** of stimuli associated with the trauma, **numbed responsiveness** (e.g., detachment, anhedonia), and ↑ **arousal** (e.g., hypervigilance, exaggerated startle) that lead to significant distress or impairment in functioning.
  - Symptoms must persist for > 1 month.
  - Survivor guilt, irritability, poor concentration, amnesia, personality change, sleep disturbance, substance abuse, depression, and suicidality may be present.
  - Some controversy exists regarding the prevalence of PTSD, which some clinicians feel is overdiagnosed. It is therefore prudent to carefully consider other diagnoses in the differential—e.g., major depressive disorder, personality disorder, or adjustment disorder.
- **Tx:**
  - SSRIs are first line; buspirone, TCAs, and MAOIs may be helpful (see Table 2.14-1).
  - Short-term agents **targeting anxiety** include β-blockers and α_2-agonists (e.g., clonidine).
  - Benzodiazepines are also used but should be avoided in light of their addictive potential, as there is a high incidence of substance abuse among individuals with PTSD.
  - **Psychotherapy** and **support groups** are useful.

Affect memory, orientation, judgment, and attention.

Dementia

An impairment in **cognitive** functioning with **global deficits. Level of consciousness is stable.** Prevalence is highest among those > 85 years of age. The course is persistent and progressive. The most common causes are **Alzheimer's disease** (50%) and **multi-infarct dementia** (25%). Other causes are outlined in the mnemonic **DEMENTIAS.**

HISTORY/PE

Diagnostic criteria include **memory impairment and one or more** of the following:

- **Aphasia:** Language impairment.
- **Apraxia:** Inability to perform motor activities.
- **Agnosia:** Inability to recognize previously known objects.
- **Impaired executive function (problems with planning, organizing, and abstracting)** in the presence of a **clear sensorium.**
- Personality, mood, and behavior changes are common (e.g., wandering and aggression).

DIAGNOSIS

- A careful history and physical are critical. Serial mini-mental status exams should be performed.
- Rule out treatable causes of dementia; obtain CBC, RPR, CMP, TFTs, HIV, B$_{12}$/folate, ESR, UA, and a head CT or MRI.
- Table 2.14-3 outlines key characteristics distinguishing dementia from delirium.

Causes of dementia—

DEMENTIAS

Degenerative diseases (Parkinson's, Huntington's)
Endocrine (thyroid, parathyroid, pituitary, adrenal)
Metabolic (alcohol, electrolytes, vitamin B$_{12}$ deficiency, glucose, hepatic, renal, Wilson's disease)
Exogenous (heavy metals, carbon monoxide, drugs)
Neoplasia
Trauma (subdural hematoma)
Infection (meningitis, encephalitis, endocarditis, syphilis, HIV, prion diseases, Lyme disease)
Affective disorders (pseudodementia)
Stroke/**S**tructure (vascular dementia, ischemia, vasculitis, normal pressure hydrocephalus)

TABLE 2.14-3. Delirium vs. Dementia

	DELIRIUM	**DEMENTIA**
Level of attention	Impaired (fluctuating).	Usually alert.
Onset	Acute.	Gradual.
Course	Fluctuating from hour to hour.	Progressive deterioration.
Consciousness	Clouded.	Intact.
Hallucinations	Present (often visual or tactile).	Occur in approximately 30% of patients in highly advanced disease.
Prognosis	Reversible.	Largely irreversible, but up to 15% of cases are due to treatable causes and are reversible.

The 4 A's of dementia:

Amnesia
Apraxia
Aphasia
Agnosia

Major causes of delirium—

I WATCH DEATH

Infection
Withdrawal
Acute metabolic/
    substance **A**buse
Trauma
CNS pathology
Hypoxia
Deficiencies
Endocrine
Acute vascular/MI
Toxins/drugs
Heavy metals

It is common for delirium to be superimposed on dementia.

TREATMENT

- Provide **environmental cues** and a rigid structure for the patient's daily life.
- **Cholinesterase inhibitors** are used to treat. Low-dose **antipsychotics** may be used for agitation. **Avoid benzodiazepines,** which may worsen disinhibition and confusion.
- Family, caregiver, and patient education and support are imperative.

Delirium

An acute **disturbance of consciousness** with **altered cognition** that develops over a short period of time (usually hours to days). Children, the elderly, and hospitalized patients (e.g., **ICU psychosis**) are particularly susceptible. Major causes are outlined in the mnemonic **I WATCH DEATH.** Symptoms are potentially reversible if the underlying cause can be treated.

HISTORY/PE

- Presents with acute onset of **waxing and waning consciousness** with lucid intervals and **perceptual disturbances** (hallucinations, illusions, delusions).
- Patients may be combative, anxious, paranoid, or stuporous.
- Also characterized by a ↓ attention span and short-term memory, a reversed sleep-wake cycle, and ↑ symptoms at night (sundowning).

DIAGNOSIS

- Check vitals, pulse oximetry, and glucose; perform physical and neurologic exams.
- Note recent medications (narcotics, anticholinergics, steroids, or benzodiazepines), substance use, prior episodes, medical problems, signs of organ failure (kidney, liver), and infection (**occult UTI is common in the elderly;** check UA).
- Order lab and radiologic studies to identify a possible underlying cause.

TREATMENT

- **Treat underlying causes** (delirium is often reversible).
- Normalize fluids and electrolytes.
- **Optimize the sensory environment.**
- Use low-dose **antipsychotics** (e.g., haloperidol) for agitation and psychotic symptoms.
- Conservative use of **physical restraints** may be necessary to prevent harm to the patient or others.

▶ MOOD DISORDERS

Also known as **affective disorders.**

Major Depressive Disorder

A mood disorder characterized by one or more major depressive episodes (MDEs). The **male-to-female ratio is 1:2;** lifetime prevalence ranges from 15% to 25%. Onset is usually in the mid-20s; in the elderly, prevalence ↑ with age. **Chronic illness and stress** ↑ risk. Up to 15% of patients die by suicide.

MDEs can be present in major depressive disorder or in bipolar disorder types I and II.

HISTORY/PE

Diagnosis requires **depressed mood or anhedonia (loss of interest/pleasure) and five or more signs/symptoms** from the **SIG E CAPS** mnemonic for a two-week period. Table 2.14-4 outlines the differential diagnosis of conditions that may be mistaken for depression. Selected depression subtypes include the following:

- **Psychotic features:** Typically **mood-congruent** delusions/hallucinations.
- **Postpartum:** Occurs within one month postpartum; has a 10% incidence and a high risk of recurrence. Psychotic symptoms are common.
- **Atypical:** Characterized by weight gain, hypersomnia, and rejection sensitivity.
- **Seasonal:** Depressive episodes tend to occur during a particular season, most commonly winter. Responds well to light therapy +/– antidepressants.
- **Double depression:** MDE in a patient with dysthymia. Has a poorer prognosis than MDE alone.

TREATMENT

- **Pharmacotherapy:** Effective in 50–70% of patients. Allow 2–6 weeks to take effect; treat for ≥ 6 months (see Table 2.14-5).
- **Psychotherapy:** Psychotherapy combined with antidepressants is more effective than either treatment alone.
- **Electroconvulsive therapy (ECT):**
  - Safe, highly effective, often lifesaving therapy that is reserved for refractory depression or psychotic depression, or if rapid improvement in mood is needed.

> **Symptoms of a depressive episode—**
>
> **SIG E CAPS**
>
> **S**leep (hypersomnia or insomnia)
> **I**nterest (loss of interest or pleasure in activities)
> **G**uilt (feelings of worthlessness or inappropriate guilt)
> **E**nergy (↓) or fatigue
> **C**oncentration (↓)
> **A**ppetite (↑ or ↓) or weight (↑ or ↓)
> **P**sychomotor agitation or retardation
> **S**uicidal ideation

> **TCA toxicity—**
>
> **Tri-C's:**
>
> **C**onvulsions
> **C**oma
> **C**ardiac arrhythmias

TABLE 2.14-4. Differential Diagnosis of Major Depression

DISORDER	DISTINGUISHING FEATURES
Mood disorder due to a medical condition	Hypothyroidism, Parkinson's disease, CNS neoplasm, other neoplasm (e.g., pancreatic cancer), stroke (especially ACA stroke), dementias, parathyroid disorders.
Substance-induced mood disorder	Illicit drugs, alcohol, antihypertensives, corticosteroids, OCPs.
Adjustment disorder with depressed mood	A constellation of symptoms resembling an MDE but not meeting the criteria for MDE. Occurs within three months of an identifiable stressor.
Normal bereavement	Occurs after the loss of a loved one. No severe impairment/suicidality; usually resolves in one year, but varies with cultural norms. May lead to major depressive disorder requiring treatment. Illusions/hallucinations of the deceased can be normal as long as the person recognizes them as such.
Dysthymia	Milder, chronic depression with depressed mood present most of the time for at least two years; often treatment resistant.

TABLE 2.14-5.   Indications and Side Effects of Common Antidepressants

Drug Class	Examples	Indications	Side Effects
SSRIs	Fluoxetine, sertraline, paroxetine, citalopram, fluvoxamine	Depression and anxiety.	Sexual side effects, GI distress, agitation, insomnia, tremor, diarrhea. **Serotonin syndrome** (fever, myoclonus, mental status changes, cardiovascular collapse) can occur if SSRIs are used with MAOIs. Paroxetine can cause pulmonary hypertension in the fetus.
Atypicals	Bupropion, venlafaxine, mirtazapine, trazodone	Depression, anxiety, and chronic pain.	**Bupropion:** ↓ seizure threshold; **minimal sexual side effects.** Contraindicated in patients with eating disorders as well as in seizure patients. **Venlafaxine:** Diastolic hypertension. **Mirtazapine:** Weight gain, sedation. **Trazodone:** Highly sedating; priapism.
TCAs	Nortriptyline, desipramine, amitriptyline, imipramine	Depression, anxiety disorder, chronic pain, migraine headaches, enuresis (imipramine).	**Lethal** with overdose owing to cardiac conduction arrhythmias (e.g., long QRS). Monitor in the ICU for 3–4 days following an OD. **Anticholinergic** effects (dry mouth, constipation, urinary retention, sedation).
MAOIs	Phenelzine, tranylcypromine, selegiline (patch form available)	Depression, especially atypical.	Hypertensive crisis if taken with high-**tyramine** foods (cheese, red wine). Sexual side effects, orthostatic hypotension, weight gain.

Discontinue SSRIs at least two weeks before starting an MAOI. Wait five weeks if the patient was on fluoxetine.

- May also be used for mania and psychosis. Usually requires 6–12 treatments.
- Adverse effects include postictal confusion, arrhythmias, headache, and **anterograde amnesia.**
- Contraindications include recent MI/stroke, intracranial mass, and high anesthetic risk (a relative contraindication).
- **Phototherapy:** Effective for patients whose depression has a seasonal pattern.
- **Transcranial magnetic stimulation (TMS):** Now approved for the treatment of major depression. TMS is about as effective as medications but is not as effective as ECT.

Mixed states and mania are psychiatric emergencies 2° to impaired judgment and great risk of harm to self and others.

Bipolar Disorders

Prevalence is approximately 1% for type I and an additional 3% for type II; males and females are affected equally. A family history of bipolar illness significantly ↑ risk. Average age of onset is 20, and the frequency of mood episodes tends to ↑ with age. Up to 10–15% of those affected die by suicide. Subtypes are as follows:

- **Bipolar I: At least one manic or mixed episode** (usually requiring hospitalization).

- **Bipolar II: At least one MDE and one hypomanic episode** (less intense than mania). Patients do not meet the criteria for full manic or mixed episodes.
- **Rapid cycling:** Four or more episodes (MDE, manic, mixed, or hypomanic) in one year.
- **Cyclothymic:** Chronic and less severe, with alternating periods of hypomania and moderate depression for > 2 years.

HISTORY/PE

- The mnemonic **DIG FAST** outlines the clinical presentation of mania.
- Patients may report excessive engagement in pleasurable activities (e.g., excessive spending or sexual activity), reckless behaviors, and/or psychotic features.
- **Antidepressant use may trigger manic episodes.**

DIAGNOSIS

- A manic episode is **one week or more of persistently elevated, expansive, or irritable mood** plus **three DIG FAST symptoms. Psychotic symptoms** are common in mania.
- Symptoms are not due to a substance or medical condition and lead to significant impairment socially, occupationally, or familially.
- Hypomania is similar but does not involve marked functional impairment or psychotic symptoms and does not require hospitalization.

TREATMENT

- **Mania:** Give mood stabilizers for maintenance therapy (see Table 2.14-6) and antipsychotics in the acute phase (see the discussion of psychotic dis-

> **Symptoms of mania—**
>
> **DIG FAST**
>
> **D**istractibility
> **I**nsomnia (↓ need for sleep)
> **G**randiosity (↑ self-esteem)/more **G**oal directed
> **F**light of ideas (or racing thoughts)
> **A**ctivities/psychomotor **A**gitation
> **S**exual indiscretions/ other pleasurable activities
> **T**alkativeness/pressured speech

TABLE 2.14-6. Mood Stabilizers

DRUG CLASS	INDICATIONS	SIDE EFFECTS
Lithium	First-line mood stabilizer. Used for acute mania (in combination with antipsychotics), for prophylaxis in bipolar disorders, and for augmentation in depression treatment.	Thirst, polyuria, diabetes insipidus, tremor, weight gain, hypothyroidism, nausea, diarrhea, seizures, teratogenicity (if used in the first trimester), acne, vomiting. Narrow therapeutic window (but blood level can be monitored). **Lithium toxicity:** > 1.5 mEq/L; presents with ataxia, dysarthria, delirium, and acute renal failure. Avoid lithium in patients with ↓ renal function.
Carbamazepine	Second-line mood stabilizer; anticonvulsant; trigeminal neuralgia.	Nausea, skin rash, leukopenia, AV block. Rarely, aplastic anemia (monitor CBC biweekly). Stevens-Johnson syndrome.
Valproic acid	Bipolar disorder; anticonvulsant.	GI (nausea, vomiting), tremor, sedation, alopecia, weight gain. Rarely, pancreatitis, thrombocytopenia, fatal hepatotoxicity, and agranulocytosis.
Lamotrigine	Second-line mood stabilizer; anticonvulsant.	Blurred vision, GI distress, Stevens-Johnson syndrome. ↑ dose slowly to monitor for rashes.

orders below). Benzodiazepines may be of benefit in refractory agitation.

- **Bipolar depression:** Mood stabilizers +/– antidepressants. **Start mood stabilizers first** (see Table 2.14-6) to avoid inducing mania. ECT may be used to treat refractory cases.
- In patients with **severe depression** or **bipolar II with predominantly depressive features,** antidepressant treatment can be augmented with low-dose lithium—e.g., at blood levels of 0.4–0.6 mEq/L.

> ► **PERSONALITY DISORDERS**

Characteristics of personality disorders—

MEDIC

Maladaptive
Enduring
Deviate from cultural norms
Inflexible
Cause impairment in social or occupational functioning

Personality can be defined as an individual's set of emotional and behavioral traits, which are generally stable and predictable. Personality disorders are defined when one's traits become chronically rigid and maladaptive and affect most aspects of one's life (see the mnemonic **MEDIC**). Onset occurs by early adulthood. Personality disorders are defined under Axis II in the DSM-IV (see definition of axes on the following page). Specific disorders are outlined in Table 2.14-7.

TABLE 2.14-7. Signs and Symptoms of Personality Disorders

CLUSTER	DISORDERS	CHARACTERISTICS	CLINICAL DILEMMA/STRATEGY
Cluster A: "weird"	Paranoid	Distrustful, suspicious; interpret others' motives as malevolent.	Patients are suspicious and distrustful of psychiatrists, making it difficult to form therapeutic relationships between patient and psychiatrist.
	Schizoid	Isolated, detached "loners." Restricted emotional expression.	
	Schizotypal	Odd behavior, perceptions, and appearance. Magical thinking; ideas of reference.	Be clear, honest, noncontrolling, and nondefensive.
Cluster B: "wild"	Borderline	Unstable mood, relationships, and self-image; feelings of emptiness. Impulsive. History of suicidal ideation or self-harm.	Patients change the rules and demand attention. They are manipulative and demanding and will split staff members.
	Histrionic	Excessively emotional and attention seeking. Sexually provocative; theatrical.	Be firm. Stick to the treatment plan.
	Narcissistic	Grandiose; need admiration; have sense of entitlement. Lack empathy.	Be fair. Do not be punitive or derogatory. Be consistent. Do not change rules.
	Antisocial	Violate rights of others, social norms, and laws. Impulsive; lack remorse. Begins in childhood as conduct disorder.	
Cluster C: "worried and wimpy"	Obsessive-compulsive	Preoccupied with perfectionism, order, and control at the expense of efficiency. Inflexible morals, values.	Patients are controlling and may sabotage their treatment. Words may be inconsistent with actions.
	Avoidant	Socially inhibited; rejection sensitive. Fear being disliked or ridiculed.	Avoid power struggles. Give clear recommendations, but do not push patients into decisions.
	Dependent	Submissive, clingy; need to be taken care of. Difficulty making decisions. Feel helpless.	

- Ask about attitudes, mood variability, activities, and reaction to stress.
- Patients have chronic problems dealing with responsibilities, roles, and stressors. They may also deny their behavior, have difficulty understanding the cause of their problems, have difficulty changing their behavior patterns, and frequently refuse psychiatric care.

TREATMENT

- **Psychotherapy** is the mainstay of therapy.
- **Pharmacotherapy** is reserved for cases with comorbid mood, anxiety, or psychotic signs/symptoms.

▶ PSYCHOTIC DISORDERS

Schizophrenia

Characterized by hallucinations, delusions, disordered thoughts, behavioral disturbances, and disrupted social functioning with a clear sensorium.

- **Epidemiology:** Prevalence is approximately 1%; males and females are affected equally. **Peak onset is earlier in males (ages 18–25)** than in **females (ages 25–35)**, and has an ↑ incidence in those born in winter or early spring. Schizophrenia in first-degree relatives also ↑ risk. **Ten percent of those affected commit suicide.**
- **Etiology:** Etiologic theories focus on neurotransmitter abnormalities such as dopamine dysregulation (frontal hypoactivity; limbic hyperactivity; efficacy of dopamine antagonists) and brain abnormalities on CT and MRI (enlarged ventricles and ↓ cortical volume). Subtypes are as follows:
  - **Paranoid:** Delusions (often of persecution of the patient) and/or hallucinations are present. Cognitive function is usually preserved. Associated with the best overall prognosis.
  - **Disorganized:** Speech and behavior patterns are highly disordered and disinhibited with flat affect. The thought disorder is pronounced, and the patient has poor contact with reality. Carries the worst prognosis.
  - **Catatonic:** A rare form characterized by psychomotor disturbance with two or more of the following: excessive motor activity, immobility, extreme negativism, mutism, waxy flexibility, echolalia, or echopraxia.

HISTORY/PE

- Two or more of the following are present continuously for **six or more months** with **social or occupational dysfunction:**
  - ⊕ **symptoms:** Hallucinations (most often auditory), delusions, disorganized speech, bizarre behavior, and thought disorder.
  - ⊖ **symptoms:** Flat affect, ↓ emotional reactivity, poverty of speech, lack of purposeful actions, and anhedonia.
- The differential includes the following:
  - **Schizophreniform disorder:** Symptoms of schizophrenia with a duration of < 6 months.
  - **Schizoaffective disorder:** Combines the symptoms of schizophrenia with a major affective disorder (major depressive disorder or bipolar disorder).

Five categories are used by the DSM-IV to classify the factors contributing to an individual's mental state:

- ***Axis I:** Psychiatric disorders.*
- ***Axis II:** Personality disorders and mental retardation.*
- ***Axis III:** Physical and medical problems.*
- ***Axis IV:** Social and environmental problems/ stressors.*
- ***Axis V:** The Global Assessment of Functioning (GAF), which rates a patient's overall level of social, occupational, and psychological functioning on a scale of 1 (nonfunctional) to 100 (extremely high functioning across several areas).*

HIGH-YIELD FACTS

PSYCHIATRY

*Terms used to describe
components of psychosis:*

- **Delusion:** *A fixed false
  idiosyncratic belief.*
- **Hallucination:** *Perception
  of an object or event
  without an existing
  external stimulus.*
- **Illusion:** *False perception
  of an actual external
  stimulus.*

TREATMENT

- **Antipsychotics** (see Table 2.14-8); **long-term follow-up.**
- Supportive psychotherapy, training in social skills, vocational rehabilitation, and illness education may help.
- ⊖ symptoms may be more difficult to treat.

▶ **CHILDHOOD AND ADOLESCENT DISORDERS**

Attention-Deficit Hyperactivity Disorder (ADHD)

A persistent pattern of excessive inattention and/or hyperactivity/impulsivity. More common in males; typically presents between ages 3 and 13. Often shows a familial pattern.

HISTORY/PE

Diagnosis requires **six or more symptoms** from each category listed below for **six or more months** in **at least two settings,** leading to significant social and academic impairment. Some symptoms must be present in patients **before age seven.**

- **Inattention: Poor attention span** in schoolwork/play; poor attention to detail or careless mistakes; does not listen when spoken to; has **difficulty**

TABLE 2.14-8. Antipsychotic Medications

DRUG CLASS	EXAMPLES	INDICATIONS	SIDE EFFECTS
Typical antipsychotics	Haloperidol, droperidol, fluphenazine, thioridazine, chlorpromazine	Psychotic disorders, acute agitation, acute mania, Tourette's syndrome. Thought to be more effective for ⊕ symptoms of schizophrenia; primarily block D2 dopamine receptors. For patients in whom compliance is a major issue, consider antipsychotics that come in depot forms (haloperidol, fluphenazine).	**Extrapyramidal symptoms** (EPS; see Table 2.14-9), **hyperprolactinemia. Anticholinergic effects** (dry mouth, urinary retention, constipation). Seizures, hypotension, sedation, and QTc prolongation. Irreversible retinal pigmentation **(thioridazine). Neuroleptic malignant syndrome:** Fever, muscle rigidity, autonomic instability, elevated CK, clouded consciousness. **Stop medication; provide supportive care in the ICU;** administer **dantrolene** or **bromocriptine** (see Table 2.14-9).
Atypical antipsychotics	Clozapine, risperidone (also available in long-acting depot injection), quetiapine, olanzapine, ziprasidone, aripiprazole	Currently first-line treatment for schizophrenia given fewer EPS and anticholinergic effects. Clozapine is reserved for severe treatment resistance and severe tardive dyskinesia.	Weight gain, type 2 DM, somnolence, sedation, and QTc prolongation. **Agranulocytosis** requiring weekly CBC monitoring **(clozapine).**

TABLE 2.14-9. Extrapyramidal Symptoms and Treatment

EPS	DESCRIPTION	TREATMENT
Acute dystonia	Involuntary muscle contraction or spasm (e.g., torticollis, oculogyric crisis).	Anticholinergics (benztropine or diphenhydramine); some patients on antipsychotics who are prone to dystonic reactions may need regular prophylactic dosing of these.
Akathisia	Subjective/objective restlessness, which is perceived as being distressing.	↓ neuroleptic and try β-blockers (propranolol). Benzodiazepines or anticholinergics may help.
Dyskinesia	Pseudoparkinsonism (e.g., shuffling gait, cogwheel rigidity).	Give an anticholinergic (benztropine) or a dopamine agonist (amantadine). ↓ the dose of neuroleptic or discontinue (if tolerated).
Tardive dyskinesia	Stereotypic oral-facial movements. Likely from dopamine receptor sensitization. Often irreversible (50%).	Discontinue or ↓ the dose of neuroleptic; attempt treatment with more appropriate drugs; and consider changing neuroleptic (e.g., to clozapine or risperidone). **Giving anticholinergics or decreasing neuroleptics may initially worsen tardive dyskinesia.**

following instructions or finishing tasks; loses items needed to complete tasks; is forgetful and **easily distracted.**

- **Hyperactivity/impulsivity:** Fidgets; leaves seat in classroom; runs around inappropriately; cannot play quietly; talks excessively; **does not wait turn; interrupts others.**

TREATMENT

- Initial treatment may be nonpharmacologic (e.g., behavior modification). Sugar and food additives are **not** considered etiologic factors.
- Pharmacologic treatment includes the following:
  - **Psychostimulants: Methylphenidate (Ritalin),** dextroamphetamine (Dexedrine), mixed salts of dextroamphetamine and amphetamine (Adderall), atomoxetine (Strattera), pemoline (Cylert). Adverse effects include insomnia, irritability, ↓ appetite, tic exacerbation, and ↓ growth velocity (normalizes when medication is stopped).
  - **Antidepressants** (e.g., SSRIs, nortriptyline, bupropion) and α₂-agonists (e.g., **clonidine**).

> *Evolution of EPS—*
>
> **4 and A**
>
> **4** hours: **A**cute dystonia
> **4** days: **A**kinesia
> **4** weeks: **A**kathisia
> **4** months: Tardive dyskinesia (often permanent)

Children must exhibit ADHD symptoms in two or more settings (e.g., home and school).

Autism Spectrum/Pervasive Developmental Disorders

More common in males. May be associated with **tuberous sclerosis and fragile X syndrome.** Symptom severity and IQ vary widely.

HISTORY/PE

- Characterized by abnormal or **impaired social interaction and communication** together with **restricted activities and interests,** evident **before age three.**

- Patients fail to develop normal social behaviors (e.g., social smile, eye contact) and lack interest in relationships.
- The development of spoken language is delayed or absent.
- Children show **stereotyped speech and behavior** (e.g., hand flapping) and restricted interests (e.g., preoccupation with parts of objects).
- Other pervasive developmental disorders include the following:
  - **Asperger's syndrome:** An autism-like disorder of social impairment and repetitive activities, behaviors, and interests **without marked language or cognitive delays.**
  - **Rett's disorder:** A genetic neurodegenerative disorder of females with progressive impairment (e.g., language, head growth, coordination) **after five months of normal development.**
  - **Childhood disintegrative disorder:** Severe developmental **regression** after > 2 years of normal development (e.g., language, motor skills, social skills, bladder/bowel control, play).

TREATMENT

- Intensive special education, **behavioral management,** and symptom-targeted medications (e.g., neuroleptics for aggression; SSRIs for stereotyped behavior).
- Family support and counseling are crucial.

Disruptive Behavioral Disorders

*Conduct disorder is seen in **C**hildren. **A**ntisocial personality disorder is seen in **A**dults.*

- Include conduct disorder and oppositional defiant disorder.
- More common among males and in patients with a history of abuse.
- Hx/PE:
  - **Conduct disorder:** A repetitive, persistent pattern of **violating the basic rights of others** or age-appropriate **societal norms or rules** for **one year or more.** Behaviors may be **aggressive** (e.g., rape, robbery, animal cruelty) or **nonaggressive** (e.g., stealing, lying, deliberately annoying people). May progress to antisocial personality disorder in adulthood.
  - **Oppositional defiant disorder:** A pattern of **negativistic, defiant, disobedient, and hostile behavior** toward authority figures (e.g., losing temper, arguing) for six or more months. **May progress to conduct disorder.**
- Tx: Individual and family therapy.

Learning Disabilities

- Occur more frequently in males and in those of low socioeconomic status (SES); often exhibit a familial pattern.
- Hx/PE:
  - **Academic functioning is substantially lower than expected for age, intelligence, and education** as measured by standardized test achievement in reading, mathematics, or written expression.
  - Learning problems significantly interfere with schooling and daily activities.
  - Always rule out physical disorders (e.g., deafness) and social factors (e.g., non–English speakers).
- Tx: Interventions include **remedial classes** or **individualized learning strategies.**

Mental Retardation

- Associated with male gender, chromosomal abnormalities, congenital infections, teratogens, inborn errors of metabolism, and alcohol/illicit substances during pregnancy.
- Hx/PE:
  - Patients have significantly subaverage intellectual functioning (**an IQ of < 70**) with **deficits in adaptive functioning** (e.g., hygiene, social skills); onset is before the age of 18.
  - Levels of severity are **mild** (IQ 50–70; **85% of cases**), moderate (**IQ 35–49**), severe (**IQ 20–34**), and profound (**IQ < 20**).
- Tx:
  - 1° prevention consists of educating the general public about possible causes of mental retardation and providing optimal prenatal screening and health care to mothers and their children.
  - Treatment measures include family counseling and support; speech and language therapy; occupational/physical therapy; behavioral intervention; educational assistance; and social skills training.

Fetal alcohol syndrome is the number one avoidable cause of mental retardation.

Tourette's Syndrome

- More common in males; shows a genetic predisposition. **Associated with ADHD, learning disorders**, and **OCD**.
- Hx/PE:
  - Begins prior to age 18.
  - Characterized by **multiple motor** (e.g., blinking, grimacing) and **vocal** (e.g., grunting, coprolalia) **tics** occurring many times per day, recurrently, for > 1 year with social or occupational impairment.
- Tx: Treatments include **dopamine receptor antagonists** (haloperidol, pimozide) or clonidine. Behavioral therapy may be of benefit, and counseling can aid in social adjustment and coping. Stimulants can worsen or precipitate tics.

Coprolalia = repetition of obscene words.

▶ MISCELLANEOUS DISORDERS

Substance Abuse/Dependence

Both substance abuse and substance dependence are maladaptive patterns of substance use that lead to clinically significant impairment. Substance abuse is distinguished from substance dependence as follows:

- **Substance abuse:** Requires one or more of the following in one year:
  - **Failure to fulfill responsibilities** at work, school, or home.
  - Use in **physically hazardous** situations (e.g., driving while intoxicated).
  - **Legal problems** during the time of substance use.
  - Continued substance use despite recurrent social or interpersonal problems 2° to the effects of such use (e.g., frequent arguments with spouse over the substance use).
- **Substance dependence:** Requires three or more of the following in one year:
  - **Tolerance** and use of progressively larger amounts to obtain the same desired effect.
  - **Withdrawal** symptoms when not taking the substance.
  - Failed attempts to cut down use or abstain from the substance.

Features of substance dependence—

WITHDraw IT

Three or more of seven within a 12-month period:
Withdrawal
Interest or Important activities given up or reduced
Tolerance
Harm (physical and psychosocial) with continued use
Desire to cut down/ control
Intended time/amount exceeded
Time spent obtaining/ using the substance is ↑

A diagnosis of substance dependence trumps a diagnosis of substance abuse.

- Significant time spent obtaining the substance (e.g., visiting many doctors to obtain a prescription for pain pills).
- Isolation from life activities.
- Taking greater amounts of the substance than intended.
- Continued substance abuse despite recurrent physical or psychological problems 2° to the effect of the substance use.

DIAGNOSIS/TREATMENT

- Substance use is often denied or underreported, so seek out collateral information from family and friends.
- Check urine and blood toxicology screens, LFTs, and serum EtOH level.
- The management of intoxication for selected drugs is described in Table 2.14-10.

TABLE 2.14-10. Signs and Symptoms of Substance Abuse

DRUG	INTOXICATION	WITHDRAWAL
Alcohol	Disinhibition, emotional lability, slurred speech, ataxia, aggression, blackouts, hallucinations, memory impairment, impaired judgment, coma.	Tremor, tachycardia, hypertension, malaise, nausea, seizures, DTs, agitation.
Opioids	Euphoria leading to apathy, CNS depression, constipation, **pupillary constriction,** and respiratory depression (life threatening in overdose). Naloxone/naltrexone will block opioid receptors and reverse effects (beware of antagonist clearing before opioids, particularly with long-acting opioids such as methadone).	Dysphoria, insomnia, anorexia, myalgias, fever, lacrimation, diaphoresis, dilated pupils, rhinorrhea, piloerection, nausea, vomiting, stomach cramps, diarrhea, yawning. Opioid withdrawal is not life threatening, "hurts all over," and does not cause seizures.
Amphetamines	Psychomotor agitation, impaired judgment, hypertension, **pupillary dilation,** tachycardia, fever, diaphoresis, anxiety, angina, euphoria, prolonged wakefulness/attention, arrhythmias, delusions, seizures, hallucinations. Haloperidol can be given for severe agitation and symptom-targeted medications (e.g., antiemetics, NSAIDs).	Postuse "crash" with anxiety, lethargy, headache, stomach cramps, hunger, fatigue, depression/dysphoria, sleep disturbance, nightmares.
Cocaine	Psychomotor agitation, euphoria, impaired judgment, tachycardia, **pupillary dilation,** hypertension, paranoia, hallucinations, sudden death. ECG changes from ischemia are often seen ("cocaine chest pain"). Treat with haloperidol for severe agitation along with symptom-specific medications (e.g., to control hypertension).	Postuse "crash" with hypersomnolence, depression, malaise, severe craving, angina, suicidality, ↑ appetite, nightmares, "cocaine bugs."

HIGH-YIELD FACTS

PSYCHIATRY

TABLE 2.14-10. Signs and Symptoms of Substance Abuse *(continued)*

DRUG	INTOXICATION	WITHDRAWAL
Phencyclidine hydrochloride (PCP)	**Assaultiveness,** belligerence, psychosis, violence, impulsiveness, psychomotor agitation, fever, tachycardia, **vertical/horizontal nystagmus,** hypertension, impaired judgment, ataxia, seizures, delirium. Give benzodiazepines or haloperidol for severe symptoms; otherwise reassure. Acidification of urine or gastric lavage can help eliminate the drug.	Recurrence of intoxication symptoms due to reabsorption in the GI tract; sudden onset of severe, random violence.
LSD	Marked anxiety or depression, delusions, visual hallucinations, flashbacks, pupillary dilation, impaired judgment, diaphoresis, tachycardia, hypertension, heightened senses (e.g., colors become more intense). Supportive counseling; traditional antipsychotics for psychotic symptoms; benzodiazepines for anxiety.	
Marijuana	Euphoria, slowed sense of time, impaired judgment, social withdrawal, ↑ appetite, dry mouth, conjunctival injection, hallucinations, anxiety, paranoia, amotivational syndrome.	
Barbiturates	Low safety margin; respiratory depression.	Anxiety, seizures, delirium, life-threatening cardiovascular collapse.
Benzodiazepines	Interactions with alcohol, amnesia, ataxia, somnolence, mild respiratory depression. (Avoid using for insomnia in the elderly; can cause paradoxical agitation even in relatively low doses.)	Rebound anxiety, seizures, tremor, insomnia, hypertension, tachycardia, **death.**
Caffeine	Restlessness, insomnia, diuresis, muscle twitching, arrhythmias, tachycardia, flushed face, psychomotor agitation.	Headache, lethargy, depression, weight gain, irritability, craving.
Nicotine	Restlessness, insomnia, anxiety, arrhythmias.	Irritability, headache, anxiety, weight gain, craving, bradycardia, difficulty concentrating, insomnia.

Alcoholism

- Occurs more often in **males** (4:1) and in those 21–34 years of age, although the incidence in females is rising. Also associated with a ⊕ family history.
- **Hx/PE:** See Table 2.14-10 for the symptoms of intoxication and withdrawal. Look for palmar erythema or telangiectasias as well as for other signs and symptoms of end-organ complications.
- **Dx:** Screen with the **CAGE questionnaire.** Monitor vital signs for evidence of withdrawal. Labs may reveal ↑ LFTs, LDH, and MCV.
- **Tx:**
  - Rule out medical complications; correct electrolyte abnormalities.
  - Start a **benzodiazepine taper** for withdrawal symptoms. Add haloperidol for hallucinations and psychotic symptoms.

Pinpoint pupils are not always a reliable sign of opioid ingestion because coingestions can lead to normal or enlarged pupils. Also look for a ↓ respiratory rate, track marks, and ↓ breath sounds.

HIGH-YIELD FACTS

PSYCHIATRY

There are two types of anorexia nervosa:

- *Restricting type*
- *Binging/purge-eating type*

- Give **multivitamins and folic acid;** administer **thiamine** before glucose (which depletes thiamine) to prevent Wernicke's encephalopathy.
- Give anticonvulsants to patients with a seizure history.
- Group therapy, disulfiram, or naltrexone can aid patients with dependence.
- Long-term rehabilitative therapy (e.g., Alcoholic Anonymous).
- **Cx:**
  - **GI bleeding from gastritis, ulcers, varices, or Mallory-Weiss tears.**
  - **Pancreatitis, liver disease,** DTs, alcoholic hallucinosis, peripheral neuropathy, Wernicke's encephalopathy, Korsakoff's psychosis, fetal alcohol syndrome, cardiomyopathy, anemia, aspiration pneumonia, ↑ risk of sustaining trauma (e.g., subdural hematoma).

Anorexia Nervosa

- Risk factors include female gender, low self-esteem, and high SES. Also associated with OCD, major depressive disorder, anxiety, and careers such as modeling, gymnastics, ballet, and running.
- **Hx/PE:** Diagnosed as follows (see also Table 2.14-11):
  - Body weight is < 85% of that expected.
  - Patients present with **refusal to maintain normal body weight,** an intense **fear of weight gain,** a distorted body image (**patients perceive themselves as fat**), and **amenorrhea.**
  - Patients **restrict** (e.g., fasting, excessive exercise) or **binge and purge** (through vomiting, laxatives, and diuretics).
  - Signs and symptoms include **lanugo,** dry skin, bradycardia, lethargy, hypotension, cold intolerance, and hypothermia (as low as 35°C).
- **Dx:** Measure height and weight; check **CBC, electrolytes,** endocrine levels, and **ECG.** Perform a **psychiatric evaluation** to screen patients for comorbid conditions.
- **Tx:**
  - Initially, monitor caloric intake to restore nutritional status and to stabilize weight; then focus on **weight gain.**
  - Hospitalize if necessary to restore nutritional status, rehydrate, and correct electrolyte imbalances.
  - Once the patient is medically stable, initiate individual, family, and group **psychotherapy.** Treat comorbid depression and anxiety.
- **Cx:** Mitral valve prolapse, arrhythmias, hypotension, bradycardia, **amenor-**

TABLE 2.14-11. Anorexia vs. Bulimia

	ANOREXIA NERVOSA	**BULIMIA NERVOSA**
Body image	Disturbed body image; use extensive measures to avoid weight gain (e.g., purging, excess exercise).	Same.
Binge eating	May occur.	Same.
Weight	Patients are underweight (≥ 15% below expected weight).	Patients are of normal weight or are overweight.
Attitude toward illness	Patients are typically not distressed by their illness and may thus be resistant to treatment.	Patients are typically distressed about their symptoms and are thus easier to treat.

rhea (missing three consecutive cycles), nephrolithiasis, osteoporosis, multiple stress fractures, pancytopenia, thyroid abnormalities (see Table 2.14-12). Mortality from **suicide** or medical complications is > **10%**.

Bulimia Nervosa

- More common among women; associated with low self-esteem, mood disorders, and OCD.
- Hx/PE: Diagnostic criteria are as follows (see also Table 2.14-11):
  - **Patients have normal weight or are overweight.** For at least two times a week for three or more months, patients have episodes of **binge eating** and **compensatory behaviors** that include **purging** or **fasting.**
  - Patients are usually **ashamed** and conceal their behaviors.
  - **Signs** include **dental enamel erosion, enlarged parotid glands,** and **scars on the dorsal hand surfaces** (from inducing vomiting). Patients usually have normal body weight.
- Tx: **Psychotherapy** focuses on behavior modification and body image. **Antidepressants** may be effective for both depressed and nondepressed patients.
- **Cx:** See Table 2.14-12.

Sexual Disorders

SEXUAL CHANGES WITH AGING

- Interest in sexual activity usually does not ↓ with aging.
- Men usually require ↑ stimulation of the genitalia for longer periods of time to reach orgasm; intensity of orgasm ↓, and the length of the refractory period before the next orgasm ↑.
- In women, estrogen levels ↓ after menopause, leading to vaginal dryness and thinning, which may result in discomfort during coitus. May be treated with HRT, estrogen vaginal suppositories, or other vaginal creams.

PARAPHILIAS

- Preoccupation with or engagement in unusual sexual fantasies, urges, or behaviors for > 6 months with clinically significant impairment in one's life. Includes criminal sex offenders (e.g., pedophilia); see Table 2.14-13. Found almost exclusively in men, and usually begins before or during puberty.
- Sexual excitement is derived from unique exposures to certain situations, individuals, or objects.

Bulimic patients tend to be more disturbed by their behavior than anorexics and are more easily engaged in therapy. Anorexic patients deny health risks associated with their behavior, making them resistant to treatment.

Bupropion should be avoided in the treatment of patients with eating disorders, as it is associated with a ↓ seizure threshold.

TABLE 2.14-12.   **Medical Complications of Eating Disorders**

CONSTITUTIONAL	CARDIAC	GI	GU	OTHER
Cachexia	Arrhythmias	Dental erosions	Amenorrhea	**Dermatologic:** Lanugo
Hypothermia	Sudden death	and decay	Nephrolithiasis	**Hematologic:** Leukopenia
Fatigue	Hypotension	Abdominal pain		**Neurologic:** Seizures
Electrolyte	Bradycardia	Delayed gastric		**Musculoskeletal:** Osteoporosis,
abnormalities	Prolonged QT interval	emptying		stress fractures

TABLE 2.14-13. Features of Common Paraphilias

DISORDER	CLINICAL MANIFESTATIONS
Exhibitionism	Sexual arousal from exposing one's genitals to a stranger.
Pedophilia	Urges or behaviors involving sexual activities with children.
Voyeurism	Observing unsuspecting persons unclothed or involved in sex.
Fetishism	Use of nonliving objects (often clothing) for sexual arousal.
Transvestic fetishism	Cross-dressing for sexual arousal.
Frotteurism	Touching or rubbing one's genitalia against a nonconsenting person (common in subways).
Sexual sadism	Sexual arousal from inflicting suffering on sexual partner.
Sexual masochism	Sexual arousal from being hurt, humiliated, bound, or threatened.

- **Tx:** Treatment includes insight-oriented psychotherapy and behavioral therapy. Antiandrogens (e.g., Depo-Provera) have been used for hypersexual paraphilic activity.

GENDER IDENTITY DISORDERS

- **Strong, persistent cross-gender identification** and **discomfort with one's assigned sex or gender role of the assigned sex** in the absence of intersexual disorders. Patients may have a history of dressing like the opposite sex, taking sex hormones, or pursuing surgeries to reassign their sex.
- More common in males than in females. Associated with depression, anxiety, substance abuse, and personality disorders, which may be addressed and treated.
- **Tx:** Treatment is complex and includes educating the patient about culturally acceptable behavior patterns. Other options include sex-reassignment surgery or hormonal treatment (e.g., estrogen for males, testosterone for females). Supportive psychotherapy is helpful.

SEXUAL DYSFUNCTION

- Problems in sexual **arousal, desire, or orgasm or pain** with sexual intercourse.
- Prevalence is 30%; one-third of cases are attributable to biological factors and another third to psychological factors.
- **Tx:** Treatment depends on the particular condition. Pharmacologic strategies include sildenafil (Viagra) and bupropion (Wellbutrin). Psychotherapeutic strategies include sensate focusing.

Sleep Disorders

Up to one-third of all American adults suffer from some type of sleep disorder during their lives. The term *dyssomnia* describes any condition that leads to a disturbance in the normal rhythm or pattern of sleep. Insomnia is the most common example. **Risk factors** include female gender, the presence of mental and medical disorders, substance abuse, and advanced age.

1° INSOMNIA

- **Affects up to 30% of the general population;** causes sleep disturbance that is not attributable to physical or mental conditions. Often exacerbated by anxiety, and patients may become preoccupied with getting enough sleep.
- **Dx:** Patients present with a history of **nonrestorative sleep** or **difficulty initiating or maintaining sleep** that is present at least three times a week for one month.
- **Tx:**
  - First-line therapy includes the initiation of **good sleep hygiene** measures, which include the following:
    - Establishment of a regular sleep schedule
    - Limiting of caffeine intake
    - Avoidance of daytime naps
    - Warm baths in the evening
    - Use of the bedroom for sleep and sexual activity only
    - Exercising early in the day
    - Relaxation techniques
    - Avoidance of large meals near bedtime
  - Pharmacotherapy is considered second-line therapy and should be **initiated with care for short periods of time** (< 2 weeks). Pharmacologic agents include diphenhydramine (Benadryl), zolpidem (Ambien), zaleplon (Sonata), and trazodone (Desyrel).

1° HYPERSOMNIA

- **Dx:** Diagnosed when a patient complains of **excessive daytime sleepiness or nighttime sleep** that occurs for > 1 month. The excessive somnolence cannot be attributable to medical or mental illness, medications, poor sleep hygiene, insufficient sleep, or narcolepsy.
- **Tx:**
  - First-line therapy includes **stimulant drugs** such as amphetamines.
  - Antidepressants such as SSRIs may be useful in some patients.

NARCOLEPSY

- May affect up to 0.16% of the population. Onset typically occurs by young adulthood, generally before the age of 30. Some forms of narcolepsy may have a genetic component.
- **Dx:**
  - Manifestations include **excessive daytime somnolence** and ↓ **REM sleep latency** on a daily basis for at least three months. **Sleep attacks** are the classic symptom; patients cannot avoid falling asleep.

- The characteristic excessive sleepiness may be associated with the following:
  - **Cataplexy:** Sudden loss of muscle tone that leads to collapse.
  - **Hypnagogic hallucinations:** Occur as the patient is falling asleep.
  - **Hypnopompic hallucinations:** Occur as the patient awakens.
  - **Sleep paralysis:** Brief paralysis upon awakening.
- **Tx:** Treat with a regimen of **scheduled daily naps** plus **stimulant drugs** such as amphetamines; give SSRIs for cataplexy.

SLEEP APNEA

- Occurs 2° to **disturbances in breathing** during sleep that lead to **excessive daytime somnolence** and **sleep disruption.** Etiologies can be either central or peripheral.
  - **Central sleep apnea (CSA):** A condition in which both airflow and respiratory effort cease. CSA is linked to **morning headaches,** mood changes, and repeated awakenings during the night.
  - **Obstructive sleep apnea (OSA):** A condition in which airflow ceases as a result of obstruction along the respiratory passages. OSA is strongly associated with **snoring.** Risk factors include **male gender, obesity,** prior upper airway surgeries, a deviated nasal septum, a large uvula or tongue, and retrognathia (recession of the mandible).
- In both forms, arousal results in cessation of the apneic event.
- Associated with **sudden death in infants and elderly,** headaches, depression, ↑ systolic blood pressure, and **pulmonary hypertension.**
- **Dx: Sleep studies (polysomnography)** document the number of arousals, obstructions, and episodes of ↓ O_2 saturation; distinguish OSA from CSA; and identify possible movement disorders, seizures, or other sleep disorders.
- **Tx:**
  - **OSA:** Nasal continuous positive airway pressure (CPAP). Weight loss if obese. In children, most cases are due to tonsillar/adenoidal hypertrophy, which is corrected surgically.
  - **CSA:** Mechanical ventilation (e.g., BPAP) with a backup rate for severe cases.

CIRCADIAN RHYTHM SLEEP DISORDER

- A spectrum of disorders characterized by a **misalignment between desired and actual sleep** periods. Subtypes include jet-lag type, shift-work type, delayed sleep-phase type, and unspecified.
- **Tx:**
  - Jet-lag type usually **resolves** within 2–7 days **without specific treatment.**
  - Shift-work type may respond to **light therapy.**
  - Oral melatonin may be useful if given 5½ hours prior to the desired bedtime.

Factitious disorders and malingering are distinct from somatoform disorders in that they involve conscious and intentional processes.

Somatoform and Factitious Disorders

Patients often present with **medically unexplained somatic symptoms,** generally with varying etiologies.

- **Somatoform disorders:** Patients have **no conscious control over symptoms.** The five main categories are outlined in Table 2.14-14.
- **Factitious disorders: Patients fabricate symptoms or cause self-injury to assume the sick role (1° gain).** More common in males.
    - **Munchausen's syndrome:** Common among **health care workers.**
    - **Munchausen's syndrome by proxy:** A "caregiver" makes someone else ill and enjoys taking on the role of concerned onlooker.
- **Malingering:** Patients **intentionally cause** or feign symptoms for **2° gain** of **financial benefit** or **housing.**

In malingering, patients intentionally simulate illness for personal gain.

Sexual and Physical Abuse

- Most frequently affects women < 35 years of age who fill the following criteria:
    - Are experiencing marital discord and are substance abusers or have a partner who is a substance abuser; or
    - Are pregnant, are of low SES, or have obtained a restraining order.

Sexual abusers are usually male and are often known to the victim (and are often family members).

TABLE 2.14-14. Somatoform Disorders

Somatization disorder	Multiple, chronic somatic symptoms from different organ systems with multiple GI, sexual, neurologic, and pain complaints. Frequent clinical contacts and/or surgeries; significant functional impairment. The male-to-female ratio is 1:20; onset is usually before age of 30. Schedule regular appointments with the identified 1° caregiver who maintains communication with consultants and specialists; psychotherapy.
Conversion disorder	Symptoms or deficits of voluntary motor or sensory function (e.g., blindness, seizure-like movements, paralysis) incompatible with medical processes. Close temporal relationship to stress or intense emotion. More common in young females and in lower socioeconomic and less educated groups. Usually resolves spontaneously, but psychotherapy may help.
Hypochondriasis	Preoccupation with or fear of having a serious disease despite medical reassurance, leading to significant distress/impairment. Often involves a history of prior physical disease. Men and women are equally affected. Onset is in adulthood. Manage with group therapy and schedule regular appointments with the patient's 1° caregiver.
Body dysmorphic disorder	Preoccupation with an imagined physical defect or abnormality that leads to significant distress/impairment. Patients often present to dermatologists or plastic surgeons. Has a slight female predominance. May be associated with depression. SSRIs may be of benefit.
Somatoform pain disorder	Intensity or profile of pain symptoms is inconsistent with physiologic processes. Close temporal relationship with psychological factors. More common in females; peak onset is at 40–50 years of age. May be associated with depression. Treatment includes rehabilitation (e.g., physical therapy), psychotherapy, and behavioral therapy. Analgesia is usually not helpful. TCAs and SNRIs (venlafaxine and duloxetine) may be therapeutic.

Suicide is the third leading cause of death (after homicide and accidents) among 15- to 24-year-olds in the United States.

Emergent inpatient hospitalization is required for patients with suicidal intentions.

- Victims of childhood abuse are more likely to become adult victims of abuse.
- Hx/PE:
  - Patients typically have **multiple somatic complaints, frequent ER** visits, and **unexplained injuries** with **delayed medical treatment.** They may also **avoid eye contact** or act afraid or hostile.
  - Children may exhibit precocious sexual behavior, **genital or anal trauma, STDs,** UTIs, and psychiatric problems.
  - Other clues include a partner who answers questions for the patient or refuses to leave the exam room.
- **Tx:** Perform a screening assessment of the patient's safety domestically and in their close personal relationships. Provide **medical care,** emotional **support, and counseling;** educate the patient about **support services** and refer appropriately. **Documentation** is crucial.

Suicidality

- Accounts for 30,000 deaths per year in the United States; the eighth overall cause of death in the United States. One suicide occurs every 20 minutes.
- Risk factors include male gender, age greater than 45 years, psychiatric disorders (major depression, presence of psychotic symptoms), a history of an admission to a psychiatric institution, a previous suicide attempt, a history of violent behavior, ethanol or substance abuse, recent severe stressors, and a family suicide history (see the mnemonic **SAD PERSONS**).
- Women are more likely to attempt suicide, whereas men are more likely to succeed by virtue of their ↑ use of more lethal methods.
- **Dx:**
  - Perform a comprehensive psychiatric evaluation.
  - Ask about family history, previous attempts, ambivalence toward death, and hopelessness.
  - Ask directly about suicidal ideation, intent, and plan, and look for available means.
- **Tx:** A patient who endorses suicidality requires emergent inpatient hospitalization even against his will. Suicide risk may ↑ after antidepressant therapy is initiated because a patient's energy to act on suicidal thoughts can return before the depressed mood lifts.

HIGH-YIELD FACTS IN

Pulmonary

> **Etiologies of obstructive pulmonary disease—**
>
> **ABCT**
>
> **A**sthma
> **B**ronchiectasis
> **C**ystic fibrosis
> **T**racheal or bronchial obstruction

Beware—all that wheezes is not asthma!

Asthma should be suspected in children with multiple episodes of croup and URIs associated with dyspnea.

Characterized by airway narrowing, obstructive lung diseases restrict air movement and often cause air trapping. The etiologies of obstructive lung disease are described in the mnemonic **ABCT**. Figure 2.15-1 illustrates the role of lung volume measurements in the diagnosis of lung disease; Table 2.15-1 and Figure 2.15-2 contrast obstructive with restrictive lung disease.

Asthma

Reversible airway obstruction 2° to **bronchial hyperreactivity,** airway **inflammation, mucous plugging,** and **smooth muscle hypertrophy.**

HISTORY/PE

- Presents with **cough, episodic wheezing,** dyspnea, and/or chest tightness. Symptoms often worsen at night or early in the morning.
- Exam reveals **wheezing, prolonged expiratory duration** ($\downarrow$ I/E ratio), **accessory muscle use,** tachypnea, tachycardia, $\downarrow$ breath sounds (late sign), $\downarrow$ O_2 saturation (late sign), hyperresonance, and possible pulsus paradoxus.

DIAGNOSIS

- **ABGs: Mild hypoxia** and **respiratory alkalosis.** Normalizing P_{CO_2}, respiratory acidosis, and more severe hypoxia in an acute exacerbation warrant close observation, as they may indicate fatigue and impending respiratory failure.

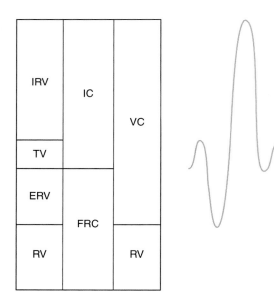

VC = vital capacity   ERV = expiratory reserve volume
RV = residual volume   IRV = inspiratory reserve volume
FRC = functional residual capacity   IC = inspiratory capacity
TV = tidal volume

FIGURE 2.15-1. **Lung volumes in the interpretation of pulmonary function tests.**

(Reproduced, with permission, from Gomella LG et al. *Clinician's Pocket Reference,* 11th ed. New York: McGraw-Hill, 2006: Fig. 18-1.)

TABLE 2.15-1. **Obstructive vs. Restrictive Lung Disease**[a]

TEST	NORMAL	MILD	MODERATE	SEVERE
Obstructive				
FEV_1 (% of forced VC)	> 75	60–75	40–60	< 40
RV (% of predicted)	80–120	120–150	150–175	> 200
Restrictive				
FVC (% of predicted)	> 80	60–80	50–60	< 50
FEV_1 (% of VC)	> 75	> 75	> 75	> 75
RV (% of predicted)	80–120	80–120	70–80	70

[a] FEV_1 = forced expiratory volume in one second; FVC = forced vital capacity.

- **Spirometry/PFTs:** ↓ FEV_1/FVC; peak flow is diminished acutely; ↑ RV and total lung capacity (TLC).
- **CBC:** Possible eosinophilia.
- **CXR:** Hyperinflation.
- **Methacholine challenge:** Tests for bronchial hyperresponsiveness; useful when PFTs are normal but asthma is still suspected.

Asthma triggers include allergens, URIs, cold air, exercise, drugs, and stress.

TREATMENT

In general, avoid allergens or any potential triggers. Management is as follows (see also Tables 2.15-2 and 2.15-3):

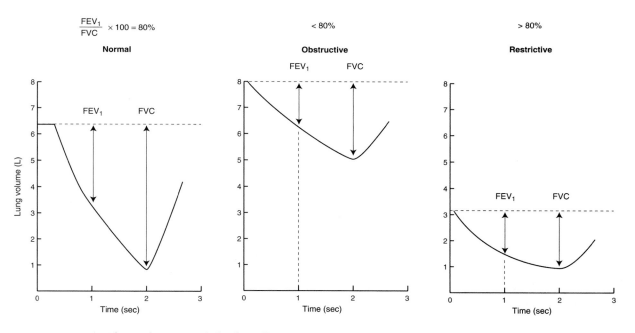

FIGURE 2.15-2. **Obstructive vs. restrictive lung disease.**

Note: Obstructive lung volumes > normal (↑ TLC, ↑ FRC, ↑ RV); restrictive lung volumes < normal. In both obstructive and restrictive disease, FEV_1 and FVC are reduced, but in obstructive disease, FEV_1 is more dramatically reduced, resulting in a ↓ FEV_1/FVC ratio.

TABLE 2.15-2.   **Common Asthma Medications and Their Mechanisms**

DRUG	MECHANISM OF ACTION
β_2-agonists	**Albuterol:** Relaxes bronchial smooth muscle (β_2-adrenoceptors). Give during acute exacerbations. **Salmeterol:** Long-acting agent for prophylaxis.
Corticosteroids	**Beclomethasone, prednisone:** Inhibit the synthesis of virtually all cytokines; inactivate NF-κB, a transcription factor for TNF-α, among other inflammatory agents. **Inhaled corticosteroids** are the first-line treatment for long-term control of asthma.
Muscarinic antagonists	**Ipratropium:** Competitively blocks muscarinic receptors, preventing bronchoconstriction.
Methylxanthines	**Theophylline:** Likely causes bronchodilation by inhibiting phosphodiesterase, thereby $\downarrow$ cAMP hydrolysis and $\uparrow$ cAMP levels. Usage is limited because of its narrow therapeutic-toxic index (cardiotoxicity, neurotoxicity).
Cromolyn	Prevents release of vasoactive mediators from mast cells. Useful for exercise-induced bronchospasm. Effective only for the prophylaxis of asthma; not effective during an acute asthmatic attack. Toxicity is rare.
Antileukotrienes	**Zileuton:** A 5-lipoxygenase pathway inhibitor. Blocks conversion of arachidonic acid to leukotrienes. **Montelukast, zafirlukast:** Blocks leukotriene receptors.

- **Acute:** O$_2$, **bronchodilating agents** (short-acting inhaled β_2-agonists are first-line therapy), **ipratropium** (never use alone for asthma), systemic **corticosteroids**, magnesium (for severe exacerbations). Maintain a low threshold for intubation in severe cases or acutely in patients with PCO$_2$ > 50 mmHg or PO$_2$ < 50 mmHg.
- **Chronic:** Measure lung function (FEV$_1$, peak flow, and sometimes ABGs) to guide management. Administer long-acting inhaled **bronchodilators** and/ or inhaled corticosteroids, systemic **corticosteroids**, cromolyn, or, rarely,

TABLE 2.15-3.   **Medications for Chronic Treatment of Asthma**

TYPE	SYMPTOMS (DAY/NIGHT)	FEV$_1$	MEDICATIONS
Mild intermittent	$\leq$ 2 days/week $\leq$ 2 nights/month	$\geq$ 80%	No daily medications. PRN short-acting bronchodilator.
Mild persistent	> 2/week but < 1/day > 2 nights/month	$\geq$ 80%	Daily low-dose inhaled corticosteroids. PRN short-acting bronchodilator.
Moderate persistent	Daily > 1 night/week	60–80%	Low- to medium-dose inhaled corticosteroids + long-acting inhaled β_2-agonists.
Severe persistent	Continual, frequent	$\leq$ 60%	High-dose inhaled corticosteroids + long-acting inhaled β_2-agonists. Possible PO corticosteroids. PRN short-acting bronchodilator.

theophylline. Montelukast and other leukotriene antagonists are oral adjuncts to inhalant therapy.

Bronchiectasis

A disease caused by cycles of infection and inflammation in the bronchi/bronchioles that lead to permanent fibrosis, remodeling, and **dilation of bronchi.**

HISTORY/PE

- Presents with chronic cough accompanied by frequent bouts of yellow or green sputum production, dyspnea, and possible hemoptysis and halitosis.
- Associated with a history of pulmonary infections (e.g., *Pseudomonas, Haemophilus*, TB), hypersensitivity (allergic bronchopulmonary aspergillosis), cystic fibrosis, immunodeficiency, localized airway obstruction (foreign body, tumor), aspiration, autoimmune disease (e.g., rheumatoid arthritis, SLE), or IBD.
- Exam reveals rales, wheezes, rhonchi, purulent mucus, and occasional hemoptysis.

DIAGNOSIS

- **CXR:** ↑ bronchovascular markings; **tram lines** (parallel lines outlining dilated bronchi as a result of peribronchial inflammation and fibrosis); areas of **honeycombing.**
- **High-resolution CT: Dilated airways** and ballooned cysts at the end of the bronchus (mostly lower lobes). Spirometry shows a ↓ FEV_1/FVC ratio.

TREATMENT

- Antibiotics for bacterial infections; consider inhaled corticosteroids.
- Maintain bronchopulmonary hygiene (cough control, postural drainage, chest physiotherapy).
- Consider lobectomy for localized disease or lung transplantation for severe disease.

Chronic Obstructive Pulmonary Disease (COPD)

Characterized by ↓ lung function with airflow obstruction. Generally 2° to chronic bronchitis or emphysema, which are distinguished as follows:

- **Chronic bronchitis**: Productive cough for > 3 months per year for two consecutive years.
- **Emphysema**: Terminal airway destruction and dilation that may be 2° to **smoking** (centrilobular) or to α_1-**antitrypsin deficiency** (panlobular).

HISTORY/PE

- Symptoms are minimal or nonspecific until the disease is advanced.
- The clinical spectrum includes the following (most patients are a combination of the two phenotypes):
    - **Emphysema ("pink puffer"): Dyspnea, pursed lips,** minimal cough, ↓ breath sounds, late hypercarbia/hypoxia. Patients often have a thin, wasted appearance. Pure emphysematous patients tend to have few reactive episodes between exacerbations.

In COPD patients with chronic hypercapnia, high concentrations of O_2 may suppress patients' hypoxic respiratory drive.

Supplemental oxygen titrated to > 90% SaO_2 for > 15 hours a day and smoking cessation are the only interventions proven to improve survival in patients with COPD.

- **Chronic bronchitis ("blue bloater"): Cyanosis with mild dyspnea;** productive cough. Patients are often overweight with peripheral edema, rhonchi, and early signs of hypercarbia/hypoxia. Look for the classic barrel chest, use of accessory chest muscles, JVD, end-expiratory wheezing, and muffled breath sounds.

DIAGNOSIS

- **CXR: Hyperinflated lungs,** ↓ lung markings with flat diaphragms, and a thin-appearing heart and mediastinum. Parenchymal **bullae** or subpleural **blebs** (pathognomonic of emphysema) are also seen (see Figure 2.15-3).
- **PFTs:** ↓ FEV_1/FVC; normal or ↓ FVC; normal or ↑ TLC (emphysema, asthma); ↓ DL_{CO} (in emphysema).
- **ABGs: Hypoxemia** with **acute** or **chronic respiratory acidosis** (↑ PCO_2).
- **Blood cultures:** Obtain if the patient is febrile.
- **Gram stain and sputum culture:** Consider in the setting of fever or productive cough, especially if infiltrate is seen on CXR.

TREATMENT

- **Acute exacerbations:** O_2, inhaled β-agonists (albuterol) and **anticholinergics** (ipratropium, tiotropium), IV +/− inhaled **corticosteroids, antibiotics.** Severe cases may benefit from noninvasive ventilation. Consider intubation in the setting of severe hypoxemia or hypercapnia, impending respiratory fatigue, or changes in mental status.
- **Chronic: Smoking cessation,** supplemental O_2 (if resting PaO_2 is ≤ 55 mmHg or SaO_2 is ≤ 89%, or in the setting of cor pulmonale, pulmonary hypertension, a hematocrit > 55%, or nocturnal hypoxia), inhaled β-agonists,

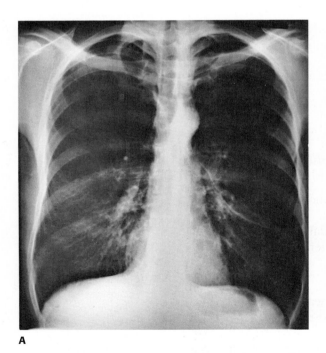
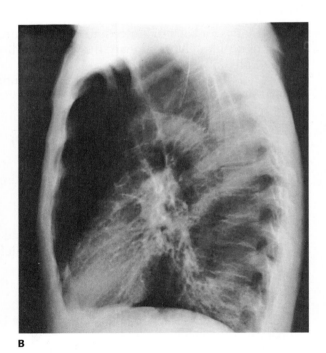

A **B**

FIGURE 2.15-3. **Chronic obstructive pulmonary disease.**

Note the hyperinflated and hyperlucent lungs, flat diaphragms, ↑ AP diameter, narrow mediastinum, and large upper bullae on (A) AP and (B) lateral CXRs. (Reproduced, with permission, from Stobo J et al. *The Principles and Practice of Medicine*, 23rd ed. Stamford, CT: Appleton & Lange, 1996: 135.)

anticholinergics (tiotropium), systemic or inhaled corticosteroids. Give **pneumococcal** and **flu vaccines.**

► **RESTRICTIVE LUNG DISEASE**

Characterized by a loss of lung compliance, restrictive lung diseases result in ↑ lung stiffness and ↓ lung expansion. Table 2.15-1 and Figure 2.15-2 contrast obstructive with restrictive lung disease. The etiologies of restrictive lung disease are shown in the mnemonic **PAINT.**

Interstitial Lung Disease

A heterogeneous group of disorders characterized by **inflammation** and/or **fibrosis** of the **interalveolar septum.** In advanced disease, cystic spaces develop in the lung periphery ("honeycombing"). Causes include idiopathic interstitial pneumonias, collagen vascular disease, granulomatous disorders, drugs, hypersensitivity disorders, pneumoconiosis, and eosinophilic pulmonary syndromes.

HISTORY/PE

Presents with **shallow, rapid breathing;** dyspnea with exercise; and a nonproductive cough. Patients may have cyanosis, inspiratory squeaks, fine or "Velcro-like" crackles, finger clubbing, or right heart failure.

DIAGNOSIS

- **CXR:** Reticular, nodular, or ground-glass pattern; "honeycomb" pattern (severe disease).
- ↓ **TLC,** ↓ **FVC,** ↓ **DL$_{CO}$** (may be normal if the cause is extrapulmonary), normal **FEV$_1$/FVC.** Serum markers of connective tissue diseases should be obtained if clinically indicated.

TREATMENT

Supportive. Avoid exposure to causative agents. Some inflammatory diseases respond to **corticosteroids** or other anti-inflammatory/immunosuppressive agents.

Systemic Sarcoidosis

A multisystem disease of unknown etiology characterized by **noncaseating granulomas.** Most commonly found in **African-American females** and northern European Caucasians; most often arises in the third or fourth decade of life.

HISTORY/PE

Presents with **fever, cough, malaise,** weight loss, dyspnea, and **arthritis.** The lungs, liver, eyes, skin (erythema nodosum, violaceous skin plaques), nervous system, heart, and kidney may be affected. Symptoms may be **GRUELING** (see mnemonic).

Causes of restrictive lung disease—

PAINT

Pleural (fibrosis, effusions, empyema, pneumothorax)
Alveolar (edema, hemorrhage, pus)
Interstitial lung disease (idiopathic interstitial pneumonias), **I**nflammatory (sarcoid, cryptogenic organizing pneumonitis), **I**diopathic
Neuromuscular (myasthenia, phrenic nerve palsy, myopathy)
Thoracic wall (kyphoscoliosis, obesity, ascites, pregnancy, ankylosing spondylitis)

Medications that can cause or contribute to interstitial lung disease include busulfan, nitrofurantoin, amiodarone, bleomycin, radiation, and long-term high O$_2$ concentration (e.g., ventilators).

DIAGNOSIS

- **CXR:** Radiographic findings are used to stage the disease.
- **Biopsy: Lymph node biopsy** or transbronchial/video-assisted thoracoscopic **lung biopsy** reveals **noncaseating granulomas.**
- **PFTs:** Restrictive or obstructive pattern and ↓ diffusion capacity.
- **Other findings:** ↑ **serum ACE levels** (neither sensitive nor specific), **hypercalcemia,** hypercalciuria, ↑ alkaline phosphatase (with liver involvement), lymphopenia, cranial nerve defects, arrhythmias.

TREATMENT

Systemic **corticosteroids** are indicated for constitutional symptoms, hypercalcemia, or extrathoracic organ involvement.

Hypersensitivity Pneumonitis

Risk factors include environmental exposure to antigens leading to alveolar thickening and granulomas. Types and etiologies are listed in Table 2.15-4.

HISTORY/PE

- **Acute:** Dyspnea, fever, malaise, shivering, and cough starting 4–6 hours after exposure.
- **Chronic:** Patients present with progressive dyspnea; exam reveals fine bilateral rales.

DIAGNOSIS

CXR is normal or shows miliary nodular infiltrate (acute); fibrosis is seen in the upper lobes (chronic).

TREATMENT

Avoid ongoing exposure to inciting agents; give corticosteroids to ↓ chronic inflammation.

TABLE 2.15-4. Antigens of Hypersensitivity Pneumonitis

DISORDER	ANTIGEN
Farmer's lung	Spores of actinomycetes from moldy hay.
Bird fancier's lung	Antigens from feathers, excreta, serum.
Mushroom worker's lung	Spores of actinomycetes from compost.
Malt worker's lung	Spores of *Aspergillus clavatus* in grain.
Grain handler's lung	Grain weevil dust.
Bagassosis	Spores of actinomycetes from sugarcane.
Air conditioner lung	Spores of actinomycetes from air conditioners.

Pneumoconiosis

Risk factors include prolonged occupational exposure and inhalation of small inorganic dust particles.

HISTORY/PE/DIAGNOSIS

Table 2.15-5 outlines the findings and diagnostic criteria associated with common pneumoconioses.

TREATMENT

Avoid triggers; supportive therapy and supplemental O_2.

Usual Interstitial Pneumonia (Idiopathic Pulmonary Fibrosis)

The most common form of **idiopathic interstitial pneumonia.** Has an unrelenting progression, with death usually occurring within 5–10 years.

Usual interstitial pneumonia is one of the most common forms of interstitial pneumonia.

HISTORY/PE

- **Exertional dyspnea** and a nonproductive **cough.**
- **Inspiratory crackles** and/or clubbing on exam.

TABLE 2.15-5. Diagnosis of Pneumoconioses

	HISTORY	DIAGNOSIS	COMPLICATIONS
Asbestosis	Work involving manufacture of tile or brake linings, insulation, construction, demolition, or shipbuilding. Presents 15–20 years after initial exposure.	**CXR:** Linear opacities at lung bases and interstitial fibrosis; calcified pleural plaques are indicative of benign pleural disease.	↑ risk of mesothelioma (rare) and lung cancer; risk of lung cancer is higher in smokers.
Coal miner's disease	Work in underground coal mines.	**CXR:** Small nodular opacities (< 1 cm) in upper lung zones. **Spirometry:** Consistent with restrictive disease.	Progressive massive fibrosis.
Silicosis	Work in mines or quarries or with glass, pottery, or silica.	**CXR:** Small (< 1-cm) nodular opacities in upper lung zones. **Eggshell calcifications. Spirometry:** Consistent with restrictive disease.	↑ risk of TB; need annual TB skin test. Progressive massive fibrosis.
Berylliosis	Work in high-technology fields such as aerospace, nuclear, and electronics plants; ceramics industries; foundries; plating facilities; dental material sites; and dye manufacturing.	**CXR:** Diffuse infiltrates; hilar adenopathy.	Requires chronic corticosteroid treatment.

DIAGNOSIS

- **High-resolution CT:** Patchy opacities at the lung bases, often with honeycombing.
- **PFTs:** Restrictive pattern.
- **Surgical biopsy** (usually required to confirm the diagnosis): Interstitial inflammation, fibrosis, and honeycombing.

TREATMENT

Options include corticosteroids, cytotoxic agents (azathioprine, cyclophosphamide), antifibrotic agents (have not been shown to improve survival), and lung transplantation.

Eosinophilic Pulmonary Syndromes

A diverse group of disorders characterized by eosinophilic **pulmonary infiltrates** and **peripheral blood eosinophilia**. Includes **allergic bronchopulmonary aspergillosis, Löffler's syndrome,** and **acute eosinophilic pneumonia.**

HISTORY/PE

Presents with dyspnea, cough, and/or fever.

DIAGNOSIS

CBC reveals peripheral eosinophilia; CXR shows pulmonary infiltrates.

TREATMENT

Removal of the extrinsic cause or treatment of underlying infection if identified. Corticosteroid treatment may be used if no cause is identified.

> ▶ **ACUTE RESPIRATORY FAILURE**

Hypoxemia

Causes include **ventilation-perfusion (V/Q) mismatch**, right-to-left shunt, hypoventilation, low inspired O_2 content (important at altitudes), and **diffusion impairment.**

HISTORY/PE

Findings depend on the etiology. ↓ **HbO_2 saturation,** cyanosis, tachypnea, shortness of breath, pleuritic chest pain, and altered mental status may be seen.

DIAGNOSIS

- **Pulse oximetry:** Demonstrates ↓ HbO_2 saturation.
- **CXR:** To rule out ARDS, atelectasis, or an infiltrative process (e.g., pneumonia) and to look for signs of pulmonary embolism.
- **ABGs:** To evaluate PaO_2 and to calculate the **alveolar-arterial (A-a) oxygen gradient** ($[(P_{atm} - 47) \times FiO_2 - (PaCO_2/0.8)] - PaO_2$). An ↑ A-a gradient suggests a V/Q mismatch or a diffusion impairment. Figure 2.15-4 summarizes the approach toward hypoxemic patients.

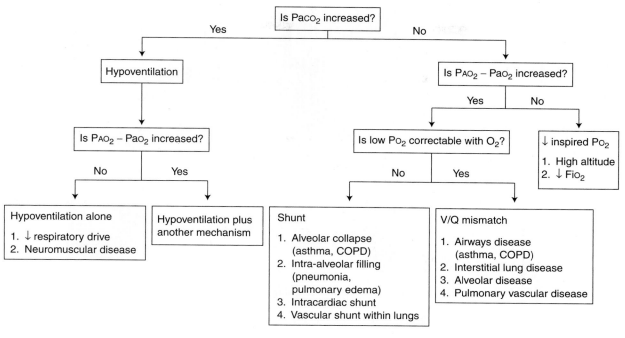

FIGURE 2.15-4. Determination of the mechanism of hypoxia.

(Reproduced, with permission, from Kasper DL et al. *Harrison's Principles of Internal Medicine*, 16th ed. New York: McGraw-Hill, 2005.)

TREATMENT

- Address the underlying etiology.
- Administer O_2 before initiating evaluation.
- **If the patient is on a ventilator,** ↑ O_2 saturation by increasing FiO_2, **positive end-expiratory pressure (PEEP),** or the I/E ratio.
- **Hypercapnic patients**: ↑ minute ventilation.

Acute Respiratory Distress Syndrome (ARDS)

Acute respiratory failure with refractory **hypoxemia, ↓ lung compliance,** and noncardiogenic **pulmonary edema.** The pathogenesis is thought to be endothelial injury. Common triggers include sepsis, pneumonia, aspiration, multiple blood transfusions, inhaled/ingested toxins, and trauma. Overall mortality is 30–40%.

HISTORY/PE

Presents with **acute-onset** (12–48 hours) tachypnea, dyspnea, and tachycardia +/− fever, cyanosis, labored breathing, diffuse high-pitched rales, and hypoxemia in the setting of one of the systemic inflammatory causes or exposure. Additional findings are as follows:

- **Phase 1 (acute injury):** Normal physical exam; possible respiratory alkalosis.
- **Phase 2 (6–48 hours):** Hyperventilation, hypocapnia, widening A-a oxygen gradient.
- **Phase 3:** Acute respiratory failure, tachypnea, dyspnea, ↓ lung compliance, scattered rales, diffuse chest infiltrates on CXR (see Figure 2.15-5).

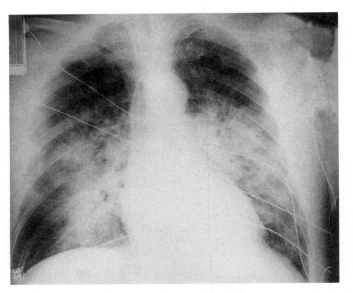

FIGURE 2.15-5. **AP CXR showing a diffuse alveolar filling pattern 2° to ARDS.**

(Reproduced, with permission, from Kasper DL et al. *Harrison's Principles of Internal Medicine*, 16th ed. New York: McGraw-Hill, 2005: 1497.)

- **Phase 4:** Severe hypoxemia unresponsive to therapy; ↑ intrapulmonary shunting; metabolic and respiratory acidosis.

DIAGNOSIS

The criteria for ARDS diagnosis (according to the American-European Consensus Conference definition) are as follows:

- Acute onset of respiratory distress.
- **PaO$_2$/FiO$_2$ ratio ≤ 200 mmHg.**
- Bilateral pulmonary infiltrates on CXR.
- **No evidence of cardiac origin** (capillary wedge pressure < 18 mmHg or no clinical evidence of elevated left atrial pressure).

TREATMENT

- There is no standard treatment.
- **Treat the underlying disease and maintain adequate perfusion to prevent end organ damage.**
- Minimize injury induced by mechanical ventilation by ventilating with **low tidal volumes.**
- Use PEEP to recruit collapsed alveoli and titrate PEEP and FiO$_2$ to achieve adequate oxygenation. Goal oxygenation is PaO$_2$ > 60 mmHg or SaO$_2$ > 90% on FiO$_2$ ≤ 0.6.
- Slowly wean patients from ventilation, and follow with extubation trials (see Table 2.15-6).

> **PULMONARY VASCULAR DISEASE**

Pulmonary Hypertension/Cor Pulmonale

Pulmonary hypertension is defined as a mean pulmonary arterial pressure of > 25 mmHg (normal = 15 mmHg). It is classified as either 1° (if the etiology

---

ARDS diagnosis:

Acute onset
Ratio (PaO$_2$/FiO$_2$) ≤ 200
Diffuse infiltration
Swan-Ganz wedge
 pressure < 18 mmHg

TABLE 2.15-6. Criteria for Extubation from Mechanical Ventilation[a]

PARAMETER	VALUE
Pulmonary mechanics	
Vital capacity	> 10–15 mL/kg
Resting minute ventilation (tidal volume × rate)	> 10 L/min
Spontaneous respiratory rate	< 33 breaths/min
Lung compliance	> 100 mL/cm water
Negative inspiratory force (NIF)	> –25 cm water
Oxygenation	
A-a gradient	< 300–500 mmHg
Shunt fraction	< 15%
Po_2 (on 40% Fio_2)	> 70 mmHg
Pco_2	< 45 mmHg

[a] Patients who meet these criteria are typically given a weaning (T-piece) trial to determine if they are ready for extubation.

is unknown) or 2°. 1° pulmonary hypertension most often occurs in young or middle-aged women. The main causes of 2° pulmonary hypertension include the following:

- ↑ pulmonary venous pressure from left-sided **heart failure** or mitral valve disease.
- ↑ pulmonary blood flow 2° to **congenital heart disease** with left-to-right shunt.
- **Hypoxic vasoconstriction** 2° to chronic lung disease (e.g., COPD).
- **Thromboembolic** disease.
- Remodeling of pulmonary vessels 2° to structural lung disease.

HISTORY/PE

- Presents with dyspnea on exertion, fatigue, lethargy, syncope with exertion, chest pain, and symptoms of right-sided CHF (edema, abdominal distention, JVD).
- Inquire about a history of COPD, interstitial lung disease, heart disease, sickle cell anemia, emphysema, and pulmonary emboli.
- Exam reveals a loud, palpable S_2 (often split), a systolic ejection murmur, an S_4, or a parasternal heave.

DIAGNOSIS

- CXR shows enlargement of central pulmonary arteries.
- ECG demonstrates RVH.
- Echocardiogram and right heart catheterization may show signs of right ventricular overload and may aid in the diagnosis of the underlying cause.

TREATMENT

Supplemental O_2, anticoagulation, vasodilators, and diuretics if symptoms of right-sided CHF are present. Treat underlying causes of 2° pulmonary hypertension.

Causes of pulmonary hypertension include left heart failure, mitral valve disease, and ↑ resistance in the pulmonary veins, including hypoxic vasoconstriction.

Pulmonary Thromboembolism

Occlusion of the pulmonary vasculature by a blood clot. Ninety-five percent of emboli originate from DVTs in the deep leg veins. Often leads to pulmonary infarction, right heart failure, and hypoxemia. **Virchow's triad** consists of the following:

- **Stasis:** Immobility, CHF, obesity, surgery, ↑ central venous pressure.
- **Endothelial injury:** Trauma, surgery, recent fracture, previous DVT.
- **Hypercoagulable states:** Pregnancy/postpartum, OCP use, coagulation disorders (e.g., protein C/protein S deficiency, factor V Leiden), malignancy, severe burns.

HISTORY/PE

- Presents with **sudden-onset dyspnea, pleuritic chest pain, low-grade fever,** cough, and, rarely, hemoptysis.
- **Pulmonary embolism:**
  - **Hypoxia and hypocarbia** with resulting respiratory alkalosis.
  - Tachypnea, tachycardia, and fever.
  - Exam may reveal a loud P_2 and prominent jugular A waves with right heart failure.
- **Venous thrombosis:** Unilateral swelling; cords on the calf.

DIAGNOSIS

- **ABGs: Respiratory alkalosis** (2° hyperventilation) with $Po_2 < 80$ mmHg.
- **CXR:** Usually normal, but may show atelectasis, pleural effusion, **Hampton's hump** (a wedge-shaped infarct), or **Westermark's sign** (oligemia in the affected lung zone).
- **ECG:** Not diagnostic; most commonly reveals **sinus tachycardia.** The classic triad of **S1Q3T3**—acute right heart strain with an S wave in lead I, a Q wave in lead III, and an inverted T wave in lead III—is uncommon.
- **Helical (spiral) CT with IV contrast:** Sensitive for pulmonary embolism.
- **V/Q scan:** May reveal segmental areas of mismatch. Results are reported with a designated probability of pulmonary embolism (low, indeterminate, or high) and are interpreted in combination with clinical suspicion.
- **Angiogram:** The gold standard, but more invasive and rarely done today (see Figure 2.15-6).
- **D-dimer:** Sensitive but not specific in patients at risk for DVT or pulmonary embolism (a useful "rule-out" test in patients with a low clinical suspicion, but it cannot rule out DVT or pulmonary embolism alone in patients with an intermediate or high clinical suspicion of clot).
- **Venous ultrasound of the lower extremity:** Can detect a clot that may have given off the pulmonary embolism. Serial ultrasounds have high diagnostic specificity.

TREATMENT

- **Heparin:** Bolus followed by weight-based continuous infusion of unfractioned heparin or low-molecular-weight heparin (LMWH) SQ.
- **Warfarin:** For long-term anticoagulation, usually given for at least six months unless the underlying predisposing factor persists (and is then given indefinitely). Follow INR (goal = 2–3).
- **IVC filter:** Indicated for patients with documented DVT in a lower extremity if anticoagulation is contraindicated or if patients experience recurrent emboli while anticoagulated.

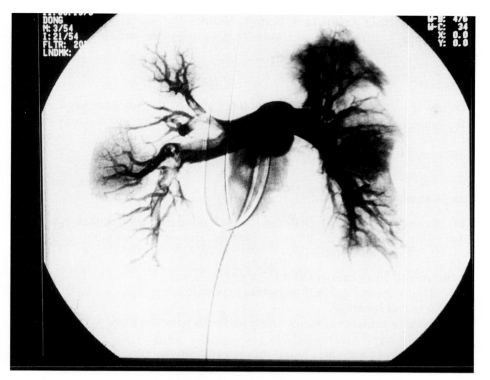

FIGURE 2.15-6. Pulmonary embolus.

A large filling defect in the pulmonary artery is evident on pulmonary angiogram.

- **Thrombolysis:** Indicated only in cases of massive DVT or pulmonary embolism causing right heart failure and hemodynamic instability (contraindicated in patients with recent surgery or bleeding).
- **DVT prophylaxis:** Treat all immobile patients; give **SQ heparin**, LMWH, intermittent pneumatic compression of the lower extremities (less effective), and **early ambulation (most effective).**

Lung Nodules

HISTORY/PE

Often asymptomatic, or patients may present with chronic cough, dyspnea, and shortness of breath. Always inquire about smoking and exposure history.

DIAGNOSIS

- **Serial CXRs:** Determine the location, progression, and extent of the nodule.
- **Chest CT:** Determine the nature, extent, and infiltrating nature of the nodule.
- **Characteristics favoring carcinoma:** Age > 45–50; smoking history; history of malignancy; new or enlarging (unless very rapidly enlarging) lesions; absence of calcification or irregular calcification; size > 2 cm; irregular margins.

Lung nodule clues based on the history:

- *Recent immigrant: Think TB.*
- *From the southwestern United States: Think coccidioidomycosis.*
- *From the Ohio River Valley: Think histoplasmosis.*

- **Characteristics favoring a benign lesion:** Age < 35; no change from old films; central/uniform/laminated/popcorn calcification; size < 2 cm; smooth margins.

TREATMENT

Surgical resection is indicated for nodules at high risk for malignancy. Low-risk nodules can be followed with CXR or CT every three months for one year and then every six months for another year. An invasive diagnostic procedure is indicated if the size of the nodule ↑.

Main locations for lung cancer metastasis—

BLAB

Bone
Liver
Adrenals
Brain

Lung Cancer

The leading cause of cancer **death** in the United States. Risk factors include tobacco smoke (except for bronchoalveolar carcinoma) and radon or asbestos exposure. Types are as follows:

- **Small cell lung cancer (SCLC):**
  - Highly correlated with **cigarette exposure.**
  - **Central location.**
  - **Neuroendocrine origin;** associated with paraneoplastic syndromes (see Table 2.15-7).
  - Metastases are often found on presentation (intrathoracic and extrathoracic sites such as brain, liver, and bone).
- **Non–small cell lung cancer (NSCLC):** Less likely to metastasize.

TABLE 2.15-7. Paraneoplastic Syndromes of Lung Cancer

CLASSIFICATION	SYNDROME	HISTOLOGIC TYPE
Endocrine/metabolic	Cushing's syndrome (ACTH)	Small cell
	SIADH leading to hyponatremia	Small cell
	Hypercalcemia (PTHrP)	Squamous cell
	Gynecomastia	Large cell
Skeletal	Hypertrophic pulmonary osteoarthropathy	Non–small cell
	Digital clubbing	Non–small cell
Neuromuscular	Peripheral neuropathy	Small cell
	Subacute cerebellar degeneration	Small cell
	Myasthenia (Eaton-Lambert syndrome)	Small cell
	Dermatomyositis	All
Cardiovascular	Thrombophlebitis	Adenocarcinoma
	Nonbacterial verrucous endocarditis	Adenocarcinoma
Hematologic	Anemia	All
	DIC	All
	Eosinophilia	All
	Thrombocytosis	All
	Hypercoagulability	Adenocarcinoma
Cutaneous	Acanthosis nigricans	All

- **Adenocarcinoma:** The most common lung cancer; **peripheral** location. Includes **bronchoalveolar carcinoma,** which is associated with multiple nodules, interstitial infiltration, and prolific sputum production but is not associated with smoking.
- **Squamous cell carcinoma:** Central location; 98% are seen in smokers.
- **Large cell/neuroendocrine carcinomas:** Least common; associated with a poor prognosis.

HISTORY/PE

- Presents with cough, hemoptysis, dyspnea, wheezing, postobstructive pneumonia, chest pain, weight loss, and possible abnormalities on respiratory exam (crackles, atelectasis).
- Other findings include **Horner's syndrome** (miosis, ptosis, anhidrosis) in patients with Pancoast's tumor at the apex of the lung; **superior vena cava syndrome** (obstruction of the SVC with supraclavicular venous engorgement); **hoarseness** (2° to recurrent laryngeal nerve involvement); and many **paraneoplastic syndromes** (see Table 2.15-7).

DIAGNOSIS

- CXR or **chest CT.**
- Fine-needle aspiration (CT guided) for peripheral lesions and **bronchoscopy** (biopsy or brushing) for central lesions.
- Thoracoscopic biopsy may be performed, with conversion to open thoracotomy if the lesion is found to be malignant.

TREATMENT

- **SCLC: Unresectable.** Often responds to radiation and chemotherapy initially but always recurs; has a lower median survival rate than NSCLC. Has usually metastasized at the time of diagnosis.
- **NSCLC: Surgical resection** in early stages (IA, IB, IIA, IIB, and possibly IIIA). The extent of resection is based on lesion size; the presence of metastases; and the patient's age, general health, and lung function. Supplement surgery with radiation or chemotherapy (depending on the stage). Palliative radiation and/or chemotherapy is appropriate for symptomatic but unresectable disease.

Chemotherapy is the mainstay of treatment for small cell lung cancer.

> ▶ **PLEURAL DISEASE**

Pleural Effusion

An abnormal **accumulation of fluid in the pleural space.** Classified as follows:

- **Transudate:** 2° to ↑ pulmonary capillary wedge pressure (PCWP) or ↓ oncotic pressure.
- **Exudate:** 2° to ↑ pleural vascular permeability.

Table 2.15-8 lists the possible causes of both transudates and exudates.

HISTORY/PE

Presents with **dyspnea,** pleuritic chest pain, and/or cough. Exam reveals **dullness to percussion** and ↓ **breath sounds** over the effusion. A pleural friction rub may be present.

TABLE 2.15-8. Causes of Pleural Effusions

TRANSUDATES	EXUDATES
CHF	Pneumonia (parapneumonic effusion)
Cirrhosis	TB
Nephrotic syndrome	Malignancy
	Pulmonary embolism
	Collagen vascular disease (rheumatoid arthritis, SLE)
	Pancreatitis
	Trauma

DIAGNOSIS

- CXR shows costophrenic angle blunting.
- **Thoracentesis** is indicated for new effusions > 1 cm in decubitus view, except with bilateral effusions and other clinical evidence of CHF.
- The effusion is an exudate if it meets Light's criteria:
  - The ratio of pleural to serum protein is > 0.5 **or**
  - The ratio of pleural to serum LDH is > 0.6 **or**
  - Pleural fluid LDH is more than two-thirds the upper normal limit of serum LDH
- A parapneumonic effusion is classified as complicated in the setting of a ⊕ Gram stain or culture **or** a pH < 7.2 (normal is 7.6) **or** a glucose level of < 60. The presence of **pus** indicates an **empyema.**

TREATMENT

Treatment is directed toward the underlying condition causing the effusion. Complicated parapneumonic effusions and empyemas require **chest tube drainage** in addition to **antibiotic therapy.**

Complicated parapneumonic effusions necessitate chest tube drainage.

Pneumothorax

A collection of air in the pleural space that can lead to pulmonary collapse. Subtypes are as follows:

- **1° spontaneous pneumothorax:** 2° to rupture of subpleural apical blebs (usually found in **tall, thin young males**).
- **2° pneumothorax:** 2° to COPD, TB, trauma, *Pneumocystis jiroveci* (formerly *P. carinii*) pneumonia, and iatrogenic factors (thoracentesis, subclavian line placement, positive-pressure mechanical ventilation, bronchoscopy).
- **Tension pneumothorax:** A pulmonary or chest wall defect acts as a **one-way valve,** drawing air into the pleural space during inspiration but trapping air during expiration. Etiologies include penetrating trauma, infection, and positive-pressure mechanical ventilation. Shock and death result unless the condition is immediately recognized and treated.

HISTORY/PE

- Presents with acute onset of **unilateral pleuritic chest pain** and **dyspnea.**
- Exam reveals tachypnea, **diminished or absent breath sounds, hyperreso-**

Presentation of pneumothorax:

P-THORAX

Pleuritic pain
Tracheal deviation
Hyperresonance
Onset sudden
Reduced breath sounds (and dyspnea)
Absent fremitus
X-ray shows collapse

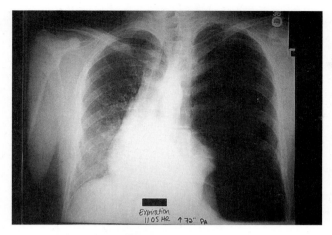

FIGURE 2.15-7.   Tension pneumothorax.

Note the hyperlucent lung field, hyperexpanded lower diaphragm, collapsed lung, tracheal deviation, mediastinal shift, and compression of the opposite lung on AP CXR.

nance, ↓ **tactile fremitus,** and JVD 2° to compression of the superior vena cava.

■ Suspect tension pneumothorax in the presence of **tracheal deviation,** respiratory distress, falling O_2 saturation, hypotension, and distended neck veins.

DIAGNOSIS

CXR shows the presence of a visceral pleural line and/or **lung retraction** from the chest wall (best seen in end-expiratory films; see Figure 2.15-7).

TREATMENT

■ Small pneumothoraces may resorb spontaneously. Supplemental O_2 therapy is helpful.
■ Large, symptomatic pneumothoraces require chest tube placement.
■ Tension pneumothorax requires immediate needle decompression (second intercostal space at the midclavicular line) followed by chest tube placement.

Renal/Genitourinary

Hypernatremia causes—

The 6 D's

Diuresis
Dehydration
Diabetes insipidus
Docs (iatrogenic)
Diarrhea
Disease (e.g., kidney, sickle cell)

Hypernatremia

Serum sodium > 145 mEq/L. Usually due to **water loss** rather than sodium gain.

HISTORY/PE

- Presents with **thirst** (due to hypertonicity) as well as with oliguria or polyuria (depending on the etiology).
- **Neurologic symptoms** include mental status changes, weakness, focal neurologic deficits, and seizures.
- Exam reveals **"doughy" skin** and signs of volume depletion.

DIAGNOSIS

- Assess volume status by conducting a clinical exam and measuring urine volume and osmolality.
  - **Hypertonic Na$^+$ gain:** Due to hypertonic saline/tube feeds or ↑ **aldosterone** (suppresses ADH).
  - **Pure water loss:** Due to central or nephrogenic **diabetes insipidus**; characterized by large volumes of dilute urine. Do not neglect dermal and respiratory insensible losses.
  - **Hypotonic fluid loss:** Due to ↓ intake, diuretics, intrinsic renal disease, GI losses **(diarrhea),** burns, and osmotic diuresis (mannitol, glucose in DKA, urea with high protein feeds).
- A minimal volume (approximately 500 ml/day) of maximally concentrated urine (> 800 mOsm/kg) suggests adequate renal response without adequate free-water replacement.

TREATMENT

- Treat the underlying causes and replace free-water deficit with hypotonic saline, D$_5$W, or oral water, depending on volume status.
- Correction of chronic hypernatremia (> 36–48 hours) should be accomplished **gradually over 48–72 hours** (≤ 0.5 mEq/L/hr) to prevent neurologic damage 2° to cerebral edema.

Hyponatremia

Serum sodium < 135 mEq/L. Almost always due to ↑ ADH.

HISTORY/PE

- May be asymptomatic or may present with **confusion, lethargy,** muscle cramps, hyporeflexia, and nausea.
- Can progress to seizures, coma, or brain stem herniation.

DIAGNOSIS

Hyponatremia can be categorized according to serum and urine osmolality as well as by volume status (i.e., by clinical exam). Osmolality is classified as follows:

- **High (> 295 mEq/L):** Hyperglycemia, hypertonic infusion (e.g., mannitol).
- **Normal (280–295 mEq/L):** Hypertriglyceridemia, paraproteinemia (pseudohyponatremia).

- **Low (< 280 mEq/L):** Applies to the majority of cases. Hypotonic etiologies are listed in Table 2.16-1.

TREATMENT

- Specific treatments are outlined in Table 2.16-1.
- Chronic hyponatremia (> 72 hours' duration) should be corrected slowly (no more than 0.5 mEq/L/hr) in order to prevent central pontine myelinolysis (symptoms include paraparesis/quadriparesis, dysarthria, and coma).

Hyperkalemia

Serum potassium > 5 mEq/L. Etiologies are as follows:

- **Spurious:** Hemolysis of blood samples, fist clenching during blood draws, delays in sample analysis, extreme leukocytosis or thrombocytosis.
- **↓ excretion:** Renal insufficiency, drugs (e.g., spironolactone, triamterene, ACEIs, trimethoprim, NSAIDs), hypoaldosteronism, type IV renal tubular acidosis (RTA).
- **Cellular shifts:** Cell lysis, tissue injury (rhabdomyolysis), insulin deficiency, acidosis, drugs (e.g., succinylcholine, digitalis, arginine, β-blockers), exercise.
- **Iatrogenic.**

HISTORY/PE

May be asymptomatic or may present with nausea, vomiting, **intestinal colic, areflexia, weakness,** flaccid paralysis, and paresthesias.

DIAGNOSIS

- Confirm hyperkalemia with a **repeat blood draw.** In the setting of extreme leukocytosis or thrombocytosis, check plasma potassium.
- ECG findings include **tall, peaked T waves;** a wide QRS; PR prolongation; and loss of P waves (see Figure 2.16-1). Can progress to **sine waves,** ventricular fibrillation, and cardiac arrest.

Consider using hypertonic saline only if a patient has seizures due to hyponatremia, and use it cautiously and briefly. In most instances, normal saline is the best replacement fluid.

What dreaded complication can arise from treating hyponatremia too rapidly? Central pontine myelinolysis.

TABLE 2.16-1. Evaluation and Treatment of Hypotonic Hyponatremia

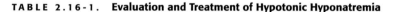

VOLUME STATUS	ETIOLOGIES	TREATMENT
Hypervolemic	Renal failure, nephrotic syndrome, cirrhosis, CHF, hypothyroidism, 2° or 3° adrenal insufficiency.	Water restriction; consider diuretics; cortisol replacement with adrenal insufficiency; thyroid replacement with hypothyroidism.
Euvolemic	**SIADH,** renal failure, drugs, psychogenic polydipsia, oxytocin use.	Water restriction.
Hypovolemic	Diuretics (especially thiazides), vomiting, diarrhea, bleeding, third spacing, dehydration, DKA, 1° adrenal insufficiency.	Replete volume with normal saline.

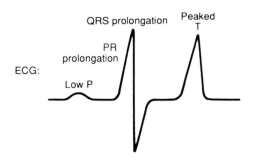

FIGURE 2.16-1. Hyperkalemia on ECG.

Electrocardiographic manifestations include peaked T waves, PR prolongation, and a widened QRS complex. (Reproduced, with permission, from Cogan MG. *Fluid and Electrolytes*, 1st ed. Stamford, CT: Appleton & Lange, 1991: 170.)

> **Treatment of hyperkalemia—**
>
> **C BIG K**
>
> **C**alcium
> **B**icarbonate
> **I**nsulin
> **G**lucose
> **K**ayexalate

TREATMENT

- Values of > 6.5 mEq/L or ECG changes (especially PR prolongation or wide QRS) require emergent treatment.
- The mnemonic **C BIG K** summarizes the treatment of hyperkalemia.
    - First give **calcium gluconate** for cardiac cell membrane stabilization.
    - Give **bicarbonate and/or insulin and glucose** to temporarily shift potassium into cells.
    - β-agonists (e.g., albuterol) promote cellular reuptake of potassium.
    - Eliminate potassium from diet and IV fluids.
    - **Kayexalate** to remove potassium from the body.
- Dialysis is appropriate for patients with renal failure or for severe, refractory cases.

Hypokalemia is usually due to renal or GI losses

Hypokalemia sensitizes the heart to digitalis toxicity because K+ and digitalis compete for the same sites on the Na+/K+ pump, so if a patient is on digitalis, potassium levels must be carefully monitored.

Hypokalemia

Serum potassium < 3.6 mEq/L. Etiologies are as follows:

- **Transcellular shifts:** Insulin, β2-agonists, alkalosis, familial hypokalemic periodic paralysis.
- **GI losses:** Diarrhea, chronic laxative abuse, vomiting, NG suction.
- **Renal losses:** Diuretics (e.g., loop or thiazide), 1° mineralocorticoid excess or 2° hyperaldosteronism, ↓ circulating volume, Bartter's and Gitelman's syndromes, drugs (e.g., gentamicin, amphotericin), DKA, hypomagnesemia, type I RTA (defective distal H+ secretion), polyuria.

HISTORY/PE

Presents with fatigue, **muscle weakness or cramps, ileus,** hypotension, hyporeflexia, paresthesias, rhabdomyolysis, and ascending paralysis.

DIAGNOSIS

- Twenty-four-hour or spot urine potassium may distinguish renal from GI losses.
- ECG may show **T-wave flattening, U waves** (an additional wave after the T wave), and ST-segment depression, leading to AV block and subsequent cardiac arrest.
- Consider RTA in the setting of metabolic acidosis.

TREATMENT

- Treat the underlying disorder.
- Oral and/or IV **potassium repletion**. Do not exceed 20 mEq/L/hr.
- Replace magnesium, as this deficiency complicates potassium repletion.
- Monitor ECG and plasma potassium levels frequently during replacement.

Hypercalcemia

Serum calcium > 10.2 mg/dL. The most common causes are **hyperparathyroidism and malignancy** (e.g., breast cancer, squamous cell carcinoma, multiple myeloma). Other causes are summarized in the mnemonic **CHIMPANZEES.**

HISTORY/PE

Usually asymptomatic and discovered by routine labs, but may present with **bones** (osteopenia, fractures), **stones** (kidney stones), abdominal **groans** (anorexia, constipation), and **psychiatric overtones** (weakness, fatigue, altered mental status).

DIAGNOSIS

Order a total/ionized calcium, albumin, phosphate, PTH, parathyroid hormone–related peptide (PTHrP), vitamin D, and ECG (may show a **short QT interval**).

TREATMENT

- **IV hydration** followed by **furosemide** to ↑ calcium excretion.
- Calcitonin, bisphosphonates (e.g., pamidronate), glucocorticoids, calcimimetics, and dialysis are used for severe or refractory cases. **Avoid thiazide diuretics,** which ↑ tubular reabsorption of calcium.

Hypocalcemia

Serum calcium < 8.5 mg/dL. Etiologies include hypoparathyroidism (postsurgical, idiopathic), malnutrition, hypomagnesemia, acute pancreatitis, vitamin D deficiency, and pseudohypoparathyroidism. In infants, consider DiGeorge's syndrome (tetany shortly after birth; absence of thymic shadow).

HISTORY/PE

- Presents with **abdominal muscle cramps,** dyspnea, **tetany, perioral and acral paresthesias,** and convulsions.
- Facial spasm elicited from tapping of the facial nerve **(Chvostek's sign)** and carpal spasm after arterial occlusion by a BP cuff **(Trousseau's sign)** are classic findings that are most commonly seen in severe hypocalcemia.

DIAGNOSIS

- Order an ionized Ca^{2+}, Mg^+, PTH, albumin, and possibly calcitonin. If the patient is post-thyroidectomy, review the operative note to determine the number of parathyroid glands removed.
- ECG may show a **prolonged QT interval.**

Loops (furosemide) Lose calcium.

A classic case of hypocalcemia is a patient who develops cramps and tetany following thyroidectomy.

Serum calcium may be falsely low in hypoalbuminemia; check ionized calcium.

HIGH-YIELD FACTS

RENAL/GENITOURINARY

TREATMENT

- Treat the underlying disorder.
- Magnesium repletion.
- Administer oral **calcium supplements;** give IV calcium for severe symptoms.

Hypomagnesemia

Serum magnesium < 1.5 mEq/L. Etiologies are as follows:

- ↓ **intake:** Malnutrition, malabsorption, short bowel syndrome, TPN.
- ↑ **loss:** Diuretics, diarrhea, vomiting, hypercalcemia, drugs (e.g., aminoglycosides, amphotericin), alcoholism, kidney losses (e.g., recovering ATN, postobstructive diuresis).
- **Miscellaneous: DKA,** pancreatitis, extracellular fluid volume expansion.

HISTORY/PE

- Symptoms are generally related to concurrent hypocalcemia and hypokalemia; they include anorexia, nausea, vomiting, muscle cramps, and weakness.
- In severe cases, symptoms may also include hyperactive reflexes, tetany, paresthesias, irritability, confusion, lethargy, seizures, and arrhythmias.

DIAGNOSIS

- Labs may show concurrent hypocalcemia and hypokalemia.
- ECG may reveal prolonged PR and QT intervals.

TREATMENT

- IV and oral supplements.
- Hypokalemia and hypocalcemia will not correct without magnesium correction.

▶ ACID-BASE DISORDERS

See Figure 2.16-2 for a diagnostic algorithm of acid-base disorders.

▶ RENAL TUBULAR ACIDOSIS (RTA)

A net ↓ in either tubular H^+ secretion or HCO_3^- reabsorption that leads to a **non–anion gap metabolic acidosis.** There are three main types of RTA; **type IV (distal)** is the **most common form** (see Table 2.16-2).

▶ ACUTE RENAL FAILURE (ARF)

An abrupt ↓ in renal function leading to the retention of creatinine and BUN. ↓ urine output (oliguria, defined as < 500 cc/day) is not required for ARF. ARF is categorized as follows (see also Table 2.16-3):

- **Prenal:** ↓ renal perfusion.
- **Intrinsic:** Injury within the nephron unit.
- **Postrenal:** Urinary outflow obstruction. Generally, both kidneys must be obstructed before one can see a significant ↑ in BUN and creatinine.

Alcoholics are the most common patient population with hypomagnesemia.

Aspirin (salicylate) overdose can cause both a metabolic acidosis and a respiratory alkalosis.

If an asthmatic patient's blood gas goes from alkalotic to normal, it can be a sign of respiratory muscle fatigue, which requires urgent intubation.

↑ **anion gap caused by–**

MUDPILES

Methanol
Uremia
DKA
Paraldehyde
Intoxication
Lactic acidosis
Ethylene glycol
Salicylates

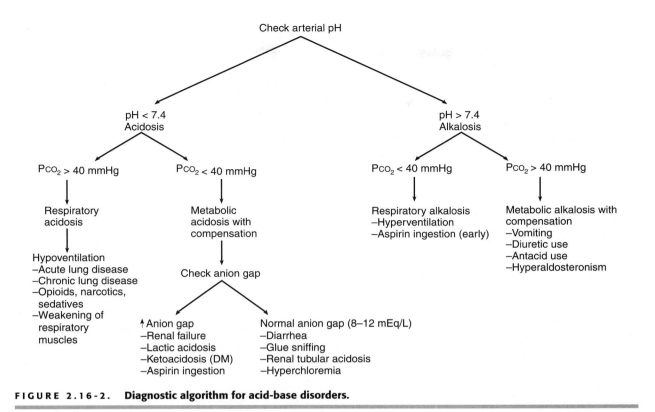

Check arterial pH

pH < 7.4
Acidosis

$P_{CO_2} > 40$ mmHg

Respiratory acidosis

Hypoventilation
–Acute lung disease
–Chronic lung disease
–Opioids, narcotics, sedatives
–Weakening of respiratory muscles

$P_{CO_2} < 40$ mmHg

Metabolic acidosis with compensation

Check anion gap

↑Anion gap
–Renal failure
–Lactic acidosis
–Ketoacidosis (DM)
–Aspirin ingestion

Normal anion gap (8–12 mEq/L)
–Diarrhea
–Glue sniffing
–Renal tubular acidosis
–Hyperchloremia

pH > 7.4
Alkalosis

$P_{CO_2} < 40$ mmHg

Respiratory alkalosis
–Hyperventilation
–Aspirin ingestion (early)

$P_{CO_2} > 40$ mmHg

Metabolic alkalosis with compensation
–Vomiting
–Diuretic use
–Antacid use
–Hyperaldosteronism

FIGURE 2.16-2. Diagnostic algorithm for acid-base disorders.

HISTORY/PE

- Symptoms of **uremia** include malaise, fatigue, confusion, oliguria, anorexia, and nausea.
- Exam may show a **pericardial rub, asterixis, hypertension,** ↓ urine output, and an ↑ respiratory rate (compensation of metabolic acidosis or from pulmonary edema 2° to volume overload)
- Category-specific symptoms are as follows:
    - **Prerenal:** Thirst, orthostatic hypotension, tachycardia, ↓ skin turgor, dry mucous membranes, reduced axillary sweating, stigmata of comorbid conditions.
    - **Intrinsic:** Associated with a history of drug exposure (aminoglycosides, NSAIDs), infection, or exposure to contrast media or toxins (e.g., myoglobin, myeloma protein). Hematuria or tea-colored urine, foamy urine (from proteinuria), hypertension, and/or edema may also be present.
    - **Atheroemboli:** Subcutaneous nodules, livedo reticularis, digital ischemia.
    - **Postrenal:** Prostatic disease, ↓ urine output leading to suprapubic pain, distended bladder and flank pain.

DIAGNOSIS

- Check serum electrolytes. Examine the urine for RBCs, WBCs, casts (see Table 2.16-4), and **urine eosinophils.**
- An $Fe_{Na} < 1\%$, a $U_{Na} < 20$, a urine specific gravity > 1.020, or a BUN/Cr ratio > 20 suggests a prerenal etiology.
- A urinary catheter and renal ultrasound can help rule out obstruction. Ultrasound can also identify kidneys that are ↓ in size, as occurs with chronic kidney disease.

Patients with ARF may have a normal urine volume.

An $Fe_{Na} < 1\%$ indicates that the kidneys are trying to conserve sodium, suggesting a prerenal etiology.

TABLE 2.16-2. Types of Renal Tubular Acidosis

	Type I (Distal)	Type II (Proximal)	Type IV (Distal)
Defect	H^+ secretion	HCO_3^- reabsorption	Aldosterone deficiency or resistance, leading to defects in Na^+ reabsorption and H^+ and K^+ excretion
Serum K^+	Low	Low	**High**
Urinary pH	> 5.3	5.3 initially; < 5.3 once serum is acidic	< 5.3
Etiologies (most common)	Hereditary, cirrhosis, autoimmune disorders (Sjögren's syndrome, SLE), hypercalciuria, sickle cell disease, drugs (lithium, amphotericin)	Hereditary (idiopathic or part of syndromes such as Fanconi's syndrome or cystinosis), drugs (carbonic anhydrase inhibitors), multiple myeloma, amyloidosis, heavy metal poisoning, vitamin D deficiency	1° aldosterone deficiency, hyporeninemic hypoaldosteronism (e.g., from kidney disease, ACEIs, NSAIDs), drugs (e.g., amiloride, spironolactone, heparin), pseudohypoaldosteronism
Treatment	Potassium citrate	Potassium citrate	Furosemide, mineralocorticoid +/− glucocorticoid replacement, and low-potassium diet in patients with aldosterone deficiency
Complications	**Nephrolithiasis**	Rickets, osteomalacia	Hyperkalemia

TABLE 2.16-3. Causes of Acute Renal Failure

Prerenal	Renal (Intrinsic)	Postrenal
Hypovolemia (hemorrhage, dehydration, burns)	Acute tubular necrosis (ATN)	Prostatic disease
Cardiogenic shock (↓ CO)	Acute/allergic interstitial nephritis	Nephrolithiasis
Systemic vasodilation (sepsis, burns)	Glomerulonephritis	Pelvic tumors
Anaphylaxis	Thromboembolism	Recent pelvic surgery
Drugs (ACEIs, ARBs, NSAIDs)	Renovascular disease (HUS/TTP, scleroderma)	Retroperitoneal fibrosis
Renal artery stenosis		
Cirrhosis with ascites (hepatorenal syndrome)		

URINE SEDIMENT	ETIOLOGY	CLASSIFICATION
Hyaline casts	Normal finding, but an ↑ amount suggests volume depletion	Prerenal
Red cell casts, dysmorphic red cells	Glomerulonephritis	Intrinsic
White cells, eosinophils	Allergic interstitial nephritis, atheroembolic disease	Intrinsic
Granular casts, renal tubular cells, "muddy-brown cast"	ATN	Intrinsic
White cells, white cell casts	Pyelonephritis	Postrenal

- In patients with oliguria, the Fe_{Na} can help identify prerenal failure and distinguish it from intrinsic renal disease.
- Obtain a renal biopsy only when the cause of intrinsic renal disease is unclear.

TREATMENT

- Balance fluids and electrolytes; avoid nephrotoxic drugs.
- In acute or allergic interstitial nephritis, adjust or discontinue offending medications.
- Dialyze if indicated (see the mnemonic **AEIOU**) using hemodialysis. Peritoneal dialysis should be considered only for long-term dialysis patients or for patients who are not hemodynamically stable.

COMPLICATIONS

- Metabolic acidosis; hyperkalemia leading to arrhythmias.
- Hypertension (from renin hypersecretion).
- Volume overload leading to CHF and pulmonary edema.
- Chronic kidney disease may result, requiring dialysis to prevent the buildup of K^+, H^+, phosphate, and **toxic metabolites.**

> *Indications for urgent dialysis—*
>
> **AEIOU**
>
> **A**cidosis
> **E**lectrolyte abnormalities (hyperkalemia)
> **I**ngestions (salicylates, theophylline, methanol, barbiturates, lithium, ethylene glycol)
> **O**verload (fluid)
> **U**remic symptoms (pericarditis, encephalopathy, bleeding, nausea, pruritus, myoclonus)

▶ CHRONIC KIDNEY DISEASE (CKD)

Most commonly due to diabetes mellitus (DM), hypertension, and glomerulonephritis. Another commonly tested etiology is polycystic kidney disease (the autosomal-dominant form is more common and is adult onset; the autosomal-recessive form is seen in children).

HISTORY/PE

Generally asymptomatic until GFR < 30, but patients gradually experience the signs and symptoms of uremia (anorexia, nausea, vomiting, uremic pericarditis, "uremic frost," delirium, seizures, coma).

DIAGNOSIS

Common metabolic derangements include the following:

- Azotemia (↑ BUN and creatinine).
- Fluid retention (hypertension, edema, CHF, pulmonary edema).

- Metabolic acidosis.
- Hyperkalemia.
- Anemia of chronic disease ($\downarrow$ erythropoietin production).
- Hypocalcemia, hyperphosphatemia ($\downarrow$ phosphate excretion; impaired vitamin D production leading to renal osteodystrophy).

TREATMENT

- ACEIs/ARBs and hypertension control have been shown to $\downarrow$ the progression of CKD.
- Additional pharmacotherapy is as follows:
    - Erythropoietin analogs for anemia of chronic disease.
    - Fluid restriction; low Na^+/K^+/phosphate intake.
    - Oral phosphate binders and calcitriol (1,25-OH vitamin D) for renal osteodystrophy.
- **Renal replacement therapy** includes hemodialysis, peritoneal dialysis, and renal transplantation.

▶ DIURETICS

Table 2.16-5 and Figure 2.16-3 summarize the mechanisms of action and side effects of commonly used diuretics.

TABLE 2.16-5. Mechanism of Action and Side Effects of Diuretics

TYPE	DRUGS	SITE OF ACTION	MECHANISM OF ACTION	SIDE EFFECTS
Carbonic anhydrase inhibitors	Acetazolamide	Proximal convoluted tubule.	Inhibit carbonic anhydrase, $\uparrow H^+$ reabsorption, block Na^+/H^+ exchange.	Hyperchloremic metabolic acidosis, sulfa allergy.
Osmotic agents	Mannitol, urea	Entire tubule.	$\uparrow$ tubular fluid osmolarity.	Pulmonary edema due to CHF and anuria.
Loop agents	Furosemide, ethacrynic acid, bumetanide, torsemide	Ascending loop of Henle.	Inhibit $Na^+/K^+/2Cl^-$ transporter.	Water loss, metabolic alkalosis, $\downarrow K^+$, $\downarrow Ca^{2+}$, **ototoxicity**, sulfa allergy (except ethacrynic acid, hyperuricemia).
Thiazide agents	HCTZ, chlorothiazide	Distal convoluted tubule.	Inhibit Na^+/Cl^- transporter.	Water loss, metabolic alkalosis, $\downarrow Na^+$, $\downarrow K^+$, $\uparrow$ glucose, $\uparrow Ca^{2+}$, $\uparrow$ uric acid, sulfa allergy, pancreatitis.
K^+-sparing agents	Spironolactone, triamterene, amiloride	Cortical collecting tubule.	Aldosterone receptor antagonist (spironolactone); block sodium channel (triamterene, amiloride).	Metabolic acidosis; $\uparrow K^+$; antiandrogenic effects, including gynecomastia (spironolactone).

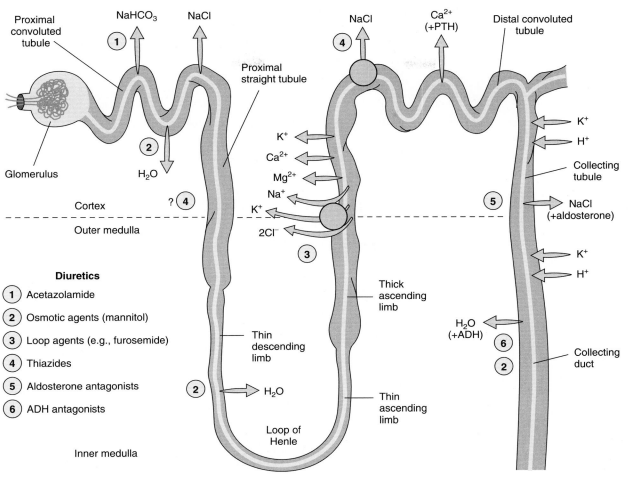

FIGURE 2.16-3. Overview of diuretics.

(Reproduced, with permission, from Katzung BG. *Basic & Clinical Pharmacology*, 10th ed. New York: McGraw-Hill, 2007: Fig. 15-1.)

▶ GLOMERULAR DISEASE

Nephritic Syndrome

A disorder of glomerular inflammation, also called glomerulonephritis. Proteinuria may be present but is usually < 1.5 g/day. Causes are summarized in Table 2.16-6.

HISTORY/PE

The classic findings are oliguria, macroscopic/microscopic hematuria (tea- or cola-colored urine), hypertension, and **edema.**

DIAGNOSIS

- UA shows hematuria and possibly mild proteinuria.
- Patients have a ↓ GFR with elevated BUN and creatinine. Complement, ANA, ANCA, and anti-GBM antibody levels should be measured to determine the underlying etiology.
- Renal biopsy may be useful for histologic evaluation.

Think nephritic syndrome if the patient has hematuria, hypertension, and oliguria.

485

TABLE 2.16-6. Causes of Nephritic Syndrome

	DESCRIPTION	HISTORY/PE	LABS/ HISTOLOGY	TREATMENT/ PROGNOSIS
Immune complex				
Postinfectious glomerulonephritis	Classically associated with recent group A β-hemolytic **streptococcal infection,** but can be seen with any infection (usually 2–6 weeks prior).	Oliguria, edema, hypertension, tea- or cola-colored urine.	Low serum C3 that normalizes 6–8 weeks after presentation; ↑ **ASO titer; lumpy-bumpy immunofluorescence.**	Supportive. Almost all children and most adults have a complete recovery.
IgA nephropathy (Berger's disease)	The **most common type;** associated with upper respiratory or GI infections. Commonly seen in young males; may be seen in Henoch-Schönlein purpura.	Episodic gross hematuria or persistent microscopic hematuria.	Normal C3.	Glucocorticoids for select patients; ACEIs in patients with proteinuria. Some 20% of cases progress to end-stage renal disease (ESRD).
Pauci-immune				
Wegener's granulomatosis	Granulomatous inflammation of the respiratory tract and kidney with necrotizing vasculitis.	Fever, weight loss, hematuria, hearing disturbances, respiratory and sinus symptoms. Cavitary pulmonary lesions bleed and lead to **hemoptysis.**	Presence of **c-ANCA** (cell-mediated immune response). Renal biopsy shows segmental necrotizing glomerulonephritis with few immunoglobulin deposits on immunofluorescence.	High-dose corticosteroids and cytotoxic agents. Patients tend to have frequent relapses.
Anti-GBH disease				
Goodpasture's syndrome	Rapidly progressing glomerulonephritis with pulmonary hemorrhage; peak incidence is in males in their mid-20s.	**Hemoptysis,** dyspnea, possible respiratory failure.	**Linear anti-GBM deposits** on immunofluorescence; iron deficiency anemia; hemosiderin-filled macrophages in sputum; pulmonary infiltrates on CXR.	Plasma exchange therapy; pulsed steroids. May progress to ESRD.
Alport's syndrome	Hereditary glomerulonephritis; presents in boys 5–20 years of age.	Asymptomatic hematuria associated with **nerve deafness** and eye disorders.	GBM splitting on electron microscopy.	Progresses to renal failure. Anti-GBM nephritis may recur after transplant.

TREATMENT

- Treat hypertension, fluid overload, and uremia with salt and water restriction, diuretics, and, if necessary, dialysis.
- In some cases, **corticosteroids** are useful in reducing glomerular inflammation.

Nephrotic Syndrome

Defined as **proteinuria (≥ 3.5 g/day), generalized edema, hypoalbuminemia,** and **hyperlipidemia.** Approximately one-third of all cases result from systemic diseases such as DM, SLE, or amyloidosis. Causes are summarized in Table 2.16-7.

TABLE 2.16-7. Causes of Nephrotic Syndrome

	DESCRIPTION	HISTORY/PE	LABS/ HISTOLOGY	TREATMENT/ PROGNOSIS
Minimal change disease	The most common cause of nephrotic syndrome in children. Idiopathic etiology; 2° causes include NSAIDs and hematologic malignancies.	Tendency toward infections and thrombotic events.	Light microscopy appears **normal;** electron microscopy shows **fusion of epithelial foot processes** with lipid-laden renal cortices.	Steroids; excellent prognosis.
Focal segmental glomerulosclerosis	Idiopathic, IV drug use, HIV infection, obesity.	The typical patient is a young African-American male with uncontrolled hypertension.	Microscopic hematuria; biopsy shows sclerosis in capillary tufts.	Prednisone, cytotoxic therapy, ACEIs/ARBs to ↓ proteinuria.
Membranous nephropathy	**The most common nephropathy in Caucasian adults.** 2° causes includes solid tumor malignancies (especially in patients > 60 years of age) and immune complex disease.	Associated with HBV, syphilis, malaria, and gold.	**"Spike-and-dome"** appearance due to granular deposits of IgG and C3 at the basement membrane.	Prednisone and cytotoxic therapy for severe disease.
Diabetic nephropathy	Two characteristic forms: diffuse hyalinization and nodular glomerulosclerosis **(Kimmelstiel-Wilson lesions).**	Generally have long-standing, poorly controlled DM with evidence of retinopathy or neuropathy.	Thickened GBM; ↑ **mesangial matrix.**	Tight control of blood sugar; ACEIs for type 1 DM and ARBs for type 2 DM.

TABLE 2.16-7.   Causes of Nephrotic Syndrome (*continued*)

	Description	History/PE	Labs/Histology	Treatment/Prognosis
Lupus nephritis	Classified as WHO types I–VI. Both nephrotic and nephritic. The severity of renal disease often determines overall prognosis.	Proteinuria or RBCs on UA may be found during evaluation of SLE patients.	Mesangial proliferation; subendothelial and/or subepithelial immune complex deposition.	Prednisone and cytotoxic therapy may slow disease progression.
Renal amyloidosis	1° (plasma cell dyscrasia) and 2° (infectious or inflammatory) are the most common.	Patients may have multiple myeloma or a chronic inflammatory disease (e.g., rheumatoid arthritis, TB).	Nodular glomerulosclerosis; EM reveals amyloid fibrils; **apple-green** birefringence with Congo red stain.	Prednisone and melphalan. Bone marrow transplant may be used for multiple myeloma.
Membrano-proliferative nephropathy	Can also be nephritic syndrome. Type I is associated with HCV, cryoglobulinemia, SLE, and subacute bacterial endocarditis.	Idiopathic form is present at 8–30 years of age. Slow progression to renal failure.	**"Tram-track,"** double-layered basement membrane. Type I has subendothelial deposits and mesangial deposits; all three types have low serum C3; type II by way of C3 nephritic factor.	Corticosteroids and cytotoxic agents may help.

Proteinuria, hypoalbuminemia, edema, hyperlipidemia, and hyperlipiduria in nephrotic syndrome are due to the initial ↑ in permeability of the glomerulus to protein.

HISTORY/PE

- Presents with **generalized edema** and **foamy urine.** In severe cases, dyspnea and ascites may develop.
- Patients have ↑ susceptibility to infection as well as a predisposition to hypercoagulable states with an ↑ risk for venous thrombosis and pulmonary embolism.

DIAGNOSIS

- UA shows **proteinuria** (≥ 3.5 g/day) and lipiduria.
- Blood chemistry shows ↓ **albumin** (< 3 g/dL) and hyperlipidemia.
- Evaluation should include workup for 2° causes.
- Renal biopsy is used to definitively diagnose the underlying etiology.

TREATMENT

- Treat with **protein and salt restriction,** judicious diuretic therapy, and antihyperlipidemics.

HIGH-YIELD FACTS

RENAL/GENITOURINARY

- Immunosuppressant medications may be useful for certain etiologies.
- **ACEIs** ↓ proteinuria and diminish the progression of renal disease in patients with renal scarring.
- Vaccinate with 23-polyvalent pneumococcus vaccine (PPV23), as patients are at ↑ risk of *Streptococcus pneumoniae* infection.

▶ NEPHROLITHIASIS

Renal calculi. Stones are most commonly calcium oxalate but may also be calcium phosphate, struvite, uric acid, or cystine (see Table 2.16-8 and Figure 2.16-4). Risk factors include a ⊕ family history, **low fluid intake**, gout, medications (allopurinol, chemotherapy, loop diuretics), postcolectomy/postileostomy, specific enzyme deficiencies, type I RTA (due to alkaline urinary pH and associated hypocitruria), and hyperparathyroidism. Most common in older males.

HISTORY/PE

- Presents with **acute onset of severe, colicky flank pain** that may **radiate to the testes or vulva** and is associated with nausea and vomiting.
- Patients are unable to get comfortable and shift position frequently (as opposed to those with peritonitis, who lie still).

DIAGNOSIS

- UA may show gross or **microscopic hematuria** (85%) and an **altered urine pH.**
- KUB (kidney/ureter/bladder radiography) identifies radiopaque stones but will miss the 10% of stones that are radiolucent.

Which bacteria are associated with "staghorn calculi"? Urease-producing organisms such as Proteus.

TABLE 2.16-8. **Types of Nephrolithiasis**

TYPE	FREQUENCY	ETIOLOGY AND CHARACTERISTICS	TREATMENT
Calcium oxalate/ calcium phosphate	83%	The most common causes are **idiopathic hypercalciuria** and 1° hyperparathyroidism. Alkaline urine. Radiopaque.	Hydration, dietary sodium and protein restriction, thiazide diuretic. Avoid ↓ calcium intake (can lead to hyperoxaluria and an ↑ risk of osteoporosis).
Struvite (Mg-NH$_4$-PO$_4$) or "triple phosphate"	9%	Associated with urease-producing organisms (e.g., *Proteus*). Form **staghorn calculi**. Alkaline urine. Radiopaque.	Hydration; treat UTI if present; surgical removal of staghorn stone.
Uric acid	7%	Associated with gout, xanthine oxidase deficiency, and high purine turnover states (e.g., chemotherapy). Acidic urine (pH < 5.5). **Radiolucent.**	Hydration; alkalinize urine with citrate, which is converted to HCO$_3^-$ in the liver; dietary purine restriction and allopurinol.
Cystine	1%	Due to a defect in renal transport of certain amino acids (COLA—cystine, ornithine, lysine, and arginine). **Hexagonal crystals**. Radiopaque.	Hydration, dietary sodium restriction, alkalinization of urine, penicillamine.

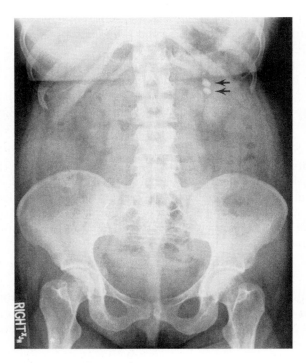

FIGURE 2.16-4. Nephrolithiasis.

KUB shows two dense 1-cm calcifications (arrows) projecting over the midportion of the left kidney, consistent with nephrolithiasis. (Reproduced, with permission, from Chen MY, Pope TL Jr., Ott DJ. *Basic Radiology*, 1st ed. New York: McGraw-Hill, 2004: 243.)

- **Noncontrast abdominal CT scans** are the **gold standard** for the diagnosis of kidney stones.
- Consider a **renal ultrasound** to look for obstruction (ultrasound is also preferred for pregnant patients, in whom radiation from CT should be avoided).
- An **IVP** can be used to confirm the diagnosis if there is a lack of contrast filling below the stone.

TREATMENT

- **Hydration and analgesia** are the initial treatment.
- Kidney stones < 5 mm in diameter can pass through the urethra; stones < 3 cm in diameter can be treated with **extracorporeal shock-wave lithotripsy (ESWL)**, percutaneous nephrolithotomy, or retrograde ureteroscopy.
- Preventive measures include hydration; additional prophylaxis is dependent on stone composition.

▶ POLYCYSTIC KIDNEY DISEASE (PKD)

Characterized by the presence of progressive cystic dilation of the renal tubules, as well as by cysts in the spleen, liver, and pancreas. The two major forms are as follows:

- **Autosomal dominant (ADPKD):**
  - Most common.
  - Usually asymptomatic until patients are > 30 years of age.

- One-half of ADPKD patients will have ESRD requiring dialysis by age 60.
- Associated with an ↑ risk of cerebral aneurysm, especially in patients with a ⊕ family history.
- **Autosomal recessive (ARPKD):** Less common but more severe. Presents in infants and young children with renal failure, liver fibrosis, and portal hypertension; may lead to death in the first few years of life.

HISTORY/PE

- **Pain and hematuria** are the most common presenting symptoms. Sharp, localized pain may result from cyst rupture, infection, or passage of renal calculi.
- Additional findings include **hypertension, hepatic cysts, cerebral berry aneurysms,** diverticulosis, and mitral valve prolapse.
- Patients may have large, palpable kidneys on abdominal exam.

DIAGNOSIS

Based on ultrasound (most common) or CT scan. Multiple bilateral cysts will be present throughout the renal parenchyma, and renal enlargement will be visualized. Genetic testing by DNA linkage analysis for *ADPKD1* and *ADPKD2* is available.

TREATMENT

- **Prevent complications and ↓ the rate of progression to ESRD.** Early management of UTIs is critical to prevent renal cyst infection. BP control (ACEIs, ARBs) is necessary to ↓ hypertension-induced renal damage.
- Dialysis and renal transplantation are used to manage patients with ESRD.

*If a patient with known ADPKD develops a sudden-onset, severe headache, you must rule out subarachnoid hemorrhage from a **ruptured berry aneurysm!***

▶ HYDRONEPHROSIS

Dilation of renal calyces. Usually occurs 2° to obstruction of the urinary tract. In pediatric patients, the obstruction is often at the ureteropelvic junction. In adults, it may be due to BPH, tumors, aortic aneurysms, or renal calculi. Can also be caused by high-output urinary flow and vesicoureteral reflux.

HISTORY/PE

May be asymptomatic, or may present with flank/back pain, ↓ urine output, abdominal pain, and UTIs.

DIAGNOSIS

- **Ultrasound** or CT scan to detect dilation of the renal calyces and/or ureter.
- ↑ BUN and creatinine provide evidence of 2° renal failure.

TREATMENT

- Surgically correct any anatomic obstruction; use laser or sound wave lithotripsy if calculi are causing obstruction.
- Ureteral stent placement across the obstructed area of the urinary tract and/or percutaneous nephrostomy tube placement to relieve pressure may be appropriate if the urinary outflow tract is not sufficiently cleared of obstruction. Foley or suprapubic catheters may be required for lower urinary tract obstruction (e.g., BPH).

Left untreated, hydronephrosis resulting from urinary obstruction leads to hypertension, acute or chronic renal failure, or sepsis, and has a very poor prognosis.

▶ VESICOURETERAL REFLUX

Retrograde projection of urine from the bladder to the ureters and kidneys. Often caused by insufficient tunneling of the ureters into submucosal bladder tissue, leading to ineffective restriction of retrograde urine flow during bladder contraction. May also be due to posterior urethral valves, urethral or meatal stenosis, or a neurogenic bladder. Classified as follows:

- **Mild reflux (grades I–II):** No ureteral or renal pelvic dilation. Often resolves spontaneously.
- **Moderate to severe reflux (grade III–V):** Ureteral dilation with associated caliceal blunting in severe cases.

HISTORY/PE

Patients present with recurrent UTIs, typically in childhood. Prenatal ultrasound may identify hydronephrosis.

DIAGNOSIS

- Obtain a **voiding cystourethrogram** (VCUG) to detect abnormalities at ureteral insertion sites and to classify the grade of reflux.
- Nuclear renal scan (DMSA or MAG-3) can be used to evaluate for renal function.

TREATMENT

- Treat infections aggressively. Treat mild reflux with daily prophylactic antibiotics (amoxicillin if < 2 months of age; otherwise TMP-SMX or nitrofurantoin) until reflux resolves.
- Surgery (ureteral reimplantation) is generally reserved for children with persistent high-grade (III to V) reflux or for those with breakthrough pyelonephritis while on prophylaxis. Inadequate treatment can lead to progressive renal scarring and ESRD.

A VCUG should be obtained in all boys presenting with their first UTI, girls < 3 years of age with their first UTI or < 5 years of age with febrile UTI, and older girls with pyelonephritis or recurrent UTIs.

▶ CRYPTORCHIDISM

Failure of one or both of the testes to fully descend into the scrotum. **Low birth weight is a risk factor.**

HISTORY/PE

Bilateral cryptorchidism is associated with prematurity, oligospermia, congenital malformation syndromes (Prader-Willi, Noonan syndromes), and infertility. Associated with an ↑ risk of testicular malignancy.

DIAGNOSIS

The testes **cannot be manipulated into the scrotal sac** with gentle pressure (vs. retractile testes) and may be palpated anywhere along the inguinal canal or in the abdomen.

TREATMENT

- **Orchiopexy** by 6–12 months of age (most testes will spontaneously descend by 3 months).
- If discovered later, treat with orchiectomy to avoid the risk of testicular cancer.

*Bringing the testes into the scrotum does **not** ↓ the risk of testicular cancer.*

▶ SCROTAL SWELLING

Table 2.16-9 outlines the etiologies, presentation, diagnosis, and treatment of scrotal swelling.

▶ ERECTILE DYSFUNCTION (ED)

Found in 10–25% of middle-aged and elderly men. Classified as failure to initiate (e.g., psychological, endocrinologic, neurologic), failure to fill (e.g., arteriogenic), or failure to store (e.g., veno-occlusive dysfunction). Risk factors include **DM, atherosclerosis, medications** (e.g., β-blockers, SSRIs, TCAs, diuretics), hypertension, heart disease, surgery or radiation for prostate cancer, and spinal cord injury.

HISTORY/PE

- Because patients rarely volunteer this complaint, physicians should make a specific inquiry.
- Ask about risk factors (diabetes, peripheral vascular disease), **medication use,** recent life changes, and psychological stressors.
- The distinction between psychological and organic ED is based on the presence of **nocturnal or early-morning erections** (if present, it is nonorganic) and on **situation dependence** (i.e., occurring with only one partner).

TABLE 2.16-9. **Differential Diagnosis of Scrotal Swelling**

DISORDER	CAUSE	HISTORY/PE	DIAGNOSIS	TREATMENT
Painless causes				
Hydrocele	Remnant of the processus vaginalis.	Usually asymptomatic; transilluminates.	Lab and radiologic workups are rarely indicated. Obtain an ultrasound if there is concern for inguinal hernia or testicular cancer.	Typically none unless hernia is present or hydrocele persists beyond 12–18 months of age (indicates patent processus vaginalis, which leads to an ↑ risk for inguinal hernia).
Varicocele	Dilation of the pampiniform venous plexus ("bag of worms").	Asymptomatic or presents with vague, aching scrotal pain. Affects the left testicle more often than the right. May disappear in the supine position. Does **not** transilluminate.	Ultrasound.	If symptomatic or if testis makes up < 40% of total volume, may be treated surgically with a varicocelectomy or ligation, or through embolization via interventional radiology.

493

TABLE 2.16-9. **Differential Diagnosis of Scrotal Swelling** (*continued*)

DISORDER	CAUSE	HISTORY/PE	DIAGNOSIS	TREATMENT
Painful causes				
Epididymitis	Infection of the epididymis, usually from STIs, prostatitis, and/or reflux.	Typically affects those > 30 years of age; presents with epididymal tenderness, tender/enlarged testicle(s), fever, scrotal thickening, erythema, and pyuria. Pain may ↓ with scrotal elevation (⊕ Prehn's sign).	UA, culture (pyuria). Culture often shows *Neisseria gonorrhoeae, E. coli,* or *Chlamydia.* Doppler ultrasound shows normal to ↑ blood flow to testes.	Antibiotics (tetracycline, fluoroquinolones); NSAIDs; scrotal support for pain.
Testicular torsion	Twisting of the spermatic cord, leading to ischemia and possible testicular infarction.	Typically affects those < 30 years of age; presents with intense, acute-onset scrotal pain that remains the same or ↑ with scrotal elevation (⊖ Prehn's sign). Pain is often accompanied by nausea/vomiting and/or dizziness. Loss of cremasteric reflex is also seen.	Doppler ultrasound shows ↓ blood flow to testes. (If there is a high clinical suspicion for testicular torsion, do not wait for ultrasound and proceed immediately to surgery!)	Attempt manual detorsion. Immediate surgery to salvage testis (the testicle is often unsalvageable after six hours of ischemia). Orchiopexy of **both** testes to prevent future torsion.

- Evaluate for **neurologic dysfunction** (e.g., anal tone, lower extremity sensation) and for **hypogonadism** (e.g., small testes, loss of 2° sexual characteristics).

DIAGNOSIS

- **Testosterone** and **gonadotropin levels** may be abnormal.
- Check prolactin levels, as elevated **prolactin** can result in ↓ androgen activity.

TREATMENT

- Patients with psychological ED may benefit from psychotherapy or sex therapy involving discussion and exercises with the appropriate partner.
- Oral **sildenafil (Viagra), vardenafil (Levitra), and tadalafil (Cialis)** are phosphodiesterase-5 (PDE5) inhibitors that result in prolonged action of cGMP-mediated smooth muscle relaxation and ↑ blood flow in the corpora cavernosa.

"Point and Shoot": The ***Parasympathetic*** *nervous system mediates erection; the* ***Sympathetic*** *nervous system mediates ejaculation.*

- **Testosterone** is a useful therapy for patients with hypogonadism of testicular or pituitary origin; it is discouraged for patients with normal testosterone levels.
- Vacuum pumps, intracavernosal prostaglandin injections, and surgical implantation of semirigid or inflatable penile prostheses are alternatives for patients who fail PDE5 therapy.

▶ BENIGN PROSTATIC HYPERPLASIA (BPH)

Enlargement of the prostate that is a normal part of the aging process and is seen in > **80% of men by age 80.** Most commonly presents in men > **50 years of age.** BPH can result in urinary retention, recurrent UTIs, bladder and renal calculi, hydronephrosis, and kidney damage over time.

History/PE

- **Obstructive symptoms:** Hesitancy, weak stream, intermittent stream, incomplete emptying, urinary retention, bladder fullness.
- **Irritative symptoms:** Nocturia, daytime frequency, urge incontinence, opening hematuria.
- On DRE, the prostate is uniformly enlarged with a rubbery texture. If the prostate is hard or has irregular lesions, cancer should be suspected.

Diagnosis

- Conduct a **DRE** to screen for masses; if findings are suspicious, evaluate for prostate cancer.
- Obtain a **UA and urine culture** to rule out infection and hematuria.
- Measure **creatinine levels** to rule out obstructive uropathy and renal insufficiency.
- PSA testing and cystoscopy are not recommended for longitudinal BPH monitoring.

Treatment

- **Medical therapy** includes α-blockers (e.g., terazosin), which relax smooth muscle in the prostate and bladder neck, as well as 5α-reductase inhibitors (e.g., finasteride), which inhibit the production of dihydrotestosterone.
- Transurethral resection of the prostate (TURP) or open prostatectomy is appropriate for patients with moderate to severe symptoms.

▶ PROSTATE CANCER

The **most common cancer in men** and the **second leading cause of cancer death** in men (after lung cancer). Risk factors include advanced age and a ⊕ family history.

History/PE

- Usually **asymptomatic,** but may present with obstructive urinary symptoms (e.g., **urinary retention,** a ↓ in the force of the urine stream) as well as with lymphedema due to obstructing metastases, constitutional symptoms, and **back pain due to bone metastases.**
- DRE may reveal a **palpable nodule** or an area of induration. Early carcinoma is usually not detectable on exam.
- A tender prostate suggests prostatitis.

What drugs are an absolute contraindication to sildenafil? Nitrates (the combined effect of ↓ BP can lead to myocardial ischemia).

BPH most commonly occurs in the central (periurethral) zone of the prostate and may not be detected on DRE.

The major side effect of α-blockers is orthostatic hypotension.

Leading causes of cancer death in men:

1. Lung cancer
2. Prostate cancer
3. Colorectal cancer
4. Pancreatic cancer
5. Leukemia

DIAGNOSIS

- Suggested by clinical findings and/or a markedly ↑ **PSA** (> 4 ng/mL).
- Definitive diagnosis is made with **ultrasound-guided transrectal** biopsy, which typically shows adenocarcinoma.
- Tumors are graded by the **Gleason histologic system,** which sums the scores (from 1 to 5) of the two most dysplastic samples (10 is the highest grade).
- Look for metastases with CXR and **bone scan** (metastatic lesions show an **osteoblastic** or ↑ bone density). Fully 40% of patients present with metastatic disease at diagnosis.

TREATMENT

- Treatment is controversial, as many cases of prostate cancer are slow to progress. Treatment choice is based on the aggressiveness of the tumor and the patient's mortality risk.
- **Watchful waiting** may be the best approach for elderly patients with low-grade tumors.
- **Radical prostatectomy** and **radiation therapy** (e.g., brachytherapy or external beam) are associated with an ↑ risk of incontinence and/or impotence.
- **PSA,** while controversial as a screening test, is used to follow patients post-treatment to evaluate for disease recurrence.
- Treat metastatic disease with **androgen ablation** (e.g., GnRH agonists, orchiectomy, flutamide) and chemotherapy.

PREVENTION

- All males > 50 years of age should have an **annual DRE.** Screening should begin earlier in African-American males and in those with a first-degree relative with prostate cancer.
- Screening with PSA is common, but its utility remains controversial.

An elevated PSA may be due to BPH, prostatitis, UTI, prostatic trauma, or carcinoma.

An annual DRE after age 50 is the recommended screening method for prostate cancer.

> **Differential for hematuria—**
>
> **S2I3T3**
>
> **S**trictures
> **S**tones
> **I**nfection
> **I**nflammation
> **I**nfarction
> **T**umor
> **T**rauma
> **T**B

▶ BLADDER CANCER

The second most common urologic cancer and the **most frequent malignant tumor of the urinary tract;** usually a **transitional cell carcinoma.** Most prevalent in males during the sixth and seventh decades. Risk factors include smoking, diets rich in meat and fat, schistosomiasis, chronic treatment with cyclophosphamide, and occupational exposure to aniline dye (a benzene derivative).

HISTORY/PE

- **Gross hematuria** is the most common presenting symptom.
- Other urinary symptoms, such as frequency, urgency, and dysuria, may also be seen, but most patients are asymptomatic in the early stages of disease.

DIAGNOSIS

- **Cystoscopy with biopsy is diagnostic.**
- **UA** often shows hematuria (macro- or microscopic); cytology may show dysplastic cells.
- **IVP** can examine the upper urinary tract as well as defects in bladder filling.

- MRI, CT, and bone scan are important tools with which to define invasion and metastases.

TREATMENT

Treatment depends on the extent of spread beyond the bladder mucosa.

- **Carcinoma in situ:** Intravesicular chemotherapy.
- **Superficial cancers:** Complete transurethral resection or intravesicular chemotherapy with mitomycin-C or BCG (the TB vaccine).
- **Large, high-grade recurrent lesions:** Intravesicular chemotherapy.
- **Invasive cancers without metastases:** Radical cystectomy or radiotherapy for patients who are deemed poor candidates for radical cystectomy as well as for those with unresectable local disease.
- **Invasive cancers with distant metastases:** Chemotherapy alone.

▶ RENAL CELL CARCINOMA

An adenocarcinoma from tubular epithelial cells (~80–90% of all malignant tumors of the kidney). Tumors can spread along the renal vein to the IVC and can metastasize to lung and bone. Risk factors include male **gender, smoking, obesity, acquired cystic kidney disease in ESRD,** and von Hippel–Lindau disease.

HISTORY/PE

- Presenting signs include **hematuria, flank pain,** and a **palpable flank mass.** Metastatic disease can present with weight loss and malaise.
- Many patients have **fever** or other constitutional symptoms. Left-sided varicocele may seen in males (due to tumor blockage of the left gonadal vein, which empties into the left renal vein; the right gonadal vein empties directly into the IVC).
- **Anemia is common at presentation,** but **polycythemia** due to ↑ erythropoietin production may be seen in 5–10% of patients.

DIAGNOSIS

Ultrasound and/or CT to characterize the renal mass (usually complex cysts or solid tumor).

TREATMENT

- **Surgical resection** may be curative in localized disease.
- Response rates from radiation or chemotherapy are only 15–30%. Newer tyrosine kinase inhibitors (sorafenib, sunitinib), which ↓ tumor angiogenesis and cell proliferation, have shown promising results and have recently been approved by the FDA for the treatment of renal cell carcinoma.

▶ TESTICULAR CANCER

A heterogeneous group of neoplasms. Some 95% of testicular tumors derive from **germ cells,** and **virtually all are malignant. Cryptorchidism** is associated with an ↑ risk of neoplasia in both testes. **Klinefelter's syndrome** is also a risk factor. Testicular cancer is the most common malignancy in males 15–34 years of age.

The classic triad of renal cell carcinoma is hematuria, flank pain, and a palpable flank mass, but only 5–10% present with all three components of the triad.

History/PE

- Patients most often present with **painless enlargement of the testes.**
- Most testicular cancers occur between ages 15 and 30, but seminomas have a peak incidence between 40 and 50 years of age.

Diagnosis

- **Testicular** ultrasound.
- CXR and abdominal/pelvic CT to evaluate for metastasis.
- **Tumor markers** are useful for diagnosis and in monitoring treatment response.
- β-hCG is always elevated in choriocarcinoma and is elevated in 10% of seminomas.
- α-fetoprotein (AFP) is often elevated in nonseminomatous germ cell tumors, particularly endodermal sinus (yolk sac) tumors. It is also elevated in hepatocellular carcinoma, hepatoblastoma, and neuroblastoma.

β-hCG in men =

choriocarcinoma.

Treatment

- Radical orchiectomy.
- Seminomas are **exquisitely radiosensitive** and also respond to chemotherapy.
- Platinum-based chemotherapy is used for nonseminomatous germ cell tumors.

Selected Topics in Emergency Medicine

1° survey of a trauma patient—

ABCDE

Airway
Breathing
Circulation
Disability
Exposure

To remember the Glasgow Coma Scale, think **4**-eyes, Jackson-**5**, V**6** engine. Four points can be assigned for eye response, five points for verbal response, and six points for motor response.

The steps underlying the acute management of a trauma patient can be remembered with the mnemonic **ABCDE. Establishing airway patency takes precedence over all other treatment,** followed by providing respiratory support and treating conditions that impair respiration, followed in turn by providing circulatory support and treating conditions that impair circulation.

1° Survey

- Airway:
  - Start with supplemental O_2 by nasal cannula or face mask for conscious patients. Use a jaw-thrust maneuver to reposition the tongue in an unconscious patient. A chin-lift maneuver can be used as a last resort but should be avoided where possible, as it requires movement of the potentially unstable C-spine. An oropharyngeal or nasopharyngeal airway may facilitate bag-mask ventilation.
  - Perform intubation in patients with apnea, significantly depressed mental status (Glasgow Coma Scale [GCS] < 8), or impending airway compromise (e.g., significant maxillofacial trauma or inhalation injury in fires).
  - Perform a surgical airway (cricothyroidotomy) in patients who cannot be intubated or in whom there is significant maxillofacial trauma, making intubation impractical.
  - Maintain cervical spine stabilization/immobilization in trauma patients until the spine is appropriately cleared through exam and radiographic studies. However, **never allow this concern to delay airway management.**
- Breathing:
  - Thorough cardiac and pulmonary exams will identify the five thoracic causes of immediate death: **tension pneumothorax, cardiac tamponade, open pneumothorax, massive hemothorax, and airway obstruction.**
  - If tension pneumothorax (absent breath sounds on the affected side in combination with shock and hypoxemia) is identified, immediate needle decompression is needed. This is accomplished by placing a 16- to 18-gauge angiocatheter into the second intercostal space at the midclavicular line, followed by placement of a chest tube.
  - If open pneumothorax is identified, an occlusive dressing must be applied immediately. This must be secured on three sides only to prevent the development of tension pneumothorax.
  - Massive hemothorax is diagnosed through chest tube placement and is defined as > 1000 cc of immediate blood return or > 200/hour for > 2–4 hours. The treatment for massive hemothorax is volume resuscitation followed by surgery to repair the site of bleeding. The treatment for flail chest is supportive, followed by surgical fixation of the chest wall.
- Circulation:
  - Apply direct pressure to any actively bleeding wounds.
  - Place a 16-gauge IV in each antecubital fossa.
  - Isotonic fluids (LR or NS) are repleted in a **3:1 ratio (fluid to blood loss).** Start with a fluid bolus of 1–2 L in adults; then recheck vitals and continue repletion as indicated.
  - If the patient remains tachycardic or hypotensive after the first 2 L of isotonic fluid, transfusion with packed RBCs may be indicated.

- Patients with chest trauma and shock may have cardiac tamponade. The relevant signs are JVD, hypotension, and muffled heart sounds. This can be diagnosed with bedside ultrasound. If tamponade is diagnosed, an immediate pericardiocentesis is necessary.
- **Disability/Exposure:**
  - Disability (CNS dysfunction) is assessed and quantified with the GCS.
  - Exposure requires that the patient be completely disrobed and assessed for injury and temperature status on both the front and back of the body. Hypothermia is a common problem in trauma and can worsen bleeding; once the exam is done, the patient should be covered with warm blankets.

2° Survey

- Once the patient is stable, conduct a full examination.
- For unstable patients with suspected hemoperitoneum or tamponade, do a focused abdominal sonography for trauma (**FAST**) scan. Four spaces are checked for blood: between the right kidney and liver (Morrison's pouch), between the left kidney and spleen (the splenorenal recess), posterior to the bladder (the pouch of Douglas), and in the pericardium. Hemoperitoneum requires immediate surgical consultation for operative management; hemopericardium requires immediate pericardiocentesis.
- Radiology studies should be ordered on the basis of the patient assessment. A CXR is needed for all patients with thoracic trauma, and a head CT should be ordered for all patients with loss of consciousness or depressed mental status. A C-spine CT is needed for all patients with neck pain or tenderness, neurologic findings, or depressed mental status.
- After urethral injury has been ruled out, place a Foley catheter if it is necessary to monitor urine output (e.g., in hemodynamically unstable patients, patients receiving fluid resuscitation, or patients undergoing major surgery).
- Pertinent labs should be ordered based on the mechanism of injury, suspicion of intoxication or OD, and past medical history.

▶ PENETRATING TRAUMA

The evaluation and treatment of penetrating trauma depend on the location and extent of the injury.

Neck

- Intubate early.
- Immediate surgical exploration is mandatory for patients with shock and active ongoing hemorrhage from neck wounds.
- All wounds that violate the platysma are considered true penetrating neck trauma. The neck is divided into three zones, and treatment varies according to which zone is injured (see Figure 2.17-1).
- Diagnostic workup is individualized based on the location of the wound, suspected injuries, and the preference of the trauma surgeon. Appropriate tests may include angiography of the aorta and carotid/cerebral arteries, CT scan of the neck with or without CT angiography, Doppler ultrasound, contrast esophagography, esophagoscopy, or bronchoscopy.

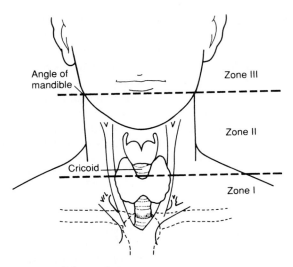

FIGURE 2.17-1. Zones of the neck.

(Reproduced, with permission, from Way LW. *Current Surgical Diagnosis & Treatment*, 10th ed. Stamford, CT: Appleton & Lange, 1994: 223.)

Immediately evaluate trauma patients for tension pneumothorax, cardiac tamponade, open pneumothorax, massive hemothorax, flail chest, and airway obstruction.

Chest

- Unstable patients with penetrating thoracic injuries require immediate **intubation** followed by assessment and treatment of the life-threatening injuries described above. Empiric placement of bilateral chest tubes may be needed if the precise nature of injury is unclear.
- Open thoracotomy may be indicated for patients with penetrating chest trauma leading to cardiac arrest, **provided that the patient arrested in the ED or shortly before arrival.**
- Leave any impaled objects in place until the patient is taken to the OR, as such objects may tamponade further blood loss.
- Beware of tension pneumothorax, open pneumothorax, massive hemothorax, flail chest, cardiac tamponade, aortic disruption, diaphragmatic tear, and esophageal injury.
- If a previously stable chest trauma patient suddenly dies, suspect **air embolism.**
- A new diastolic murmur after chest trauma suggests aortic dissection.

Abdomen

- The absence of pain does not rule out an abdominal injury.
- Gunshot wounds usually require immediate exploratory laparotomy, although stable patients can be managed conservatively in select cases.
- Stab wounds in a hemodynamically unstable patient or in a patient with peritoneal signs or evisceration require immediate exploratory laparotomy.
- Stab wounds in a hemodynamically stable patient warrant a CT or FAST scan followed by close inpatient observation.

Musculoskeletal

- Complete neurovascular assessment is critical; check pulses, motor function, and sensory function.

- Arteriography and surgical management are required for patients with suspected vascular injuries.
- Nerve injuries generally require surgical repair.
- **Early wound irrigation** and **tissue debridement,** not antibiotic therapy, are the most important steps in the treatment of contaminated wounds. However, do administer antibiotics and tetanus prophylaxis.

▶ BLUNT AND DECELERATION TRAUMA

Head

- A rapid deceleration head injury causes **coup-contrecoup** injuries, in which a bleed is noted both at the site of impact and across from the point of impact.
- **Epidural hematomas:** Lenticular in shape on head CT. Bleed is from the medial meningeal artery (the higher arterial pressure is able to push the dura away from the skull, causing the lens shape on imaging). These bleeds **cannot cross suture lines** but can expand rapidly and cause herniation and death. Patients classically have loss of consciousness immediately after the injury and then have a "lucid interval" after which they become comatose.
- **Subdural hematomas:** Follow the curve of the skull and result from shearing of the dural bridging veins. These bleeds **can cross suture lines.** In a pediatric patient, a subdural hematoma coupled with **retinal hemorrhages** constitutes child abuse until proven otherwise. These bleeds accumulate more slowly than epidural hematomas but can still cause death. They may present acutely (immediate), subacutely (days), or chronically (weeks).

Other signs of suspected child abuse are spiral fractures in the limbs, bucket-handle fractures, bruises, and rib fractures.

Chest

AORTIC DISRUPTION

The classic cause is a **rapid deceleration injury** (e.g., high-speed motor vehicle accidents, ejection from vehicles, and falls from heights). Since complete aortic rupture is rapidly fatal (85% die at the scene), patients with aortic disruption who are seen in the ED usually have a contained hematoma within the adventitia. Laceration is most common just proximal to the ligamentum arteriosum.

Marfan's syndrome, syphilis, and Ehlers-Danlos syndrome all predispose to a weak aortic wall.

DIAGNOSIS

- **Immediate CXR** reveals a **widened mediastinum** (> 8 cm), **loss of aortic knob, pleural cap,** deviation of the trachea and esophagus to the right, and depression of the left main stem bronchus.
- CT evaluation and/or transesophageal echocardiography (TEE) prior to surgery.
- **Aortography is the gold standard for evaluation.**

TREATMENT

Basic trauma management (ABCs); emergent surgery for defect repair.

Aortic disruption is often associated with first and second rib, scapular, and sternal fractures.

FLAIL CHEST

- Three or more adjacent ribs fractured at two points, causing paradoxical inward movement of the flail segment with inspiration.

- **Hx/PE:** Presents with crepitus and abnormal chest wall movement. Abnormal chest wall movement may not be appreciated if the patient is splinting because of pain.
- **Dx:** Primarily clinical, although CXR, O_2 saturation, and blood gases may help.
- **Tx:** O_2, narcotic analgesia. Respiratory support, including intubation and mechanical ventilation, may be needed to treat hypoxemia in severe cases. Surgical fixation of the chest wall is generally needed.
- **Cx: Respiratory compromise** is a complication due to underlying pulmonary contusion.

Abdomen/Pelvis

- The **spleen** and **liver** are the **most commonly injured organs following blunt abdominal trauma.** Symptoms are consistent with signs of blood loss and include hypotension, tachycardia, and peritonitis. Suspect spleen or liver injury when lower rib fractures are present.
- Pancreatic rupture should be suspected after a direct epigastric blow (handlebar injury).
- **Diaphragmatic rupture** may occur with blunt or penetrating trauma. It is difficult to diagnose and often missed. **Kehr's sign** may be present; radiographs may demonstrate abdominal viscera in the thorax.
- The **kidneys** are the **most commonly injured GU organ in trauma,** with injuries including renal contusion, laceration, fracture, and pedicle injury.
- In hemodynamically stable patients, abdominal blunt trauma can be diagnosed with FAST scan (see the 2° Survey section), CT scan, and serial abdominal exams.
- In hemodynamically unstable patients, abdominal blunt trauma should be treated with immediate exploratory laparotomy to look for organ injury or intra-abdominal bleeding.

***Kehr's sign:** Referred shoulder pain due to diaphragmatic irritation (classically on the left due to spleen rupture).*

PELVIC FRACTURES

Most commonly occur after high-speed traumas such as motor vehicle accidents or falls from heights. Require immediate attention by the orthopedist owing to their life-threatening potential.

DIAGNOSIS

- May present with an unstable pelvis upon compression.
- Pelvic x-rays may confirm the fracture; in a stable patient, a CT scan of the pelvis will better define the extent of injury.
- If hypotension and shock are present, an exsanguinating hemorrhage is likely. In the field, MAST (military antishock trousers; rarely used today) can be used to maintain adequate BP and organ perfusion.

TREATMENT

- Consider embolization of bleeding vessels, emergent external pelvic fixation, or, in a hemodynamically stable patient, internal fixation. Give blood early. Hemorrhage results in death in 50% of patients.
- Pelvic injuries can be associated with urethral injury. It is suggested by **blood at the urethral meatus; a high-riding, "ballotable" prostate;** or **lack of a prostate.**

- If present, a **retrograde urethrogram** must be performed to rule out injury before a Foley catheter is placed.
- **Never explore a pelvic or retroperitoneal hematoma. Follow with serial hemoglobin and hematocrit.**

▶ CARDIAC LIFE SUPPORT BASICS

Table 2.17-1 summarizes the basic management of cardiac arrhythmias in an acute setting.

*Updated in 2005, CPR is **30 compressions to every two breaths** for all arrest victims after puberty.*

TABLE 2.17-1. **Management of Cardiac Arrhythmias**[a,b]

ARRHYTHMIA	TREATMENT
Asystole	Epinephrine and atropine.
Ventricular fibrillation or pulseless ventricular tachycardia	Unsynchronized shock with 360 J → 360-J shock → epinephrine → 360-J shock → amiodarone or lidocaine → 360-J shock → epinephrine. Vasopressin may be given in place of the first or second dose of epinephrine. Amiodarone, lidocaine, procainamide, or sotalol may be used for stable ventricular tachycardia.
Pulseless electrical activity (PEA)	Epinephrine or vasopressin; simultaneously search for the underlying cause (see the **5 H's and 5 T's** mnemonic) and provide empiric treatment. Give atropine for bradycardic PEA only.
Supraventricular tachycardia (SVT)	If unstable, perform synchronized electrical cardioversion. If stable, control rate with vagal maneuvers (Valsalva maneuver, carotid sinus massage, or cold stimulus). If resistant to maneuvers, give up to three doses of adenosine followed by other AV-nodal blocking agents (calcium channel blockers [CCBs] or β-blockers).
Atrial fibrillation/flutter	If unstable, perform synchronized electrical cardioversion starting at 100 J. If stable, control rate with diltiazem or β-blockers and anticoagulate if duration is > 48 hours. Elective cardioversion may be performed if duration is < 48 hours; otherwise, the clinician must anticoagulate or perform TEE prior to conversion. Do not give nodal blockers if there is evidence of Wolff-Parkinson-White syndrome (δ waves) on ECG.
Bradycardia	If symptomatic, give atropine and consider dopamine, epinephrine, and glucagon. If Mobitz II or third-degree heart block is present, place transcutaneous pacemaker pads, and have atropine at the bedside. A temporary transvenous pacemaker may be required for hemodynamically unstable patients.

[a] In all cases, disruptions of CPR should be minimized. After a shock or administration of a drug, CPR should be resumed immediately, and five cycles of CPR should be given before checking for a pulse or rhythm.

[b] Doses of electricity listed above assume a monophasic defibrillator. Maximum energy output on more modern biphasic defibrillators is usually 150–200 J.

HIGH-YIELD FACTS

EMERGENCY MEDICINE

> **Possible causes of PEA—**
>
> **The 5 H's and 5 T's**
>
> **H**ypovolemia
> **H**ypoxia
> **H**ydrogen ion: Acidosis
> **H**yper/**H**ypo: K+, other metabolic
> **H**ypothermia
> **T**ablets: Drug OD, ingestion
> **T**amponade: Cardiac
> **T**ension pneumothorax
> **T**hrombosis: Coronary
> **T**hrombosis: Pulmonary embolism

Acute-onset abdominal pain has many potential etiologies and may require immediate medical or surgical intervention. Sharp, focal pain generally implies a parietal (peritoneal) etiology; dull, diffuse pain is commonly of visceral (organ) origin. Figure 2.17-2 identifies the common causes of acute abdomen.

HISTORY/PE

- Obtain a complete history, including the elements indicated in the mnemonic **OPQRST.**
- Obtain a full gynecologic history for females (including last menstrual period, pregnancy, and any STD symptoms). If a female has abdominal pain with cervical motion tenderness, there should be a low threshold to treat for **pelvic inflammatory disease (PID).**
- **Perforation** leads to sudden onset of diffuse, severe pain, usually with abdominal rigidity on exam.
- **Obstruction** leads to acute onset of severe, radiating, colicky pain. Patients may complain of obstipation or bilious emesis.
- **Inflammation** leads to gradual onset (over 10–12 hours) of constant, ill-defined pain.
- **Associated symptoms** include the following:
  - Anorexia, nausea, vomiting, changes in bowel habits, hematochezia, and melena suggest GI etiologies.

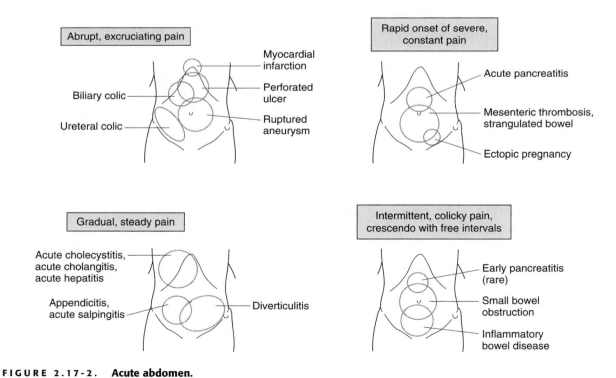

FIGURE 2.17-2. Acute abdomen.

The location and character of pain are helpful in the differential diagnosis of the acute abdomen. (Reproduced, with permission, from Way LW. *Current Surgical Diagnosis & Treatment*, 10th ed. Stamford, CT: Appleton & Lange, 1994: 444.)

- Fever and cough suggest pneumonia.
- Hematuria, pyuria, and costovertebral angle tenderness point to a GU etiology.
- If associated with meals, consider mesenteric ischemia, PUD, biliary disease, pancreatitis, or bowel pathology.
- A family history of abdominal pain may indicate familial Mediterranean fever or acute intermittent porphyria.

DIAGNOSIS

- If peritoneal signs, shock, or impending shock is present, emergent exploratory laparotomy is necessary. **A positive β-hCG in the setting of shock is a ruptured ectopic pregnancy until proven otherwise. Abdominal pain plus syncope or shock in an older patient is a ruptured abdominal aortic aneurysm (AAA) until proven otherwise.**
- If the patient is stable, a complete physical exam—including a **rectal exam** and, in women, a **pelvic exam**—is mandatory.
- Obtain electrolytes, LFTs, amylase, lipase, **urine or serum β-hCG**, UA, and a CBC with differential.
- Consider a CXR for suspected perforation or pulmonary pathology. AXR may be useful for obstruction, but CT is more sensitive and specific. CT is used to diagnose appendicitis, diverticulitis, abscess, renal stones, AAA, obstruction, and other pathology. Ultrasound is the best tool for diagnosing gallstones and gynecologic pathology. Bedside ultrasound (FAST and aortic views) can diagnose hemoperitoneum and AAA in unstable patients.

TREATMENT

- Hemodynamically unstable patients must have **emergent surgical management.**
- In stable patients, expectant management may include NPO status, NG tube placement, IV fluids, placement of a Foley catheter (to monitor urine output and fluid status), and vital sign monitoring with serial abdominal exams and serial labs.
- Give broad-spectrum antibiotics to all patients with perforation or signs of sepsis. Antibiotics may also be indicated for patients with infectious processes such as cholecystitis, diverticulitis, and pyelonephritis.
- Type and cross all unstable patients.

▶ ACUTE APPENDICITIS

The inciting event is obstruction of the appendiceal lumen with subsequent inflammation and infection. Rising intraluminal pressure leads to vascular compromise of the appendix, ischemia, necrosis, and possible perforation. Etiologies include hypertrophied lymphoid tissue (55–65%), fecalith (35%), foreign body, tumor (e.g., carcinoid tumor), and parasites. Incidence peaks in the early teens (most patients are between 10 and 30 years of age), and the male-to-female ratio is 2:1.

HISTORY/PE

- Presents with dull periumbilical pain lasting 1–12 hours that leads to sharp RLQ pain at McBurney's point.
- Also presents with nausea, vomiting, anorexia ("hamburger sign"), and low-grade fever.
- Psoas, obturator, and Rovsing's signs are insensitive tests that may be ⊕.

If the patient remembers the exact moment of pain onset, think perforation.

Pneumonia can present as right or left upper quadrant abdominal pain.

All female patients with an acute abdomen require a pelvic exam and a pregnancy test to rule out PID, ectopic pregnancy, and ovarian torsion.

McBurney's point is located one-third of the distance from the anterior superior iliac spine to the umbilicus.

■ **"Hamburger sign":** If
a patient wants to eat,
consider a diagnosis
other than appendicitis.
Anorexia is 80% specific
for appendicitis.

■ **Psoas sign:** Passive
extension of the hip
leading to RLQ pain.

■ **Obturator sign:** Passive
internal rotation of the
flexed hip leading to
RLQ pain.

■ **Rovsing's sign:** Deep
palpation of the LLQ
leading to RLQ pain.

■ In **perforated appendix,** partial pain relief is possible, but peritoneal signs (e.g., rebound, guarding, hypotension, ↑ WBC count, fever) will ultimately develop.

■ Children, the elderly, pregnant women, and those with retrocecal appendices may have atypical presentations that may result in misdiagnosis and ↑ mortality.

DIAGNOSIS

■ Diagnosed by clinical impression.

■ Look for fever, mild leukocytosis (11,000–15,000 cells/μL) with left shift, and UA with a few RBCs and/or WBCs.

■ If the clinical diagnosis is unequivocal, no imaging studies are necessary. Otherwise, studies include the following:
  ■ **KUB:** Fecalith or loss of psoas shadow.
  ■ **Ultrasound:** Enlarged, noncompressible appendix.
  ■ **CT scan with contrast (95–98% sensitive):** Periappendiceal stranding or fluid; enlarged appendix.

TREATMENT

■ The patient should be NPO and should receive IV hydration and antibiotics with anaerobic and gram-⊖ coverage.

■ Immediate open or laparoscopic appendectomy is the definitive treatment. If appendicitis is not found, complete exploration of the abdomen is performed.

■ **Perforation:** Administer antibiotics until the patient is afebrile with a normalized WBC count; the wound should be closed by delayed 1° closure.

■ **Abscess:** Treat with broad-spectrum antibiotics and percutaneous drainage; an elective appendectomy should be performed 6–8 weeks later.

▶ BURNS

The **second leading cause of death in children.** Serious burn patients should be treated in an ICU setting. Burns can be chemical, electrical, or thermal and are categorized by depth of tissue destruction:

■ **First degree:** Only the epidermis is involved. The area is painful and erythematous, but blisters are not present, and capillary refill is intact. Looks like a sunburn.

■ **Second degree:** The epidermis and partial thickness of the dermis are involved. The area is painful, and blisters are present.

■ **Third degree:** The epidermis, the full thickness of the dermis, and potentially deeper tissues are involved. The area is painless, white, and charred.

HISTORY/PE

■ Patients may present with obvious skin wounds, but significant deep destruction may not be visible, especially with electrical burns.

■ Conduct a thorough airway and lung exam to assess for inhalation injury.

■ Always assume carbon monoxide poisoning in patients with inhalation injury.

■ Consider cyanide poisoning in closed-space fires with burning carpets and textiles.

DIAGNOSIS

- Assess the ABCs. If airway compromise is impending, intubate.
- Be vigilant for shock, inhalation injury, and carbon monoxide poisoning. Obtain a CXR and a carboxyhemoglobin level.
- Evaluate the percentage of body surface area (% BSA) involved.

TREATMENT

- Supportive measures; tetanus, stress ulcer prophylaxis, and IV narcotic analgesia.
- For second- and third-degree burns, fluid repletion using the **Parkland formula** is critical; adjust repletion on the basis of additional insensible losses to maintain at least 1 cc/kg/hr of urine output.
- Topical silver sulfadiazine and mafenide may be used prophylactically; however, there is no proven benefit associated with the use of PO/IV antibiotics or corticosteroids.

COMPLICATIONS

- Shock and superinfection, with the latter most likely due to *Pseudomonas* or gram-⊕ cocci.
- Criteria for transfer to a burn center include the following:
    - Full-thickness burn > 5% of BSA.
    - Partial-thickness burn > 10% BSA.
    - Any full- or partial-thickness burn over critical areas (face, hands, feet, genitals, perineum, major joints).
    - Circumferential burns; chemical, electrical, or lightning injury; inhalation injury.
    - Any special psychosocial or rehabilitative care needs.

▶ POSTOPERATIVE FEVER

- Occurs in 40% of all postoperative patients. Remember the mnemonic "Wind, Water, Wounds, Walking, and Wonder drugs."
- ↓ the risk of postoperative fever with incentive spirometry, pre- and postoperative antibiotics when indicated, short-term Foley catheter use, early ambulation, and DVT prophylaxis (e.g., anticoagulation, compression stockings).
- Fevers before postoperative day 3 are unlikely to be infectious unless *Clostridium* or β-hemolytic streptococci are involved.

▶ SHOCK

Defined as **inadequate tissue-level oxygenation to maintain vital organ function.** The multiple etiologies are differentiated by their cardiovascular effects and treatment options (see Table 2.17-2).

▶ THERMAL DYSREGULATION

Hypothermia

- A body temperature < 95° F (35° C) accompanied by mental status and neurologic deficits.

Parkland formula: *Fluids for the first 24 hours = 4 × patient's weight in kg × % BSA. Give 50% of fluids over the first eight hours and the remaining 50% over the following 16 hours.*

Use the "rule of 9's" to estimate % BSA in adults:

Head and each arm = 9%
Back and chest each = 18%
Each leg = 18%
Perineum = 1%

The 5 W's of postoperative fever:

Wind: Atelectasis, pneumonia
Water: UTI
Wounds: Wound infection, abscess
Walking: DVT
Wonder drugs: Drug reaction

A sixth "W" of postoperative fever is "Womb" in OB/GYN.

TABLE 2.17-2.   **Types of Shock**

Type of Shock	Major Causes	Cardiac Output	PCWP[a]	PVR[b]	Treatment
Hypovolemic	Trauma, blood loss, dehydration with inadequate fluid repletion, third spacing, burns.	↓	↓	↑	Replete with isotonic solution (e.g., LR or NS) and blood in a 3:1 (fluid-to-blood) ratio.
Cardiogenic	CHF, arrhythmia, structural heart disease (severe mitral regurgitation, VSD), MI (> 40% of left ventricular function).	↓	↑	↑	Identify the cause and treat if possible. Give inotropic support with pressors such as dopamine (if hypotensive) or dobutamine (if not hypotensive).
Obstructive	Cardiac tamponade, tension pneumothorax, massive pulmonary embolism.	↓	↑	↑	Treat the underlying cause: pericardiocentesis, decompression of pneumothorax, thrombolysis.
Septic	Bacteremia, especially gram-⊖ organisms.	↑	↓	↓	Administer broad-spectrum antibiotics. Measure central venous pressure (CVP) and give fluid until CVP = 8. Then give pressors (dopamine or norepinephrine). Obtain cultures prior to administration of antibiotics if possible.
Anaphylactic	Bee stings, medication, food allergies.	↑	↓	↓	Give diphenhydramine. If severe, administer 1:1000 epinephrine.

[a] PCWP = pulmonary capillary wedge pressure.

[b] PVR = peripheral vascular resistance.

- Remove the patient from the cold or windy environment and remove wet clothing. In mild cases, rewarm the patient with blankets or warm water. In more severe cases, the patient may need a heating blanket, warmed oxygen, or warm IV fluids. In unstable patients, invasive rewarming may be necessary (e.g., NG or bladder lavage, pleural lavage, or cardiac bypass). If the patient has frostbite, thaw the affected areas with the same methods. Patients will need narcotic analgesia for thawing.
- Monitor the ECG for arrhythmias such as bradycardia and slow atrial fibrillation. The stereotypic sign is the **J wave** (aka Osborn wave). Also monitor electrolytes and acid-base balance.
- Do not stop resuscitation efforts until the patient has been warmed.

Hyperthermia

- A body temperature $> 104°$ F ($40°$ C), possibly from heat stroke.
- Cool the patient with cold water, wet blankets, and ice. Consider a benzo-diazepine to prevent convulsions. Rule out causes of fever such as infection or drug reaction.

▶ TOXICOLOGY

Carbon Monoxide Poisoning

A **hypoxemic poisoning syndrome** seen in patients who have been exposed to automobile exhaust, smoke inhalation, barbecues, or old appliances in poorly ventilated locations.

HISTORY/PE

- Presents with hypoxemia, **cherry-red skin** (rare), confusion, and **headaches.** Coma or seizures occur in severe cases.
- Chronic low-level exposure may cause **flulike symptoms** with generalized myalgias, nausea, and headaches. Ask about symptoms in others living in the same house.
- **Suspect smoke inhalation** in the presence of **singed nose hairs, facial burns, hoarseness, wheezing,** or **carbonaceous sputum.**

DIAGNOSIS

- Check an ABG and serum carboxyhemoglobin level (normal is $< 5\%$ in nonsmokers and $< 10\%$ in smokers).
- Check an ECG in the elderly and in patients with a history of cardiac disease.

TREATMENT

- Treat with 100% O_2 until asymptomatic and carboxyhemoglobin falls to normal levels.
- Use **hyperbaric O_2** for pregnant patients, nonresponders, those with signs of CNS or cardiac ischemia, or those with severely $\uparrow$ carboxyhemoglobin to facilitate displacement of carbon monoxide from hemoglobin.
- Patients with **airway burns** or **smoke inhalation** may require early intubation, since upper airway edema can rapidly lead to complete obstruction.

Common Drug Interactions/Reactions

Table 2.17-3 outlines drug interactions and reactions that are commonly encountered in a clinical setting.

Drug Overdose

Table 2.17-4 summarizes antidotes and treatments for substances commonly encountered in overdoses and intoxications. If a patient is unresponsive, it is common to empirically treat with a dose of Narcan.

Malignant hyperthermia and neuroleptic malignant syndrome (NMS) should be ruled out in any suspected case of hyperthermia. Malignant hyperthermia would be seen after halothane exposure, and NMS after a neuroleptic. Both conditions are treated with dantrolene.

In carbon monoxide poisoning, the patient's oxygen saturation is usually normal. This is because carboxyhemoglobin is read by the pulse oximeter as a normal saturated hemoglobin molecule.

HIGH-YIELD FACTS

EMERGENCY MEDICINE

TABLE 2.17-3. Drug Interactions and Reactions

INTERACTION/REACTION	DRUGS
Induction of P-450 enzymes	Barbiturates, phenytoin, carbamazepine, rifampin, quinidine, griseofulvin.
Inhibition of P-450 enzymes	Cimetidine, ketoconazole, INH, grapefruit, erythromycin, sulfonamides.
Metabolism by P-450 enzymes	Benzodiazepines, amide anesthetics, metoprolol, propranolol, nifedipine, phenytoin, quinidine, theophylline, warfarin, barbiturates.
↑ risk of digoxin toxicity	Quinidine, cimetidine, amiodarone, CCBs.
Competition for albumin-binding sites	Warfarin, ASA, phenytoin.
Blood dyscrasias	Ibuprofen, quinidine, methyldopa, chemotherapeutic agents.
Hemolysis in G6PD-deficient patients	Sulfonamides, isoniazid (INH), ASA, ibuprofen, nitrofurantoin, primaquine, pyrimethamine, chloramphenicol.
Gynecomastia	**S**pironolactone, **E**strogens, **D**igitalis, **C**imetidine, chronic **A**lcohol use, **K**etoconazole: "**S**ome **E**xcellent **D**rugs **C**reate **A**wesome **K**nockers."
Stevens-Johnson syndrome	Ethosuximide, sulfonamides.
Photosensitivity	Tetracycline, amiodarone, sulfonamides.
Drug-induced SLE	Procainamide, hydralazine, INH, penicillamine, chlorpromazine, methyldopa, quinidine.

TABLE 2.17-4. Specific Antidotes

TOXIN	ANTIDOTE/TREATMENT
Acetaminophen	*N*-acetylcysteine.
Acid/alkali ingestion	Upper endoscopy to evaluate for stricture.
Anticholinesterases, organophosphates	Atropine, pralidoxime.
Antimuscarinic/anticholinergic agents	Physostigmine.
Arsenic, mercury, gold	Succimer, dimercaprol.
β-blockers	Glucagon.
Barbiturates (phenobarbital)	Urine alkalinization, dialysis, activated charcoal, supportive care.
Benzodiazepines	Flumazenil (can precipitate withdrawal).

TABLE 2.17-4. Specific Antidotes (*continued*)

Toxin	Antidote/Treatment
Black widow bite	Calcium gluconate, methocarbamol.
Carbon monoxide	100% O_2, hyperbaric O_2.
Copper, arsenic, lead, gold	Penicillamine.
Cyanide	Amyl nitrate, sodium nitrate, sodium thiosulfate.
Digitalis	Normalize K^+ but avoid giving Ca^{++}, Mg^{++}, or lidocaine (for torsades), antidigitalis Fab.
Heparin	Protamine sulfate.
INH	Pyridoxine.
Iron salts	Deferoxamine.
Lead	Succimer, CaEDTA, dimercaprol.
Methanol, ethylene glycol (antifreeze)	EtOH, fomepizole, dialysis, calcium gluconate for ethylene glycol.
Methemoglobin	Methylene blue.
Opioids	Naloxone.
Salicylates	Urine alkalinization, dialysis, activated charcoal.
TCAs	Sodium bicarbonate for QRS prolongation; diazepam or lorazepam for seizures; cardiac monitor for arrhythmias.
Theophylline	Activated charcoal. Consider repeat doses.
tPA, streptokinase	Aminocaproic acid.
Warfarin	Vitamin K, FFP.

Major Drug Side Effects

Table 2.17-5 outlines the major side effects of select drugs.

Management of Drug Withdrawal

Table 2.17-6 summarizes common drug withdrawal symptoms and treatment.

▶ VITAMIN DEFICIENCIES

Table 2.17-7 summarizes the signs and symptoms of key vitamin deficiencies.

TABLE 2.17-5. **Drug Side Effects**

DRUG	SIDE EFFECTS
ACEIs	**Cough,** rash, proteinuria, angioedema, taste changes, teratogenic effects.
Amantadine	Ataxia, **livedo reticularis.**
Aminoglycosides	Ototoxicity, nephrotoxicity (acute tubular necrosis).
Amiodarone	Acute: AV block, hypotension, bradycardia. Chronic: pulmonary fibrosis, peripheral deposition leading to bluish discoloration, arrhythmias, hypo-/hyperthyroidism, corneal deposition.
Amphotericin	Fever/rigors, nephrotoxicity, bone marrow suppression, anemia.
Antipsychotics	Sedation, acute dystonic reaction, akathisia, parkinsonism, tardive dyskinesia, **NMS.**
Azoles (e.g., fluconazole)	Inhibition of P-450 enzymes.
AZT	Thrombocytopenia, megaloblastic anemia.
β-blockers	Asthma exacerbation, masking of hypoglycemia, impotence, bradycardia, AV block, CHF.
Benzodiazepines	Sedation, dependence, respiratory depression.
Bile acid resins	GI upset, malabsorption of vitamins and medications.
CCBs	Peripheral edema, constipation, cardiac depression.
Carbamazepine	Induction of P-450 enzymes, **agranulocytosis,** aplastic anemia, liver toxicity.
Chloramphenicol	**Gray baby syndrome**, aplastic anemia.
Cisplatin	Nephrotoxicity, acoustic nerve damage.
Clonidine	Dry mouth; **severe rebound headache and hypertension.**
Clozapine	Agranulocytosis.
Corticosteroids	Mania, hyperglycemia (acute), immunosuppression, bone mineral loss, thinning of skin, easy bruising, myopathy, cataracts (chronic).
Cyclophosphamide	Myelosuppression, **hemorrhagic cystitis.**
Digoxin	GI disturbance, **yellow visual changes, arrhythmias** (e.g., junctional tachycardia or SVT).
Doxorubicin	**Cardiotoxicity (cardiomyopathy).**
Ethyl alcohol	Renal dysfunction, CNS depression.
Fluoroquinolones	Cartilage damage in children; Achilles tendon rupture in adults.
Furosemide	Ototoxicity, hypokalemia, nephritis, gout.
Gemfibrozil	Myositis, reversible ↑ in LFTs.

TABLE 2.17-5. Drug Side Effects (*continued*)

DRUG	SIDE EFFECTS
Halothane	Hepatotoxicity, **malignant hyperthermia.**
HCTZ	Hypokalemia, hyponatremia, hyperuricemia, hyperglycemia, hypercalcemia.
HMG-CoA reductase inhibitors	Myositis, reversible ↑ in LFTs.
Hydralazine	Drug-induced SLE.
Hydroxychloroquine	Retinopathy.
INH	Peripheral neuropathy **(prevent with pyridoxine/vitamin B₆),** hepatotoxicity, inhibition of P-450 enzymes, seizures with overdose, hemolysis in G6PD deficiency.
MAOIs	**Hypertensive tyramine reaction, serotonin syndrome** (with meperidine).
Methanol	Blindness.
Methotrexate	Hepatic fibrosis, pneumonitis, anemia.
Methyldopa	⊕ Coombs' test, drug-induced SLE.
Metronidazole	Disulfiram reaction, vestibular dysfunction, **metallic taste.**
Niacin	**Cutaneous flushing.**
Nitroglycerin	Hypotension, tachycardia, headache, tolerance.
Penicillamine	Drug-induced SLE.
Penicillin/β-lactams	Hypersensitivity reactions.
Phenytoin	Nystagmus, diplopia, ataxia, arrhythmia (in toxic doses), **gingival hyperplasia,** hirsutism, teratogenic effects.
Prazosin	First-dose hypotension.
Procainamide	Drug-induced SLE.
Propylthiouracil	Agranulocytosis, aplastic anemia.
Quinidine	Cinchonism (headache, tinnitus), thrombocytopenia, arrhythmias (e.g., **torsades de pointes**).
Reserpine	Depression.
Rifampin	Induction of P-450 enzymes; **orange-red body secretions**.
Salicylates	Fever; hyperventilation with **respiratory alkalosis and metabolic acidosis;** dehydration, diaphoresis, hemorrhagic gastritis.
SSRIs	Anxiety, **sexual dysfunction,** serotonin syndrome if taken with MAOIs.

HIGH-YIELD FACTS

EMERGENCY MEDICINE

TABLE 2.17-5. Drug Side Effects (*continued*)

DRUG	SIDE EFFECTS
Succinylcholine	**Malignant hyperthermia,** hyperkalemia.
TCAs	Sedation, coma, anticholinergic effects, seizures and arrhythmias.
Tetracyclines	Tooth discoloration, photosensitivity, Fanconi's syndrome, GI distress.
Trimethoprim	Megaloblastic anemia, leukopenia, granulocytopenia.
Valproic acid	Teratogenicity leads to neural tube defects; rare fatal hepatotoxicity.
Vancomycin	Nephrotoxicity, ototoxicity, **"red man syndrome"** (histamine release; not an allergy).
Vinblastine	Severe myelosuppression.
Vincristine	Peripheral neuropathy, paralytic ileus.

TABLE 2.17-6. Symptoms and Treatment of Drug Withdrawal

DRUG	WITHDRAWAL SYMPTOMS	TREATMENT
Alcohol	Tremor (6–12 hours). Tachycardia, hypertension, agitation, seizures (within 48 hours). Hallucinations, **DTs**—severe autonomic instability leading to tachycardia, hypertension, delirium, and possibly death (within 2–7 days). Mortality is 15–20%.	**Benzodiazepines** (can require massive doses); haloperidol for hallucinations; **thiamine,** folate, and multivitamin replacement (do not affect withdrawal, but most alcoholics are deficient).
Barbiturates	Anxiety, seizures, delirium, tremor; cardiac and respiratory depression.	**Benzodiazepines.**
Benzodiazepines	Rebound anxiety, seizures, tremor, insomnia.	**Benzodiazepines.** Monitor for DTs.
Cocaine/ amphetamines	Depression, hyperphagia, hypersomnolence.	Supportive treatment. Avoid pure β-blockers (may lead to unopposed α activity, causing hypertension).
Opioids	Anxiety, insomnia, flulike symptoms, piloerection, fever, rhinorrhea, lacrimation, yawning, nausea, stomach cramps, diarrhea, mydriasis.	Antiemetics, muscle relaxers, and NSAIDs for mild symptoms; clonidine, buprenorphine, or methadone for moderate to severe symptoms.

TABLE 2.17-7. Vitamin Functions and Deficiencies

VITAMIN	SIGNS/SYMPTOMS OF DEFICIENCY
Vitamin A	Night blindness, dry skin.
Vitamin B$_1$ (thiamine)	Beriberi (polyneuritis, dilated cardiomyopathy, high-output CHF, edema), Wernicke-Korsakoff syndrome.
Vitamin B$_2$ (riboflavin)	Angular stomatitis, cheilosis, corneal vascularization.
Vitamin B$_3$ (niacin)	Pellagra (diarrhea, dermatitis, dementia).
Vitamin B$_5$ (pantothenate)	Dermatitis, enteritis, alopecia, adrenal insufficiency.
Vitamin B$_6$ (pyridoxine)	Convulsions, hyperirritability; required during administration of INH.
Vitamin B$_{12}$ (cobalamin)	Macrocytic, megaloblastic anemia; neurologic symptoms (e.g., optic neuropathy, subacute combined degeneration, paresthesias); glossitis.
Vitamin C	Scurvy (e.g., swollen gums, bruising, anemia, poor wound healing).
Vitamin D	Rickets in children (bending bones), osteomalacia in adults (soft bones), hypocalcemic tetany.
Vitamin E	↑ fragility of RBCs.
Vitamin K	Neonatal hemorrhage; ↑ PT and aPTT, normal BT.
Biotin	Dermatitis, enteritis. Can be caused by ingestion of **raw eggs** or antibiotic use.
Folic acid	The **most common vitamin deficiency in the United States.** Sprue; macrocytic, megaloblastic anemia without neurologic symptoms.
Magnesium	Weakness, muscle cramps, exacerbation of hypocalcemic tetany, CNS hyperirritability leading to tremors, choreoathetoid movement.
Selenium	Keshan disease (cardiomyopathy).

HIGH-YIELD FACTS

EMERGENCY MEDICINE

HIGH-YIELD FACTS IN

Rapid Review

Classic ECG finding in atrial flutter.	"Sawtooth" P waves.
Definition of unstable angina.	Angina is new, is worsening, or occurs at rest.
Antihypertensive for a diabetic patient with proteinuria.	ACEI.
Beck's triad for cardiac tamponade.	Hypotension, distant heart sounds, and JVD.
Drugs that slow AV node transmission.	β-blockers, digoxin, calcium channel blockers.
Hypercholesterolemia treatment that leads to flushing and pruritus.	Niacin.
Murmur—hypertrophic obstructive cardiomyopathy (HOCM).	Systolic ejection murmur heard along the lateral sternal border that ↑ with Valsalva maneuver and standing.
Murmur—aortic insufficiency.	Diastolic, decrescendo, high-pitched, blowing murmur that is best heard sitting up; ↑ with ↓ preload (handgrip maneuver).
Murmur—aortic stenosis.	Systolic crescendo/decrescendo murmur that radiates to the neck; ↑ with ↑ preload (Valsalva maneuver).
Murmur—mitral regurgitation.	Holosystolic murmur that radiates to the axillae or carotids.
Murmur—mitral stenosis.	Diastolic, mid- to late, low-pitched murmur.
Treatment for atrial fibrillation and atrial flutter.	If unstable, cardiovert. If stable or chronic, rate control with calcium channel blockers or β-blockers.
Treatment for ventricular fibrillation.	Immediate cardioversion.
Autoimmune complication occurring 2–4 weeks post-MI.	Dressler's syndrome: fever, pericarditis, ↑ ESR.
IV drug use with JVD and holosystolic murmur at the left sternal border. Treatment?	Treat existing heart failure and replace the tricuspid valve.
Diagnostic test for hypertrophic cardiomyopathy.	Echocardiogram (showing thickened left ventricular wall and outflow obstruction).
A fall in systolic BP of > 10 mmHg with inspiration.	Pulsus paradoxus (seen in cardiac tamponade).
Classic ECG findings in pericarditis.	Low-voltage, diffuse ST-segment elevation.
Definition of hypertension.	BP > 140/90 on three separate occasions two weeks apart.
Eight surgically correctable causes of hypertension.	Renal artery stenosis, coarctation of the aorta, pheochromocytoma, Conn's syndrome, Cushing's syndrome, unilateral renal parenchymal disease, hyperthyroidism, hyperparathyroidism.

Evaluation of a pulsatile abdominal mass and bruit.	Abdominal ultrasound and CT.
Indications for surgical repair of abdominal aortic aneurysm.	> 5.5 cm, rapidly enlarging, symptomatic, or ruptured.
Treatment for acute coronary syndrome.	Morphine, O_2, sublingual nitroglycerin, ASA, IV β-blockers, heparin.
What is metabolic syndrome?	Abdominal obesity, high triglycerides, low HDL, hypertension, insulin resistance, prothrombotic or proinflammatory states.
Appropriate diagnostic test? ■ A 50-year-old man with angina can exercise to 85% of maximum predicted heart rate. ■ A 65-year-old woman with left bundle branch block and severe osteoarthritis has unstable angina.	Exercise stress treadmill with ECG. Pharmacologic stress test (e.g., dobutamine echo).
Target LDL in a patient with diabetes.	< 70.
Signs of active ischemia during stress testing.	Angina, ST-segment changes on ECG, or ↓ BP.
ECG findings suggesting MI.	ST-segment elevation (depression means ischemia), flattened T waves, and Q waves.
Coronary territories in MI.	Anterior wall (LAD/diagonal), inferior (PDA), posterior (left circumflex/oblique, RCA/marginal), septum (LAD/diagonal).
A young patient has angina at rest with ST-segment elevation. Cardiac enzymes are normal.	Prinzmetal's angina.
Common symptoms associated with silent MIs.	CHF, shock, and altered mental status.
The diagnostic test for pulmonary embolism.	V/Q scan.
An agent that reverses the effects of heparin.	Protamine.
The coagulation parameter affected by warfarin.	PT.
A young patient with a family history of sudden death collapses and dies while exercising.	Hypertrophic cardiomyopathy.
Endocarditis prophylaxis regimens.	Oral surgery—amoxicillin; GI or GU procedures—ampicillin and gentamicin before and amoxicillin after.
The 6 P's of ischemia due to peripheral vascular disease.	Pain, pallor, pulselessness, paralysis, paresthesia, poikilothermia.
Virchow's triad.	Stasis, hypercoagulability, endothelial damage.
The most common cause of hypertension in young women.	OCPs.
The most common cause of hypertension in young men.	Excessive EtOH.

"Stuck-on" appearance.	Seborrheic keratosis.
Red plaques with silvery-white scales and sharp margins.	Psoriasis.
The most common type of skin cancer; the lesion is a pearly-colored papule with a translucent surface and telangiectasias.	Basal cell carcinoma.
Honey-crusted lesions.	Impetigo.
A febrile patient with a history of diabetes presents with a red, swollen, painful lower extremity.	Cellulitis.
⊕ Nikolsky's sign.	Pemphigus vulgaris.
⊖ Nikolsky's sign.	Bullous pemphigoid.
A 55-year-old obese patient presents with dirty, velvety patches on the back of the neck.	Acanthosis nigricans. Check fasting blood glucose to rule out diabetes.
Dermatomal distribution.	Varicella zoster.
Flat-topped papules.	Lichen planus.
Iris-like target lesions.	Erythema multiforme.
A lesion characteristically occurring in a linear pattern in areas where skin comes into contact with clothing or jewelry.	Contact dermatitis.
Presents with a herald patch, Christmas-tree pattern.	Pityriasis rosea.
A 16-year-old presents with an annular patch of alopecia with broken-off, stubby hairs.	Alopecia areata (an autoimmune process).
Pinkish, scaling, flat lesions on the chest and back; KOH prep has a "spaghetti-and-meatballs" appearance.	Pityriasis versicolor.
Four characteristics of a nevus suggestive of melanoma.	Asymmetry, border irregularity, color variation, and large diameter.
A premalignant lesion from sun exposure that can lead to squamous cell carcinoma.	Actinic keratosis.
"Dewdrops on a rose petal."	Lesions of 1° varicella.
"Cradle cap."	Seborrheic dermatitis. Treat with antifungals.
Associated with *Propionibacterium acnes* and changes in androgen levels.	Acne vulgaris.

A painful, recurrent vesicular eruption of mucocutaneous surfaces.	Herpes simplex.
Inflammation and epithelial thinning of the anogenital area, predominantly in postmenopausal women.	Lichen sclerosus.
Exophytic nodules on the skin with varying degrees of scaling or ulceration; the second most common type of skin cancer.	Squamous cell carcinoma.

► ENDOCRINOLOGY

The most common cause of hypothyroidism.	Hashimoto's thyroiditis.
Lab findings in Hashimoto's thyroiditis.	High TSH, low T_4, antimicrosomal antibodies.
Exophthalmos, pretibial myxedema, and ↓ TSH.	Graves' disease.
The most common cause of Cushing's syndrome.	Iatrogenic corticosteroid administration. The second most common cause is Cushing's disease.
A patient presents with signs of hypocalcemia, high phosphorus, and low PTH.	Hypoparathyroidism.
"Stones, bones, groans, psychiatric overtones."	Signs and symptoms of hypercalcemia.
A patient complains of headache, weakness, and polyuria; exam reveals hypertension and tetany. Labs reveal hypernatremia, hypokalemia, and metabolic alkalosis.	1° hyperaldosteronism (due to Conn's syndrome or bilateral adrenal hyperplasia).
A patient presents with tachycardia, wild swings in BP, headache, diaphoresis, altered mental status, and a sense of panic.	Pheochromocytoma.
Should α- or β-antagonists be used first in treating pheochromocytoma?	α-antagonists (phentolamine and phenoxybenzamine).
A patient with a history of lithium use presents with copious amounts of dilute urine.	Nephrogenic diabetes insipidus (DI).
Treatment of central DI.	Administration of DDAVP ↓ serum osmolality and free water restriction.
A postoperative patient with significant pain presents with hyponatremia and normal volume status.	SIADH due to stress.
An antidiabetic agent associated with lactic acidosis.	Metformin.
A patient presents with weakness, nausea, vomiting, weight loss, and new skin pigmentation. Labs show hyponatremia and hyperkalemia. Treatment?	1° adrenal insufficiency (Addison's disease). Treat with replacement glucocorticoids, mineralocorticoids, and IV fluids.

Goal HbA_{1c} for a patient with DM.	< 7.0.
Treatment of DKA.	Fluids, insulin, and aggressive replacement of electrolytes (e.g., K^+).
Why are β-blockers contraindicated in diabetics?	They can mask symptoms of hypoglycemia.

▶ EPIDEMIOLOGY

Bias introduced into a study when a clinician is aware of the patient's treatment type.	Observational bias.
Bias introduced when screening detects a disease earlier and thus lengthens the time from diagnosis to death.	Lead-time bias.
If you want to know if geographical location affects infant mortality rate but most variation in infant mortality is predicted by socioeconomic status, then socioeconomic status is a _____.	Confounding variable.
The number of true positives divided by the number of patients with the disease is _____.	Sensitivity.
Sensitive tests have few false negatives and are used to rule _____ a disease.	Out.
PPD reactivity is used as a screening test because most people with TB (except those who are anergic) will have a ⊕ PPD. Highly sensitive or specific?	Highly sensitive for TB.
Chronic diseases such as SLE—higher prevalence or incidence?	Higher prevalence.
Epidemics such as influenza—higher prevalence or incidence?	Higher incidence.
Cross-sectional survey—incidence or prevalence?	Prevalence.
Cohort study—incidence or prevalence?	Incidence and prevalence.
Case-control study—incidence or prevalence?	Neither.
Describe a test that consistently gives identical results, but the results are wrong.	High reliability, low validity.
Difference between a cohort and a case-control study.	Cohort studies can be used to calculate relative risk (RR), incidence, and/or odds ratio (OR). Case-control studies can be used to calculate an OR.

Attributable risk?	The incidence rate (IR) of a disease in exposed – the IR of a disease in unexposed.
Relative risk?	The IR of a disease in a population exposed to a particular factor ÷ the IR of those not exposed.
Odds ratio?	The likelihood of a disease among individuals exposed to a risk factor compared to those who have not been exposed.
Number needed to treat?	1 ÷ (rate in untreated group – rate in treated group).
In which patients do you initiate colorectal cancer screening early?	Patients with IBD; those with familial adenomatous polyposis (FAP)/hereditary nonpolyposis colorectal cancer (HNPCC); and those who have first-degree relatives with adenomatous polyps (< 60 years of age) or colorectal cancer.
The most common cancer in men and the most common cause of death from cancer in men.	Prostate cancer is the most common cancer in men, but lung cancer causes more deaths.
The percentage of cases within one SD of the mean? Two SDs? Three SDs?	68%, 95.4%, 99.7%.
Birth rate?	Number of live births per 1000 population in one year.
Fertility rate?	Number of live births per 1000 females (15–44 years of age) in one year.
Mortality rate?	Number of deaths per 1000 population in one year.
Neonatal mortality rate?	Number of deaths from birth to 28 days per 1000 live births in one year.
Postnatal mortality rate?	Number of deaths from 28 days to one year per 1000 live births in one year.
Infant mortality rate?	Number of deaths from birth to one year of age per 1000 live births (neonatal + postnatal mortality) in one year.
Fetal mortality rate?	Number of deaths from 20 weeks' gestation to birth per 1000 total births in one year.
Perinatal mortality rate?	Number of deaths from 20 weeks' gestation to one month of life per 1000 total births in one year.
Maternal mortality rate?	Number of deaths during pregnancy to 90 days postpartum per 100,000 live births in one year.

True or false: Once patients sign a statement giving consent, they must continue treatment.	False. Patients may change their minds at any time. Exceptions to the requirement of informed consent include emergency situations and patients without decision-making capacity.
A 15-year-old pregnant girl requires hospitalization for preeclampsia. Is parental consent required?	No. Parental consent is not necessary for the medical treatment of pregnant minors.
A doctor refers a patient for an MRI at a facility he/she owns.	Conflict of interest.
Involuntary psychiatric hospitalization can be undertaken for which three reasons?	The patient is a danger to self, a danger to others, or gravely disabled (unable to provide for basic needs).
True or false: Withdrawing a nonbeneficial treatment is ethically similar to withholding a nonindicated one.	True.
When can a physician refuse to continue treating a patient on the grounds of futility?	When there is no rationale for treatment, maximal intervention is failing, a given intervention has already failed, and treatment will not achieve the goals of care.
An eight-year-old child is in a serious accident. She requires emergent transfusion, but her parents are not present.	Treat immediately. Consent is implied in emergency situations.
Conditions in which confidentiality must be overridden.	Real threat of harm to third parties; suicidal intentions; certain contagious diseases; elder and child abuse.
Involuntary commitment or isolation for medical treatment may be undertaken for what reason?	When treatment noncompliance represents a serious danger to public health (e.g., active TB).
A 10-year-old child presents in status epilepticus, but her parents refuse treatment on religious grounds.	Treat because the disease represents an immediate threat to the child's life. Then seek a court order.
A son asks that his mother not be told about her recently discovered cancer.	A physician can withhold information from the patient only in the rare case of therapeutic privilege or if the patient requests not to be told. A patient's family cannot require the physician to withhold information from the patient.

▶ GASTROINTESTINAL

A patient presents with sudden onset of severe, diffuse abdominal pain. Exam reveals peritoneal signs, and AXR reveals free air under the diaphragm. Management?	Emergent laparotomy to repair perforated viscus.
The most likely cause of acute lower GI bleed in patients > 40 years of age.	Diverticulosis.

Diagnostic modality used when ultrasound is equivocal for cholecystitis.	HIDA scan.
Risk factors for cholelithiasis.	Fat, female, fertile, forty, flatulent.
Inspiratory arrest during palpation of the RUQ.	Murphy's sign, seen in acute cholecystitis.
The most common cause of SBO in patients with no history of abdominal surgery.	Hernia.
The most common cause of SBO in patients with a history of abdominal surgery.	Adhesions.
Identify key organisms causing diarrhea: ■ Most common organism ■ Recent antibiotic use ■ Camping ■ Traveler's diarrhea ■ Church picnics/mayonnaise ■ Uncooked hamburgers ■ Fried rice ■ Poultry/eggs ■ Raw seafood ■ AIDS ■ Pseudoappendicitis	 *Campylobacter* *Clostridium difficile* *Giardia* ETEC *S. aureus* *E. coli* O157:H7 *Bacillus cereus* *Salmonella* *Vibrio*, HAV *Isospora, Cryptosporidium, Mycobacterium avium* complex (MAC) *Yersinia*
A 25-year-old Jewish man presents with pain and watery diarrhea after meals. Exam shows fistulas between the bowel and skin and nodular lesions on his tibias.	Crohn's disease.
Inflammatory disease of the colon with ↑ risk of colon cancer.	Ulcerative colitis (greater risk than Crohn's).
Extraintestinal manifestations of IBD.	Uveitis, ankylosing spondylitis, pyoderma gangrenosum, erythema nodosum, 1° sclerosing cholangitis.
Medical treatment for IBD.	5-ASA agents and steroids during acute exacerbations.
Difference between Mallory-Weiss and Boerhaave tears.	Mallory-Weiss—superficial tear in the esophageal mucosa; Boerhaave—full-thickness esophageal rupture.
Charcot's triad.	RUQ pain, jaundice, and fever/chills in the setting of ascending cholangitis.
Reynolds' pentad.	Charcot's triad plus shock and mental status changes, with suppurative ascending cholangitis.
Medical treatment for hepatic encephalopathy.	↓ protein intake, lactulose, rifaximin.

First step in the management of a patient with an acute GI bleed.	Establish the ABCs.
A four-year-old child presents with oliguria, petechiae, and jaundice following an illness with bloody diarrhea. Most likely diagnosis and cause?	Hemolytic-uremic syndrome (HUS) due to *E. coli* O157: H7.
Post-HBV exposure treatment.	HBV immunoglobulin.
Classic causes of drug-induced hepatitis.	TB medications (INH, rifampin, pyrazinamide), acetaminophen, and tetracycline.
A 40-year-old obese woman with elevated alkaline phosphatase, elevated bilirubin, pruritus, dark urine, and clay-colored stools.	Biliary tract obstruction.
Hernia with highest risk of incarceration—indirect, direct, or femoral?	Femoral hernia.
A 50-year-old man with a history of alcohol abuse presents with boring epigastric pain that radiates to the back and is relieved by sitting forward. Management?	Confirm the diagnosis of acute pancreatitis with elevated amylase and lipase. Make the patient NPO and give IV fluids, O_2, analgesia, and "tincture of time."

► HEMATOLOGY/ONCOLOGY

Four causes of microcytic anemia.	**TICS**—**T**halassemia, **I**ron deficiency, anemia of **C**hronic disease, and **S**ideroblastic anemia.
An elderly man with hypochromic, microcytic anemia is asymptomatic. Diagnostic tests?	Fecal occult blood test and sigmoidoscopy; suspect colorectal cancer.
Precipitants of hemolytic crisis in patients with G6PD deficiency.	Sulfonamides, antimalarial drugs, fava beans.
The most common inherited cause of hypercoagulability.	Factor V Leiden mutation.
The most common inherited bleeding disorder.	von Willebrand's disease.
The most common inherited hemolytic anemia.	Hereditary spherocytosis.
Diagnostic test for hereditary spherocytosis.	Osmotic fragility test.
Pure RBC aplasia.	Diamond-Blackfan anemia.
Anemia associated with absent radii and thumbs, diffuse hyperpigmentation, café au lait spots, microcephaly, and pancytopenia.	Fanconi's anemia.
Medications and viruses that lead to aplastic anemia.	Chloramphenicol, sulfonamides, radiation, HIV, chemotherapeutic agents, hepatitis, parvovirus B19, EBV.

How to distinguish polycythemia vera from 2° polycythemia.	Both have ↑ hematocrit and RBC mass, but polycythemia vera should have normal O_2 saturation and low erythropoietin levels.
Thrombotic thrombocytopenic purpura (TTP) pentad?	**"FAT RN":** **F**ever, **A**nemia, **T**hrombocytopenia, **R**enal dysfunction, **N**eurologic abnormalities.
HUS triad?	Anemia, thrombocytopenia, and acute renal failure.
Treatment for TTP.	Emergent large-volume plasmapheresis, corticosteroids, antiplatelet drugs.
Treatment for idiopathic thrombocytopenic purpura (ITP) in children.	Usually resolves spontaneously; may require IVIG and/or corticosteroids.
Which of the following are ↑ in DIC: fibrin split products, D-dimer, fibrinogen, platelets, and hematocrit.	Fibrin split products and D-dimer are elevated; platelets, fibrinogen, and hematocrit are ↓.
An eight-year-old boy presents with hemarthrosis and ↑ PTT with normal PT and bleeding time. Diagnosis? Treatment?	Hemophilia A or B; consider desmopressin (for hemophilia A) or factor VIII or IX supplements.
A 14-year-old girl presents with prolonged bleeding after dental surgery and with menses, normal PT, normal or ↑ PTT, and ↑ bleeding time. Diagnosis? Treatment?	von Willebrand's disease; treat with desmopressin, FFP, or cryoprecipitate.
A 60-year-old African-American man presents with bone pain. Workup for multiple myeloma might reveal?	Monoclonal gammopathy, Bence Jones proteinuria, "punched-out" lesions on x-ray of the skull and long bones.
Reed-Sternberg cells.	Hodgkin's lymphoma.
A 10-year-old boy presents with fever, weight loss, and night sweats. Exam shows an anterior mediastinal mass. Suspected diagnosis?	Non-Hodgkin's lymphoma.
Microcytic anemia with ↓ serum iron, ↓ total iron-binding capacity (TIBC), and normal or ↑ ferritin.	Anemia of chronic disease.
Microcytic anemia with ↓ serum iron, ↓ ferritin, and ↑ TIBC.	Iron deficiency anemia.
An 80-year-old man presents with fatigue, lymphadenopathy, splenomegaly, and isolated lymphocytosis. Suspected diagnosis?	Chronic lymphocytic leukemia (CLL).
The lymphoma equivalent of CLL.	Small lymphocytic lymphoma.
A late, life-threatening complication of chronic myelogenous leukemia (CML).	Blast crisis (fever, bone pain, splenomegaly, pancytopenia).
Auer rods on blood smear.	Acute myelogenous leukemia (AML).
AML subtype associated with DIC.	M3.

Electrolyte changes in tumor lysis syndrome.	$\downarrow$ Ca^{2+}, $\uparrow$ K$^+$, $\uparrow$ phosphate, $\uparrow$ uric acid.
Treatment for AML M3.	Retinoic acid.
A 50-year-old man presents with early satiety, splenomegaly, and bleeding. Cytogenetics show t(9,22). Diagnosis?	CML.
Heinz bodies?	Intracellular inclusions seen in thalassemia, G6PD deficiency, and postsplenectomy.
An autosomal-recessive disorder with a defect in the GPIIbIIIa platelet receptor and $\downarrow$ platelet aggregation.	Glanzmann's thrombasthenia.
Virus associated with aplastic anemia in patients with sickle cell anemia.	Parvovirus B19.
A 25-year-old African-American man with sickle cell anemia has sudden onset of bone pain. Management of pain crisis?	O$_2$, analgesia, hydration, and, if severe, transfusion.
A significant cause of morbidity in thalassemia patients. Treatment?	Iron overload; use deferoxamine.

▶ INFECTIOUS DISEASE

The three most common causes of fever of unknown origin (FUO).	Infection, cancer, and autoimmune disease.
Four signs and symptoms of streptococcal pharyngitis.	Fever, pharyngeal erythema, tonsillar exudate, lack of cough.
A nonsuppurative complication of streptococcal infection that is not altered by treatment of 1° infection.	Postinfectious glomerulonephritis.
Asplenic patients are particularly susceptible to these organisms.	Encapsulated organisms—pneumococcus, meningococcus, *Haemophilus influenzae, Klebsiella.*
The number of bacteria on a clean-catch specimen to diagnose a UTI.	10^5 bacteria/mL.
Which healthy population is susceptible to UTIs?	Pregnant women. Treat this group aggressively because of potential complications.
A patient from California or Arizona presents with fever, malaise, cough, and night sweats. Diagnosis? Treatment?	Coccidioidomycosis. Amphotericin B.
Nonpainful chancre.	1° syphilis.
A "blueberry muffin" rash is characteristic of what congenital infection?	Rubella.

Meningitis in neonates. Causes? Treatment?	Group B strep, *E. coli, Listeria.* Treat with gentamicin and ampicillin.
Meningitis in infants. Causes? Treatment?	Pneumococcus, meningococcus, *H. influenzae.* Treat with cefotaxime and vancomycin.
What should always be done prior to LP?	Check for ↑ ICP; look for papilledema.
CSF findings: ▪ Low glucose, PMN predominance ▪ Normal glucose, lymphocytic predominance ▪ Numerous RBCs in serial CSF samples ▪ ↑ gamma globulins	 Bacterial meningitis Aseptic (viral) meningitis Subarachnoid hemorrhage (SAH) MS
Initially presents with a pruritic papule with regional lymphadenopathy; evolves into a black eschar after 7–10 days. Treatment?	Cutaneous anthrax. Treat with penicillin G or ciprofloxacin.
Findings in 3° syphilis.	Tabes dorsalis, general paresis, gummas, Argyll Robertson pupil, aortitis, aortic root aneurysms.
Characteristics of 2° Lyme disease.	Arthralgias, migratory polyarthropathies, Bell's palsy, myocarditis.
Cold agglutinins.	*Mycoplasma.*
A 24-year-old man presents with soft white plaques on his tongue and the back of his throat. Diagnosis? Workup? Treatment?	Candidal thrush. Workup should include an HIV test. Treat with nystatin oral suspension.
Begin *Pneumocystis jiroveci* (formerly *P. carinii*) pneumonia prophylaxis in an HIV-positive patient at what CD4 count? *Mycobacterium avium–intracellulare* (MAI) prophylaxis?	≤ 200 for *P. jiroveci* (with TMP-SMX); ≤ 50–100 for MAI (with clarithromycin/azithromycin).
Risk factors for pyelonephritis.	Pregnancy, vesicoureteral reflux, anatomic anomalies, indwelling catheters, kidney stones.
Neutropenic nadir postchemotherapy.	7–10 days.
Erythema migrans.	Lesion of 1° Lyme disease.
Classic physical findings for endocarditis.	Fever, heart murmur, Osler's nodes, splinter hemorrhages, Janeway lesions, Roth's spots.
Aplastic crisis in sickle cell disease.	Parvovirus B19.
Ring-enhancing brain lesion on CT with seizures.	*Taenia solium* (cysticercosis).

Name the organism:

▪ Branching rods in oral infection	*Actinomyces israelii*
▪ Painful chancroid	*Haemophilus ducreyi*
▪ Dog or cat bite	*Pasteurella multocida*
▪ Gardener	*Sporothrix schenckii*
▪ Pregnant women with pets	*Toxoplasma gondii*
▪ Meningitis in adults	*Neisseria meningitidis*
▪ Meningitis in elderly	*Streptococcus pneumoniae*
▪ Alcoholic with pneumonia	*Klebsiella*
▪ "Currant jelly" sputum	*Klebsiella*
▪ Infection in burn victims	*Pseudomonas*
▪ Osteomyelitis from foot wound puncture	*Pseudomonas*
▪ Osteomyelitis in a sickle cell patient	*Salmonella*

A 55-year-old man who is a smoker and a heavy drinker presents with a new cough and flulike symptoms. Gram stain shows no organisms; silver stain of sputum shows gram-negative rods. What is the diagnosis?	*Legionella* pneumonia.
A middle-aged man presents with acute-onset monoarticular joint pain and bilateral Bell's palsy. What is the likely diagnosis, and how did he get it? Treatment?	Lyme disease, *Ixodes* tick, doxycycline.
A patient develops endocarditis three weeks after receiving a prosthetic heart valve. What organism is suspected?	*S. aureus* or *S. epidermidis*.

▶ MUSCULOSKELETAL

Back pain that is exacerbated by standing and walking and relieved with sitting and hyperflexion of the hips.	Spinal stenosis.
Joints in the hand affected in rheumatoid arthritis.	MCP and PIP joints; DIP joints are spared.
Joint pain and stiffness that worsen over the course of the day and are relieved by rest.	Osteoarthritis.
Genetic disorder associated with multiple fractures and commonly mistaken for child abuse.	Osteogenesis imperfecta.
Hip and back pain along with stiffness that improves with activity over the course of the day and worsens at rest. Diagnostic test?	Suspect ankylosing spondylitis. Check HLA-B27.
Arthritis, conjunctivitis, and urethritis in young men. Associated organisms?	Reactive (Reiter's) arthritis. Associated with *Campylobacter, Shigella, Salmonella, Chlamydia,* and *Ureaplasma*.
A 55-year-old man has sudden, excruciating first MTP joint pain after a night of drinking red wine. Diagnosis, workup, and chronic treatment?	Gout. Needle-shaped, negatively birefringent crystals are seen on joint fluid aspirate. Chronic treatment with allopurinol or probenecid.

Rhomboid-shaped, positively birefringent crystals on joint fluid aspirate.	Pseudogout.
An elderly woman presents with pain and stiffness of the shoulders and hips; she cannot lift her arms above her head. Labs show anemia and ↑ ESR.	Polymyalgia rheumatica.
An active 13-year-old boy has anterior knee pain. Diagnosis?	Osgood-Schlatter disease.
Bone is fractured in a fall on an outstretched hand.	Distal radius (Colles' fracture).
Complication of scaphoid fracture.	Avascular necrosis.
Signs suggesting radial nerve damage with humeral fracture.	Wrist drop, loss of thumb abduction.
A young child presents with proximal muscle weakness, waddling gait, and pronounced calf muscles.	Duchenne muscular dystrophy.
A first-born female who was born in breech position is found to have asymmetric skin folds on her newborn exam. Diagnosis? Treatment?	Developmental dysplasia of the hip. If severe, consider a Pavlik harness to maintain abduction.
An 11-year-old obese African-American boy presents with sudden onset of limp. Diagnosis? Workup?	Slipped capital femoral epiphysis. AP and frog-leg lateral view.
The most common 1° malignant tumor of bone.	Multiple myeloma.

▶ NEUROLOGY

Unilateral, severe periorbital headache with tearing and conjunctival erythema.	Cluster headache.
Prophylactic treatment for migraine.	Antihypertensives, antidepressants, anticonvulsants.
The most common pituitary tumor. Treatment?	Prolactinoma. Dopamine agonists (e.g., bromocriptine).
A 55-year-old patient presents with acute "broken speech." What type of aphasia? What lobe and vascular distribution?	Broca's aphasia. Frontal lobe, left MCA distribution.
The most common cause of SAH.	Trauma; the second most common is berry aneurysm.
A crescent-shaped hyperdensity on CT that does not cross the midline.	Subdural hematoma—bridging veins torn.
A history significant for initial altered mental status with an intervening lucid interval. Diagnosis? Most likely source? Treatment?	Epidural hematoma. Middle meningeal artery. Neurosurgical evacuation.
CSF findings with SAH.	Elevated ICP, RBCs, xanthochromia.

Albuminocytologic dissociation.	Guillain-Barré syndrome (↑ protein in CSF without a significant ↑ in cell count).
Cold water is flushed into a patient's ear, and the fast phase of the nystagmus is toward the opposite side. Normal or pathologic?	Normal.
The most common 1° sources of metastases to the brain.	Lung, breast, skin (melanoma), kidney, GI tract.
May be seen in children who are accused of inattention in class and confused with ADHD.	Absence seizures.
The most frequent presentation of intracranial neoplasm.	Headache.
The most common cause of seizures in children (2–10 years).	Infection, febrile seizures, trauma, idiopathic.
The most common cause of seizures in young adults (18–35 years).	Trauma, alcohol withdrawal, brain tumor.
First-line medication for status epilepticus.	IV benzodiazepine.
Confusion, confabulation, ophthalmoplegia, ataxia.	Wernicke's encephalopathy due to a deficiency of thiamine.
What % lesion is an indication for carotid endarterectomy?	Seventy percent if the stenosis is symptomatic.
The most common causes of dementia.	Alzheimer's and multi-infarct.
Combined UMN and LMN disorder.	ALS.
Rigidity and stiffness with resting tremor and masked facies.	Parkinson's disease.
The mainstay of Parkinson's therapy.	Levodopa/carbidopa.
Treatment for Guillain-Barré syndrome.	IVIG or plasmapheresis.
Rigidity and stiffness that progress to choreiform movements, accompanied by moodiness and altered behavior.	Huntington's disease.
A six-year-old girl presents with a port-wine stain in the V_2 distribution as well as with mental retardation, seizures, and ipsilateral leptomeningeal angioma.	Sturge-Weber syndrome. Treat symptomatically. Possible focal cerebral resection of the affected lobe.
Café au lait spots on skin.	Neurofibromatosis type 1.
Hyperphagia, hypersexuality, hyperorality, and hyperdocility.	Klüver-Bucy syndrome (amygdala).
May be administered to a symptomatic patient to diagnose myasthenia gravis.	Edrophonium.

1° causes of third-trimester bleeding.	Placental abruption and placenta previa.
Classic ultrasound and gross appearance of complete hydatidiform mole.	Snowstorm on ultrasound. "Cluster-of-grapes" appearance on gross examination.
Chromosomal pattern of a complete mole.	46,XX.
Molar pregnancy containing fetal tissue.	Partial mole.
Symptoms of placental abruption.	Continuous, painful vaginal bleeding.
Symptoms of placenta previa.	Self-limited, painless vaginal bleeding.
When should a vaginal exam be performed with suspected placenta previa?	Never.
Antibiotics with teratogenic effects.	Tetracycline, fluoroquinolones, aminoglycosides, sulfonamides.
Shortest AP diameter of the pelvis.	Obstetric conjugate: between the sacral promontory and the midpoint of the symphysis pubis.
Medication given to accelerate fetal lung maturity.	Betamethasone or dexamethasone × 48 hours.
The most common cause of postpartum hemorrhage.	Uterine atony.
Treatment for postpartum hemorrhage.	Uterine massage; if that fails, give oxytocin.
Typical antibiotics for group B streptococcus (GBS) prophylaxis.	IV penicillin or ampicillin.
A patient fails to lactate after an emergency C-section with marked blood loss.	Sheehan's syndrome (postpartum pituitary necrosis).
Uterine bleeding at 18 weeks' gestation; no products expelled; membranes ruptured; cervical os open.	Inevitable abortion.
Uterine bleeding at 18 weeks' gestation; no products expelled; cervical os closed.	Threatened abortion.

► GYNECOLOGY

The first test to perform when a woman presents with amenorrhea.	β-hCG; the most common cause of amenorrhea is pregnancy.
Term for heavy bleeding during and between menstrual periods.	Menometrorrhagia.

Cause of amenorrhea with normal prolactin, no response to estrogen-progesterone challenge, and a history of D&C.	Asherman's syndrome.
Therapy for polycystic ovarian syndrome.	Weight loss and OCPs.
Medication used to induce ovulation.	Clomiphene citrate.
Diagnostic step required in a postmenopausal woman who presents with vaginal bleeding.	Endometrial biopsy.
Indications for medical treatment of ectopic pregnancy.	Stable, unruptured ectopic pregnancy of < 3.5 cm at < 6 weeks' gestation.
Medical options for endometriosis.	OCPs, danazol, GnRH agonists.
Laparoscopic findings in endometriosis.	"Chocolate cysts," powder burns.
The most common location for an ectopic pregnancy.	Ampulla of the oviduct.
How to diagnose and follow a leiomyoma.	Ultrasound.
Natural history of a leiomyoma.	Regresses after menopause.
A patient has ↑ vaginal discharge and petechial patches in the upper vagina and cervix.	*Trichomonas* vaginitis.
Treatment for bacterial vaginosis.	Oral or topical metronidazole.
The most common cause of bloody nipple discharge.	Intraductal papilloma.
Contraceptive methods that protect against PID.	OCPs and barrier contraception.
Unopposed estrogen is contraindicated in which cancers?	Endometrial or estrogen receptor–⊕ breast cancer.
A patient presents with recent PID with RUQ pain.	Consider Fitz-Hugh–Curtis syndrome.
Breast malignancy presenting as itching, burning, and erosion of the nipple.	Paget's disease.
Annual screening for women with a strong family history of ovarian cancer.	CA-125 and transvaginal ultrasound.
A 50-year-old woman leaks urine when laughing or coughing. Nonsurgical options?	Kegel exercises, estrogen, pessaries for stress incontinence.
A 30-year-old woman has unpredictable urine loss. Examination is normal. Medical options?	Anticholinergics (oxybutynin) or β-adrenergics (metaproterenol) for urge incontinence.
Lab values suggestive of menopause.	↑ serum FSH.
The most common cause of female infertility.	Endometriosis.

Two consecutive findings of atypical squamous cells of undetermined significance (ASCUS) on Pap smear. Follow-up evaluation?	Colposcopy and endocervical curettage.
Breast cancer type that ↑ the future risk of invasive carcinoma in both breasts.	Lobular carcinoma in situ.

Nontender abdominal mass associated with elevated VMA and HVA.	Neuroblastoma.
The most common type of tracheoesophageal fistula (TEF). Diagnosis?	Esophageal atresia with distal TEF (85%). Unable to pass NG tube.
Not contraindications to vaccination.	Mild illness and/or low-grade fever, current antibiotic therapy, and prematurity.
Tests to rule out shaken baby syndrome.	Ophthalmologic exam, CT, and MRI.
A neonate has meconium ileus.	CF or Hirschsprung's disease.
Bilious emesis within hours after the first feeding.	Duodenal atresia.
A two-month-old baby presents with nonbilious projectile emesis. What are the appropriate steps in management?	Correct metabolic abnormalities. Then correct pyloric stenosis with pyloromyotomy.
The most common 1° immunodeficiency.	Selective IgA deficiency.
An infant has a high fever and onset of rash as fever breaks. What is he at risk for?	Febrile seizures (roseola infantum).
What is the immunodeficiency? ■ A boy has chronic respiratory infections. Nitroblue tetrazolium test is ⊕. ■ A child has eczema, thrombocytopenia, and high levels of IgA. ■ A four-month-old boy has life-threatening *Pseudomonas* infection.	Chronic granulomatous disease Wiskott-Aldrich syndrome Bruton's X-linked agammaglobulinemia
Acute-phase treatment for Kawasaki disease.	High-dose aspirin for inflammation and fever; IVIG to prevent coronary artery aneurysms.
Treatment for mild and severe unconjugated hyperbilirubinemia.	Phototherapy (mild) or exchange transfusion (severe).
Sudden onset of mental status changes, emesis, and liver dysfunction after taking aspirin.	Reye's syndrome.
A child has loss of red light reflex. Diagnosis?	Suspect retinoblastoma.

Vaccinations at a six-month well-child visit.	HBV, DTaP, Hib, IPV, PCV.
Tanner stage 3 in a six-year-old girl.	Precocious puberty.
Infection of small airways with epidemics in winter and spring.	RSV bronchiolitis.
Cause of neonatal RDS.	Surfactant deficiency.
A condition associated with red "currant-jelly" stools.	Intussusception.
A congenital heart disease that causes 2° hypertension.	Coarctation of the aorta.
First-line treatment for otitis media.	Amoxicillin × 10 days.
The most common pathogen causing croup.	Parainfluenza virus type 1.
A homeless child is small for his age and has peeling skin and a swollen belly.	Kwashiorkor (protein malnutrition).
Defect in an X-linked syndrome with mental retardation, gout, self-mutilation, and choreoathetosis.	Lesch-Nyhan syndrome (purine salvage problem with HGPRTase deficiency).
A newborn girl has a continuous "machinery murmur."	Patent ductus arteriosus (PDA).

▶ PSYCHIATRY

First-line pharmacotherapy for depression.	SSRIs.
Antidepressants associated with hypertensive crisis.	MAOIs.
Galactorrhea, impotence, menstrual dysfunction, and ↓ libido.	Patient on dopamine antagonist.
A 17-year-old girl has left arm paralysis after her boyfriend dies in a car crash. No medical cause is found.	Conversion disorder.
Name the defense mechanism: ■ A mother who is angry at her husband yells at her child. ■ A pedophile enters a monastery. ■ A woman calmly describes a grisly murder. ■ A hospitalized 10-year-old begins to wet his bed.	Displacement Reaction formation Isolation Regression
Life-threatening muscle rigidity, fever, and rhabdomyolysis.	Neuroleptic malignant syndrome.
Amenorrhea, bradycardia, and abnormal body image in a young female.	Anorexia.

A 35-year-old man has recurrent episodes of palpitations, diaphoresis, and fear of going crazy.	Panic disorder.
The most serious side effect of clozapine.	Agranulocytosis.
A 21-year-old man has three months of social withdrawal, worsening grades, flattened affect, and concrete thinking.	Schizophreniform disorder (diagnosis of schizophrenia requires ≥ 6 months of symptoms).
Key side effects of atypical antipsychotics.	Weight gain, type 2 DM, QT prolongation.
A young weight lifter receives IV haloperidol and complains that his eyes are deviated sideways. Diagnosis? Treatment?	Acute dystonia (oculogyric crisis). Treat with benztropine or diphenhydramine.
Medication to avoid in patients with a history of alcohol withdrawal seizures.	Neuroleptics.
A 13-year-old boy has a history of theft, vandalism, and violence toward family pets.	Conduct disorder.
A five-month-old girl has ↓ head growth, truncal dyscoordination, and ↓ social interaction.	Rett's disorder.
A patient hasn't slept for days, lost $20,000 gambling, is agitated, and has pressured speech. Diagnosis? Treatment?	Acute mania. Start a mood stabilizer (e.g., lithium).
After a minor fender bender, a man wears a neck brace and requests permanent disability.	Malingering.
A nurse presents with severe hypoglycemia; blood analysis reveals no elevation in C-peptide.	Factitious disorder (Munchausen syndrome).
A patient continues to use cocaine after being in jail, losing his job, and not paying child support.	Substance abuse.
A violent patient has vertical and horizontal nystagmus.	Phencyclidine hydrochloride (PCP) intoxication.
A woman who was abused as a child frequently feels outside of or detached from her body.	Depersonalization disorder.
A man has repeated, intense urges to rub his body against unsuspecting passengers on a bus.	Frotteurism (a paraphilia).
A schizophrenic patient takes haloperidol for one year and develops uncontrollable tongue movements. Diagnosis? Treatment?	Tardive dyskinesia. ↓ or discontinue haloperidol and consider another antipsychotic (e.g., risperidone, clozapine).
A man unexpectedly flies across the country, takes a new name, and has no memory of his prior life.	Dissociative fugue.

Risk factors for DVT.	Stasis, endothelial injury, and hypercoagulability (Virchow's triad).
Criteria for exudative effusion.	Pleural/serum protein > 0.5; pleural/serum LDH > 0.6.
Causes of exudative effusion.	Think of leaky capillaries. Malignancy, TB, bacterial or viral infection, pulmonary embolism with infarct, and pancreatitis.
Causes of transudative effusion.	Think of intact capillaries. CHF, liver or kidney disease, and protein-losing enteropathy.
Normalizing P_{CO_2} in a patient having an asthma exacerbation may indicate?	Fatigue and impending respiratory failure.
Dyspnea, lateral hilar lymphadenopathy on CXR, noncaseating granulomas, ↑ ACE, and hypercalcemia.	Sarcoidosis.
PFTs showing ↓ FEV_1/FVC.	Obstructive pulmonary disease (e.g., asthma).
PFTs showing ↑ FEV_1/FVC.	Restrictive pulmonary disease.
Honeycomb pattern on CXR. Diagnosis? Treatment?	Diffuse interstitial pulmonary fibrosis. Supportive care. Steroids may help.
Treatment for SVC syndrome.	Radiation.
Treatment for mild, persistent asthma.	Inhaled β-agonists and inhaled corticosteroids.
Treatment for COPD exacerbation.	O_2, bronchodilators, antibiotics, corticosteroids with taper, smoking cessation.
Treatment for chronic COPD.	Smoking cessation, home O_2, β-agonists, anticholinergics, systemic or inhaled corticosteroids, flu and pneumococcal vaccines.
Acid-base disorder in pulmonary embolism.	Hypoxia and hypocarbia (respiratory alkalosis).
Non–small cell lung cancer (NSCLC) associated with hypercalcemia.	Squamous cell carcinoma.
Lung cancer associated with SIADH.	Small cell lung cancer (SCLC).
Lung cancer highly related to cigarette exposure.	SCLC.
A tall white male presents with acute shortness of breath. Diagnosis? Treatment?	Spontaneous pneumothorax. Spontaneous regression. Supplemental O_2 may be helpful.
Treatment of tension pneumothorax.	Immediate needle thoracostomy.

Characteristics favoring carcinoma in an isolated pulmonary nodule.	Age > 45–50 years; lesions new or larger in comparison to old films; absence of calcification or irregular calcification; size > 2 cm; irregular margins.
Hypoxemia and pulmonary edema with normal pulmonary capillary wedge pressure.	ARDS.
Sequelae of asbestos exposure.	Pulmonary fibrosis, pleural plaques, bronchogenic carcinoma (mass in lung field), mesothelioma (pleural mass).
↑ risk of what infection with silicosis?	*Mycobacterium tuberculosis.*
Causes of hypoxemia.	Right-to-left shunt, hypoventilation, low inspired O_2 tension, diffusion defect, V/Q mismatch.
Classic CXR findings for pulmonary edema.	Cardiomegaly, prominent pulmonary vessels, Kerley B lines, "bat's-wing" appearance of hilar shadows, and perivascular and peribronchial cuffing.

▶ RENAL/GENITOURINARY

Renal tubular acidosis (RTA) associated with abnormal H+ secretion and nephrolithiasis.	Type I (distal) RTA.
RTA associated with abnormal HCO_3^- and rickets.	Type II (proximal) RTA.
RTA associated with aldosterone defect.	Type IV (distal) RTA.
"Doughy" skin	Hypernatremia.
Differential of hypervolemic hyponatremia.	Cirrhosis, CHF, nephritic syndrome.
Chvostek's and Trousseau's signs.	Hypocalcemia.
The most common causes of hypercalcemia.	Malignancy and hyperparathyroidism.
T-wave flattening and U waves.	Hypokalemia.
Peaked T waves and widened QRS.	Hyperkalemia.
First-line treatment for moderate hypercalcemia.	IV hydration and loop diuretics (furosemide).
Type of ARF in a patient with $Fe_{Na} < 1\%$.	Prerenal.
A 49-year-old man presents with acute-onset flank pain and hematuria.	Nephrolithiasis.
The most common type of nephrolithiasis.	Calcium oxalate.
A 20-year-old man presents with a palpable flank mass and hematuria. Ultrasound shows bilateral enlarged kidneys with cysts. Associated brain anomaly?	Cerebral berry aneurysms (autosomal-dominant PCKD).

Hematuria, hypertension, and oliguria.	Nephritic syndrome.
Proteinuria, hypoalbuminemia, hyperlipidemia, hyperlipiduria, and edema.	Nephrotic syndrome.
The most common form of nephritic syndrome.	Membranous glomerulonephritis.
The most common form of glomerulonephritis.	IgA nephropathy (Berger's disease).
Glomerulonephritis with deafness.	Alport's syndrome.
Glomerulonephritis with hemoptysis.	Wegener's granulomatosis and Goodpasture's syndrome.
Presence of red cell casts in urine sediment.	Glomerulonephritis/nephritic syndrome.
Eosinophils in urine sediment.	Allergic interstitial nephritis.
Waxy casts in urine sediment and Maltese crosses (seen with lipiduria).	Nephrotic syndrome.
Drowsiness, asterixis, nausea, and a pericardial friction rub.	Uremic syndrome seen in patients with renal failure.
A 55-year-old man is diagnosed with prostate cancer. Treatment options?	Wait, surgical resection, radiation and/or androgen suppression.
Low urine specific gravity in the presence of high serum osmolality.	Diabetes insipidus.
Treatment of SIADH?	Fluid restriction, demeclocycline.
Hematuria, flank pain, and palpable flank mass.	Renal cell carcinoma (RCC).
Testicular cancer associated with β-hCG, AFP.	Choriocarcinoma.
The most common type of testicular cancer.	Seminoma, a type of germ cell tumor.
The most common histology of bladder cancer.	Transitional cell carcinoma.
Complication of overly rapid correction of hyponatremia.	Central pontine myelinolysis.
Salicylate ingestion occurs in what type of acid-base disorder?	Anion gap acidosis and 1° respiratory alkalosis due to central respiratory stimulation.
Acid-base disturbance commonly seen in pregnant women.	Respiratory alkalosis.
Three systemic diseases that lead to nephrotic syndrome.	DM, SLE, and amyloidosis.
Elevated erythropoietin level, elevated hematocrit, and normal O_2 saturation suggest?	RCC or other erythropoietin-producing tumor; evaluate with CT scan.
A 55-year-old male presents with irritative and obstructive urinary symptoms. Treatment options?	Likely BPH. Options include no treatment, terazosin, finasteride, or surgical intervention (TURP).

Class of drugs that may cause syndrome of muscle rigidity, hyperthermia, autonomic instability, and extrapyramidal symptoms.	Antipsychotics (neuroleptic malignant syndrome).
Side effects of corticosteroids.	Acute mania, immunosuppression, thin skin, osteoporosis, easy bruising, myopathies.
Treatment for DTs.	Benzodiazepines.
Treatment for acetaminophen overdose.	*N*-acetylcysteine.
Treatment for opioid overdose.	Naloxone.
Treatment for benzodiazepine overdose.	Flumazenil.
Treatment for neuroleptic malignant syndrome and malignant hyperthermia.	Dantrolene.
Treatment for malignant hypertension.	Nitroprusside.
Treatment of atrial fibrillation.	Rate control, rhythm conversion, and anticoagulation.
Treatment of supraventricular tachycardia.	If stable, rate control with carotid massage or other vagal stimulation; if unsuccessful, consider adenosine.
Causes of drug-induced SLE.	INH, penicillamine, hydralazine, procainamide, chlorpromazine, methyldopa, quinidine.
Macrocytic, megaloblastic anemia with neurologic symptoms.	B_{12} deficiency.
Macrocytic, megaloblastic anemia without neurologic symptoms.	Folate deficiency.
A burn patient presents with cherry-red flushed skin and coma. Sao_2 is normal, but carboxyhemoglobin is elevated. Treatment?	Treat CO poisoning with 100% O_2 or with hyperbaric O_2 if poisoning is severe or the patient is pregnant.
Blood in the urethral meatus or high-riding prostate.	Bladder rupture or urethral injury.
Test to rule out urethral injury.	Retrograde cystourethrogram.
Radiographic evidence of aortic disruption or dissection.	Widened mediastinum (> 8 cm), loss of aortic knob, pleural cap, tracheal deviation to the right, depression of left main stem bronchus.
Radiographic indications for surgery in patients with acute abdomen.	Free air under the diaphragm, extravasation of contrast, severe bowel distention, space-occupying lesion (CT), mesenteric occlusion (angiography).

HIGH-YIELD FACTS

RAPID REVIEW

The most common organism in burn-related infections.	*Pseudomonas.*
Method of calculating fluid repletion in burn patients.	Parkland formula.
Acceptable urine output in a trauma patient.	50 cc/hr.
Acceptable urine output in a stable patient.	30 cc/hr.
Cannon "a" waves.	Third-degree heart block.
Signs of neurogenic shock.	Hypotension and bradycardia.
Signs of ↑ ICP (Cushing's triad).	Hypertension, bradycardia, and abnormal respirations.
↓ CO, ↓ pulmonary capillary wedge pressure (PCWP), ↑ peripheral vascular resistance (PVR).	Hypovolemic shock.
↓ CO, ↑ PCWP, ↑ PVR.	Cardiogenic (or obstructive) shock.
↑ CO, ↓ PCWP, ↓ PVR.	Septic or anaphylactic shock.
Treatment of septic shock.	Fluids and antibiotics.
Treatment of cardiogenic shock.	Identify cause; pressors (e.g., dopamine).
Treatment of hypovolemic shock.	Identify cause; fluid and blood repletion.
Treatment of anaphylactic shock.	Diphenhydramine or epinephrine 1:1000.
Supportive treatment for ARDS.	Continuous positive airway pressure.
Signs of air embolism.	A patient with chest trauma who was previously stable suddenly dies.
Trauma series.	AP chest, AP/lateral C-spine, AP pelvis.

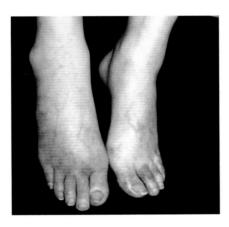

Cutaneous findings in atheromatous embolism. Typical appearance of blue toes due to multiple atheromatous emboli to the lower limbs in a patient with extensive atheromatous disease of the aorta. (Reproduced, with permission, from Wolff K et al. *Fitzpatrick's Dermatology in General Medicine,* 7th ed. New York: McGraw-Hill, 2008: Fig. 174-5A.)

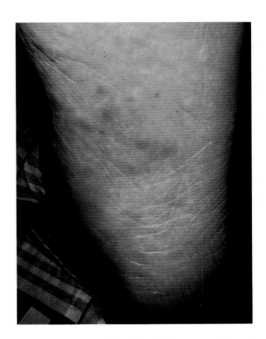

Janeway lesions. Peripheral embolization to the sole leads to a cluster of erythematous macules known as Janeway lesions. (Courtesy of the Department of Dermatology, Wilford Hall USAF Medical Center and Brooke Army Medical Center, San Antonio, TX, as published in Knoop KJ et al. *Atlas of Emergency Medicine,* 2nd ed. New York: McGraw-Hill, 2002: 384.)

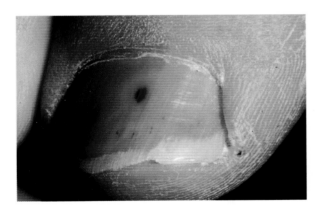

Splinter hemorrhages. Note the splinter hemorrhages along the distal aspect of the nail plate, due to emboli from subacute bacterial endocarditis. (Courtesy of the Armed Forces Institute of Pathology, Bethesda, MD, as published in Knoop KJ et al. *Atlas of Emergency Medicine,* 2nd ed. New York: McGraw-Hill, 2002: 384.)

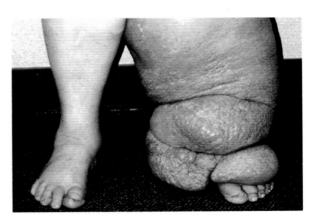

Left leg lymphedema with typical skin changes. Note that the toes are edematous and the skin is thickened in a classic *peau d'orange* pattern with verrucous changes. (Reproduced, with permission, from Fuster V et al. *Hurst's The Heart,* 12th ed. New York: McGraw-Hill, 2008: Fig. 108-1.)

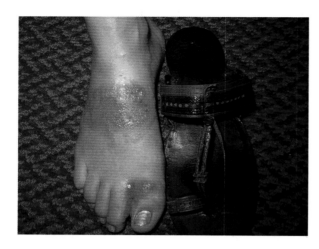

Contact dermatitis. Erythematous papules, vesicles, and serous weeping localized to areas of contact with the offending agent are characteristic. (Reproduced, with permission, from Hurwitz RM. *Pathology of the Skin: Atlas of Clinical–Pathological Correlation,* 2nd ed. Stamford, CT: Appleton & Lange, 1998: 3.)

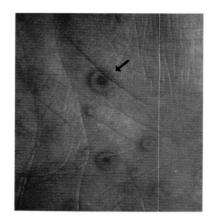

Erythema multiforme. The classic target lesion has a dull red center, pale zone, and darker outer ring (arrow). This acute self-limited reaction may occur with infection, antibiotic use, exposure to radiation or chemicals, or malignancy. (Reproduced, with permission, from Bondi EE. *Dermatology: Diagnosis and Therapy,* 1st ed. Stamford, CT: Appleton & Lange, 1991: 392.)

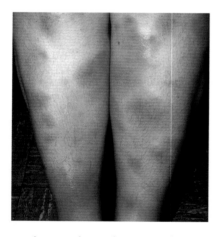

Erythema nodosum. The erythematous plaques and nodules are commonly located on pretibial areas. Lesions are painful and indurated and heal spontaneously without ulceration. (Reproduced, with permission, from Hurwitz RM. *Pathology of the Skin: Atlas of Clinical–Pathological Correlation,* 2nd ed. Stamford, CT: Appleton & Lange, 1998: 132.)

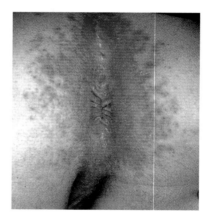

Candidal intertrigo. Erythematous areas surrounded by satellite pustules are restricted to warm, moist intertriginous areas. (Reproduced, with permission, from Bondi EE. *Dermatology: Diagnosis and Therapy,* 1st ed. Stamford, CT: Appleton & Lange, 1991: 390.)

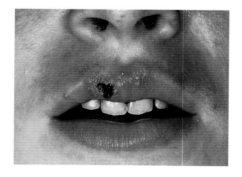

A

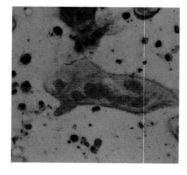

B

Herpes simplex. (A) Primary infection. Grouped vesicles on an erythematous base on the patient's lips and oral mucosa may progress to pustules before resolving. (B) Tzanck smear. The multinucleated giant cells from vesicular fluid provide a presumptive diagnosis of HSV infection. However, the Tzanck smear cannot distinguish between HSV and VZV infection. (Reproduced, with permission, from Hurwitz RM. *Pathology of the Skin: Atlas of Clinical–Pathological Correlation,* 2nd ed. Stamford, CT: Appleton & Lange, 1998: 145; and Bondi EE. *Dermatology: Diagnosis and Therapy,* 1st ed. Stamford, CT: Appleton & Lange, 1991: 396.)

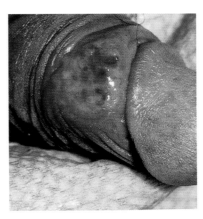

Primary syphilis. The chancre, which appears at the site of infection, is an ulcerated papule with a smooth, clean base; raised, indurated borders; and scant discharge. (Reproduced, with permission, from Bondi EE. *Dermatology: Diagnosis and Therapy,* 1st ed. Stamford, CT: Appleton & Lange, 1991: 394.)

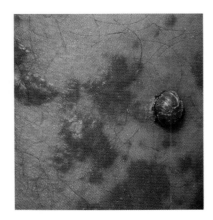

Kaposi's sarcoma. Manifests as red to purple nodules and surrounding pink to red macules. The latter appear most often in immunosuppressed patients. (Reproduced, with permission, from Bondi EE. *Dermatology: Diagnosis and Therapy,* 1st ed. Stamford, CT: Appleton & Lange, 1991: 393.)

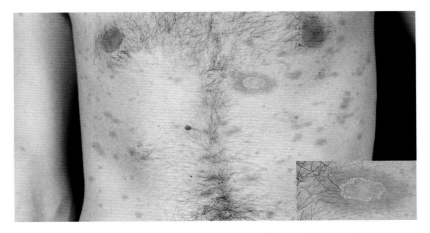

Pityriasis rosea. Pink plaques with an oval configuration are seen that follow the lines of cleavage. Inset: Herald patch. The collarette of scale is more obvious on this magnification. (Reproduced, with permission, from Wolff K et al. *Fitzpatrick's Color Atlas & Synopsis of Clinical Dermatology,* 5th ed. New York: McGraw-Hill, 2005: 119.)

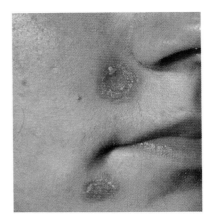

Impetigo. Dried pustules with superficial golden-brown crust are most commonly found around the nose and mouth. (Reproduced, with permission, from Bondi EE. *Dermatology: Diagnosis and Therapy,* 1st ed. Stamford, CT: Appleton & Lange, 1991: 390.)

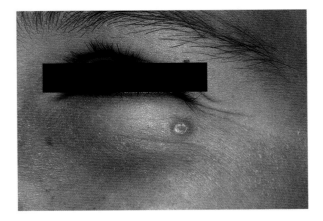

Molluscum contagiosum. The dome-shaped, fleshy, umbilicated papule on the child's eyelid is characteristic. (Reproduced, with permission, from Hurwitz RM. *Pathology of the Skin: Atlas of Clinical–Pathological Correlation,* 2nd ed. Stamford, CT: Appleton & Lange, 1998: 149.)

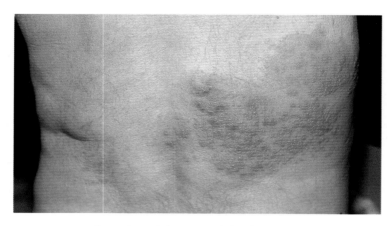

Herpes zoster. The unilateral dermatomal distribution of the grouped vesicles on an erythematous base is characteristic. (Reproduced, with permission, from Wolff K et al. *Fitzpatrick's Color Atlas & Synopsis of Clinical Dermatology,* 5th ed. New York, McGraw-Hill, 2005: 823.)

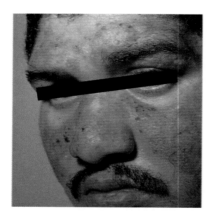

Malar rash of systemic lupus erythematosus. The malar rash is a red to purple, continuous plaque extending across the bridge of the nose and to both cheeks. (Reproduced, with permission, from Bondi EE. *Dermatology: Diagnosis and Therapy,* 1st ed. Stamford, CT: Appleton & Lange, 1991: 395.)

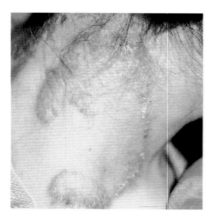

Tinea corporis. Ring-shaped, erythematous, scaling macules with central clearing are characteristic. (Reproduced, with permission, from Bondi EE. *Dermatology: Diagnosis and Therapy,* 1st ed. Stamford, CT: Appleton & Lange, 1991: 389.)

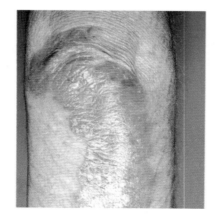

A

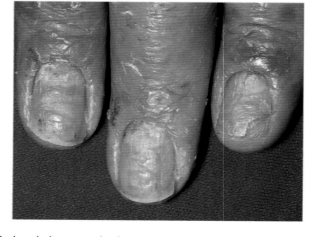

B

Psoriasis. (A) Skin changes. The classic sharply demarcated dark red plaques with silvery scales are commonly located on extensor surfaces (e.g., elbows, knees). (B) Nail changes. Note the pitting, onycholysis, and oil spots. (Reproduced, with permission, from Bondi EE. *Dermatology: Diagnosis and Therapy,* 1st ed. Stamford, CT: Appleton & Lange, 1991: 389; and Hurwitz RM. *Pathology of the Skin: Atlas of Clinical–Pathological Correlation,* 1st ed. Stamford, CT: Appleton & Lange, 1991.)

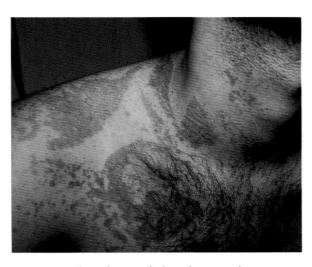

Tinea versicolor. These pinkish scaling macules commonly appear on the chest and back. Lesions may also be lightly pigmented or hypopigmented depending on the patient's skin color and sun exposure. (Courtesy of the Department of Dermatology, Wilford Hall USAF Medical Center and Brooke Army Medical Center, San Antonio, TX, as published in Knoop KJ et al. *Atlas of Emergency Medicine,* 2nd ed. New York: McGraw-Hill, 2002: 406.)

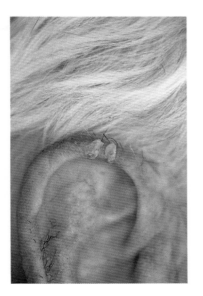

Actinic keratosis. The discrete patch has an erythematous base and rough white scaling. Actinic keratosis is a premalignant lesion that may progress to squamous cell carcinoma. It is most commonly found in sun-exposed areas. (Reproduced, with permission, from Hurwitz RM. *Pathology of the Skin: Atlas of Clinical–Pathological Correlation,* 2nd ed. Stamford, CT: Appleton & Lange, 1998: 359.)

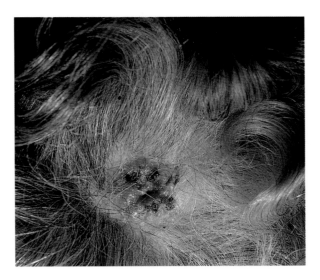

Squamous cell carcinoma. Note the crusting and ulceration of this erythematous plaque. Most lesions are exophytic nodules with erosion or ulceration. (Reproduced, with permission, from Hurwitz RM. *Pathology of the Skin: Atlas of Clinical–Pathological Correlation,* 2nd ed. Stamford, CT: Appleton & Lange, 1998: 360.)

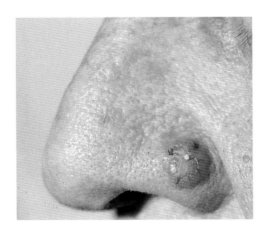

Nodular basal cell carcinoma. A smooth, pearly nodule with telangiectasias. (Reproduced, with permission, from Wolff K et al. *Fitzpatrick's Color Atlas & Synopsis of Clinical Dermatology,* 5th ed. New York: McGraw-Hill, 2005: 283.)

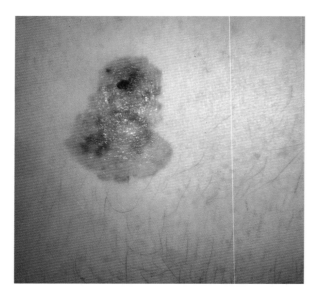

Melanoma. Note the **a**symmetry, **b**order irregularity, **c**olor variation, and large **d**iameter of this plaque. (Reproduced, with permission, from Hurwitz RM. *Pathology of the Skin: Atlas of Clinical–Pathological Correlation,* 1st ed. Stamford, CT: Appleton & Lange, 1991: 432.)

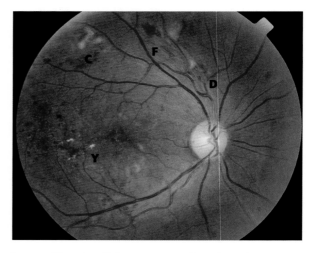

Nonproliferative diabetic retinopathy. Flame hemorrhages (F), dot-blot hemorrhages (D), cotton-wool spots (C), and yellow exudate (Y) result from small vessel damage and occlusion.

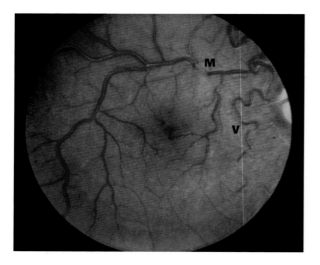

Hypertensive retinopathy. Note the tortuous retinal veins (V) and venous microaneurysms (M). Other findings include hemorrhages, retinal infarcts, detachment of the retina, and disk edema.

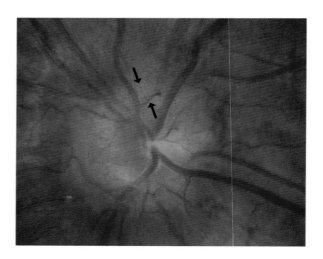

Papilledema. Look for blurred disk margins due to edema of the optic disk (arrows).

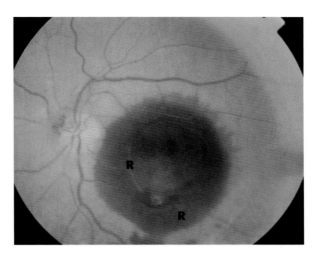

Subretinal hemorrhage. Note the preretinal blood and overlying retinal vessels (R). Subretinal hemorrhages may be seen in any condition with abnormal vessel proliferation (e.g., diabetes, hypertension) or in trauma.

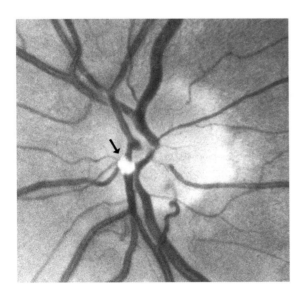

Cholesterol emboli. Cholesterol emboli (Hollenhorst plaque; arrow) usually arise in atherosclerotic carotid arteries and often lodge at the bifurcation of retinal arteries. (Reproduced, with permission, from Vaughan D. *General Ophthalmology,* 14th ed. Stamford, CT: Appleton & Lange, 1995: 299.)

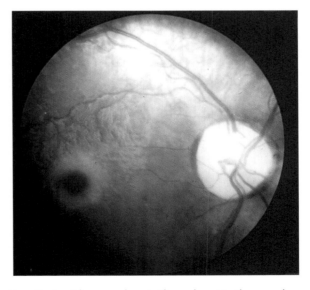

Tay–Sachs. Cherry-red spot. The red spot in the macula may be seen in Tay–Sachs disease, Niemann–Pick disease, central retinal artery occlusion, and methanol toxicity. (Reproduced, with permission, from Vaughan D. *General Ophthalmology,* 14th ed. Stamford, CT: Appleton & Lange, 1995: 293.)

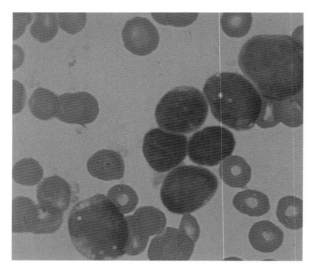

Acute lymphoblastic leukemia. Peripheral blood smear reveals numerous large, uniform lymphoblasts, which are large cells with a high nuclear-to-cytoplasmic ratio. Some lymphoblasts have visible clefts in their nuclei. (Courtesy of Dr. Peter McPhedran, Yale Department of Hematology.)

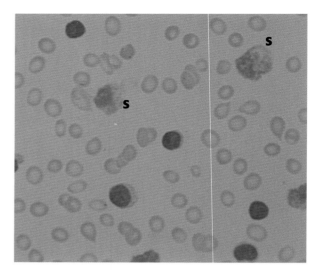

Chronic lymphocytic leukemia. The numerous, small, mature lymphocytes and smudge cells (S; fragile malignant lymphocytes are disrupted during blood smear preparation) are characteristic. (Courtesy of Dr. Peter McPhedran, Yale Department of Hematology.)

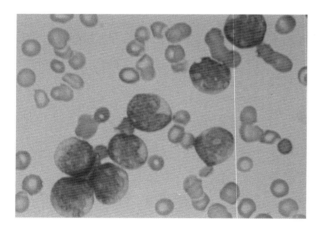

Acute myelocytic leukemia. Large, uniform myeloblasts with round or kidney-shaped nuclei and prominent nucleoli are characteristic. (Courtesy of Dr. Peter McPhedran, Yale Department of Hematology.)

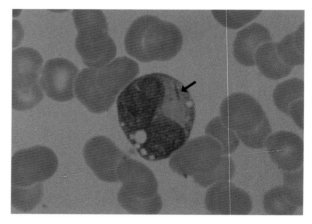

Auer rod in acute myelocytic leukemia. The red rod-shaped structure (arrow) in the cytoplasm of the myeloblast is pathognomonic. (Courtesy of Dr. Peter McPhedran, Yale Department of Hematology.)

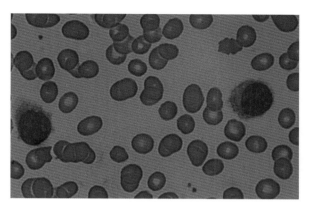

Hairy cell leukemia. Note the hairlike cytoplasmic projections from neoplastic lymphocytes. Villous lymphoma can also look like this. (Courtesy of Dr. Peter McPhedran, Yale Department of Hematology.)

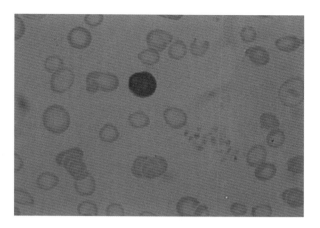

Iron deficiency anemia. Note the microcytic, hypochromic RBCs ("doughnut cells") with enlarged areas of central pallor. (Courtesy of Dr. Peter McPhedran, Yale Department of Hematology.)

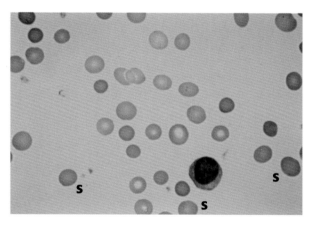

Spherocytes. These RBCs (S) lack areas of central pallor. Spherocytes are seen in autoimmune hemolysis and hereditary spherocytosis. (Courtesy of Dr. Peter McPhedran, Yale Department of Hematology.)

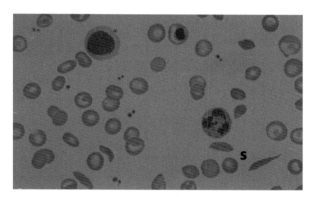

Sickle cells. Sickle-shaped RBCs (S) are almost always seen on the blood smear, regardless of whether the patient is having a sickle cell crisis or not. Anisocytosis, poikilocytosis, target cells, and nucleated RBCs can also be seen. (Courtesy of Dr. Peter McPhedran, Yale Department of Hematology.)

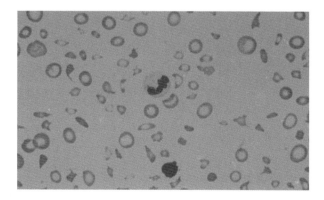

Schistocytes. These fragmented RBCs may be seen in microangiopathic hemolytic anemia and mechanical hemolysis. (Courtesy of Dr. Peter McPhedran, Yale Department of Hematology.)

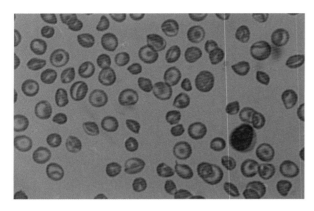

Target cells. The dense zone of hemoglobin in the RBC center is characteristic. Target cells are seen in hemoglobin C or S disease, thalassemia, severe liver disease, and severe iron deficiency anemia as well as postsplenectomy. (Courtesy of Dr. Peter McPhedran, Yale Department of Hematology.)

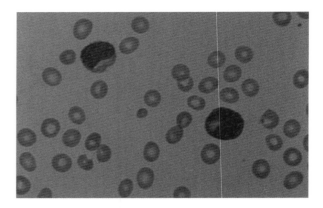

Mononucleosis. These atypical lymphocytes, with abundant blue cytoplasm, no granules, and variably shaped nuclei, are classically seen in EBV and CMV infections. (Courtesy of Dr. Peter McPhedran, Yale Department of Hematology.)

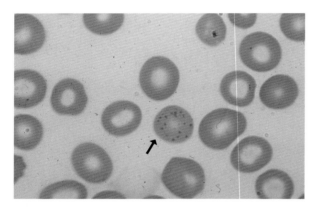

Basophilic stippling. The basophilic granules (arrow) within the RBCs are a nonspecific finding that may suggest megaloblastic anemia, lead poisoning, or reticulocytes. (Reproduced, with permission, from Lichtman MA et al. *Williams Hematology,* 7th ed. New York: McGraw-Hill, 2006, Plate IV-3.)

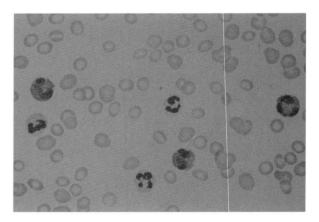

Eosinophilia. Eosinophils have red-staining cytoplasmic granules. Eosinophilia may be seen in atopic diseases, parasitic infections, collagen vascular diseases, medications, malignancies such as Hodgkin's disease, and endocrinopathies like adrenal insufficiency. (Courtesy of Dr. Peter McPhedran, Yale Department of Hematology.)

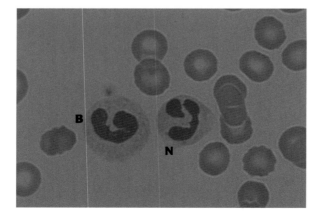

Neutrophil (N) and band (B). The more immature band form has a stretched, nonlobulated nucleus rather than a segmented nucleus. Bands are nonspecific markers of stress. (Courtesy of Dr. Peter McPhedran, Yale Department of Hematology.)

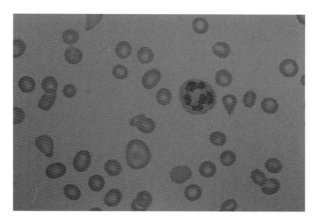

Hypersegmentation. The nucleus of this hypersegmented neutrophil has six lobes (six or more nuclear lobes are required). This is a characteristic finding of megaloblastic anemia. (Courtesy of Dr. Peter McPhedran, Yale Department of Hematology.)

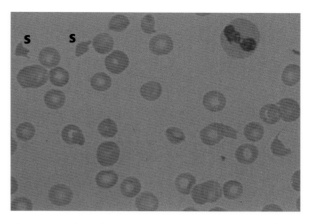

Thrombotic thrombocytopenic purpura (TTP). Note the schistocytes (S) and paucity of platelets. TTP is characterized by microangiopathic hemolytic anemia, thrombocytopenia, fever, neurologic abnormalities, and renal failure. (Courtesy of Dr. Peter McPhedran, Yale Department of Hematology.)

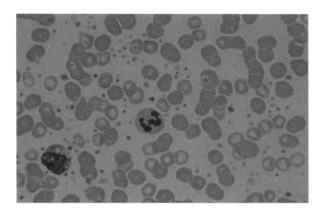

Thrombocytosis. Numerous platelets are seen in myeloproliferative disorders, severe iron deficiency anemia, inflammation, and postsplenectomy states. (Courtesy of Dr. Peter McPhedran, Yale Department of Hematology.)

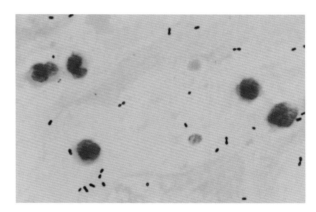

Streptococcus pneumoniae. This is a sputum sample from a patient with pneumonia. Note the characteristic lancet-shaped gram-positive diplococci.

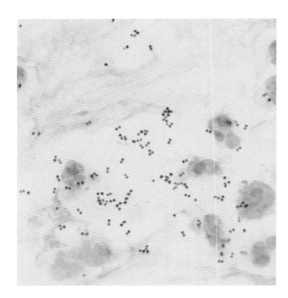

Staphylococcus aureus. These clusters of gram-positive cocci were isolated from the sputum of a patient with pneumonia.

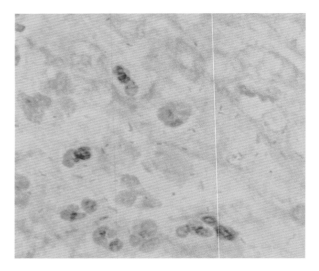

Pseudomonas aeruginosa. This sputum sample from a patient with pneumonia revealed gram-negative rods. The large number of neutrophils and relative paucity of epithelial cells indicate that this sample is not contaminated with oropharyngeal flora.

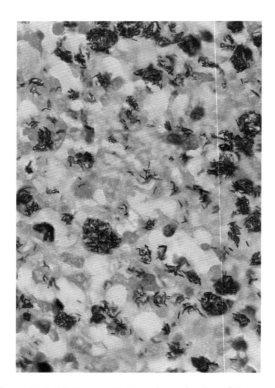

Tuberculosis (AFB smear). Note the red color of the tubercle bacilli an acid-fast staining of a sputum sample ("red snappers"). (Reproduced, with permission, from Milikowski C. *Color Atlas of Basic Histopathology,* 1st ed. Stamford, CT: Appleton & Lange, 1997: 193.)

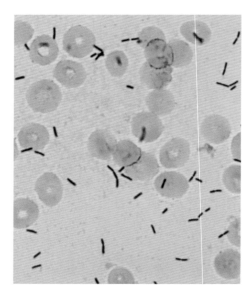

Listeria. These numerous rod-shaped bacilli were isolated from the blood of a patient with *Listeria* meningitis.

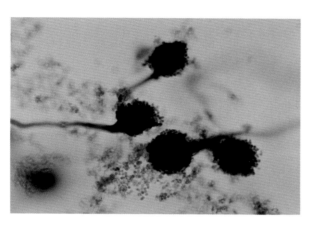

Aspergillosis. Note the characteristic appearance of *Aspergillus* spores in radiating columns.

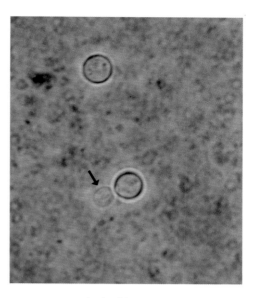

Cryptococcus. Note the budding yeast (arrow) and wide capsule of *Cryptococcus* isolated from CSF.

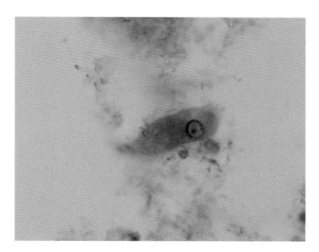

Entamoeba. *Entamoeba* cysts have large nuclei. This is a sample from diarrheal stool.

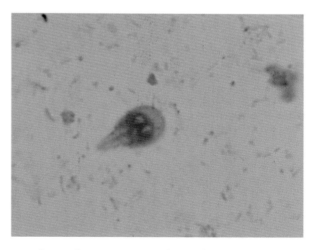

Giardia trophozoite in stool. The trophozoite exhibits a classic pear shape with two nuclei imparting an owl's-eye appearance.

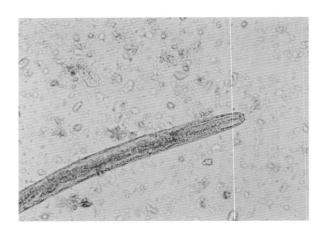

Strongyloides. These filarial larvae were found in the stool of a patient with watery diarrhea.

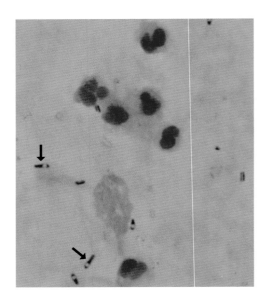

Clostridium wound infection. The lucency at the end of each gram-positive bacillus is the terminal spore (arrow). This sample was isolated from an infected wound site.

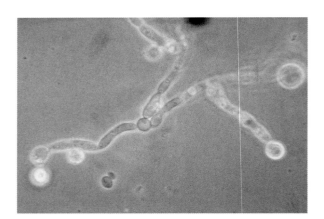

KOH mount of Candida albicans. (Reproduced, with permission, from Wolff K et al. *Fitzpatrick's Color Atlas & Synopsis of Clinical Dermatology,* 5th ed. New York: McGraw-Hill, 2005: 717.)

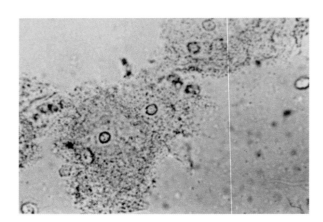

Gardnerella vaginalis. Note the granular epithelial cells ("clue cells") and indistinct cell margins. (Reproduced, with permission, from Kasper DL et al. *Harrison's Principles of Internal Medicine,* 16th ed. New York: McGraw-Hill, 2005: 767.)

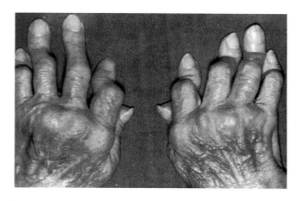

Rheumatoid arthritis. The swan-neck deformities of the digits and severe involvement of the proximal interphalangeal joints are characteristic. (Reproduced, with permission, from Chandrasoma P. *Concise Pathology*, 3rd ed. Stamford, CT: Appleton & Lange, 1998: 978.)

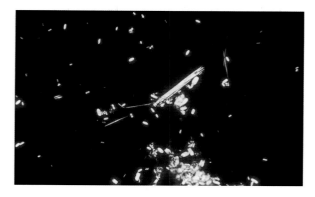

Gout. Negatively birefringent crystals. (Reproduced, with permission, from Milikowski C. *Color Atlas of Basic Histopathology*, 1st ed. Stamford, CT: Appleton & Lange, 1997: 546.)

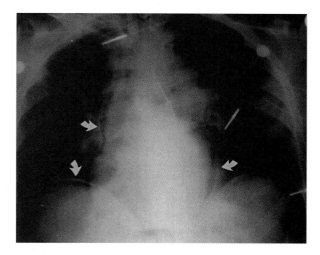

Pneumomediastinum. The lucency outlining the left heart border on chest x-ray suggests air in the mediastinum. (Reproduced, with permission, from Goldfrank LR. *Toxic Emergencies*, 6th ed. Stamford, CT: Appleton & Lange, 1998: 285.)

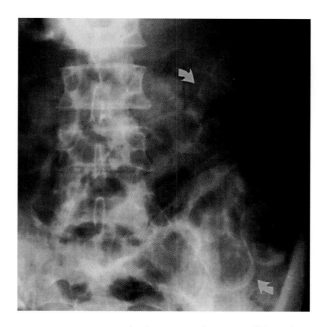

Pneumoperitoneum. The lucency outlining small bowel on abdominal x-ray indicated the abnormal presence of air. (Reproduced, with permission, from Goldfrank LR. *Toxic Emergencies*, 6th ed. Stamford, CT: Appleton & Lange, 1998: 285.)

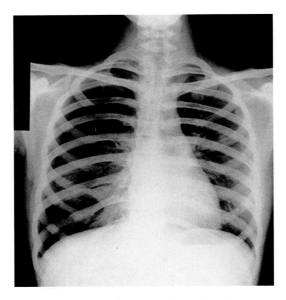

Spontaneous pneumothorax on the right side. (Reproduced, with permission, from Doherty GM, Way LW. *Current Surgical Diagnosis & Treatment,* 12th ed. New York: McGraw-Hill, 2006: Fig. 18-16.)

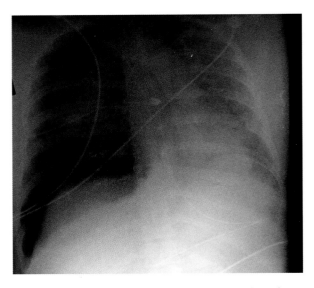

CXR demonstrating tension pneumothorax. Clinical signs alone should be sufficient to diagnose this condition and avert the life-threatening delay involved in obtaining an x-ray. (Reproduced, with permission, from Stone CK, Humphries RL. *Current Diagnosis & Treatment: Emergency Medicine,* 6th ed. New York: McGraw-Hill, 2008: Fig. 22-1.)

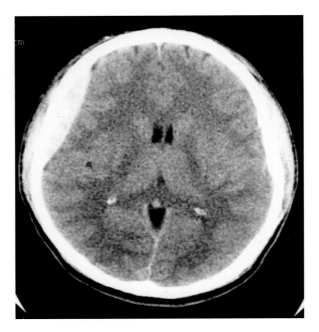

Acute epidural hematoma. Unenhanced CT scan shows a typical lens-shaped frontal epidural clot. (Reproduced, with permission, from Ropper AH, Brown RH. *Adams and Victor's Principles of Neurology,* 8th ed. New York: McGraw-Hill, 2005: Fig. 35-8.)

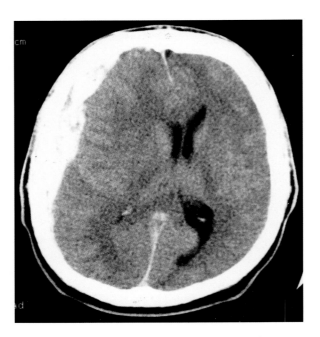

Acute subdural hematoma. Note the substantial mass effect (displacement) of brain tissue but little edema. (Reproduced, with permission, from Ropper AH, Brown RH. *Adams and Victor's Principles of Neurology,* 8th ed. New York: McGraw-Hill, 2005: Fig. 35-9.)

SECTION 3

Top-Rated Review Resources

This section is a database of recommended clinical science review books, sample examination books, and commercial review courses marketed to medical students studying for the USMLE Step 2 CK. For each book, we list the **Title** of the book, the **First Author** (or editor), the **Current Publisher,** the **Copyright Year**, the **Edition**, the **Number of Pages**, the **ISBN Code**, the **Approximate List Price,** the **Format** of the book, and the **Number of Test Questions.** Most entries also include Summary Comments that describe the style and utility of each book for studying. Finally, each book receives a **Rating.** The books are sorted into a comprehensive section as well as into sections corresponding to the six clinical disciplines (internal medicine, neurology, OB/GYN, pediatrics, psychiatry, and surgery). Within each section, books are arranged first by Rating, then by Author, and finally by Title.

For this seventh edition of *First Aid for the USMLE Step 2 CK,* the database of review books has been completely revised, with in-depth summary comments on more than 100 books and software. A letter rating scale with six different grades reflects the detailed student evaluations. Each book receives a rating as follows:

A+	Excellent for boards review.
A	
A–	Very good for boards review; choose among the group.

B+	
B	Good, but use only after exhausting better sources.
B–	

The **Rating** is meant to reflect the overall usefulness of the book in preparing for the USMLE Step 2 CK exam. This is based on a number of factors, including:

- The cost of the book
- The readability of the text
- The appropriateness and accuracy of the book
- The quality and number of sample questions
- The quality of written answers to sample questions
- The quality and appropriateness of the illustrations (e.g., graphs, diagrams, photographs)
- The length of the text (longer is not necessarily better)
- The quality and number of other books available in the same discipline
- The importance of the discipline on the USMLE Step 2 CK exam

Please note that **the rating does not reflect the quality of the book for purposes other than reviewing for the USMLE Step 2 CK exam.** Many books with low ratings are well written and informative but are not ideal for boards preparation. We have also avoided listing or commenting on the wide variety of general textbooks available in the clinical sciences.

Evaluations are based on the cumulative results of formal and informal surveys of hundreds of medical students from medical schools across the country. The summary comments and overall ratings represent a consensus opinion, but there may have been a large range of opinions or limited student feedback on any particular book.

Please note that the data listed are subject to change because:

- Publishers' prices change frequently.
- Individual bookstores often charge an additional markup.
- New editions come out frequently, and the quality of updating varies.
- The same book may be reissued through another publisher.

We actively encourage medical students and faculty to submit their opinions and ratings of these clinical science review books so that we may update our database (see "How to Contribute," p. xv). In addition, we ask that publishers and authors submit review copies of clinical science review books, including new editions and books not included in our database, for evaluation. We also solicit reviews of new books or suggestions for alternate modes of study that may be useful in preparing for the examination, such as flash cards, computer-based tutorials, commercial review courses, and Internet Web sites.

DISCLAIMER/CONFLICT-OF-INTEREST STATEMENT

No material in this book, including the ratings, reflects the opinion or influence of the publisher. All errors and omissions will gladly be corrected if brought to the attention of the authors through the publisher.

A

Boards & Wards $39.95 Review

AYALA

**Lippincott Williams & Wilkins, 2006, 3rd ed., 546 pages,
ISBN 9781405105095**

A concise book presented in outline format, packed with key information across the various fields of medicine. **Pros:** Very high yield. Makes nice use of tables and charts. Good for quick study and last-minute review. Useful on the wards as well, and fits in a pocket. **Cons:** Small print. Not tremendously detailed, but covers many topics. More in-depth books are required for further explanation. **Summary:** A good, comprehensive review, but lacks some detail.

A

USMLE Step 2 Mock Exam $35.95 Test/750 q

BROCHERT

Hanley & Belfus, 2004, 2nd ed., 350 pages, ISBN 9781560536109

Includes 750 vignette-style questions in 15 test blocks. **Pros:** Questions are case based and offer a good approximation of real boards questions. Questions cover high-yield topics, and explanations are terse but adequate. Many questions also include images and associated laboratory findings. **Cons:** Explanations may not be adequate for those who require an in-depth review of certain topics. **Summary:** Excellent vignette-type questions in mock exam format.

A⁻

USMLE Step 2 Secrets $39.95 Review

BROCHERT

Hanley & Belfus, 2004, 2nd ed., 250 pages, ISBN 9781560536086

Typical Secrets-series format, with questions and answers organized by specialty. **Pros:** A concise review of many high-yield topics. Makes good use of clinical images, including patient photos, blood smears, and radiographs. Gives clinical pearls that help differentiate and diagnose common clinical presentations. **Cons:** Contains no clinical vignettes; simply lists questions that might be posed on the wards. Does not follow Step 2 CK format. Expensive. Content overlaps with that of other books by Brochert. **Summary:** An excellent book to page through during brief periods of "downtime." Does not substitute for a formal review or practice tests. A portable book that stresses relevant topics in a quick, easy format.

REVIEW RESOURCES

COMPREHENSIVE

A⁻

First Aid Cases for the USMLE Step 2 CK
$41.95   Review

Le

McGraw-Hill, 2006, 1st ed., 272 pages, ISBN 9780071464116

A review of high-yield clinical vignettes for the Step 2 CK exam. **Pros:** Cases provide detailed answers to high-yield topics and are arranged in an easy-to-follow format. Emphasizes the most likely diagnosis, the next step, and initial management answers. **Cons:** Some topics are either not covered or given only brief treatment. **Summary:** A good review with emphasis on vignette-style case presentations and boards-relevant answers, but not sufficient as a stand-alone text for review.

B⁺

Crush Step 2
$39.95   Review

Brochert

Mosby, 2007, 3rd ed., 352 pages, ISBN 9781416029762

A comprehensive review of many high-yield topics, organized by specialty. **Pros:** Places good emphasis on key points. The conversational style is easy to read. Makes good use of charts and diagrams. Covers surgical topics in more depth than similar books. **Cons:** Not comprehensive. Contains no practice questions or vignettes. Not sufficiently detailed to be used alone for Step 2 CK preparation. **Summary:** A solid review of key points and frequently tested topics. Should probably be supplemented with other review material and practice tests.

B⁺

Lange Q&A: USMLE Step 2
$44.95   Test/1000+ q

Chan

McGraw-Hill, 2008, 6th ed., 440 pages, ISBN 9780071494007

Review questions organized by specialty along with two comprehensive practice exams. **Pros:** Overall question content is good, with broad coverage of high-yield topics. Well illustrated. **Cons:** Vignettes are brief, with short explanations. Some questions are more detailed than actual Step 2 CK questions. **Summary:** Well suited to focused specialty review by virtue of overall review questions on high-yield topics. A good buy for the number of questions.

B⁺

Lange Practice Tests: USMLE Step 2
$44.95   Test/900 q

Goldberg

McGraw-Hill, 2005, 3rd ed., 288 pages, ISBN 9780071446167

Comprehensive test questions. **Pros:** A great source of high-yield questions covering all topics. Many questions include clinically relevant radiographs and photographs of pathology. Offers adequate explanations. **Cons:** Some questions are not vignette style and do not reflect boards format. **Summary:** A good compilation of test questions that focus on high-yield material, but some questions still do not reflect boards style. A good source of supplemental questions.

550

B+

NMS Review for USMLE Step 2 CK
IBSEN

$46.95   Test/900 q

Lippincott Williams & Wilkins, 2006, 3rd ed., 654 pages,
ISBN 9780781765220

A comprehensive review book in question-and-answer format. **Pros:** Offers clear, concise, and broad coverage of high-yield topics, presented in a format similar to that of the actual Step 2 CK exam. Complete explanations. **Cons:** Questions are more detailed than needed for the boards. Lacks illustrations or images. **Summary:** A good source of Step 2 CK–style questions with appropriate format and content, but questions may be more detailed than those on the actual exam.

 B+

Underground Clinical Vignettes: Step 2 Bundle
KIM

$159.95   Review

Lippincott Williams & Wilkins; 2007, 4th ed., 256 pages,
ISBN 9780781763639

A set containing clinical case scenarios of the various specialties, including OB/GYN, neurology, internal medicine, surgery, emergency medicine, psychiatry, and pediatrics, along with an extensive color atlas supplement. **Pros:** Well organized by focus points: pathogenesis, epidemiology, management, complications, and associated diseases. Small, portable texts. **Cons:** Not comprehensive; best used as a supplement for review. **Summary:** Organized and easy-to-read clinical vignettes. Excellent as a supplement to studying, but not sufficient by itself. More economical to purchase the nine-volume set than individual volumes.

 B+

Step-Up to USMLE Step 2
VAN KLEUNEN

$39.95   Review

Lippincott Williams & Wilkins, 2007, 2nd ed., 352 pages,
ISBN 9780781771566

A Step 2 CK test review typical of the Step-Up series format, organized by system. **Pros:** A concise boards review resource with many tables organizing the information and quick facts isolated in the page margins. **Cons:** Not very detailed, but covers most boards exam topics and serves as a good source of study organization. **Summary:** A good, comprehensive review for the Step 2 CK exam with many quick-study features.

Lange Outline Review: USMLE Step 2
$41.95   Review

GOLDBERG

McGraw-Hill, 2006, 5th ed., 650 pages, ISBN 9780071451925

A comprehensive boards review book with chapters organized by clinical discipline. **Pros:** A comprehensive review source with extensive coverage of clinical topics and an organized, in-depth review of each. **Cons:** Covers some low-yield topics. Includes relatively few images, figures, or tables. **Summary:** A solid, single-source, comprehensive review for the Step 2 CK exam.

USMLE Step 2 Made Ridiculously Simple
$29.95   Review

CARL

MedMaster, 2006, 3rd ed., 356 pages, ISBN 9780940780729

A general review of topics for the Step 2 CK exam. Presented in outline format with tables and brief discussions. **Pros:** A quick review. Useful in areas that might otherwise be overlooked—e.g., ophthalmology, dermatology, and ENT. Helpful for last-minute review. **Cons:** The tabular format does not provide substantive details but aids in the memorization of lists. Some have found it too simple. **Summary:** Highlights most high-yield topics, but should not be used alone for review.

Kaplanmedical.com   *$149–$499*
KAPLAN

A compilation of online programs for Step 2 CK review, including a large test bank. **Pros:** Questions can be arranged by topic or randomly to simulate the real exam. Tests are timed to simulate boards conditions. Includes an extensive number of questions in vignette format. The content level of questions reflects the boards test. Explanations are thorough, and the text now reports the national average for each question. Allows students to identify strong and weak points. **Cons:** Very expensive. Online lectures can be difficult to watch for extensive periods of time. **Summary:** A good source of questions with thorough explanations, but the price may be prohibitive for many.

USMLERx.com   *$68–$298*
Step 2 CK Qmax

A test bank with more than 2600 questions. **Pros:** Written by students who have done well on the Step 2 CK exam; then reviewed by faculty experts. Offers highly comprehensive explanations. **Cons:** A newer resource that is still evolving. **Summary:** A great question bank source. New, but feedback from students has been excellent thus far.

USMLEWorld.com   *$90–$175*
USMLE World

A test bank with more than 2000 questions. Similar to the Kaplan test bank. **Pros:** Features well-written questions with explanations. Cheaper than Kaplan. Questions tend to be more difficult than those on the actual exam, but many students find this an advantage during preparation. **Cons:** Some questions are overly picky. **Summary:** An excellent source of questions that is cheaper than Kaplan.

USMLEasy.com   *$99–$199*
McGraw-Hill

A comprehensive test bank with more than 3300 questions and explanations. Similar in style to the Kaplan question bank described above. **Pros:** Features a large number of questions. Mimics the CBT format. Cheaper than Kaplan. Access is often free through medical libraries. **Cons:** Questions can be more obscure than those appearing on the actual exam. Questions overlap with those of the PreTest series of review books. **Summary:** A fair source of questions that may be good for supplemental review, especially in preparation for clerkship shelf exams.

REVIEW RESOURCES

ONLINE REVIEW

Step-Up to Medicine
AGABEGI

$42.95   Review

Lippincott Williams & Wilkins, 2008, 2nd ed., 560 pages,
ISBN 9780781771535

A comprehensive review of commonly tested diseases and topics in internal medicine, organized in an outline format. Includes a color atlas and an appendix on interpreting x-rays, ECGs, and physical exam findings. **Pros:** Very comprehensive, with informative tables and diagrams to help synthesize information. Includes occasional clinical vignettes that correlate with the topic being discussed. Quick facts to remember are included in the margins of each page. **Cons:** Very lengthy. Geared more toward clerkship preparation than Step 2 CK review. **Summary:** A good book that is packed with useful information for the wards, but may be too lengthy and detailed for the Step 2 CK exam.

High-Yield Internal Medicine
NIRULA

$26.95   Review

Lippincott Williams & Wilkins, 2006, 3rd ed., 128 pages,
ISBN 9780781781695

A core review of internal medicine in outline format. **Pros:** Focuses on high-yield diseases and symptoms. A quick and easy read. **Cons:** Not comprehensive. Lacks many illustrations and has no index. **Summary:** A good, fast review presented in a format that allows for quick and repetitive reading. Best used as a supplement, not as a primary study source.

First Aid for the Medicine Clerkship
STEAD

$42.95   Review

McGraw-Hill, 2005, 2nd ed., 416 pages, ISBN 9780071448758

A high-yield review of symptoms and diseases. **Pros:** A comprehensive review that is well organized by symptom with good illustrations, scenarios, diagrams, algorithms, and mnemonics. **Cons:** May not be suited to readers who prefer information arranged in text form. May be too basic for certain topics. **Summary:** An excellent, concise review of medicine for those who prefer its format.

REVIEW RESOURCES

INTERNAL MEDICINE

554

B+

Underground Clinical Vignettes: Emergency Medicine
KIM

$22.95   Review

Lippincott Williams & Wilkins, 2007, 4th ed., 256 pages,
ISBN 9780781768344

A clinical vignette–based review of emergency medicine topics. **Pros:** Well organized by focus points: pathogenesis, epidemiology, management, complications, and associated diseases. Well illustrated, and includes high-yield "minicases" and links to the Underground Clinical Vignettes' Clinical and Basic Science Color Atlases. **Cons:** Not comprehensive; best used as a supplement. **Summary:** An organized and easy-to-read supplement to studying.

B+

Underground Clinical Vignettes: Internal Medicine, Vols. I and II
KIM

$22.95 each   Review

Lippincott Williams & Wilkins, 2007, 4th ed., 256 pages each,
ISBN 9780781768351, 9780781768368

A clinical vignette–based review of common topics in internal medicine. **Pros:** Well organized by focus points: pathogenesis, epidemiology, management, complications, and associated diseases. Vignettes mirror the boards-style presentation of questions. **Cons:** Not comprehensive; best used as a supplement. **Summary:** An organized and easy-to-read supplement to studying.

B+

Blueprints Clinical Cases in Medicine
LI

$29.95   Test/200 q

Lippincott Williams & Wilkins, 2006, 2nd ed., 425 pages,
ISBN 9781405104913

A compendium of vignette-type cases arranged by symptom, followed by related questions and answers. **Pros:** An excellent companion to the Blueprints series. Focuses on high-yield cases. Easy to read with nice illustrations and a good review of management. **Cons:** Not comprehensive; use as a supplement for review. Better suited to clerkship preparation than to the Step 2 CK exam. **Summary:** An organized and easy-to-read supplement. Adds clinical correlates to the Blueprints series. Best used with the Blueprints text.

B+

Medical Secrets
ZOLLO

$39.95   Review

Hanley & Belfus, 2004, 4th ed., 608 pages, ISBN 9781560533870

A question-and-answer text typical of the Secrets series. **Pros:** Covers a great deal of clinically relevant information. Concise answers are given with pearls, tips, and memory aids. **Cons:** Too lengthy and detailed for USMLE review. **Summary:** Not a focused review. May be more appropriate for wards use.

Medicine Recall

$39.95   Review

BERGIN

Lippincott Williams & Wilkins, 2007, 3rd ed., 832 pages,
ISBN 9780781794145

A review book presented in standard Recall-series question-and-answer format, organized by medical specialty. **Pros:** Addresses a broad range of high-yield clinical topics. Presented in a format that is good for self-quizzing. Appropriate level of detail. **Cons:** Contains no vignettes or images; requires significant time commitment. Style simulates questions asked on rounds, not those on the Step 2 CK exam. **Summary:** Written in a style that may be more conducive to wards than to boards preparation. Best used as a supplement to other resources.

In A Page Emergency Medicine

$34.95   Review

CATERINO

Blackwell Publishing, 2003, 1st ed., 344 pages,
ISBN 9781405103572

A collection of short, one-page summaries of 250 medical emergencies discussed in terms of etiology, differential diagnosis, presentation, diagnostic tests, treatment, and disposition. **Pros:** Concise and high yield. Covers a wide variety of emergencies seen in the ER. **Cons:** The text is crowded and somewhat confusing. Contains no images or diagrams. **Summary:** Good for use during the emergency medicine clerkship, but may not be appropriate for Step 2 CK review.

Blueprints Clinical Cases in Family Medicine

$34.95   Test/200 q

CHANG

Lippincott Williams & Wilkins, 2006, 2nd ed., 437 pages,
ISBN 9781405104951

A compendium of vignette-type cases arranged by symptom, followed by related questions and answers. **Pros:** An excellent companion to the Blueprints series. Focuses on high-yield cases. Easy to read with nice illustrations and a good review of management. **Cons:** Not comprehensive; best used as a supplement for review. **Summary:** An organized and easy-to-read supplement. Adds clinical correlates to the Blueprints series. Best if used with the Blueprints text.

B

Internal Medicine Pearls

$41.95   Review

HEFFNER

Elsevier, 2001, 2nd ed., 249 pages, ISBN 9781560534044

One-page reviews of more than 200 diseases discussed by etiology, epidemiology, signs/symptoms, differential diagnosis, diagnostic tests, treatment, and prognosis. **Pros:** A fast and concise review of high-yield information on common diseases. **Cons:** Text is crowded onto one page without any images or diagrams. **Summary:** Useful for quick study on the wards, but may not be comprehensive enough for the Step 2 CK exam.

B

Blueprints Q & A Step 2 Medicine

$19.95   Test/200 q

SHINAR

Lippincott Williams & Wilkins, 2004, 2nd ed., 276 pages, ISBN 9781405103893

Two hundred vignette-style questions. **Pros:** A nice companion to the Blueprints series. Focuses on high-yield topics. Explanations are easy to follow. **Cons:** Not comprehensive; best used as a supplement for review. Expensive; includes few questions given the cost of the book. **Summary:** An organized and easy-to-read supplement. Adds clinical correlates to the Blueprints series.

B

First Aid for the Emergency Medicine Clerkship

$42.95   Review

STEAD

McGraw-Hill, 2006, 2nd ed., 416 pages, ISBN 9780071448734

A high-yield review of symptoms and diseases. **Pros:** A comprehensive review; well organized by symptom with good illustrations, scenarios, diagrams, algorithms, and mnemonics. **Cons:** May not be suited to the reader who prefers information arranged in text form. **Summary:** An excellent review of emergency medicine and a nice presentation of high-yield topics for Step 2 CK preparation, but not sufficient for stand-alone review for the Step 2 CK exam.

B

Blueprints in Medicine

$38.95   Review/Test/100 q

YOUNG

Lippincott Williams & Wilkins, 2009, 5th ed., 448 pages, ISBN 9780781788700

A text review of internal medicine, organized by common diseases and common symptoms. Includes a question-and-answer section with explanations. **Pros:** A well-organized, concise review that makes for easy reading. Differential diagnoses for symptoms are helpful. Contains good charts and diagrams. **Cons:** Offers few illustrations. Contains some superfluous details, and some areas are too broad and simplistic to be useful for testing purposes. **Summary:** Poorly illustrated, but a good primary boards review for internal medicine.

PreTest Medicine

BERK

$26.95   Test/500 q

McGraw-Hill, 2006, 11th ed., 356 pages, ISBN 9780071455534

A question-and-answer format organized by medical subspecialty. **Pros:** Organization by subspecialty helps readers pinpoint weak areas. Offers a substantial number of vignette-style questions with detailed explanations. **Cons:** Many questions are more detailed than needed for the boards and are geared more toward the shelf exam. Few illustrations. **Summary:** A solid source of challenging review questions.

A⁻

Blueprints in Neurology $37.95   Review
DRISLANE
Lippincott Williams & Wilkins, 2009, 3rd ed., 256 pages,
ISBN 9780781796859
A review of neurology by disease and symptom with a brief exam. **Pros:**
Reviews high-yield topics of a complex discipline while remaining easy
to follow. Makes good use of tables, images, and diagrams. Questions
in the exam are similar to those found on both the shelf exam and Step
2 CK. **Cons:** Lengthy. **Summary:** An excellent review of high-yield
material for the wards and the Step 2 CK exam.

B⁺

PreTest Neurology $26.95   Test/500 q
ANSCHEL
McGraw-Hill, 2009, 7th ed., 352 pages, ISBN 9780071597920
A question-and-answer review of neurology. **Pros:** Offers thorough coverage of neurology topics with a good number of clinical vignettes.
Places appropriate emphasis on common topics and thorough explanations of answers. Good practice for interpreting common head CTs/
MRIs that might be tested. **Cons:** Some questions may be more detailed than needed for the boards. **Summary:** A good source of test
questions for rapid review of neurology, but may be too detailed for
boards review.

B⁺

Underground Clinical Vignettes: Neurology $22.95   Review
KIM
Lippincott Williams & Wilkins, 2007, 4th ed., 256 pages,
ISBN 9780781768375
A clinical vignette–based review of high-yield topics in neurology.
Pros: Well organized by focus points: pathogenesis, epidemiology,
management, complications, and associated diseases. Well illustrated,
and includes "minicases," links to a color atlas supplement, and updated treatments. **Cons:** Not comprehensive; best used as a supplement for review. **Summary:** An organized and easy-to-read supplement
to studying. Lengthy for a dedicated review of neurology.

B

Neurology Recall $36.95   Review
MILLER
Lippincott Williams & Wilkins, 2003, 2nd ed., 377 pages,
ISBN 9780781745888
Brief question-and-answer format. **Pros:** Reviews many important facts,
making it useful for self-quizzing. **Cons:** Not a comprehensive review.
Lengthy and lacks illustrations. Concepts are not integrated. **Sum-
mary:** Good for review of some high-yield concepts, but not a stand-
alone resource for this topic.

REVIEW RESOURCES

NEUROLOGY

Neurology Secrets

$45.95   Review

ROLAK

Elsevier, 2004, 4th ed., 480 pages, ISBN 9781560536215

A review book presented in Secrets-series question-and-answer format. **Pros:** A concise review of many high-yield topics. Makes good use of clinical images. **Cons:** Contains no clinical vignettes; instead, offers lists of questions that might be posed on the wards. Lacks a structured format, and leaves out important information. Relatively expensive and lengthy. Not a reference book. **Summary:** Overall, good content for self-quizzing and study, but does not substitute for a formal review or practice tests. More appropriate for clerkship than for boards review.

Blueprints Clinical Cases in Neurology

$29.95   Review

SHETH

Lippincott Williams & Wilkins, 2006, 2nd ed., 390 pages, ISBN 9781405104944

Vignette-type cases organized by symptom, followed by related question and answers. **Pros:** An excellent companion to the Blueprints subspecialty series. Focuses on high-yield cases. Easy to read, with nice illustrations and a good review of management. **Cons:** Not comprehensive; best used as a supplement. Offers few illustrations. **Summary:** Organized and easy to read. Adds clinical correlates to the Blueprints series.

A⁻ ***Blueprints in Obstetrics and Gynecology*** $38.95 Review/Test/100 q
CALLAHAN
Lippincott Williams & Wilkins, 2008, 5th ed., 368 pages,
ISBN 9780781782494
A text review with tables and illustrations. Includes a short exam with explanations. **Pros:** Places strong emphasis on high-yield topics with concise text, clear diagrams, and many classic illustrations. Makes for easy reading. Appropriate for both clinical clerkship and Step 2 CK preparation. **Cons:** Some topics are overly detailed, while some are not detailed enough. **Summary:** Overall, a good choice for boards and wards preparation.

A⁻ ***Blueprints Clinical Cases in Obstetrics and Gynecology*** $29.95 Test/200 q
CAUGHEY
Lippincott Williams & Wilkins, 2006, 2nd ed., 418 pages,
ISBN 9781405104906
Vignette-type cases arranged by symptom, followed by related questions and answers. **Pros:** An excellent companion to the Blueprints series. Focuses on high-yield cases. Easy to read, with nice illustrations and a good review of management. **Cons:** Not comprehensive; best used as a supplement. **Summary:** An organized and easy-to-read supplement. Adds clinical correlates to the Blueprints series.

A⁻ ***Underground Clinical Vignettes: OB/GYN*** $22.95 Review
KIM
Lippincott Williams & Wilkins, 2007, 4th ed., 256 pages,
ISBN 9780781768405
A clinical vignette–style review of frequently tested diseases in obstetrics and gynecology. **Pros:** Well organized by focus points: pathogenesis, epidemiology, management, complications, and associated diseases. Well illustrated. An easy read that stresses high-yield facts. **Cons:** Not comprehensive; best used as a supplement. **Summary:** Well-organized and easy-to-read practice vignettes.

REVIEW RESOURCES

OB/GYN

NMS Obstetrics and Gynecology
PFEIFER

$48.95   Review/Test/500 q

Lippincott Williams & Wilkins, 2007, 6th ed., 496 pages,
ISBN 9780781770712

A detailed outline of OB/GYN with few tables and diagrams. **Pros:** A comprehensive review for both wards and boards. The final exam is relatively good and offers complete explanations. **Cons:** The OB/GYN review is dense and lengthy. Many questions do not reflect the boards format. Lacks illustrations. **Summary:** A complete review with questions and discussions. Better for clerkship studying than for boards review.

High-Yield Obstetrics and Gynecology
SAKALA

$26.95   Review

Lippincott Williams & Wilkins, 2005, 2nd ed., 208 pages,
ISBN 9780781796309

A review of high-yield topics in outline format. Clinical scenarios at the end of each chapter highlight key points. **Pros:** Easy to read, with a good discussion of high-yield topics. **Cons:** Lacks depth and contains no practice questions. **Summary:** A quick but superficial review.

First Aid for the OB/GYN Clerkship
STEAD

$42.95   Review

McGraw-Hill, 2006, 2nd ed., 304 pages, ISBN 9780071448741

A high-yield review of symptoms and diseases. **Pros:** A comprehensive review with nice diagrams, images, charts, algorithms, and mnemonics. **Cons:** Lengthy review. **Summary:** An excellent review of OB/GYN, but too lengthy for boards review.

Case Files: Obstetrics and Gynecology
TOY

$32.95   Review

McGraw-Hill, 2009, 3rd ed., 456 pages, ISBN 9780071605809

A review of OB/GYN in case format with questions and answers following each vignette. **Pros:** Cases reflect high-yield topics and are arranged in an easy-to-follow format. **Cons:** Some topics are either not covered or given only brief treatment. Contains few diagrams and images. Lengthy and time-consuming for one topic. Explanations are terse. **Summary:** A good review of the subject in clinical vignette format, but may be too detailed for Step 2 CK review.

B+

Blueprints Q & A Step 2 Obstetrics & Gynecology

TRAN

$19.95   Test/200 q

Lippincott Williams & Wilkins, 2004, 2nd ed., 168 pages,
ISBN 9781405103909

One hundred vignette-style questions. **Pros:** A nice companion to the Blueprints series. Focuses on high-yield topics. Explanations are easy to follow. **Cons:** Not comprehensive; best used as a supplement for review. Sparse images. Some questions are esoteric and not boards-like. **Summary:** A well-organized and easy-to-read supplement. Adds clinical correlates to the Blueprints series.

B

Obstetrics and Gynecology Secrets

BADER

$31.95   Review

Mosby, 2004, 3rd ed., 448 pages, ISBN 9780323034159

A review book presented in Secrets-series question-and-answer format, organized by topic within OB/GYN. **Pros:** Offers good coverage of many high-yield, clinically relevant topics. **Cons:** Too detailed to be useful for rapid review. Contains no vignettes and few illustrations or images. **Summary:** Good clinical content, but does not serve as a formal topic review. Better for use during clerkship than for Step 2 CK preparation.

B

PreTest Obstetrics and Gynecology

SCHNEIDER

$26.95   Test/500 q

McGraw-Hill, 2009, 12th ed., 355 pages, ISBN 9780071599795

A question-and-answer review with detailed explanations for OB/GYN. **Pros:** Organization by subtopic may be useful for studying weak areas. Good content emphasis. Generally well illustrated. **Cons:** Some questions are too difficult or detailed. Vignette-based questions are shorter and more simplistic than those on the Step 2 CK. **Summary:** A decent source of questions to supplement topic study, especially for addressing specific areas of weakness.

B–

Obstetrics and Gynecology Recall

BOURGEOIS

$36.95   Review/Test/350 q

Lippincott Williams & Wilkins, 2007, 3rd ed., 608 pages,
ISBN 9780781770699

A review book presented in standard Recall-series question-and-answer style. **Pros:** The two-column format makes the text useful for self-quizzing. Reviews many high-yield concepts and facts. **Cons:** Questions emphasize individual facts but do not integrate concepts. Contains no vignettes or images. Coverage of some topics is spotty. **Summary:** Useful for review of selected concepts, but not a comprehensive source for Step 2 CK preparation. More appropriate for clerkship than for boards.

A⁻

Platinum Vignettes: Pediatrics   *$29.95*   Review

BROCHERT

Hanley & Belfus, 2002, 1st ed., 104 pages, ISBN 9781560535331

A clinical vignette–based review of common topics in pediatrics. **Pros:**
Well-written cases are similar to boards-type vignettes. Well illustrated.
The discussion is organized by pathophysiology, diagnosis and treatment, and more high-yield facts. **Cons:** Expensive for the amount of
material. Not comprehensive; best used as a supplement. Has not
been updated since 2002. **Summary:** An organized and easy-to-read
supplement to studying.

A⁻

Underground Clinical Vignettes: Pediatrics   *$22.95*   Review

KIM

Lippincott Williams & Wilkins, 2007, 4th ed., 256 pages,
ISBN 9780781768443

A clinical vignette review of frequently tested topics in pediatrics. **Pros:**
Well organized by focus points: pathogenesis, epidemiology, management, complications, and associated diseases. Well illustrated, and the
new edition includes "minicases" to broaden subject material and
present more high-yield information. **Cons:** Not comprehensive; best
used as a supplement to text review. **Summary:** Well organized and
easy to read, but intended as a supplement for review.

A⁻

PreTest Pediatrics   *$26.95*   Test/500 q

YETMAN

McGraw-Hill, 2006, 11th ed., 464 pages, ISBN 9780071455527

A question-and-answer review with detailed discussion. **Pros:** Organization by organ system is useful for pinpointing weaknesses. Gives
strong, thorough explanations. Includes a fair number of vignette-style
questions. Well illustrated. **Cons:** Some questions are too detailed or
emphasize low-yield topics. **Summary:** A good source of questions and
review for pediatrics. Solid content with good illustrations, although
not entirely in Step 2 CK format.

REVIEW RESOURCES

PEDIATRICS

Blueprints Q & A Step 2 Pediatrics   *$17.95*   Test/100 q

FOTI

Lippincott Williams & Wilkins, 2004, 2nd ed., 176 pages,
ISBN 9781405103916

Vignette-style questions. **Pros:** A nice companion to the Blueprints series. Focuses on high-yield topics. Explanations are easy to follow. **Cons:** Not comprehensive; best used as a supplement for review. Sparse images. **Summary:** An organized and easy-to-read supplement. Adds clinical correlates to the Blueprints series.

In A Page Pediatrics   *$34.95*   Review

KAHAN

Lippincott Williams & Wilkins, 2008, 2nd ed., 384 pages,
ISBN 9780781770453

One-page reviews of 228 diseases/topics discussed by etiology, epidemiology, signs/symptoms, differential diagnosis, diagnostic tests, treatment, and prognosis. **Pros:** A fast and concise review of high-yield information on common diseases. **Cons:** Each topic is crowded onto one page without any images or diagrams. Includes low-yield topics. **Summary:** Useful for quick study on the wards, but too time intensive for Step 2 CK review.

Blueprints Clinical Cases in Pediatrics   *$29.95*   Test/200 q

LONDHE

Lippincott Williams & Wilkins, 2006, 2nd ed., 426 pages,
ISBN 9781405104920

Vignette-type cases arranged by symptom followed by related questions and answers. **Pros:** An excellent companion to the Blueprints series. Focuses on high-yield cases. Easy to read with nice illustrations and a good review of management. **Cons:** Not comprehensive; best used as a supplement for review. **Summary:** An organized and easy-to-read supplement. Adds clinical correlates to the Blueprints series.

Blueprints in Pediatrics   *$38.95*   Review/Test/100 q

MARINO

Lippincott Williams & Wilkins, 2008, 5th ed., 384 pages,
ISBN 9780781782517

A text review of pediatrics with tables and diagrams. Includes a question-and-answer section with explanations. **Pros:** Appropriate focus on high-yield topics. **Cons:** A relatively dense text with few illustrations. Overly detailed. **Summary:** Good for a more comprehensive review.

Case Files: Pediatrics

TOY

$29.95   Review

McGraw-Hill, 2006, 2nd ed., 576 pages,
ISBN 9780071463027

A review of pediatrics in case format with questions and answers following each vignette. **Pros:** Cases reflect high-yield topics and are arranged in an easy-to-follow format. Emphasizes the next step and the most likely diagnosis. **Cons:** Not suited for high-yield rapid review. **Summary:** An excellent review with emphasis on vignette-style case presentation and important boards-type answers, but may be too detailed for a stand-alone boards review book. Excellent for clerkship preparation.

A&L's Review of Pediatrics

VIESSMAN

$41.95   Test/1000+ q

McGraw-Hill, 2004, 6th ed., 250 pages, ISBN 9780838503034

A question-and-answer review of pediatrics with detailed explanations. **Pros:** Questions focus on boards-relevant content. The last chapter includes excellent vignette-based questions. Offers thorough, well-written explanations. Includes a nice primer on test-taking strategies. **Cons:** Non-vignette-based questions are shorter and more straightforward than those on the Step 2 CK exam. Some questions may be too detailed for Step 2 CK preparation. Poorly illustrated. **Summary:** An excellent, concise review with appropriate content and good discussions, but the majority of questions do not reflect Step 2 CK style.

NMS Pediatrics

DWORKIN

$42.95   Review/Test/100+ q

Lippincott Williams & Wilkins, 2008, 5th ed., 480 pages,
ISBN 9780781770750

A general review of pediatrics in outline format. Includes questions at the end of each chapter. **Pros:** A thorough, detailed review of pediatrics. Boldfacing highlights key points. Case studies and a comprehensive exam at the end of the book (also provided on CD-ROM) are helpful. Includes a good discussion. **Cons:** A dense, lengthy text. Lacks good illustrations of any kind. **Summary:** A thorough review, but more appropriate for clerkships than for Step 2 CK review, in large part because of its depth.

B⁻ | ***Pediatrics Recall*** | **$36.95** | Review

McGahren

Lippincott Williams & Wilkins, 2007, 3rd ed., 508 pages, ISBN 9780781771184

A review book presented in a concise question-and-answer format typical of the Recall series. **Pros:** The two-column format makes self-quizzing easy. Emphasis is placed on diagnosis and management. **Cons:** Requires time commitment, and not all topics are covered thoroughly. Contains no vignettes. **Summary:** Useful material, but does not provide a systematic review or a substitute for practice tests. Better suited to clerkship review.

B⁻ | ***Pediatric Secrets*** | **$39.95** | Review

Polin

Elsevier, 2005, 4th ed., 688 pages, ISBN 9781560536277

A question-and-answer text typical of the Secrets series, organized by pediatric subspecialty. **Pros:** Includes a thorough discussion of a wide variety of clinical topics. **Cons:** Detailed content is geared toward the wards and requires significant time investment. Contains no images or illustrations. **Summary:** Too detailed for USMLE review; better suited to clerkship.

A

Blueprints in Psychiatry   *$29.95*   Review/Test/74 q
MURPHY
Lippincott Williams & Wilkins, 2007, 2nd ed., 304 pages,
ISBN 9781405104968
A brief text review of psychiatry with DSM-IV criteria. Includes a brief
question-and-answer section at the end of the book. **Pros:** A clear, concise review of psychiatry with helpful tables. Offers good coverage of
high-yield topics, including pharmacology. A quick read. **Cons:** Too
general in certain areas; requires some supplementation. **Summary:** A
rapid review with appropriate coverage of high-yield topics.

A⁻

Blueprints Clinical Cases in Psychiatry   *$29.95*   Test/200 q
HOBLYN
Lippincott Williams & Wilkins, 2007, 2nd ed., 304 pages,
ISBN 9781405104968
Vignette-type cases arranged by symptom, followed by related questions and answers. **Pros:** An excellent companion to the Blueprints series. Focuses on high-yield cases. Easy to read with nice illustrations
and a good review of management. **Cons:** Not comprehensive; best
used as a supplement for review. **Summary:** An organized and easy-to-
read supplement. Adds clinical correlates to the Blueprints series.

A⁻

Underground Clinical Vignettes: Psychiatry   *$22.95*   Review
KIM
Lippincott Williams & Wilkins, 2007, 4th ed., 256 pages,
ISBN 9780781768467
A clinical vignette–based review of frequently tested topics in psychiatry. **Pros:** Well organized by focus points: pathogenesis, epidemiology,
management, and associated diseases. Well illustrated, and includes
"minicases" that present high-yield information. **Cons:** Not comprehensive; best used as a supplement. **Summary:** Offers organized and
easy-to-read practice vignettes.

PreTest Psychiatry

$26.95   Test/500 q

KLAMEN

McGraw-Hill, 2006, 11th ed., 355 pages, ISBN 9780071455541

A question-and-answer review of topics in psychiatry. **Pros:** Questions are well written and organized. Most questions have appropriate content level. Offers good explanations. **Cons:** Includes too few vignette-type questions. Some questions are too detailed. **Summary:** A good source of questions and review for psychiatry and the Step 2 CK exam, although the format may not reflect the actual test.

High-Yield Psychiatry

$28.95   Review

FADEM

Lippincott Williams & Wilkins, 2003, 2nd ed., 150 pages, ISBN 9780781742689

A brief outline-format review of psychiatry. **Pros:** A quick read, with clinical vignettes scattered throughout. Offers concise tables. **Cons:** Not sufficiently detailed for in-depth review. **Summary:** An excellent, quick review of psychiatry for use as an additional study source. Similar to *High-Yield Behavioral Sciences* by the same author.

A&L's Review of Psychiatry

$34.95   Test/900+ q

ORANSKY

McGraw-Hill, 2003, 7th ed., 304 pages, ISBN 9780071402538

A general review of psychiatry with questions and answers. **Pros:** Includes 114 vignette-style questions appropriate for boards review. Appropriate content emphasis; thorough explanations. The new edition features updated treatment and management sections. **Cons:** Questions are shorter and more straightforward than those of the boards. **Summary:** A decent source of boards review for psychiatry, but does not reflect boards format.

Case Files: Psychiatry

$29.95   Review

TOY

McGraw-Hill, 2006, 2nd ed., 408 pages, ISBN 9780071462822

A review of psychology in case format with questions and answers following each vignette. **Pros:** Cases reflect high-yield topics and are arranged in an easy-to-follow format. Emphasizes the next step, the most likely diagnosis, and the best initial treatment. **Cons:** Not suited to high-yield rapid review, and may be too detailed for Step 2 CK review. **Summary:** An excellent subject review that places emphasis on vignette-style case presentation and important boards-type answers. Great for the wards, and a good supplement for the boards.

Platinum Vignettes: Psychiatry

$29.95   Review

BROCHERT

Hanley & Belfus, 2002, 1st ed., 102 pages, ISBN 9781560535348

A clinical vignette review of common topics in psychiatry. **Pros:** Well-written cases are similar to boards-type vignettes. Well illustrated. Discussion is organized by pathophysiology, diagnosis and treatment, and more high-yield facts. **Cons:** Not comprehensive; best used as a supplement. **Summary:** An organized and easy-to-read supplement to studying. Needs updating.

Blueprints Q & A Step 2 Psychiatry

$17.95   Test/200 q

MCLOONE

Lippincott Williams & Wilkins, 2004, 2nd ed., 96 pages, ISBN 9781405103923

Vignette-style questions. **Pros:** A nice companion to the Blueprints series. Focuses on high-yield topics. Explanations are easy to follow. **Cons:** Not comprehensive; best used as a supplement for review. Sparse images. Some questions are esoteric and not boards-like. **Summary:** An organized and easy-to-read supplement. Adds clinical correlates to the Blueprints series.

NMS Psychiatry

$42.95   Review/Test/500 q

SCULLY

Lippincott Williams & Wilkins, 2007, 5th ed., 300 pages, ISBN 9780781765145

A general review of topics in outline format with questions at the end of each chapter and a comprehensive final exam. **Pros:** A well-written text with concise disease discussions. Includes an expanded pharmacology section. Questions test appropriate content and have complete explanations, and the new edition offers more vignette-style questions. A good companion text for the clerkship. **Cons:** Does not contain enough vignette-style questions. Lengthy for purposes of boards review. **Summary:** A detailed review that requires time commitment. A good single choice for clerkship study, but may be too long for Step 2 CK review.

First Aid for the Psychiatry Clerkship

$42.95   Review

STEAD

McGraw-Hill, 2005, 2nd ed., 208 pages, ISBN 9780071448727

A high-yield review of symptoms and diseases. **Pros:** A comprehensive review that includes DSM-IV criteria with nice mnemonics and scenarios. Includes high-yield tear-out cards. **Cons:** May not appeal to readers who prefer information in text format. **Summary:** A good review of high-yield topics in psychiatry, but better suited to clerkship than to Step 2 CK study.

Psychiatry Recall

$36.95   Review

FADEM

Lippincott Williams & Wilkins, 2009, 3rd ed., 210 pages,
ISBN 9780781776981

A review book presented in the quick question-and-answer format typical of the Recall series. **Pros:** The two-column format is conducive to self-quizzing. Covers many high-yield facts and concepts necessary for the USMLE. **Cons:** Lacks vignettes, so does not substitute for practice tests. **Summary:** Requires time commitment. Some topics are glossed over. Best used as a supplement to other resources.

Psychiatry Made Ridiculously Simple

$13.95   Review

GOOD

MedMaster, 2005, 4th ed., 98 pages, ISBN 9780940780682

Part of the "Made Ridiculously Simple" series. **Pros:** A comprehensive, fast read with nice tables and entertaining illustrations to highlight key points. **Cons:** Some areas are not detailed enough, while others are too verbose. Not boards oriented. **Summary:** A good, fast review, but more helpful for clerkship than for the boards.

Psychiatric Secrets

$39.95   Review

JACOBSON

Hanley & Belfus, 2000, 2nd ed., 536 pages, ISBN 9781560534181

A review book presented in the question-and-discussion format typical of the Secrets series, organized by topic. **Pros:** Offers clear explanations of important concepts in psychiatry. Makes for good wards reading. **Cons:** Too detailed and lengthy for review purposes. Lacks vignettes. **Summary:** Requires significant time commitment; not for rapid, focused review. Best suited to clerkship review.

BRS Psychiatry

$37.95   Review/400 q

SHANER

Lippincott Williams & Wilkins, 2000, 2nd ed., 419 pages,
ISBN 9780683307665

A comprehensive review of psychiatry in outline format. Vignette-style questions follow each chapter. **Pros:** A thorough, systematic review of clinical psychiatry. Clear, concise definitions are provided. **Cons:** Great deal of information for single-topic review. The pharmacology section is out of date. **Summary:** Good material, but requires a large time investment; needs updating.

A⁻

Underground Clinical Vignettes: Surgery
KIM

Lippincott Williams & Wilkins, 2007, 4th ed., 256 pages,
ISBN 9780781768474

$22.95   Review

A clinical vignette–based review of frequently tested surgical topics. **Pros:** Well organized by focus points: pathogenesis, epidemiology, management, complications, and associated diseases. Well illustrated and includes "minicases" that present high-yield information. **Cons:** Not comprehensive; best used as a supplement to review. **Summary:** Well-organized and easy-to-read practice vignettes.

A⁻

Case Files: Surgery
TOY

McGraw-Hill, 2006, 2nd ed., 504 pages, ISBN 9780071463041

$29.95   Review

A review of surgery in case format with questions and answers following each vignette. **Pros:** Cases reflect high-yield topics and are arranged in an easy-to-follow format. Emphasizes the next step and the most likely diagnosis. **Cons:** Not suited to high-yield rapid review, and may be too detailed for Step 2 CK preparation. **Summary:** An excellent review with emphasis on vignette-style case presentation and important boards-type answers. Great for clerkship study, and a good supplement for boards study.

B⁺

Platinum Vignettes: Surgery and Trauma
BROCHERT

Hanley & Belfus, 2002, 1st ed., 102 pages, ISBN 9781560535355

$29.95   Review

A clinical vignette–based review of common topics in surgery and trauma medicine. **Pros:** Well-written cases are similar to boards-type vignettes. Well illustrated. Discussion is organized by pathophysiology, diagnosis and treatment, and more high-yield facts. **Cons:** Expensive for the amount of material. Not comprehensive; best used as a supplement. **Summary:** An organized and easy-to-read supplement to studying.

B⁺

PreTest Surgery
KAO

McGraw-Hill, 2009, 12th ed., 373 pages, ISBN 9780071598637

$26.95   Test/500 q

A review of topics in general surgery in question-and-answer format. **Pros:** Predominantly case based. Well organized by subspecialty. **Cons:** Many questions are too detailed or esoteric and do not reflect boards style. Some explanations are overly detailed. **Summary:** A thorough review, but questions may be beyond the level needed for Step 2 CK preparation.

NMS Surgery
JARRELL
Lippincott Williams & Wilkins, 2007, 5th ed., 645 pages,
ISBN 9780781759014

$42.95   Review/Test/350 q

An outline review of general surgery and surgical subspecialties. **Pros:** Well organized and thorough. Vignette-style questions are included after each chapter with good explanations. **Cons:** Dense, detailed text. Few tables or illustrations. **Summary:** A comprehensive surgery review, but very time consuming. More appropriate for clerkship than for boards review.

In A Page Surgery
KAHAN
Lippincott Williams & Wilkins, 2003, 1st ed., 288 pages,
ISBN 9781405103657

$34.95   Review

One-page reviews of diseases/topics discussed by etiology, epidemiology, signs/symptoms, differential diagnosis, diagnostic tests, treatment, and prognosis. **Pros:** A fast and concise review of high-yield information on common diseases. **Cons:** Text is crowded onto one page without any images or diagrams. Includes low-yield topics. **Summary:** Useful for quick study on the wards, but too time intensive for Step 2 CK review.

Blueprints in Surgery
KARP
Lippincott Williams & Wilkins, 2009, 5th ed., 320 pages,
ISBN 9780781788687

$38.95   Review/Test/100 q

A short text review of general surgery with tables and diagrams. A brief question-and-answer section is included. **Pros:** Well organized. Easy to read, with a strong focus on high-yield topics. Includes clear diagrams. **Cons:** Some sections are overly detailed (e.g., anatomy), while others are occasionally too simplistic. Too few illustrations. **Summary:** A good review of surgery, but not ideal for Step 2 CK preparation.

Blueprints Clinical Cases in Surgery
LI
Lippincott Williams & Wilkins, 2006, 2nd ed., 304 pages,
ISBN 9781405104937

$29.95   Test/200 q

Vignette-type cases arranged by symptom followed by related questions and answers. **Pros:** A excellent companion to the Blueprints series. Focuses on high-yield cases. Easy to read with nice illustrations and a good review of management. **Cons:** Not comprehensive; best used as a supplement for review. **Summary:** An organized and easy-to-read supplement. Adds clinical correlates to the Blueprints series.

B

High-Yield Surgery
NIRULA

$26.95   Review

Lippincott Williams & Wilkins, 2005, 2nd ed., 160 pages,
ISBN 9780781776561

An outline review of most common general surgery topics. **Pros:** Concise; useful for quick topic review. Well organized. **Cons:** Information can be superficial. Some topics are omitted. Offers no practice questions. **Summary:** A lean text for rapid review.

B

A&L's Review of Surgery
WAPNICK

$34.95   Test/1000+ q

McGraw-Hill, 2003, 4th ed., 320 pages, ISBN 9780071378147

A general review of surgery with questions and answers. **Pros:** Good clinical emphasis. Includes many vignette-style questions. Explanations are thorough. **Cons:** Some questions are too short, and the style does not reflect that of the Step 2 CK exam. Questions are highly variable in difficulty and are often far too detailed. Offers few illustrations. **Summary:** Good content for the exam, but much too detailed for clerkship and Step 2 CK review.

B⁻

Surgical Recall
BLACKBOURNE

$44.95   Review

Lippincott Williams & Wilkins, 2008, 5th ed., 800 pages,
ISBN 9780781770767

A review book presented in standard Recall-series question-and-answer format. **Pros:** Questions emphasize important, high-yield clinical concepts. Columns allow for self-testing. Fast review. Good preparation for "pimping" on rounds. **Cons:** Does not feature boards-type questions. Poorly organized. Coverage of some topics is spotty. **Summary:** A useful adjunct to a more organized topic review. Much more appropriate for clerkship than for boards review.

B⁻

Abernathy's Surgical Secrets
HARKEN

$47.95   Review

Elsevier, 2008, 6th ed., 534 pages, ISBN 9780323057110

A review book presented in a question-and-answer format typical of the Secrets series. **Pros:** Discussions are up to date and thorough. **Cons:** Too detailed for the purposes of the Step 2 CK, yet not comprehensive. **Summary:** Not a well-organized review. Better suited to clerkship than to boards preparation.

B−

Pocket Surgery   ***$36.95***   Review

MOSCA

Lippincott Williams & Wilkins, 2001, 1st ed., 160 pages,
ISBN 9780781735797

A review of high-yield surgical material in outline format. **Pros:** A fast, easy read. Portable. Highlights high-yield information in "fact boxes." **Cons:** Some material is not detailed enough. Offers no illustrations. **Summary:** Good for rapid review during clerkship. Does not contain enough detailed information to be used as a single study source for the boards.

B

First Aid for the International Medical Graduate $39.95 Review
CHANDER

McGraw-Hill, 2002, 2nd ed., 313 pages, ISBN 9780071385329

A high-yield review for the IMG on how to pass the USMLE boards and adapt to medical culture in the United States. **Pros:** A comprehensive, well-organized review. **Cons:** Some readers may need to obtain additional information from other sources. Immigration and visa information is outdated. **Summary:** An excellent review of material for the IMG. Best used as a primer for boards review.

Commercial preparation courses can be helpful for some students, but such courses are typically expensive and require significant time commitment. They are usually effective in organizing study material for students who feel overwhelmed by the sheer volume of material involved in Step 2 CK preparation. Note that multiweek courses may be quite intense and may thus leave limited time for independent study. Also note that some commercial courses are designed for first-time test takers while others focus on students who are repeating the exam. In addition, some courses are geared toward IMGs who want to take all three Steps in a limited amount of time.

Student experience and satisfaction with review courses are highly variable. We suggest that you discuss options with recent graduates of the review courses you are considering. In addition, course content and structure can change rapidly. Some student opinions can be found in discussion groups on the World Wide Web. Listed below is contact information for some Step 2 CK commercial review courses.

Falcon Physician Reviews
440 Wrangler Drive, Suite 100
Coppell, TX 75019
(214) 632-5466
Fax: (214) 292.8568
info@falconreviews.com
www.falconreviews.com

Kaplan Medical
700 South Flower Street
Los Angeles, CA 90017
(800) KAP-TEST (800-527-8378)
www.kaptest.com

Northwestern Medical Review
P.O. Box 22174
East Lansing, MI 48909-2174
(866) MedPass (866-633-7277)
Fax: (517) 347-7005
contactus@northwesternmedicalreview.com
http://northwesternmedicalreview.com

Postgraduate Medical Review Education (PMRE)
1909 Tyler Street, Suite 305
Hollywood, FL 33020
(877) 662-2005
Fax: (954) 926-3333
sales@pmre.com
www.pmre.com

Youel's Prep, Inc.
P.O. Box 31479
Palm Beach Gardens, FL 33420
(800) 645-3985
Fax: (561) 622-4858
info@youelsprep.com
www.youelsprep.com

APPENDIX I

Abbreviations and Symbols

Abbreviation	Meaning
A-a	alveolar-arterial (oxygen gradient)
AAA	abdominal aortic aneurysm
AAMC	Association of American Medical Colleges
ABG	arterial blood gas
ABI	ankle-brachial index
ABVD	Adriamycin (doxorubicin), bleomycin, vinblastine, dacarbazine
AC	abdominal circumference
ACA	anterior cerebral artery
ACC	American College of Cardiology
ACE	angiotensin-converting enzyme
ACEI	angiotensin-converting enzyme inhibitor
ACh	acetylcholine
ACL	anterior cruciate ligament
ACLS	advanced cardiac life support (protocol)
ACTH	adrenocorticotropic hormone
AD	Alzheimer's disease
ADA	American Diabetes Association, Americans with Disabilities Act
ADH	antidiuretic hormone
ADHD	attention-deficit hyperactivity disorder
ADPKD	autosomal-dominant polycystic kidney disease
AF	atrial fibrillation
AFB	acid-fast bacillus
AFI	amniotic fluid index
AFP	α-fetoprotein
AGC	atypical glandular cell
AHA	American Heart Association
AI	adrenal insufficiency
AICA	anterior inferior cerebellar artery
AIDS	acquired immunodeficiency syndrome
ALL	acute lymphocytic leukemia
ALS	amyotrophic lateral sclerosis
ALT	alanine aminotransferase
AMD	age-related macular degeneration

Abbreviation	Meaning
AML	acute myelogenous leukemia
ANA	antinuclear antibody
ANC	absolute neutrophil count
ANCA	antineutrophil cytoplasmic antibody
AOA	American Osteopathic Association
AP	anteroposterior
APC	activated protein C
APL	acute promyelocytic leukemia
aPTT	activated partial thromboplastin time
ARB	angiotensin receptor blocker
ARC	Appalachian Regional Commission
ARDS	acute respiratory distress syndrome
ARF	acute renal failure
ARPKD	autosomal-recessive polycystic kidney disease
5-ASA	5-aminosalicylic acid
ASA	acetylsalicylic acid
ASC	atypical squamous cells
ASC-H	atypical squamous cells suspicious of high-grade dysplasia
ASC-US	atypical squamous cells of undetermined significance
ASD	atrial septal defect
ASO	antistreptolysin O
AST	aspartate aminotransferase
ATN	acute tubular necrosis
ATRA	all-*trans* retinoic acid
AV	atrioventricular
AVM	arteriovenous malformation
AVN	avascular necrosis
AVNRT	atrioventricular nodal reentry tachycardia
AVRT	atrioventricular reciprocating tachycardia
AXR	abdominal x-ray
BAL	British anti-Lewisite (dimercaprol), bronchoalveolar lavage
BCC	basal cell carcinoma
BCG	bacille Calmette-Guérin
β-hCG	β-human chorionic gonadotropin

Abbreviation	Meaning
BID	twice a day
BMI	body mass index
BMZ	basement membrane zone
BP	blood pressure
BPD	biparietal diameter
BPH	benign prostatic hyperplasia
bpm	beats per minute
BPP	biophysical profile
BPPV	benign paroxysmal positional vertigo
BSA	body surface area
BT	bleeding time
BUN	blood urea nitrogen
BW	birth weight
CABG	coronary artery bypass graft
CAD	coronary artery disease
CaEDTA	calcium disodium edetate
CAH	congenital adrenal hyperplasia
cAMP	cyclic adenosine monophosphate
c-ANCA	cytoplasmic antineutrophil cytoplasmic antibody
CBC	complete blood count
CBT	cognitive-behavioral therapy, computer-based testing
CCB	calcium channel blocker
CCS	computer-based case simulation
CD	cluster of differentiation
CEA	carcinoembryonic antigen
CF	cystic fibrosis
CFU	colony-forming unit
CGD	chronic granulomatous disease
cGMP	cyclic guanosine monophosphate
CHF	congestive heart failure
CHOP	cyclophosphamide (Cytoxan), hydroxydaunorubicin (Adriamycin), Oncovin (vincristine), prednisone
CI	confidence interval
CIN	candidate identification number, cervical intraepithelial neoplasia
CJD	Creutzfeldt-Jakob disease
CK	clinical knowledge, creatine kinase
CKD	chronic kidney disease
CK-MB	creatine kinase, MB fraction
CLL	chronic lymphocytic leukemia
CML	chronic myelogenous leukemia
CMP	comprehensive metabolic panel
CMV	cytomegalovirus
CN	cranial nerve
CNS	central nervous system
CO	carbon monoxide
COGME	Council on Graduate Medical Education
COMT	catechol-O-methyltransferase

Abbreviation	Meaning
COPD	chronic obstructive pulmonary disease
CPAP	continuous positive airway pressure
CPR	cardiopulmonary resuscitation
CPS	child protective services
Cr	creatinine
CRL	crown-rump length
CRP	C-reactive protein
CS	clinical skills
CSA	central sleep apnea
CSD	combined system disease
CSF	cerebrospinal fluid
CST	contraction stress test
CT	computed tomography
CTS	carpal tunnel syndrome
CVA	cerebrovascular accident
CVP	central venous pressure
CVS	chorionic villus sampling
CXR	chest x-ray
D&C	dilation and curettage
D&E	dilation and evacuation
DA	developmental age
DBP	diastolic blood pressure
DDAVP	desmopressin acetate
DES	diethylstilbestrol
DEXA	dual-energy x-ray absorptiometry
DFA	direct fluorescent antibody
DHEA	dehydroepiandrosterone
DHEAS	dehydroepiandrosterone sulfate
DHS	Department of Homeland Security
DI	diabetes insipidus
DIC	disseminated intravascular coagulation
DIP	distal interphalangeal (joint)
DKA	diabetic ketoacidosis
DL_{CO}	diffusion capacity of carbon monoxide
DM	diabetes mellitus
DMARD	disease-modifying antirheumatic drug
DMD	Duchenne muscular dystrophy
DMSA	dimercaptosuccinic acid
DNA	deoxyribonucleic acid
DNI	do not intubate
DNR	do not resuscitate
DPOAHC	durable power of attorney for health care
DRE	digital rectal exam
dsDNA	double-stranded deoxyribonucleic acid
DSM	Diagnostic and Statistical Manual (of mental disorders)
DTaP	diphtheria, tetanus, acellular pertussis (vaccine)
DTRs	deep tendon reflexes

Abbreviation	Meaning
DTs	delirium tremens
DVT	deep venous thrombosis
EBV	Epstein-Barr virus
EC	emergency contraception
ECC	endocervical curettage
ECFMG	Educational Commission for Foreign Medical Graduates
ECG	electrocardiography
ECT	electroconvulsive therapy
ED	erectile dysfunction
EEG	electroencephalography
EF	ejection fraction
EFW	estimated fetal weight
EGD	esophagogastroduodenoscopy
ELISA	enzyme-linked immunosorbent assay
EM	electron microscopy
EMG	electromyography
ENT	ear, nose, and throat
EOM	extraocular movement
E/P	estrogen/progesterone
EPS	extrapyramidal symptoms
ER	emergency room, estrogen receptor
ERAS	Electronic Residency Application Service
ERCP	endoscopic retrograde cholangiopancreatography
ERV	expiratory reserve volume
ESR	erythrocyte sedimentation rate
ESRD	end-stage renal disease
ESWL	extracorporeal shock-wave lithotripsy
EtOH	ethanol
FAM-M	familial atypical mole and melanoma (syndrome)
FAST	focused abdominal sonography for trauma (scan)
FDP	fibrin degradation product
Fe_{Na}	fractional excretion of sodium
FEV_1	forced expiratory volume in 1 second
FFP	fresh frozen plasma
FHR	fetal heart rate
FiO_2	fraction of inspired oxygen
FIT	fecal immunochemical test
FL	femur length
FLAIR	fluid-attenuated inversion recovery (imaging)
FMG	foreign medical graduate
FNA	fine-needle aspiration
FOBT	fecal occult blood test
FSH	follicle-stimulating hormone
FSMB	Federation of State Medical Boards
FTA-ABS	fluorescent treponemal antibody absorption (test)
FTT	failure to thrive

Abbreviation	Meaning
5-FU	5-fluorouracil
FUO	fever of unknown origin
FVC	forced vital capacity
G6PD	glucose-6-phosphate dehydrogenase
GA	gestational age
GABA	gamma-aminobutyric acid
GAF	global assessment of functioning
GAS	group A streptococcus
GBM	glioblastoma multiforme, glomerular basement membrane
GBS	group B streptococcus, Guillain-Barré syndrome
GCS	Glasgow Coma Scale
G-CSF	granulocyte colony-stimulating factor
GERD	gastroesophageal reflux disease
GFR	glomerular filtration rate
GGT	gamma-glutamyl transferase
GH	growth hormone
GI	gastrointestinal
GLP	glucagon-like peptide
GM-CSF	granulocyte-macrophage colony-stimulating factor
GNR	gram-negative rod
GnRH	gonadotropin-releasing hormone
GTD	gestational trophoblastic disease
GU	genitourinary
GVHD	graft-versus-host disease
H&E	hematoxylin and eosin
HAART	highly active antiretroviral therapy
HAV	hepatitis A virus
HbA_{1c}	hemoglobin A_{1c}
HBcAb	hepatitis B core antibody
HBcAg	hepatitis B core antigen
HBsAb	hepatitis B surface antibody
HBsAg	hepatitis B surface antigen
HBV	hepatitis B virus
hCG	human chorionic gonadotropin
HCL	hairy cell leukemia
HCTZ	hydrochlorothiazide
HCV	hepatitis C virus
HD	Huntington's disease, Hodgkin's disease
HDL	high-density lipoprotein
HDV	hepatitis D virus
HES	hypereosinophilic syndrome
HEV	hepatitis E virus
HHNK	hyperosmolar hyperglycemic nonketotic (coma)
HHS	hyperosmolar hyperglycemic state, Health and Human Services
HHV	human herpesvirus
5-HIAA	5-hydroxyindoleacetic acid
Hib	*Haemophilus influenzae* type b

Abbreviation	Meaning
HIDA	hepato-iminodiacetic acid (scan)
HIV	human immunodeficiency virus
HLA	human leukocyte antigen
HMG-CoA	hydroxymethylglutaryl coenzyme A
HNPCC	hereditary nonpolyposis colorectal cancer
HOCM	hypertrophic obstructive cardiomyopathy
17-HP	17-hydroxyprogesterone
HPA	human placental antigen, hypothalamic-pituitary-adrenal (axis)
hpf	high-power field
HPSA	Health Professional Shortage Area
HPV	human papillomavirus
HRT	hormone replacement therapy
HSIL	high-grade squamous intraepithelial lesion
HSV	herpesvirus
HTLV	human T-cell lymphotropic virus
HUS	hemolytic-uremic syndrome
HVA	homovanillic acid
IBD	inflammatory bowel disease
IBS	irritable bowel syndrome
IC	inspiratory capacity
ICD	implantable cardiac defibrillator
ICP	intracranial pressure
ICSI	intracytoplasmic sperm injection
ICU	intensive care unit
I/E	inspiratory to expiratory (ratio)
IFN-α	α-interferon
Ig	immunoglobulin
IGF	insulin-like growth factor
IM	intramuscular
IMED	International Medical Education Directory
IMG	international medical graduate
INH	isoniazid
INR	International Normalized Ratio
I/O	intake and output
IOP	intraocular pressure
IPV	inactivated polio vaccine
IRB	institutional review board
IRV	inspiratory reserve volume
ITP	idiopathic thrombocytopenic purpura
IUD	intrauterine device
IUGR	intrauterine growth restriction
IUI	intrauterine insemination
IV	intravenous
IVC	inferior vena cava
IVF	in vitro fertilization
IVIG	intravenous immunoglobulin
IVP	intravenous pyelography

Abbreviation	Meaning
JIA	juvenile idiopathic arthritis
JNC	Joint National Committee on Prevention, Detection, Evaluation, and Treatment of High Blood Pressure
JRA	juvenile rheumatoid arthritis
JVD	jugular venous distention
JVP	jugular venous pulse
KOH	potassium hydroxide
KS	Kaposi's sarcoma
KSHV	Kaposi's sarcoma–related herpesvirus
KUB	kidney, ureter, bladder
LAD	left anterior descending (artery)
LAE	left atrial enlargement
LBBB	left bundle branch block
LBO	large bowel obstruction
LBP	low back pain
LCL	lateral collateral ligament
LDH	lactate dehydrogenase
LDL	low-density lipoprotein
LEEP	loop electrosurgical excision procedure
LES	lower esophageal sphincter
LFT	liver function test
LGV	lymphogranuloma venereum
LH	luteinizing hormone
LLQ	left lower quadrant
LMN	lower motor neuron
LMP	last menstrual period
LMWH	low-molecular-weight heparin
LP	lumbar puncture
LR	lactated Ringer's, likelihood ratio
LSIL	low-grade squamous intraepithelial lesion
LTBI	latent tuberculosis infection
LUQ	left upper quadrant
LVH	left ventricular hypertrophy
MAC	membrane attack complex, *Mycobacterium avium* complex
MAG-3	mercaptoacetyltriglycine (scan)
MALT	mucosa-associated lymphoid tissue
MAOI	monoamine oxidase inhibitor
MAST	military antishock trousers
mBPP	modified biophysical profile
MCA	middle cerebral artery
MCHC	mean corpuscular hemoglobin concentration
MCL	medial collateral ligament
MCP	metacarpophalangeal (joint)
MCV	mean corpuscular volume, meningococcal vaccine
MDE	major depressive episode
MEN	multiple endocrine neoplasia

Abbreviation	Meaning
$MgSO_4$	magnesium sulfate
MGUS	monoclonal gammopathy of undetermined significance
MHPSA	Mental Health Professional Shortage Area
MI	myocardial infarction
MIBG	metaiodobenzylguanidine (scan)
MMA	methylmalonic acid
MMF	mycophenolate mofetil
MMR	measles, mumps, rubella (vaccine)
MoM	multiple of the median
MOPP	mechlorethamine, Oncovin (vincristine), procarbazine, prednisone
MPTP	1-methyl-4-phenyl-1,2,3,6-tetrahydropyridine
MRA	magnetic resonance angiography
MRCP	magnetic resonance cholangiopancreatography
MRI	magnetic resonance imaging
MRSA	methicillin-resistant S. aureus
MS	multiple sclerosis
MSAFP	maternal serum α-fetoprotein
MSSA	methicillin-susceptible S. aureus
MTP	metatarsophalangeal (joint)
MUA	manual uterine aspiration
MUA/P	Medically Underserved Area and Population
MuSK	muscle-specific kinase
MVA	motor vehicle accident
$NaHCO_3$	sodium bicarbonate
NBME	National Board of Medical Examiners
NEC	necrotizing enterocolitis
NF	neurofibromatosis
NF-κB	nuclear factor κB
NG	nasogastric
NH_3	ammonia
NHL	non-Hodgkin's lymphoma
NIF	negative inspiratory force
NK	natural killer (cell)
NMDA	N-methyl-D-aspartate
NMS	neuroleptic malignant syndrome
NNRTI	non-nucleoside reverse transcriptase inhibitor
NPO	nil per os (nothing by mouth)
NPV	negative predictive value
NS	normal saline
NSAID	nonsteroidal anti-inflammatory drug
NSCLC	non–small cell lung cancer
NST	nonstress test
NSTEMI	non-ST-elevation myocardial infarction

Abbreviation	Meaning
NYHA	New York Heart Association
O&P	ova and parasites
OA	osteoarthritis
OCD	obsessive-compulsive disorder
OCPD	obsessive-compulsive personality disorder
OCPs	oral contraceptive pills
OD	overdose
OR	operating room
ORIF	open reduction and internal fixation
OSA	obstructive sleep apnea
OTC	over the counter
$PaCO_2$	partial pressure of carbon dioxide in arterial blood
PAN	polyarteritis nodosa
p-ANCA	perinuclear antineutrophil cytoplasmic antibody
PaO_2	partial pressure of oxygen in arterial blood
PAPP-A	pregnancy-associated plasma protein A
PAS	period acid–Schiff
PCA	posterior cerebral artery
PCI	percutaneous coronary intervention
PCKD	polycystic kidney disease
PCL	posterior cruciate ligament
PCO_2	partial pressure of carbon dioxide
PCOS	polycystic ovarian syndrome
PCP	phencyclidine hydrochloride
PCR	polymerase chain reaction
PCV	polycythemia vera, pneumococcal vaccine
PCWP	pulmonary capillary wedge pressure
PDA	patent ductus arteriosus
PDE	phosphodiesterase
PEA	pulseless electrical activity
PEEP	positive end-expiratory pressure
PET	positron emission tomography
PFT	pulmonary function test
PG	prostaglandin
PI	protease inhibitor
PICA	posterior inferior cerebellar artery
PID	pelvic inflammatory disease
PIP	proximal interphalangeal (joint)
PKD	polycystic kidney disease
PKU	phenylketonuria
PMI	point of maximal impulse
PML	promyelocytic leukemia
PMN	polymorphonuclear (leukocyte)
PND	paroxysmal nocturnal dyspnea
PO	per os (by mouth)
PO_2	partial pressure of oxygen
POC	product of conception

Abbreviation	Meaning
PPD	purified protein derivative (of tuberculin)
PPI	proton pump inhibitor
PPROM	preterm premature rupture of membranes
PPV	pneumococcal polysaccharide vaccine, positive predictive value
PR	per rectum, progesterone receptor
PRBC	packed red blood cell
PRN	pro re nata (as needed)
PROM	premature rupture of membranes
PSA	prostate-specific antigen
PT	prothrombin time
PTCA	percutaneous transluminal coronary angioplasty
PTH	parathyroid hormone
PTHrP	parathyroid hormone–related protein
PTSD	post-traumatic stress disorder
PTT	partial thromboplastin time
PUD	peptic ulcer disease
PUVA	psoralen plus ultraviolet A
PVC	premature ventricular contraction
PVR	peripheral vascular resistance
PVS	persistent vegetative state
QD	once a day
RA	rheumatoid arthritis
RAIU	radioactive iodine uptake
RBBB	right bundle branch block
RBC	red blood cell
RDS	respiratory distress syndrome
RDW	red cell distribution width
REM	rapid eye movement
RF	rheumatoid factor
RLQ	right lower quadrant
ROM	range of motion, rupture of membranes
RPR	rapid plasma reagin
RS	Reed-Sternberg (cell)
RSV	respiratory syncytial virus
RTA	renal tubular acidosis
RTI	reverse transcriptase inhibitor
RUQ	right upper quadrant
RV	residual volume
RVH	right ventricular hypertrophy
SAAG	serum-ascites albumin gradient
SAB	spontaneous abortion
SAH	subarachnoid hemorrhage
SaO_2	oxygen saturation in arterial blood
SARS	severe acute respiratory syndrome
SBO	small bowel obstruction
SBP	systolic blood pressure
SBS	shaken baby syndrome
SCC	squamous cell carcinoma

Abbreviation	Meaning
SCD	sickle cell disease
SCFE	slipped capital femoral epiphysis
SCID	severe combined immunodeficiency
SCLC	small cell lung cancer
SD	standard deviation
SES	socioeconomic status
SEVIS	Student and Exchange Visitor Information System
SEVP	Student and Exchange Visitor Program
SIADH	syndrome of inappropriate secretion of antidiuretic hormone
SIDS	sudden infant death syndrome
SIRS	systemic inflammatory response syndrome
SJS	Stevens-Johnson syndrome
SLE	systemic lupus erythematosus
SMA	superior mesenteric artery
SMV	superior mesenteric vein
SNRI	serotonin-norepinephrine reuptake inhibitor
SQ	subcutaneous
SRP	sponsoring residency program
SSRI	selective serotonin reuptake inhibitor
SSS	sick sinus syndrome
SSSS	staphylococcal scalded-skin syndrome
STD	sexually transmitted disease
STEMI	ST-elevation myocardial infarction
SVC	superior vena cava
SVT	supraventricular tachycardia
T_3	triiodothyronine
T_3RU	T_3 resin uptake
T_4	thyroxine
TA	temporal arteritis
TAB	therapeutic abortion
TAH/BSO	total abdominal hysterectomy/bilateral salpingo-oophorectomy
TB	tuberculosis
TBG	thyroxine-binding globulin
TCA	tricyclic antidepressant
TEE	transesophageal echocardiography
TEF	tracheoesophageal fistula
TEN	toxic epidermal necrolysis
TENS	transcutaneous electrical nerve stimulation
TFT	thyroid function test
TIA	transient ischemic attack
TIBC	total iron-binding capacity
TID	three times a day
TIMI	Thrombosis in Myocardial Infarction (study)
TLC	total lung capacity
TM	tympanic membrane

Abbreviation	Meaning
TMJ	temporomandibular joint
TMP-SMX	trimethoprim-sulfamethoxazole
TMS	transcranial magnetic stimulation
TNF	tumor necrosis factor
TNM	tumor, node, metastasis (staging)
TOEFL	Test of English as a Foreign Language
tPA	tissue plasminogen activator
TPN	total parenteral nutrition
TPO	thyroid peroxidase
TPPA	*T. pallidum* particle agglutination (test)
TRAP	tartrate-resistant acid phosphatase
TSH	thyroid-stimulating hormone
TSS	toxic shock syndrome
TTP	thrombotic thrombocytopenic purpura
TURP	transurethral resection of the prostate
TV	tidal volume
UA	urinalysis
UMN	upper motor neuron
URI	upper respiratory infection
USDA	United States Department of Agriculture
USIA	United States Information Agency

Abbreviation	Meaning
USMLE	United States Medical Licensing Examination
UTI	urinary tract infection
UV	ultraviolet
VA	Department of Veterans Affairs
VC	vital capacity
VCUG	voiding cystourethrography
VDRL	Venereal Disease Research Laboratory
VEGF	vascular endothelial growth factor
VF	ventricular fibrillation
VIN	vulvar intraepithelial neoplasia
VLDL	very low density lipoprotein
VMA	vanillylmandelic acid
VOC	vaso-occlusive crisis
VOR	vestibulo-ocular reflex
VP	ventriculoperitoneal
V/Q	ventilation/perfusion (scan)
VRSA	vancomycin-resistant *S. aureus*
VSD	ventricular septal defect
VT	ventricular tachycardia
vWD	von Willebrand's disease
vWF	von Willebrand factor
VZV	varicella-zoster virus
WBC	white blood cell
WHO	World Health Organization

▶ NOTES

Common Laboratory Values

* = Included in the Biochemical Profile (SMA-12)

Blood, Plasma, Serum	Reference Range	SI Reference Intervals
* Alanine aminotransferase (ALT, GPT at 30°C)	8–20 U/L	8–20 U/L
Amylase, serum	25–125 U/L	25–125 U/L
* Aspartate aminotransferase (AST, GOT at 30°C)	8–20 U/L	8–20 U/L
Bilirubin, serum (adult)		
Total // Direct	0.1–1.0 mg/dL // 0.0–0.3 mg/dL	2–17 μmol/L // 0–5 μmol/L
* Calcium, serum (Total)	8.4–10.2 mg/dL	2.1–2.8 mmol/L
* Cholesterol, serum	140–250 mg/dL	3.6–6.5 mmol/L
* Creatinine, serum (Total)	0.6–1.2 mg/dL	53–106 μmol/L
Electrolytes, serum		
Sodium	135–147 mEq/L	135–147 mmol/L
Chloride	95–105 mEq/L	95–105 mmol/L
* Potassium	3.5–5.0 mEq/L	3.5–5.0 mmol/L
Bicarbonate	22–28 mEq/L	22–28 mmol/L
Gases, arterial blood (room air)		
P_{O_2}	75–105 mmHg	10.0–14.0 kPa
P_{CO_2}	33–44 mmHg	4.4–5.9 kPa
pH	7.35–7.45	[H^+] 36–44 nmol/L
* Glucose, serum	Fasting: 70–110 mg/dL	3.8–6.1 mmol/L
	2-h postprandial: < 120 mg/dL	< 6.6 mmol/L
Growth hormone - arginine stimulation	Fasting: < 5 ng/mL	< 5 μg/L
	provocative stimuli: > 7 ng/mL	> 7 μg/L
Osmolality, serum	275–295 mOsm/kg	275–295 mOsm/kg
* Phosphatase (alkaline), serum (p-NPP at 30°C)	20–70 U/L	20–70 U/L
* Phosphorus (inorganic), serum	3.0–4.5 mg/dL	1.0–1.5 mmol/L
* Proteins, serum		
Total (recumbent)	6.0–7.8 g/dL	60–78 g/L
Albumin	3.5–5.5 g/dL	35–55 g/L
Globulins	2.3–3.5 g/dL	23–35 g/L
* Urea nitrogen, serum (BUN)	7–18 mg/dL	1.2–3.0 mmol urea/L
* Uric acid, serum	3.0–8.2 mg/dL	0.18–0.48 mmol/L
Cerebrospinal Fluid		
Glucose	40–70 mg/dL	2.2–3.9 mmol/L
Hematologic		
Erythrocyte count	Male: 4.3–5.9 million/mm³	$4.3\text{–}5.9 \times 10^{12}$/L
	Female: 3.5–5.5 million/mm³	$3.5\text{–}5.5 \times 10^{12}$/L
Hematocrit	Male: 41–53%	0.41–0.53
	Female: 36–46%	0.36–0.46
Hemoglobin, blood	Male: 13.5–17.5 g/dL	2.09–2.71 mmol/L
	Female: 12.0–16.0 g/dL	1.86–2.48 mmol/L

(continues)

Hematologic (continued)

Hemoglobin, plasma	1–4 mg/dL	0.16–0.62 μmol/L
Leukocyte count and differential		
Leukocyte count	4500–11,0 00/mm³	4.5–11.0 × 10⁹/L
Segmented neutrophils	54–62%	0.54–0.62
Band forms	3–5%	0.03–0.05
Eosinophils	1–3%	0.01–0.03
Basophils	0–0.75%	0–0.0075
Lymphocytes	25–33%	0.25–0.33
Monocytes	3–7%	0.03–0.07
Mean corpuscular hemoglobin	25.4–34.6 pg/cell	0.39–0.54 fmol/cell
Platelet count	150,000–400,000/mm³	150–400 × 10⁹/L
Prothrombin time	11–15 seconds	11–15 seconds
Reticulocyte count	0.5–1.5% of red cells	0.005–0.015
Sedimentation rate, erythrocyte	Male: 0–15 mm/h	0–15 mm/h
(Westergren)	Female: 0–20 mm/h	0–20 mm/h
Proteins, total	< 150 mg/24 h	< 0.15 g/24 h

Index

Fifth disease (erythema infectiosum), 420
Fitz-Hugh–Curtis syndrome, 236, 536
Flail chest, 503–504
Flumazenil, 432
Focal segmental glomerulosclerosis, 487
Folate deficiency, 196, 210, 314, 542
Folliculitis, 93–94
Fournier gangrene, 93
Fractures, 257–258
  pediatric, 273
Fragile X syndrome, 405, 443
Friedreich's ataxia, 284
Frontotemporal dementia (Pick's disease), 305
Frotteurism, 450, 539
Furosemide, 51
Fusobacterium, 222

G

G6PD deficiency, 197
Galleazzi's fracture, 258
Galleazzi's sign, 274
Gallstone ileus, 176
Gallstones, 173–174
Gangrene, 99
Gardnerella vaginalis, 377
Gastric cancer, 157
Gastritis, 156–157
  chronic atrophic, 213
Gastroenterology, pediatric, 407–410
  Hirschsprung's disease, 409
  intussusception, 407
  malrotation with volvulus, 409–410
  Meckel's diverticulum, 408–409
  necrotizing enterocolitis (NEC), 410
  pyloric stenosis, 408
Gastroesophageal reflux disease (GERD), 155–156
Gastrointestinal bleeding, 170, 171, 528
  features of upper and lower, 171
Gastroschisis, 423
Gaucher's disease, 210, 406
Gender identity disorders, 450
Generalized anxiety disorder, 432
Genetic disease, 404–407
  cystic fibrosis (CF), 405–407
Genital lesions, sexually transmitted, 239, 240, 241

Genital warts, 90–91
Genitourinary infections, 239, 241–242
  pyelonephritis, 241–242
  urinary tract infections (UTIs), 239, 241
Gestational diabetes, 338, 340
Gestational trophoblastic disease (GTD), 346–348
Giant cell arteritis, 271
Giardia, 159, 527
Giemsa stain, 90
Gilbert's syndrome, 178
Glanzmann's thrombasthenia, 530
Glaucoma, 314–316
  closed-angle, 315
  open-angle, 315–316
Gleason histologic system, 496
Glioblastoma multiforme, 309
Glomerular disease, 485–489
  nephritic syndrome, 485–487
    causes of, 486
  nephrotic syndrome, 487–489
    causes of, 487–488
Glomerulonephritis
  membranous, 542
  postinfectious, 486, 530
Glucose metabolism, disorders of, 114–117
  diabetes mellitus (DM)
    complications of, 115
    type 1, 114–115
    type 2, 115–116
  metabolic syndrome, 117
Gonorrhea, 236, 237
Goodpasture's syndrome, 486, 542
Gottron's papules, 267
Gout, 265–266, 532
  vs. pseudogout, 266
Graft-versus-host disease (GVHD), 212
Graft-versus-leukemia effect, 213
Grain handler's lung, 462
Granuloma inguinale-donovanosis, 240
Graves' disease, 117, 118, 119, 268, 523
  physical signs of, 118
Greenstick fracture, 273
Gullain-Barré syndrome, 245, 302–303, 534
Gynecologic infections, 374–379
  cyst and abscess of Bartholin's duct, 374–375
  pelvic inflammatory disease (PID), 377–379

toxic shock syndrome (TSS), 379
vaginitis, 375–377
  causes of, 376, 377
Gynecologic neoplasms, 379–388
  cervical cancer, 381–385
    cervical intraepithelial neoplasia, 383
    Pap smears, classification systems for, 382
    staging of, 384
  endometrial cancer, 380–381
    types of, 381
  ovarian cancer, 386–388
    pelvic masses, benign vs. malignant, 387
    tumor markers, 387
  uterine leiomyoma (fibroids), 379–380
  vaginal cancer, 385–386
  vulvar cancer, 385

H

Haemophilus ducreyi, 240, 532
Haemophilus influenzae, 217, 219, 222, 225, 226, 227, 242, 248, 412, 413, 414, 417, 530, 531
Haemophilus parainfluenzae, 250
HAIR-AN syndrome, 99, 372
"Hamburger sign," 508
Hand-foot-and-mouth disease, 421
Hashimoto's thyroiditis, 119, 523
  lab findings in, 523
Head lice, 97
Headaches, 291–294
  cavernous sinus thrombosis, 293–294
  cluster, 293, 533
  migraine, 292, 533
    prophylactic treatment for, 533
  tension-type, 293
Health screening recommendations, 141–142
  by age, 142
  by modality, 142
Hearing and vision screening, 429
Heinz bodies, 530
Helicobacter pylori, 157, 158
HELLP syndrome, 192, 193, 340
Hematologic infections, 242–245
  infectious mononucleosis, 244–245
  malaria, 243–244
  sepsis, 242–243

Rheumatoid arthritis (RA), 268, 269, 532
Rhizopus, 248
Rickettsia, 227
Rickettsia rickettsii, 227
Right bundle branch block (RBBB), 42
Ringworm (tinea capitis), 97
Rocky Mountain spotted fever, 247–48
Rosacea, 100–101
Roseola infantum, 421, 537
Roth's spots, 250, 531
Rotor's syndrome, 178
Rovsing's sign, 508
Rubella, 326, 328, 421, 530

S

Sadism, sexual, 450
Salmonella, 159, 160, 253, 266, 527, 532
Salmonella typhi, 92
Salter-Harris fracture, 273
Sarcoidosis, 54, 210, 282, 461–462, 540
Sarcoma botryoides, 364
Sarcoptes scabiei, 97
Scabies, 97–98
Scale (dermatologic), 76
Scaphoid fracture, 257, 533
Scar, 76
Scarlet fever, 92
Schilling test, 196
Schizoaffective disorder, 441
Schizophrenia, 441–442, 539
Schizophreniform disorder, 441, 539
Schwannoma, 309
Scleroderma, 268, 269–270
Scoliosis, 277
Scrotal swelling, 493–494
Seborrheic dermatitis, 80–81, 522
Seborrheic keratosis, 103, 104, 522
Seizure disorders, 294–297
    absence (petit mal) seizures, 296
    infantile spasms (West syndrome), 297
    partial seizures, 295
    status epilepticus, 296–297
    tonic-clonic (grand mal) seizures, 295–296
Seizures, febrile, 425–426, 534, 537
Selective serotonin reuptake inhibitors (SSRIs), 432–433, 438, 538

Sensitivity, 524
Sepsis, 242–243
Serratia, 239
Serum-ascites albumin gradient (SAAG), 180, 181
Serum sickness, 77
Severe combined immunodeficiency (SCID), 411, 426
Sexual assault, 361, 363–364
Sexual disorders, 449–450
    aging, sexual changes with, 449
    gender identity disorders, 450
    paraphilias, 449–450
    sexual dysfunction, 450
Sexual and physical abuse, 453–454
Sexually transmitted diseases (STDs), 235–239
    chlamydia, 235–236
    genital lesions, 239, 240, 241
    gonorrhea, 236, 237
    syphilis, 236–239
        diagostic tests for, 238
Sézary cells, 111
Shagreen patch, 310
Sheehan's syndrome (postpartum pituitary necrosis), 353, 354, 535
Shigella, 159, 160, 266, 532
Shock, 509, 510, 544
    treatment of, 544
    types of, 510
Shoulder dislocation, 257
Shoulder dystocia, 348
Shwachan-Diamond-Oski syndrome, 210
SIADH. *See* Syndrome of inappropriate antidiuretic hormone secretion
Sick sinus syndrome (SSS), 45
Sickle cell disease (SCD), 198, 287, 482
Silicosis, 463, 541
Sinus bradycardia, 45
Sinus tachycardia, 46
Sinusitis, 222–223
Sipple's syndrome (MEN type 2A), 121
Sjögren's syndrome, 268, 482
Skin, layers of, 75, 76
    components of, 76
Skin lesions, common terms used to describe, 76
Sleep disorders, 451–452
    circadian rhythm sleep disorder, 452
    hypersomnia, primary, 451

insomnia, primary, 451
narcolepsy, 451–452
sleep apnea, 452
Sleep paralysis, 452
Slipped capital femoral epiphysis (SCFE), 275–277, 533
Small bowel, disorders of, 159–166, 167
    appendicitis, 166
    carcinoid syndrome, 162
    diarrhea, 159–161
        chronic, decision diagram for, 161
        infectious, causes of, 160
    ileus, 164–165
    irritable bowel syndrome (IBS), 162–163
    lactose intolerance, 162
    mesenteric ischemia, 165–166
    small bowel obstruction (SBO), 163–164
        characteristics of, 167
Small lymphocytic lymphoma, 529
Social phobia, 434
Sokolow-Lyon criteria, 43
Somatization disorder, 4653
Somatoform and factitious disorders, 452–454
Somatoform pain disorder, 453
Somogyi effect, 116
Spherocytosis, hereditary, 528
Spinal cord lesions, 284
Spinal stenosis, 261–262, 532
Spinal tract functions, 282
Spironolactone, 51
Splinter hemorrhages, 250, 251, 531
Spontaneous abortion (SAB), 328–329
    types of, 330
Spontaneous bacterial peritonitis, 181
Sporothrix schenckii, 532
Squamous cell carcinoma (SCC), 105–106, 523, 540
ST-elevation myocardial infarction (STEMI), 56–59
ST-segment elevation, causes of, 57
Stanford system of classification for aortic dissection, 69
Staphylococcal scalded-skin syndrome (SSSS), 84, 91
Staphylococcus, 93, 217, 218, 242, 250
    coagulase-negative, 250

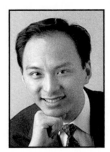
Tao Le, MD, MHS

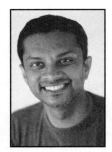
Vikas Bhushan, MD

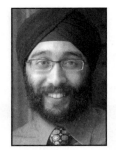
Herman Bagga, MD

Tao Le, MD, MHS

Tao has been a well-recognized figure in medical education for the past 16 years. As senior editor, he has led the expansion of *First Aid* into a global educational series. In addition, he is the founder of the *USMLERx* online learning system as well as a cofounder of the *Underground Clinical Vignettes* series. As a medical student, he was editor-in-chief of the University of California, San Francisco *Synapse,* a university newspaper with a weekly circulation of 9000. Tao earned his medical degree from the University of California, San Francisco in 1996 and completed his residency training in internal medicine at Yale University and allergy and immunology fellowship training at Johns Hopkins University. At Yale, he was a regular guest lecturer on the USMLE review courses and an adviser to the Yale University School of Medicine curriculum committee. Tao subsequently went on to cofound Medsn and served as its chief medical officer. He is currently pursuing research in asthma education at the University of Louisville.

Vikas Bhushan, MD

Vikas is an author, editor, entrepreneur, and roaming teleradiologist who divides his days between Los Angeles, Maui, and balmy remote locales with abundant bandwidth. In 1992 he conceived and authored the original *First Aid for the USMLE Step 1*, and in 1998 he originated and coauthored the *Underground Clinical Vignettes* series. His entrepreneurial adventures include a successful software company; a medical publishing enterprise (S2S); an e-learning company (Medsn); and, most recently, an ER teleradiology venture (24/7 Radiology). His eclectic interests include medical informatics, independent film, humanism, Urdu poetry, world music, South Asian diasporic culture, and avoiding a day job. He has also coproduced a music documentary on qawwali; coproduced and edited *Shabash 2.0: The Hip Guide to All Things South Asian in North America;* and is now completing a CD/book project on Sufi poetry translated into four languages. Vikas completed a bachelor's degree in biochemistry from the University of California, Berkeley; an MD with thesis from the University of California, San Francisco; and a radiology residency from the University of California, Los Angeles.

Herman Singh Bagga, MD

Herman is a Urology resident at the University of California, San Francisco. He has been involved in multiple *First Aid* projects since his time in medical school at the Johns Hopkins University School of Medicine. He was raised in New York City (which explains his rough and tough exterior) until moving to Erie, Pennsylvania (a small, quiet city responsible for cultivating his soft side), for the rest of his youth. As an undergraduate at Case Western Reserve University, he studied economics and biology before committing to medicine as his career path. His academic interests include outcomes research and medical education.

ABOUT THE AUTHORS

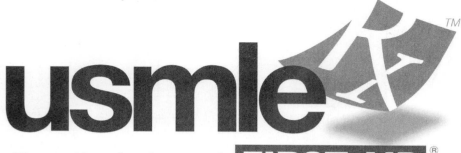
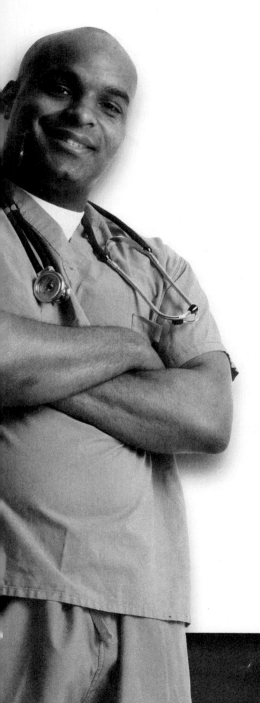